Advanced Materials for Oral Application (Volume II)

Advanced Materials for Oral Application (Volume II)

Guest Editors

Laura-Cristina Rusu
Lavinia Cosmina Ardelean

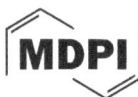

Basel • Beijing • Wuhan • Barcelona • Belgrade • Novi Sad • Cluj • Manchester

Guest Editors

Laura-Cristina Rusu
University Clinic of Oral Pathology
"Victor Babes" University of Medicine and Pharmacy
Timisoara
Romania

Lavinia Cosmina Ardelean
Academic Department of Technology of Materials and Devices in Dental Medicine
"Victor Babes" University of Medicine and Pharmacy
Timisoara
Romania

Editorial Office
MDPI AG
Grosspeteranlage 5
4052 Basel, Switzerland

This is a reprint of the Special Issue, published open access by the journal *Materials* (ISSN 1996-1944), freely accessible at: www.mdpi.com/journal/materials/special_issues/mater_oral_volume_II.

For citation purposes, cite each article independently as indicated on the article page online and using the guide below:

Lastname, A.A.; Lastname, B.B. Article Title. *Journal Name* **Year**, *Volume Number*, Page Range.

ISBN 978-3-7258-3528-7 (Hbk)
ISBN 978-3-7258-3527-0 (PDF)
https://doi.org/10.3390/books978-3-7258-3527-0

© 2025 by the authors. Articles in this book are Open Access and distributed under the Creative Commons Attribution (CC BY) license. The book as a whole is distributed by MDPI under the terms and conditions of the Creative Commons Attribution-NonCommercial-NoDerivs (CC BY-NC-ND) license (https://creativecommons.org/licenses/by-nc-nd/4.0/).

Contents

About the Editors vii

Laura-Cristina Rusu and Lavinia Cosmina Ardelean
Advanced Materials for Oral Application (Volume 2)
Reprinted from: *Materials* 2025, *18*, 1042, https://doi.org/10.3390/ma18051042 1

Shiri Livne, Sapir Simantov, Arkadi Rahmanov, Uziel Jeffet and Nir Sterer
Hydroxyethyl Cellulose Promotes the Mucin Retention of Herbal Extracts Active against *Streptococcus mutans*
Reprinted from: *Materials* 2022, *15*, 4652, https://doi.org/10.3390/ma15134652 8

Alexandra-Diana Florea, Cristina Teodora Dobrota, Rahela Carpa, Csaba-Pal Racz, Gheorghe Tomoaia and Aurora Mocanu et al.
Optimization of Functional Toothpaste Formulation Containing Nano-Hydroxyapatite and Birch Extract for Daily Oral Care
Reprinted from: *Materials* 2023, *16*, 7143, https://doi.org/10.3390/ma16227143 14

Ekta Varma Sengar, Sanjyot Mulay, Lotika Beri, Archana Gupta, Thamer Almohareb and Sultan Binalrimal et al.
Comparative Evaluation of Microleakage of Flowable Composite Resin Using Etch and Rinse, Self-Etch Adhesive Systems, and Self-Adhesive Flowable Composite Resin in Class V Cavities: Confocal Laser Microscopic Study
Reprinted from: *Materials* 2022, *15*, 4963, https://doi.org/10.3390/ma15144963 31

Jordan Maximov, Tsanka Dikova, Galya Duncheva and Georgi Georgiev
Influence of Factors in the Photopolymerization Process on Dental Composites Microhardness
Reprinted from: *Materials* 2022, *15*, 6459, https://doi.org/10.3390/ma15186459 42

Leszek Klimek, Karolina Kopacz, Beata Śmielak and Zofia Kula
An Evaluation of the Mechanical Properties of a Hybrid Composite Containing Hydroxyapatite
Reprinted from: *Materials* 2023, *16*, 4548, https://doi.org/10.3390/ma16134548 57

Mannaa K. Aldowsari, Fatimah Alfawzan, Alanoud Alhaidari, Nada Alhogail, Reema Alshargi and Saad Bin Saleh et al.
Comparison of Shear Bond Strength of Three Types of Adhesive Materials Used in the Restoration of Permanent Molars after Treatment with Silver Diamine Fluoride: An In Vitro Study
Reprinted from: *Materials* 2023, *16*, 6831, https://doi.org/10.3390/ma16216831 72

Francesco De Angelis, Simonetta D'Ercole, Mara Di Giulio, Mirco Vadini, Virginia Biferi and Matteo Buonvivere et al.
In Vitro Evaluation of *Candida albicans* Adhesion on Heat-Cured Resin-Based Dental Composites
Reprinted from: *Materials* 2023, *16*, 5818, https://doi.org/10.3390/ma16175818 82

Jeeth Janardhan Rai, Saurabh Chaturvedi, Shankar T. Gokhale, Raghavendra Reddy Nagate, Saad M. Al-Qahtani and Mohammad Al. Magbol et al.
Effectiveness of a Single Chair Side Application of NovaMin® [Calcium Sodium Phosphosilicate] in the Treatment of Dentine Hypersensitivity Following Ultrasonic Scaling—A Randomized Controlled Trial
Reprinted from: *Materials* 2023, *16*, 1329, https://doi.org/10.3390/ma16041329 94

Demet Sahin, Ceren Deger, Burcu Oglakci, Metehan Demirkol, Bedri Onur Kucukyildirim and Mehtikar Gursel et al.
The Effects of a Novel Nanohydroxyapatite Gel and Er: YAG Laser Treatment on Dentin Hypersensitivity
Reprinted from: *Materials* 2023, 16, 6522, https://doi.org/10.3390/ma16196522 109

Keerthika Rajamanickam, Kavalipurapu Venkata Teja, Sindhu Ramesh, Abdulaziz S. AbuMelha, Mazen F. Alkahtany and Khalid H. Almadi et al.
Comparative Study Assessing the Canal Cleanliness Using Automated Device and Conventional Syringe Needle for Root Canal Irrigation—An Ex-Vivo Study
Reprinted from: *Materials* 2022, 15, 6184, https://doi.org/10.3390/ma15186184 119

Saulius Drukteinis, Goda Bilvinaite and Simas Sakirzanovas
The Impact of Citric Acid Solution on Hydraulic Calcium Silicate-Based Sealers and Root Dentin: A Preliminary Assessment
Reprinted from: *Materials* 2024, 17, 1351, https://doi.org/10.3390/ma17061351 128

Tarek Ashi, Raphaël Richert, Davide Mancino, Hamdi Jmal, Sleman Alkhouri and Frédéric Addiego et al.
Do the Mechanical Properties of Calcium-Silicate-Based Cements Influence the Stress Distribution of Different Retrograde Cavity Preparations?
Reprinted from: *Materials* 2023, 16, 3111, https://doi.org/10.3390/ma16083111 139

Syed Rashid Habib, Abdul Sadekh Ansari, Aleshba Saba Khan, Nawaf M. Alamro, Meshari A. Alzaaqi and Yazeed A. Alkhunefer et al.
Push-Out Bond Strength of Endodontic Posts Cemented to Extracted Teeth: An In-Vitro Evaluation
Reprinted from: *Materials* 2022, 15, 6792, https://doi.org/10.3390/ma15196792 148

Mhd Ayham Darwich, Abeer Aljareh, Nabil Alhouri, Szabolcs Szávai, Hasan Mhd Nazha and Fabian Duvigneau et al.
Biomechanical Assessment of Endodontically Treated Molars Restored by Endocrowns Made from Different CAD/CAM Materials
Reprinted from: *Materials* 2023, 16, 764, https://doi.org/10.3390/ma16020764 161

Susi Zara, Giulia Fioravanti, Angelo Ciuffreda, Ciro Annicchiarico, Raimondo Quaresima and Filiberto Mastrangelo
Evaluation of Human Gingival Fibroblasts (HGFs) Behavior on Innovative Laser Colored Titanium Surfaces
Reprinted from: *Materials* 2023, 16, 4530, https://doi.org/10.3390/ma16134530 178

Luca Comuzzi, Margherita Tumedei, Natalia Di Pietro, Tea Romasco, Hamid Heydari Sheikh Hossein and Lorenzo Montesani et al.
A Comparison of Conical and Cylindrical Implants Inserted in an In Vitro Post-Extraction Model Using Low-Density Polyurethane Foam Blocks
Reprinted from: *Materials* 2023, 16, 5064, https://doi.org/10.3390/ma16145064 195

Barbara Illing, Leila Mohammadnejad, Antonia Theurer, Jacob Schultheiss, Evi Kimmerle-Mueller and Frank Rupp et al.
Biological Performance of Titanium Surfaces with Different Hydrophilic and Nanotopographical Features
Reprinted from: *Materials* 2023, 16, 7307, https://doi.org/10.3390/ma16237307 211

Nurulhuda Mohd, Masfueh Razali, Mariyam Jameelah Ghazali and Noor Hayaty Abu Kasim
Current Advances of Three-Dimensional Bioprinting Application in Dentistry: A Scoping Review
Reprinted from: *Materials* **2022**, *15*, 6398, https://doi.org/10.3390/ma15186398 225

Shweta Narwani, Naveen S. Yadav, Puja Hazari, Vrinda Saxena, Abdulrahman H. Alzahrani and Ahmed Alamoudi et al.
Comparison of Tensile Bond Strength of Fixed-Fixed Versus Cantilever Single- and Double-Abutted Resin-Bonded Bridges Dental Prosthesis
Reprinted from: *Materials* **2022**, *15*, 5744, https://doi.org/10.3390/ma15165744 250

Hemavardhini Addugala, Vidyashree Nandini Venugopal, Surya Rengasamy, Pradeep Kumar Yadalam, Nassreen H. Albar and Ahmed Alamoudi et al.
Marginal and Internal Gap of Metal Copings Fabricated Using Three Types of Resin Patterns with Subtractive and Additive Technology: An In Vitro Comparison
Reprinted from: *Materials* **2022**, *15*, 6397, https://doi.org/10.3390/ma15186397 261

Konstantinos Tzimas, Christos Rahiotis and Eftychia Pappa
Biofilm Formation on Hybrid, Resin-Based CAD/CAM Materials for Indirect Restorations: A Comprehensive Review
Reprinted from: *Materials* **2024**, *17*, 1474, https://doi.org/10.3390/ma17071474 273

Po-Hsu Chen, Esra Elamin, Akram Sayed Ahmed, Daniel A. Givan, Chin-Chuan Fu and Nathaniel C. Lawson
The Effect of Restoration Thickness on the Fracture Resistance of 5 mol% Yttria-Containing Zirconia Crowns
Reprinted from: *Materials* **2024**, *17*, 365, https://doi.org/10.3390/ma17020365 290

Grzegorz Sokolowski, Agata Szczesio-Wlodarczyk, Małgorzata Iwona Szynkowska-Jóźwik, Wioleta Stopa, Jerzy Sokolowski and Karolina Kopacz et al.
The Shear Bond Strength of Resin-Based Luting Cement to Zirconia Ceramics after Different Surface Treatments
Reprinted from: *Materials* **2023**, *16*, 5433, https://doi.org/10.3390/ma16155433 300

Naziratul Adirah Nasarudin, Masfueh Razali, Victor Goh, Wen Lin Chai and Andanastuti Muchtar
Expression of Interleukin-1β and Histological Changes of the Three-Dimensional Oral Mucosal Model in Response to Yttria-Stabilized Nanozirconia
Reprinted from: *Materials* **2023**, *16*, 2027, https://doi.org/10.3390/ma16052027 312

Martin Rosentritt, Thomas Strasser, Maerit-Martha Mueller and Michael Benno Schmidt
Cutting Efficiency of Diamond Grinders on Composite and Zirconia
Reprinted from: *Materials* **2024**, *17*, 2596, https://doi.org/10.3390/ma17112596 324

Beata Śmielak, Leszek Klimek and Kamil Krześniak
Effect of Sandblasting Parameters and the Type and Hardness of the Material on the Number of Embedded Al_2O_3 Grains
Reprinted from: *Materials* **2023**, *16*, 4783, https://doi.org/10.3390/ma16134783 335

About the Editors

Laura-Cristina Rusu

Professor Laura Cristina Rusu, DMD, Ph.D., is a full-time professor and the head of the Oral Pathology Department, Faculty of Dental Medicine, "Victor Babes" University of Medicine and Pharmacy, Timisoara, Romania. Her Ph.D. thesis was centered on allergens in dental materials. In 2017, she obtained a Dr. Habil and was confirmed as a Ph.D. coordinator in the field of dental medicine. She took part in 11 research projects, including FP7 COST Action MP 1005, and authored more than 140 peer-reviewed papers. She has published ten books and book chapters as an author and a co-author. She has guest-edited seven special issues in different journals and edited or co-edited five books. Moreover, she has one ongoing book-editing project. She currently holds four patents. Dr. Rusu is a member of the editorial board of the *Journal of Science* and *Art and Medicine in Evolution* and a topic editor for the journal *Materials*. Her main scientific interests are oral pathology and oral diagnosis in dental medicine, focusing on oral cancer.

Lavinia Cosmina Ardelean

Professor Lavinia Cosmina Ardelean, DMD, Ph.D., is the head of the Department of Technology of Materials and Devices in Dental Medicine, "Victor Babes" University of Medicine and Pharmacy, Timisoara, Romania. She has authored/co-authored 20 books, 15 book chapters, and over 120 peer-reviewed papers. With a current H-index of 13, she is an editorial board member of numerous journals, including Scientific Reports, and a member of the reviewer/topic boards of MDPI journals *Materials, Prosthesis, Metals, Coatings, Polymers, Journal of Functional Biomaterials, Dentistry*, and *Biomedicines*. She has guest-edited ten Special Issues in different journals and seven books, plus she has one ongoing book-editing project. Being an active reviewer, with more than 290 reviews to her credit thus far, she was awarded the Top Reviewers in Cross-Field award in 2019 and the Top Reviewers in Materials Science award in 2019. She currently holds three patents. Her research interest includes most areas of dentistry, with a focus on dental materials/biomaterials, dental alloys, resins, ceramics/bioceramics, CAD/CAM milling, 3D printing/bioprinting in dentistry, welding, scanning, prosthodontics, and oral health care.

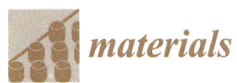

Editorial

Advanced Materials for Oral Application (Volume 2)

Laura-Cristina Rusu [1] and Lavinia Cosmina Ardelean [2,*]

[1] University Clinic of Oral Pathology, Multidisciplinary Center for Research, Evaluation, Diagnosis and Therapies in Oral Medicine, "Victor Babes" University of Medicine and Pharmacy, 300041 Timisoara, Romania; laura.rusu@umft.ro

[2] Academic Department of Technology of Materials and Devices in Dental Medicine, Multidisciplinary Center for Research, Evaluation, Diagnosis and Therapies in Oral Medicine, "Victor Babes" University of Medicine and Pharmacy, 300041 Timisoara, Romania

* Correspondence: lavinia_ardelean@umft.ro

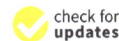

Received: 31 January 2025
Accepted: 11 February 2025
Published: 26 February 2025

Citation: Rusu, L.-C.; Ardelean, L.C. Advanced Materials for Oral Application (Volume 2). *Materials* 2025, 18, 1042. https://doi.org/10.3390/ma18051042

Copyright: © 2025 by the authors. Licensee MDPI, Basel, Switzerland. This article is an open access article distributed under the terms and conditions of the Creative Commons Attribution (CC BY) license (https://creativecommons.org/licenses/by/4.0/).

This editorial aims to present the contributions published in the second volume of the Special Issue "Advanced Materials for Oral Application", journal *Materials*. Volume 2 aimed to focus on the recent advances in this attractive field of research, encouraging a multidisciplinary approach to the subject.

Compared to the first volume, which consisted of fourteen papers, the second volume gathered twenty-six valuable manuscripts: twenty-four original research articles and two review papers, authored by leading scientists and scholars across the world with expertise in materials for dental application. These articles explore a wide variety of dental materials for direct and indirect restorations, for endodontic use, and for dental implants, as well as their properties and interactions with the oral environment. Three-dimensional bioprinting in dentistry was also assessed, and two new dentifrices were presented.

Prevention in dentistry is of the utmost importance, as it helps in maintaining good oral health. Novel formulations of more effective dentifrices are constantly being attempted. The study by Livne et al. aimed to test the effect of adding a mucoadhesive agent, namely hydroxyethyl cellulose, to an herbal extract solution containing lavender, echinacea, sage, and mastic gum, attempting to increase its bioavailability and efficacy. This formulation provides a platform for the future development of a caries-preventing toothpaste, aiming to reducing biofilm formation and the virulence of the cariogenic bacterium Streptococcus mutans [1]. Florea et al. attempted to develop functional toothpastes with combined enamel remineralization and antibacterial effects using nano-hydroxyapatites and birch extract, and they obtained the most suitable formulation out of eleven choices [2].

Materials used in restorative dentistry are being also subjected to continuous improvement in term of physical properties, aesthetic appearance, and durability, with direct composite materials being the first choice for most patients. The essential factor in providing a long-lasting restoration is the marginal seal. Restoring cervical lesions with composite resins has always been a challenge, as stated by Sengar et al. Their study aimed to evaluate and compare the microleakage of a flowable composite resin using an etch and rinse adhesive system, a self-etch adhesive system, and a self-adhesive flowable composite resin in Class V cavities. Despite the fact that none of the of the tested adhesive systems were free from microleakage, the etch and rinse adhesive showed the lowest microleakage values [3]. Different irradiation times and light intensities have been proven to affect the mechanical properties of direct composite restorations. Their successful polymerization can be evaluated by their hardness; the study of Maximov et al. aimed to investigate the influence of different photopolymerization parameters, such as light intensity, irradiation time, and layer thickness, on the microhardness of three types of dental composites (conventional, bulk-fill, and flowable). The study has shown that the significance of the factors influencing the microhardness is defined mainly by the composite resin composition, which is similar for the conventional and flowable composites, but different for the bulk-fill [4]. Another study involving direct composite resins was authored by Klimek et al. who aimed to compare the properties of a commercial hybrid composite with experimental composites doped with different amounts of hydroxyapatite. After determining the hardness, static strength properties (compression and bending), dynamic properties (impact strength and fracture toughness), and wear resistance, they concluded that the hydroxyapatite content had a great impact on the mechanical properties of the composite resin, with the best results being obtained when adding up to 5% wt [5]. The in-vitro study by Aldowsari et al. aimed to assess the shear bond strength of a new self-adhesive restorative material to the dentin of extracted permanent teeth previously treated with 38% silver diamine fluoride and to compare it with a resin-based composite and a resin-modified glass ionomer cement. The best results were obtained when using the resin-based composite, but the shear bond strength of the new self-adhesive restorative material was within the clinical acceptable limits, making it suitable for masking the discoloration caused by silver diamine fluoride application [6]. Microbial adhesion on dental restorative materials may jeopardize the long-term outcomes of restorative treatment. The goal of the in vitro study of De Angelis et al. was to assess the capability of *Candida albicans* to adhere to and form biofilms on the surfaces of dental composites with different formulations which were subjected to same surface treatments and polymerization protocols. Based on the results, the conclusion was that different formulations of commercially available composite resins may interact differently with *C. albicans* [7].

Dentinal hypersensitivity is a painful condition which may affect patients of any age, and is usually associated with exposed dentinal surfaces. Due to its negative effects on psychological and emotional wellbeing, there is continuous interest in finding new and efficient means of treating it. The randomized controlled trial of Rai et al. aimed to evaluate the effectiveness of a single chair-side application of NovaMin®, a bioactive glass containing calcium sodium phosphosilicate, in reducing dentin hypersensitivity following ultrasonic scaling. The study, carried out over a one-month period, concluded that NovaMin® is efficient in providing rapid relief from dentinal hypersensitivity [8]. Sahin et al. evaluated the effects of a novel nanohydroxyapatite gel and Er: YAG laser on the surface roughness, surface morphology, and elemental content after dentin hypersensitivity treatment, and concluded that these treatment methods could provide promising results in terms of tubular occlusion efficiency. Laser treatment resulted in significantly lower surface roughness, which could help in preventing dental plaque accumulation [9].

One dental field which has undergone great development within the recent time period is endodontics. The ultimate goal of endodontic treatment is to obtain a three-dimensional, tight canal seal. To achieve a good three-dimensional seal, the removal of the smear layer becomes mandatory, as stated by Rajamanickam et al. Their study aimed to assess the difference in debris accumulation and smear layer formation while using automated root canal irrigation and conventional syringe needle irrigation, and they observed no significant difference between the results of the two irrigation techniques [10]. The quality of the three-dimensional seal highly depends on the materials used. Over the years, various endodontic sealers have been developed. Hydraulic calcium silicate-based sealers significantly changed the fundamental principles of root canal fillings due to the lack of shrinkage and long-term dimensional stability. However, their drawback resides in the difficulty of removing them from the root canal system, even mechanically, in case of retreatment. Drukteinis et al. tested the ability of citric acid to dissolve hydraulic calcium silicate-based sealers and demonstrated its efficacy with no adverse effects on root canal dentine [11]. Characterized by high biocompatibility, low cytotoxicity, and viscosity, calcium silicate-based sealers have been considered to improve canal filling quality. The aim of the study of Ashi et al. was to investigate the influence of the mechanical properties of three different calcium-silicate-based cements on the stress distribution of three different retrograde cavity preparations. Their conclusions were that the apical preparation design influences stress distribution and that stiffer cements offer an optimal retrograde treatment with less stress in the root [12]. Following endodontic treatment, the teeth need reconstruction, which is carried out by using different post systems made of different materials, with different characteristics. Treatment failure in teeth restored with endodontic posts is frequently due to the loss of bond between the post and the tooth structure. Push-out strength tests, used by Habib et al. in their study, are widely accepted to evaluate adhesive strength. They aimed to assess the push-out strength of different sizes of fiber and metal posts, which were luted with a dual-cure resin-based cement to natural dentin. They also analyzed the type of failure and concluded that fiber and metal posts showed almost similar values of bond strength, while increasing the size of the post resulted in better retention due to the wider bonding surface area. However, the post size should be carefully chosen to avoid weakening of the root structure. Adhesive failure was the most prevalent type [13]. Endocrowns had been introduced as a more conservative approach to rehabilitate endodontically treated teeth with significant losses in coronal structure, avoiding further weakening of the root. Endocrowns are associated with lower stress concentration and higher fracture strength compared to post-supported conventional crowns. Darwel et al. aimed to assess the stress distribution in molars restored by CAD/CAM manufactured endocrowns from translucent zirconia, as well as to evaluate the biomechanical behavior of translucent zirconia endocrowns compared to endocrowns made of zirconia-reinforced lithium silicate ceramic, lithium disilicate glass ceramic, polymer-infiltrated ceramic, and resin nanoceramic. Their conclusion was that resin nanoceramic caused high stress concentrations and displacement in dental structures, thus being a less suitable material for endocrowns. Translucent zirconia was shown to be the best for endocrowns, as it absorbed stresses and showed low displacement within them as well as in the dental tissues [14].

Dental implants represent one of the greatest advances in oral rehabilitation. Titanium implants are considered the most common type of implant because of their durability and functionality. However, aesthetic failure of implant rehabilitation is quite frequent, being related to the specific color of the titanium screws. This is the reason why several technologies have been developed for the production of colored titanium surfaces, including laser. Zara et al. aimed to investigate the relationship between novel laser-colored surfaces and peri-implant soft tissues and confirmed the innovative physical titanium improvements due to laser treatment, which is biocompatible and allows a wide color palette to be obtained while maintaining the roughness of the titanium surface and being able to promote the growth of soft tissues [15]. Immediate implant placement eliminates the need for multiple surgeries and reduces treatment time. Thus, the study of Comuzzi et al. aimed to compare the stability of two conical implants and a cylindrical one inserted into low-density polyurethane blocks with or without a cortical lamina, which potentially mimicked the post-extraction condition. They concluded that the conical implant shape could be considered the best-performing one in artificial post-extraction conditions due to the higher primary stability values [16]. The micro- and nanostructures and wettability of titanium implant surfaces are essential for osseointegration. Improved cell response and shorter healing time are the results of combining hydrophilicity and nanostructure. The study of Illing et al. aimed to investigate the biological response to different wettability levels and nanostructure modifications in titanium surfaces. The additional nanostructures created by plasma etching with fluorine gas demonstrated improved fibroblast cell viability, but did not lead to improved early osseointegration. They concluded that other factors besides surface roughness and wettability play decisive roles in cell attachment, cell viability, and osseointegration [17].

The main goal of dental treatment concerns either the regeneration of diseased tissues or their replacement with prosthesis. Three-dimensional bioprinting uses bioinks to fabricate complex organ structures and functional tissues that can support live cells and other biological factors. By means of 3D bioprinting, tailored tissue-engineered constructs with customized complex architecture and properties can be speedily manufactured [18]. The scoping review of Mohd et al. aimed to explore the 3D bioprinting technologies, biomaterials, and cells used for dental applications. According to the authors, 3D bioprinting has shown promising results for periodontal ligament, dentin, dental pulp, and bone regeneration applications, but, regrettably, is not yet close to being a clinical reality [19].

Edentulism is a worldwide phenomenon with both esthetic and functional repercussions, being considered a reflection of the patient's history of dental conditions and treatments. The field of prosthetic rehabilitation has changed drastically as a result of advancements in materials and digital technology, aiming to preserving tooth structure and offering the best treatment option. Adhesive techniques need less invasive tooth preparation. Three different designs (one fixed-fixed and two cantilever designs) of resin-bonded bridges were compared and evaluated by Narwani et al. according to tensile bond strength. All designs used both the Rochette and Maryland types of retainers. The fixed–fixed design proved superior, while Maryland bridges showed higher bond strengths across all framework designs, implying that they may demonstrate lower clinical failure than cantilever designs and Rochette bridges [20].

Among the most recent and performant technologies used in prosthetic dentistry, computer-aided design and computer-aided manufacturing (CAD/CAM) enables subtractive or additive fabrication of various types of dental prostheses and appliances. Addugala et al. analyzed the marginal discrepancy and internal adaptation of copings fabricated using three types of resin patterns with subtractive (milling) and additive technology (3D printing), namely, milled polymethyl methacrylate resin and digital light-processed acrylonitrile–butadiene–styrene and polylactic acid patterns. The patterns were subsequently casted with a Co-Cr alloy, and the internal and marginal gaps of the copings were microscopically observed. Copings fabricated from the milled PMMA group had the best marginal fit, while copings fabricated with the PLA 3D printed group had the best internal fit [21].

Recent advances in CAD/CAM technologies have allowed for the manufacturing of different types of materials for the CAD/CAM milling process: metal-based, ceramic-based, and resin-based.

Biofilm formation on hybrid resin-based CAD/CAM materials was evaluated by Tzimas et al. in a comprehensive review. As biofilms play an important role in restoration failure, by facilitating secondary caries appearance at the restoration's margins and by altering the restorative material's surface characteristics, the current literature describes a possible interaction between biofilm formation and the surface of the restorative material [22].

Zirconia-based ceramic CAD/CAM blocks are a frequent choice because of their versatility, combining high strength with improved esthetics. Their lack of translucency has been overcome by the latest generations of Y-TZP zirconia, with improved properties and wider indications for both monolithic and veneered restorations. The interest for zirconia-based ceramics is highlighted by six articles published in this Special Issue, assessing this type of block [14,23–27]. Chen et al. investigated the effect of restoration thickness on the fracture resistance of translucent 5-YZP crowns cemented with different cements and subjected to different surface treatments compared to 3-YZP crowns, with detailed results available in the manuscript [23]. Sokolowski et al. investigated the shear bond strength of resin-based luting cement to zirconia ceramics after different surface treatments, aiming to determine the effect of a new etching technique on zirconia and assessing the effect of using primers on the bond strength of zirconia luted with resin cement. Their study concluded that etching of zirconia caused changes in its surface structure and a significant increase in the shear bond strength between zirconia and the resin cement. The use of primers positively affected the adhesion between the resin cement and zirconia [24]. The study of Nasarudin et al. explored the biocompatibility of 3-YZP on three-dimensional oral mucosal models constructed using human gingival fibroblasts and an immortalized human oral keratinocyte cell line co-cultured on an acellular dermal matrix. The study proved the excellent biocompatibility of 3-YZP, indicating its high potential for clinical application as a restorative material [25]. The in vitro study of Rosentritt et al. aimed to compare the cutting efficiency of diamond grinders on zirconia and resin-based composite materials by weight measurements of the material before and after grinding. The grinders showed significantly different initial wear removal and durability. With grinding on zirconia, it took five times as long to remove comparable weight [26]. Smielak et al. aimed to determine whether sandblasting was accompanied by the phenomenon of driving abrasive particles into the conditioned material. Their study assessed disks made of chromium/cobalt, chromium/nickel, titanium, and sintered zirconium dioxide, sandblasted with three different grain sizes of aluminum oxide at three different pressures. After sandblasting, abrasive particles were found on the surfaces of the materials, with the amount being dependent on the hardness of the processed material. Increased grain size and pressure led to an increased amount of embedded grain [27].

In summary, this Special Issue of *Materials*, titled "Advanced Materials for Oral Application-Volume 2", represents a valuable collection of twenty-six cutting-edge research and extensive review articles from across the world, demonstrating the great potential of novel, durable, and high aesthetic dental materials and informing the readers of the current challenges and future directions in this domain.

The Guest Editors would like to thank all contributing authors for the success of the Special Issue. This Special Issue would not have been of such quality without the constructive criticism of the Reviewers. Special thanks and appreciation go to the MDPI *Materials* Section Managing Editor for her most valuable support and collaboration.

Author Contributions: The authors had equal contributions. All authors have read and agreed to the published version of the manuscript.

Conflicts of Interest: The authors declare no conflicts of interest.

References

1. Livne, S.; Simantov, S.; Rahmanov, A.; Jeffet, U.; Sterer, N. Hydroxyethyl Cellulose Promotes the Mucin Retention of Herbal Extracts Active against *Streptococcus mutans*. *Materials* **2022**, *15*, 4652. [CrossRef]
2. Florea, A.-D.; Dobrota, C.T.; Carpa, R.; Racz, C.-P.; Tomoaia, G.; Mocanu, A.; Avram, A.; Soritau, O.; Pop, L.C.; Tomoaia-Cotisel, M. Optimization of Functional Toothpaste Formulation Containing Nano-Hydroxyapatite and Birch Extract for Daily Oral Care. *Materials* **2023**, *16*, 7143. [CrossRef]
3. Sengar, E.V.; Mulay, S.; Beri, L.; Gupta, A.; Almohareb, T.; Binalrimal, S.; Robaian, A.; Bahammam, M.A.; Bahammam, H.A.; Bahammam, S.A.; et al. Comparative Evaluation of Microleakage of Flowable Composite Resin Using Etch and Rinse, Self-Etch Adhesive Systems, and Self-Adhesive Flowable Composite Resin in Class V Cavities: Confocal Laser Microscopic Study. *Materials* **2022**, *15*, 4963. [CrossRef]
4. Maximov, J.; Dikova, T.; Duncheva, G.; Georgiev, G. Influence of Factors in the Photopolymerization Process on Dental Composites Microhardness. *Materials* **2022**, *15*, 6459. [CrossRef]

5. Klimek, L.; Kopacz, K.; Śmielak, B.; Kula, Z. An Evaluation of the Mechanical Properties of a Hybrid Composite Containing Hydroxyapatite. *Materials* **2023**, *16*, 4548. [CrossRef] [PubMed]
6. Aldowsari, M.K.; Alfawzan, F.; Alhaidari, A.; Alhogail, N.; Alshargi, R.; Bin Saleh, S.; Sulimany, A.M.; Alturki, M. Comparison of Shear Bond Strength of Three Types of Adhesive Materials Used in the Restoration of Permanent Molars after Treatment with Silver Diamine Fluoride: An In Vitro Study. *Materials* **2023**, *16*, 6831. [CrossRef]
7. De Angelis, F.; D'Ercole, S.; Di Giulio, M.; Vadini, M.; Biferi, V.; Buonvivere, M.; Vanini, L.; Cellini, L.; Di Lodovico, S.; D'Arcangelo, C. In Vitro Evaluation of *Candida albicans* Adhesion on Heat-Cured Resin-Based Dental Composites. *Materials* **2023**, *16*, 5818. [CrossRef]
8. Rai, J.J.; Chaturvedi, S.; Gokhale, S.T.; Nagate, R.R.; Al-Qahtani, S.M.; Magbol, M.A.; Bavabeedu, S.S.; Elagib, M.F.A.; Venkataram, V.; Chaturvedi, M. Effectiveness of a Single Chair Side Application of NovaMin® [Calcium Sodium Phosphosilicate] in the Treatment of Dentine Hypersensitivity following Ultrasonic Scaling—A Randomized Controlled Trial. *Materials* **2023**, *16*, 1329. [CrossRef] [PubMed]
9. Sahin, D.; Deger, C.; Oglakci, B.; Demirkol, M.; Kucukyildirim, B.O.; Gursel, M.; Eliguzeloglu Dalkilic, E. The Effects of a Novel Nanohydroxyapatite Gel and Er: YAG Laser Treatment on Dentin Hypersensitivity. *Materials* **2023**, *16*, 6522. [CrossRef] [PubMed]
10. Rajamanickam, K.; Teja, K.V.; Ramesh, S.; AbuMelha, A.S.; Alkahtany, M.F.; Almadi, K.H.; Bahammam, S.A.; Janani, K.; Choudhari, S.; Jose, J.; et al. Comparative Study Assessing the Canal Cleanliness Using Automated Device and Conventional Syringe Needle for Root Canal Irrigation—An Ex-Vivo Study. *Materials* **2022**, *15*, 6184. [CrossRef]
11. Drukteinis, S.; Bilvinaite, G.; Sakirzanovas, S. The Impact of Citric Acid Solution on Hydraulic Calcium Silicate-Based Sealers and Root Dentin: A Preliminary Assessment. *Materials* **2024**, *17*, 1351. [CrossRef] [PubMed]
12. Ashi, T.; Richert, R.; Mancino, D.; Jmal, H.; Alkhouri, S.; Addiego, F.; Kharouf, N.; Haïkel, Y. Do the Mechanical Properties of Calcium-Silicate-Based Cements Influence the Stress Distribution of Different Retrograde Cavity Preparations? *Materials* **2023**, *16*, 3111. [CrossRef] [PubMed]
13. Habib, S.R.; Ansari, A.S.; Khan, A.S.; Alamro, N.M.; Alzaaqi, M.A.; Alkhunefer, Y.A.; AlHelal, A.A.; Alnassar, T.M.; Alqahtani, A.S. Push-Out Bond Strength of Endodontic Posts Cemented to Extracted Teeth: An In-Vitro Evaluation. *Materials* **2022**, *15*, 6792. [CrossRef]
14. Darwich, M.A.; Aljareh, A.; Alhouri, N.; Szávai, S.; Nazha, H.M.; Duvigneau, F.; Juhre, D. Biomechanical Assessment of Endodontically Treated Molars Restored by Endocrowns Made from Different CAD/CAM Materials. *Materials* **2023**, *16*, 764. [CrossRef]
15. Zara, S.; Fioravanti, G.; Ciuffreda, A.; Annicchiarico, C.; Quaresima, R.; Mastrangelo, F. Evaluation of Human Gingival Fibroblasts (HGFs) Behavior on Innovative Laser Colored Titanium Surfaces. *Materials* **2023**, *16*, 4530. [CrossRef]
16. Comuzzi, L.; Tumedei, M.; Di Pietro, N.; Romasco, T.; Heydari Sheikh Hossein, H.; Montesani, L.; Inchingolo, F.; Piattelli, A.; Covani, U. A Comparison of Conical and Cylindrical Implants Inserted in an In Vitro Post-Extraction Model Using Low-Density Polyurethane Foam Blocks. *Materials* **2023**, *16*, 5064. [CrossRef]
17. Illing, B.; Mohammadnejad, L.; Theurer, A.; Schultheiss, J.; Kimmerle-Mueller, E.; Rupp, F.; Krajewski, S. Biological Performance of Titanium Surfaces with Different Hydrophilic and Nanotopographical Features. *Materials* **2023**, *16*, 7307. [CrossRef] [PubMed]
18. Tigmeanu, C.V.; Ardelean, L.C.; Rusu, L.-C.; Negrutiu, M.-L. Additive Manufactured Polymers in Dentistry, Current State-of-the-Art and Future Perspectives-A Review. *Polymers* **2022**, *14*, 3658. [CrossRef]
19. Mohd, N.; Razali, M.; Ghazali, M.J.; Abu Kasim, N.H. Current Advances of Three-Dimensional Bioprinting Application in Dentistry: A Scoping Review. *Materials* **2022**, *15*, 6398. [CrossRef]
20. Narwani, S.; Yadav, N.S.; Hazari, P.; Saxena, V.; Alzahrani, A.H.; Alamoudi, A.; Zidane, B.; Albar, N.H.M.; Robaian, A.; Kishnani, S.; et al. Comparison of Tensile Bond Strength of Fixed-Fixed Versus Cantilever Single- and Double-Abutted Resin-Bonded Bridges Dental Prosthesis. *Materials* **2022**, *15*, 5744. [CrossRef] [PubMed]
21. Addugala, H.; Venugopal, V.N.; Rengasamy, S.; Yadalam, P.K.; Albar, N.H.; Alamoudi, A.; Bahammam, S.A.; Zidane, B.; Bahammam, H.A.; Bhandi, S.; et al. Marginal and Internal Gap of Metal Copings Fabricated Using Three Types of Resin Patterns with Subtractive and Additive Technology: An In Vitro Comparison. *Materials* **2022**, *15*, 6397. [CrossRef] [PubMed]
22. Tzimas, K.; Rahiotis, C.; Pappa, E. Biofilm Formation on Hybrid, Resin-Based CAD/CAM Materials for Indirect Restorations: A Comprehensive Review. *Materials* **2024**, *17*, 1474. [CrossRef] [PubMed]
23. Chen, P.-H.; Elamin, E.; Sayed Ahmed, A.; Givan, D.A.; Fu, C.-C.; Lawson, N.C. The Effect of Restoration Thickness on the Fracture Resistance of 5 mol% Yttria-Containing Zirconia Crowns. *Materials* **2024**, *17*, 365. [CrossRef] [PubMed]
24. Sokolowski, G.; Szczesio-Wlodarczyk, A.; Szynkowska-Jóźwik, M.I.; Stopa, W.; Sokolowski, J.; Kopacz, K.; Bociong, K. The Shear Bond Strength of Resin-Based Luting Cement to Zirconia Ceramics after Different Surface Treatments. *Materials* **2023**, *16*, 5433. [CrossRef] [PubMed]
25. Nasarudin, N.A.; Razali, M.; Goh, V.; Chai, W.L.; Muchtar, A. Expression of Interleukin-1β and Histological Changes of the Three-Dimensional Oral Mucosal Model in Response to Yttria-Stabilized Nanozirconia. *Materials* **2023**, *16*, 2027. [CrossRef] [PubMed]

26. Rosentritt, M.; Strasser, T.; Mueller, M.-M.; Schmidt, M.B. Cutting Efficiency of Diamond Grinders on Composite and Zirconia. *Materials* **2024**, *17*, 2596. [CrossRef] [PubMed]
27. Śmielak, B.; Klimek, L.; Krześniak, K. Effect of Sandblasting Parameters and the Type and Hardness of the Material on the Number of Embedded Al_2O_3 Grains. *Materials* **2023**, *16*, 4783. [CrossRef]

Disclaimer/Publisher's Note: The statements, opinions and data contained in all publications are solely those of the individual author(s) and contributor(s) and not of MDPI and/or the editor(s). MDPI and/or the editor(s) disclaim responsibility for any injury to people or property resulting from any ideas, methods, instructions or products referred to in the content.

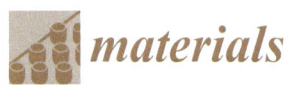

Article

Hydroxyethyl Cellulose Promotes the Mucin Retention of Herbal Extracts Active against *Streptococcus mutans*

Shiri Livne, Sapir Simantov, Arkadi Rahmanov, Uziel Jeffet and Nir Sterer *

Department of Prosthodontics, Goldschleger School of Dental Medicine, Sackler Faculty of Medicine, Tel-Aviv University, Ramat-Aviv, Tel Aviv 6997801, Israel; dr.livne@yahoo.com (S.L.); sapirs3@mail.tau.ac.il (S.S.); phenomenar18@gmail.com (A.R.); uzieljef@gmail.com (U.J.)
* Correspondence: drsterer@gmail.com; Tel.: +972-3-6409303

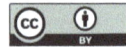

Citation: Livne, S.; Simantov, S.; Rahmanov, A.; Jeffet, U.; Sterer, N. Hydroxyethyl Cellulose Promotes the Mucin Retention of Herbal Extracts Active against *Streptococcus mutans*. *Materials* **2022**, *15*, 4652. https://doi.org/10.3390/ma15134652

Academic Editors: Lavinia Cosmina Ardelean and Laura-Cristina Rusu

Received: 13 June 2022
Accepted: 30 June 2022
Published: 1 July 2022

Publisher's Note: MDPI stays neutral with regard to jurisdictional claims in published maps and institutional affiliations.

Copyright: © 2022 by the authors. Licensee MDPI, Basel, Switzerland. This article is an open access article distributed under the terms and conditions of the Creative Commons Attribution (CC BY) license (https://creativecommons.org/licenses/by/4.0/).

Abstract: *Streptococcus mutans* is considered a major cariogenic bacterium. Most anti-cariogenic dentifrices are limited by a short exposure time. The aim of the present study was to test the hypothesis that adding a mucoadhesive agent to the formulation may increase its bioavailability and efficacy. We tested the effect of adding hydroxyethyl cellulose (HEC) to an herbal extract solution containing lavender, echinacea, sage, and mastic gum, which have been previously shown to be effective against *Streptococcus mutans*. Mucin-coated wells were treated with four test solutions: saline, herbal extracts, herbal extracts with HEC, and chlorhexidine. The wells were incubated with *Streptococcus mutans* and studied for biofilm formation (Crystal violet assay), acid production (lactate assay), acid tolerance (ATPase assay), and exopolysaccharide (EPS) production using fluorescent microscopy. The results showed that the addition of HEC to the herbal extract solution caused a significant reduction in *Streptococcus mutans* biofilm formation, lactic acid production, and EPS quantity ($p < 0.001$). These results suggest that HEC may be a beneficial added excipient to herbal extracts in an anti-cariogenic formulation.

Keywords: extracellular polysaccharide; hydroxyethyl cellulose; *Streptococcus mutans*

1. Introduction

Dental caries is a prevalent disease among youth, affecting some 45% of the population between ages 6–19 years [1]. This disease is caused by the metabolism of sugars by the saccharolytic oral bacteria that breakdown carbohydrates and dietary sugars, which are energy source yielding acidic by-products such as lactic acid that can dissolve the hydroxyapatite crystals constructing the tooth's hard tissues in a process known as demineralization [2], which, if left untreated, may result in cavitation, pain, dental infection, and tooth loss.

Streptococcus mutans is considered the main cariogenic pathogen [3] due to its enhanced abilities (i) to produce highly adhesive extracellular matrix polysaccharides in a biofilm configuration, (ii) to prolong acid production (i.e., acidogenic) facilitated by the intracellular storage of polysaccharide molecules, and (iii) to survive acidic environmental conditions (i.e., aciduric). Therefore, it is often used as the test bacterium in the evaluation of preventive treatments for caries.

Preventive dentifrices for caries are often limited in efficacy due to their short exposure time. Mucoadhesive polymers such as hydroxyethyl cellulose (HEC) have been added as excipient binders to liquid formulations in order to promote the mucosal retention of their active ingredients, thus improving their bioavailability and efficacy [4]. Other researchers have demonstrated the benefits of using mucoadhesive polymers such as HEC and HPMC as sustained-release delivery systems for antibacterial agents in a mucin-coated environment that is similar to the oral cavity, such as for eye infection treatment [5].

In a previous study, we demonstrated the antibacterial activity of four herbal extracts: lavender, echinacea, sage, and mastic gum against *Streptococcus mutans* [6]. The aim of the present study was to test the in vitro effect of adding the mucoadhesive polymer HEC to a liquid-phase herbal extract formulation on the mucoadhesive retention of the active ingredients and their effect against the cariogenic properties of *Streptococcus mutans*.

2. Materials and Methods

2.1. Bacterial Strain and Growth Conditions

Streptococcus mutans (ATCC 27351) was cultured in BHI media supplemented with sucrose (5% w/v) at 37 °C under anaerobic conditions.

2.2. Mucoadhesion Bioassay

Mucin solution was prepared by stirring and dissolving commercially available pig gastric mucin (type III, Sigma, Rehovot, Israel) in saline (1% w/v) over night at 4 °C. The mucin solution was centrifuged (6500× g, 30 min) and filter-sterilized using a vacuum-driven disposable filtration system (0.2 μm, StericupTM, Millipore, Burlington, MA, USA). The filtered mucin (40 μL) was placed on the bottoms of 96-well microplates (Nunc) and fixated over night at 37 °C by allowing the solvent to evaporate and the mucin coating to form a gel.

Four treatment solutions were tested: (i) saline as a negative control; (ii) a herbal extract formulation (NovaBreathTM, Tree of Life) without HEC; (iii) herbal extracts formulated with HEC (0.15% w/v); and (iv) chlorhexidine (0.2% w/v) as a positive control. Tested solutions and controls (40 μL) were placed on the bottoms of the mucin-coated wells for 2 min, and the wells were washed three times with saline to remove any non-adhered materials. Following washing, a bacterial suspension (0.4 OD, 40 μL) was placed in the bottoms of the treated wells, and BHI media (0.2 mL) supplemented with sucrose (5%) was gently added to each well. Microplates were incubated anaerobically at 37 °C for 24 h (end of Log phase) to allow for biofilm formation. Biofilms were studied for biomass, lactic acid production, ATPase activity, and extracellular polysaccharide formation, as described below.

2.3. Colorimetric Analysis for Biomass, Lactate and ATPase

Biofilm growth was quantified using crystal violet assay [7]. Supernatant was discarded, and 200 μL of crystal violet solution (0.1%) was added to the biofilms for 1 min. Stained biofilms were washed three times with saline to remove any unbound stain, and the stain was eluted using decolorizing solution and quantified colorimetrically. Lactate production was measured using a colorimetric lactate assay kit (abcam), and the ATPase activity in the biofilms was quantified using a colorimetric ATPase assay kit (abcam). Both kits were used as instructed in their manuals. All three colorimetric assays were performed at 600 nm using a microplate reader.

2.4. Extra-Cellular Polysaccharide (EPS) Production Assay

In a separate experiment, biofilms were grown under the same experimental conditions as stated above using a chamber slide well system (Lab TakTM, Nunc, Goteborg, Sweden). Following growth, the supernatant was discarded, and the wells were detached from their glass base without removing the silicone gasket. The gasket was used as a reservoir and filled with 40 μL of saline with 2 μL of a green fluorescent dye that stains both live and dead bacteria (DMAO, Promokine, Heidelberg, Germany) followed by 5 μL of Congo red solution (0.1%). The glass slabs with the stained biofilms were studied using fluorescent microscopy (×400, L3201LED, MRC, Rehovot, Israel) with an excitation wavelength of 460–470 nm and a blue LED filter with a cutoff of 500 nm. EPS production in the biofilms was quantified by analyzing digital images from each biofilm using morphometric software (ImageJ, NIH, Stapleton, NY, USA).

2.5. Statistical Analysis

To compare the effect of the different treatments on the various parameters, ANOVA was applied. Two-tailed tests were applied, and $p \leq 0.05$ was considered statistically significant. Experiments were performed in six replicates (n = 6).

3. Results

3.1. Biomass, Lactate and ATPase

The mean results of biomass formation, lactic acid production, and ATPase activity in the various treated samples are presented in Figures 1–3. These results show that the addition of hydroxyethyl cellulose (HEC) significantly increased the effect of the treatment in reducing biomass formation and lactic acid production compared to herbal extracts alone ($p < 0.001$). The addition of HEC also caused an 18% reduction in the ATPase activity; however, this was not statistically significant.

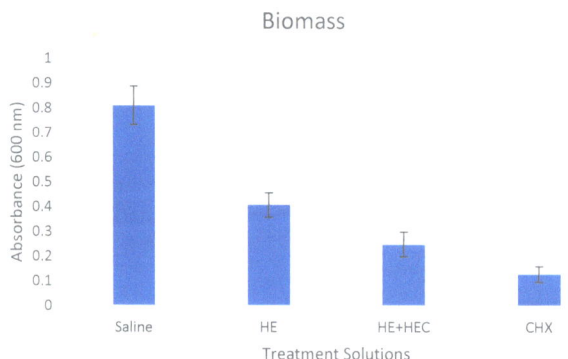

Figure 1. Effect of the various treatment solutions on *Streptococcus mutans* biofilm formation: saline as negative control; herbal extracts (HE); combined herbal extracts and hydroxyethyl cellulose (HE + HEC); and chlorhexidine (CHX) as positive control. Results (±standard deviation) are presented as absorbance at 600 nm.

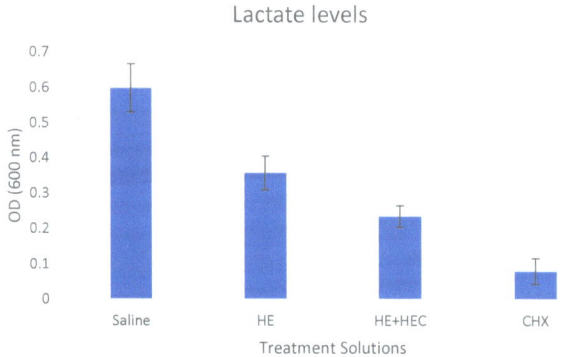

Figure 2. Effect of the various treatment solutions on *Streptococcus mutans* lactic acid production: saline as negative control; herbal extracts (HE); combined herbal extracts and hydroxyethyl cellulose (HE + HEC); and chlorhexidine (CHX) as positive control. Results (±standard deviation) measured using a colorimetric assay are presented as OD (600 nm) units.

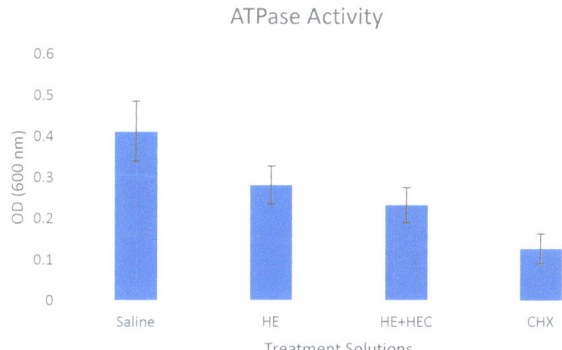

Figure 3. Effect of the various treatment solutions on *Streptococcus mutans* ATPase activity: saline as negative control; herbal extracts (HE); combined herbal extracts and hydroxyethyl cellulose (HE + HEC); and chlorhexidine (CHX) as positive control. Results (±standard deviation) measured using a colorimetric assay are presented as OD (600 nm) units.

3.2. Extra-Cellular Polysaccharide (EPS) Production Levels

The results of the fluorescent microscopy and EPS quantification are presented in Figures 4 and 5. These results show a significant 30% reduction in the EPS content in the biofilm following the addition of HEC to the treatment solution compared to the non-added herbal extract solution alone ($p < 0.001$).

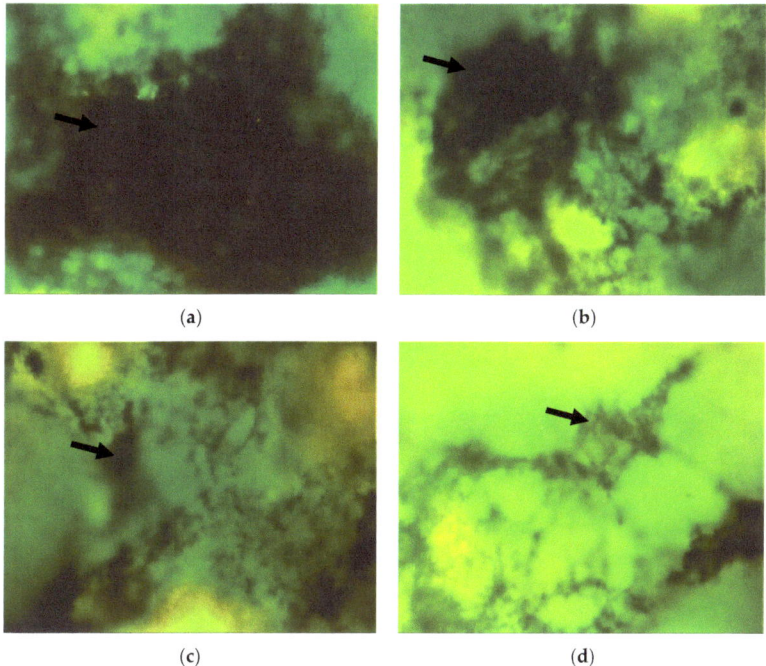

Figure 4. Fluorescent microscopy images showing EPS production (maroon-stained indicated by arrow) in the biofilms of the various treated samples: (**a**) saline; (**b**) herbal extracts; (**c**) combined herbal extracts and hydroxyethyl cellulose; and (**d**) chlorhexidine.

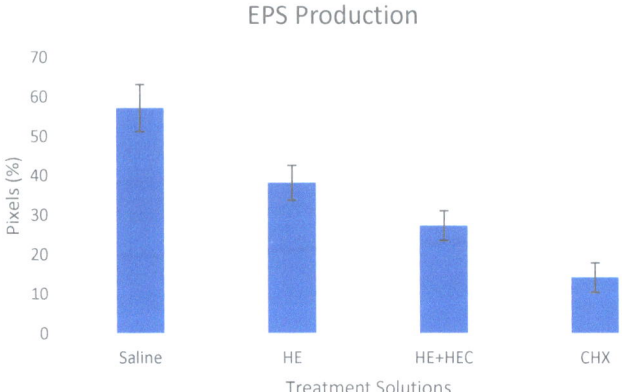

Figure 5. Effect of the various treatment solutions on *Streptococcus mutans* EPS production: saline as negative control; herbal extracts (HE); combined herbal extracts and hydroxyethyl cellulose (HE + HEC); and chlorhexidine (CHX) as positive control. Results (±standard deviation) are presented as percentage of maroon-stained pixels measured from digitally analyzed (Image J, NIH) fluorescent microscopy images.

4. Discussion

We previously showed that the antibacterial effect of four herbal extracts against the cariogenic bacterium *Streptococcus mutans* [6]. The results of the current study demonstrated that adding a mucoadhesive polymer (HEC) to the herbal formulation significantly increased its mucin-retained efficacy against *Streptococcus mutans* by hindering the bacterium's ability to form a biofilm and express its cariogenicity compared to the no-addition control. This suggests that the addition of HEC may increase the mucoadhesive binding of the herbal formulation's active ingredients without impairing their anti-cariogenic activities.

Streptococcus mutans has been implicated as a major cariogenic bacterium that is responsible for the initiation and propagation [8] of carious lesions mainly through its enhanced insoluble EPS production and cariogenic biofilm formation abilities followed by its acidogenic and aciduric properties [9,10]. Therefore, antimicrobial agents play an important part in dental caries prevention and management [11]. These agents are commonly applied to the oral cavity by means of various dentifrices such as toothpastes and mouth rinses. However, due to their limited exposure time (i.e., 1–2 min), their efficacy might also be limited [12]. Hence, prolonging the exposure time is an important goal in the development of these formulations.

The use of porcine gastric mucin (PGM) as a commercially available substitute for human mucin is common in oral microbiology studies due to its considerable overall similarity to the O-linked carbohydrate sidechains of human mucins [13]. Previous studies have shown the mucoadhesive properties of HEC using PGM [14]. These mucoadhesive properties may be beneficial in prolonging the retention time and bioavailability of active ingredients used in mouthwash formulations.

The mucoadhesive properties of the HEC that was added to the liquid herbal extract in the present study combined with the increase in efficacy compared to the non-added samples suggest that some of the active ingredients in the extracts may have been bound to the mucin coating via the mucoadhesive polymer, thus preventing them from being washed and increasing their bioavailability and efficacy. This is in agreement with other researchers showing the sustained release pattern of antibacterial agents bound to HEC in an eye drop formulation [5].

Taken together, the results of the present study suggest that within the limitations of an in vitro study, adding HEC to an herbal extract formulation that is active against the cariogenic properties of *Streptococcus mutans* may increase the bioavailability and efficacy of its active ingredients via HEC's mucoadhesive properties, thus providing a platform for the development of a caries-preventing formulation that is more efficient in reducing biofilm formation and the virulence of the cariogenic bacterium *Streptococcus mutans*. However, additional clinical investigation is warranted.

Author Contributions: Conceptualization, N.S.; methodology, N.S. and U.J.; validation, S.L., S.S. and A.R.; formal analysis, A.R.; investigation, S.L. and S.S.; resources, U.J.; data curation, A.R.; writing—original draft preparation, N.S.; writing—review and editing, S.L.; visualization, S.S.; supervision, N.S.; project administration, U.J. All authors have read and agreed to the published version of the manuscript.

Funding: This research received no external funding.

Institutional Review Board Statement: Not applicable.

Informed Consent Statement: Not applicable.

Data Availability Statement: Not applicable.

Conflicts of Interest: The authors declare no conflict of interest.

References

1. Fleming, E.; Afful, J. Prevalence of Total and Untreated Dental Caries among Youth: United States, 2015–2016. *NCHS Data Brief* **2018**, *307*, 1–8.
2. Touger-Decker, R.; van Loveren, C. Sugars and dental caries. *Am. J. Clin. Nutr.* **2003**, *78*, 881S–892S. [CrossRef] [PubMed]
3. Krzyściak, W.; Jurczak, A.; Kościelniak, D.; Bystrowska, B.; Skalniak, A. The virulence of Streptococcus mutans and the ability to form biofilms. *Eur. J. Clin. Microbiol. Infect. Dis.* **2014**, *33*, 499–515. [CrossRef] [PubMed]
4. Klemetsrud, T.; Kjøniksen, A.L.; Hiorth, M.; Jacobsen, J.; Smistad, G. Polymer coated liposomes for use in the oral cavity—A study of the in vitro toxicity, effect on cell permeability and interaction with mucin. *J. Liposome Res.* **2018**, *28*, 62–73. [CrossRef] [PubMed]
5. Taghe, S.; Mirzaeei, S.; Alany, R.G.; Nokhodchi, A. Polymeric Inserts Containing Eudragit® L100 Nanoparticle for Improved Ocular Delivery of Azithromycin. *Biomedicines* **2020**, *8*, 466. [CrossRef] [PubMed]
6. Sterer, N.; Nuas, S.; Mizrahi, B.; Goldenberg, C.; Weiss, E.I.; Domb, A.; Davidi, M.P. Oral malodor reduction by a palatal mucoadhesive tablet containing herbal formulation. *J. Dent.* **2008**, *36*, 535–539. [CrossRef] [PubMed]
7. Kaminski, K.; Syrek, K.; Grudzień, J.; Obloza, M.; Adamczyk, M.; Sulka, G.D. Physicochemical Investigation of Biosynthesis of a Protein Coating on Glass That Promotes Mammalian Cell Growth Using *Lactobacillus rhamnosus* GG Bacteria. *Coatings* **2021**, *11*, 1410. [CrossRef]
8. Gross, E.L.; Leys, E.J.; Gasparovich, S.R.; Firestone, N.D.; Schwartzbaum, J.A.; Janies, D.A.; Asnani, K.; Griffen, A.L. Bacterial 16S sequence analysis of severe caries in young permanent teeth. *J. Clin. Microbiol.* **2010**, *48*, 4121–4128. [CrossRef] [PubMed]
9. Hwang, G.; Liu, Y.; Kim, D.; Sun, V.; Aviles-Reyes, A.; Kajfasz, J.K.; Lemos, J.A.; Koo, H. Simultaneous spatiotemporal mapping of in situ pH and bacterial activity within an intact 3D microcolony structure. *Sci. Rep.* **2016**, *6*, 32841. [CrossRef] [PubMed]
10. Kim, D.; Barraza, J.P.; Arthur, R.A.; Hara, A.; Lewis, K.; Liu, Y.; Scisci, E.L.; Hajishengallis, E.; Whiteley, M.; Koo, H. Spatial mapping of polymicrobial communities reveals a precise biogeography associated with human dental caries. *Proc. Natl. Acad. Sci. USA* **2020**, *117*, 12375–12386. [CrossRef] [PubMed]
11. Balasubramanian, A.R.; Vasudevan, S.; Shanmugam, K.; Lévesque, C.M.; Solomon, A.P.; Neelakantan, P. Combinatorial effects of trans-cinnamaldehyde with fluoride and chlorhexidine on Streptococcus mutans. *J. Appl. Microbiol.* **2021**, *130*, 382–393. [CrossRef] [PubMed]
12. Borden, L.C.; Chaves, E.S.; Bowman, J.P.; Fath, B.M.; Hollar, G.L. The effect of four mouthrinses on oral malodor. *Compend. Contin. Educ. Dent.* **2002**, *23*, 531–548. [PubMed]
13. Sterer, N.; Rosenberg, M. Streptococcus salivarius promotes mucin putrefaction and malodor production by Porphyromonas gingivalis. *J. Dent. Res.* **2006**, *85*, 910–914. [CrossRef] [PubMed]
14. Ivarsson, D.; Wahlgren, M. Comparison of in vitro methods of measuring mucoadhesion: Ellipsometry, tensile strength and rheological measurements. *Colloids Surf. B Biointerfaces* **2012**, *92*, 353–359. [CrossRef]

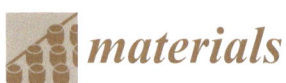 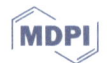

Article

Optimization of Functional Toothpaste Formulation Containing Nano-Hydroxyapatite and Birch Extract for Daily Oral Care

Alexandra-Diana Florea [1,†], Cristina Teodora Dobrota [1,2,†], Rahela Carpa [2], Csaba-Pal Racz [1], Gheorghe Tomoaia [3,4], Aurora Mocanu [1], Alexandra Avram [1], Olga Soritau [5], Lucian Cristian Pop [1] and Maria Tomoaia-Cotisel [1,4,*]

1. Research Center of Physical Chemistry, Faculty of Chemistry and Chemical Engineering, Babeş-Bolyai University, 11 Arany Janos Str., 400028 Cluj-Napoca, Romania; diana_florea03@yahoo.com (A.-D.F.); cristina.dobrota@ubbcluj.ro (C.T.D.); csaba.racz@ubbcluj.ro (C.-P.R.); aurora.mocanu@ubbcluj.ro (A.M.); alexandra.avram@ubbcluj.ro (A.A.); lucian.pop@ubbcluj.ro (L.C.P.)
2. Department of Molecular Biology and Biotechnology, Faculty of Biology and Geology, Babeş-Bolyai University, 44 Republicii Str., 400015 Cluj-Napoca, Romania; rahela.carpa@ubbcluj.ro
3. Department of Orthopedics and Traumatology, Iuliu Hatieganu University of Medicine and Pharmacy, 47 Gen. Traian Mosoiu Str., 400132 Cluj-Napoca, Romania; tomoaia2000@yahoo.com
4. Academy of Romanian Scientists, 3 Ilfov Str., 050044 Bucharest, Romania
5. Oncology Institute of Cluj-Napoca, 34-36 Republicii Str., 400015 Cluj-Napoca, Romania; olgasoritau@yahoo.com
* Correspondence: maria.tomoaia@ubbcluj.ro or mcotisel@gmail.com
† These authors contributed equally to this work.

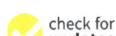

Citation: Florea, A.-D.; Dobrota, C.T.; Carpa, R.; Racz, C.-P.; Tomoaia, G.; Mocanu, A.; Avram, A.; Soritau, O.; Pop, L.C.; Tomoaia-Cotisel, M. Optimization of Functional Toothpaste Formulation Containing Nano-Hydroxyapatite and Birch Extract for Daily Oral Care. *Materials* **2023**, *16*, 7143. https://doi.org/10.3390/ma16227143

Academic Editors: Laura-Cristina Rusu and Lavinia Cosmina Ardelean

Received: 10 October 2023
Revised: 1 November 2023
Accepted: 8 November 2023
Published: 13 November 2023

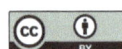

Copyright: © 2023 by the authors. Licensee MDPI, Basel, Switzerland. This article is an open access article distributed under the terms and conditions of the Creative Commons Attribution (CC BY) license (https://creativecommons.org/licenses/by/4.0/).

Abstract: This research work aims to develop functional toothpastes with combined enamel remineralization and antibacterial effects using nano-hydroxyapatites (nHAPs) and birch extract. Eleven toothpastes (notated as P1–P11) were designed featuring different concentrations of birch extract and a constant concentration of pure nHAPs or substituted nHAPs (HAP-5%Zn, HAP-0.23%Mg-3.9%Zn-2%Si-10%Sr, and HAP-2.5%Mg-2.9%Si-1.34%Zn). In vitro assessments involved treating artificially demineralized enamel slices and analyzing surface repair and remineralization using Atomic Force Microscopy (AFM). The Agar Disk Diffusion method was used to measure antibacterial activity against *Enterococcus faecalis*, *Escherichia coli*, *Porphyromonas gingivalis*, *Streptococcus mutans*, and *Staphylococcus aureus*. Topographic images of enamel structure and surface roughness, as well as the ability of nHAP nanoparticles to form self-assembled layers, revealed excellent restorative properties of the tested toothpastes, with enamel nanostructure normalization occurring as soon as 10 days after treatment. The outcomes highlighted enamel morphology improvements due to the toothpaste treatment also having various efficacious antibacterial effects. Promising results were obtained using P5 toothpaste, containing HAP-5%Zn (3.4%) and birch extract (1.3%), indicating notable remineralization and good antibacterial properties. This study represents a significant advancement in oral care by introducing toothpaste formulations that simultaneously promote enamel health through effective remineralization and bacterial inhibition.

Keywords: AFM; antibacterial activity; birch extract; enamel remineralization; nano-hydroxyapatites; oral care

1. Introduction

Biomaterials are intentionally designed to engage with biological entities and hold significant relevance within the realms of medical and biological pursuits, including but not limited to antibacterial interventions, regenerative medicine, and immunomodulation [1,2]. Notably, plant extracts sourced from renewable natural reservoirs have recently gained substantial attention due to their inherent attributes such as biocompatibility and therapeutic potential. These plant-derived extracts exhibit noteworthy qualities such as bioactivity, adaptability, and biodegradability. However, in contrast to synthetic materials, biomaterials derived from plant extracts face certain challenges, including inconsistencies between batches, potential allergenicity, and limitations in mechanical properties. Consequently, when endeavoring to create biomaterials based on plant extracts for medical applications, it becomes imperative to undertake comprehensive characterization, establish standardization protocols, and enforce stringent quality control measures [3].

Advanced formulations of toothpastes incorporate different active ingredients capable of providing a comprehensive oral cleansing experience while protecting the enamel surface. The chemical composition of toothpaste should be carefully determined so that the components do not affect the dental enamel and manifest their potential optimally [4]. Contemporary toothpaste formulations encompass an array of diverse active constituents which possess the capacity to facilitate a comprehensive oral hygiene regimen, concurrently safeguarding the integrity of dental enamel. The meticulous determination of toothpaste's chemical constituents is imperative to ensure that said constituents neither compromise the structural integrity of dental enamel nor fail to fully realize their inherent therapeutic potential. The chemical composition of toothpaste typically mirrors its envisaged clinical utility, encompassing various applications, including but not limited to antibacterial, anti-inflammatory, desensitizing, remineralizing, and whitening properties [4].

Antimicrobial agents of various types have been produced to treat dental plaque formed by biofilms. Antimicrobial agents can be categorized into three groups according to the materials they are made of: organic, biological, and inorganic [5]. Nano-calcium fluoride, which reduces caries and increases labile fluoride concentration [6], silver nanoparticles (AgNPs) with antimicrobial and anti-inflammatory properties [7], and nano-hydroxyapatite (n-HAP) containing different metal ions [8–10] are among the inorganic compounds used in toothpaste formulation.

Because of their minimal toxicity and antibacterial action, various pharmacological features, and low cost, plant secondary metabolites have attracted the interest of many researchers as naturally produced organic antimicrobial agents [11,12]. Based on their chemical contents, many plant extracts have been shown to have significant pharmacological effects. Crude extracts and distillates, comprising phenols, alkaloids, terpenoids, glycosylated compounds, vitamins, and sterols, exhibit a wide spectrum of pharmacological activity in both in vitro and in vivo contexts [13]. Products containing these plant secondary metabolites are widely embraced for their perceived safety, health benefits, and environmental friendliness when juxtaposed with synthetic chemical additives [14].

The formulation of toothpaste is straightforward, and it remains cost-effective. Moreover, toothpaste composition can be customized using a diverse array of inorganic and organic components. Birch extract, derived from various parts of birch trees, contains a plethora of bioactive constituents, such as phenolic compounds, flavonoids, and lignans, which possess noteworthy biological properties that hold promise for applications in biomaterials [15].

Some of the pharmacological actions of the secondary metabolites in birch can be found in Table 1.

To address affected enamel healing more successfully, researchers typically combine antibacterial agents with various matrix materials to create toothpastes with varying qualities. Nanomaterials, which are attractive due to their biocompatibility, are among the most common matrix materials. Research investigations into the effectiveness of nano-hydroxyapatite (nHAP) crystals within toothpaste formulations have revealed notable enhancements in the microhardness properties of human enamel following the application of toothpaste containing nHAPs [46]. Additionally, there is evidence of the proficient occlusion of dentinal tubules by nHAP particles, which adhere to the tooth surface and impede mineral dissolution processes [47].

Table 1. Pharmacological activity of birch secondary metabolites.

Plant Part	Chemical Constituents	Pharmacological Effects	References
Roots	Essential oils, ascorbic acid, coumarins, sterols, saponins, tannins, potassium, sodium	Antiscorbutic, antiarthritic, anticancer, antidiabetic, anti-inflammatory, antimicrobial, antioxidant, antiviral, gastroprotective, hepatoprotective, immunomodulatory	[15–22]
Outer bark	Pentacyclic triterpenes (mainly betulin up to 34%) terpenes, methylsalicylate, creosol, guaiacol	Antibacterial effect against *Streptococcus, Porphyromonas gingivalis, Streptococcus pyogenes, Escherichia coli, Staphylococcus aureus,* and *Enterococcus faecalis*; and antifungal, anticarcinogenic, antiperiodontic, anticancer, anti-inflammatory, antiviral, antibiofilm activities.	[17,18,23–33]
Bark extracts	Phenols, terpenoids, alkaloids, glycosylated molecules, organic acids, cathecol, oleuro-pein-aglycone, acacetin, kaempferide, dimethylquercetin, pentacosyl, resorcinol	Anti-inflammatory, antimicrobial, antioxidant, antiviral, immunomodulatory, antiarthritic, anticancer, antidiabetic, gastroprotective, hepatoprotective, prevention of degenerative diseases.	[16,23,34–36]
Birch buds	Essential oil (up to 3.8%) triterpenoids, diarylheptanoids, phenylbutanoids, lignans, phenolics and flavonoids Sesquiterpene	Antiarthritic, anticancer, antidiabetic, anti-inflammatory, antimicrobial, antioxidant, antiviral, gastroprotective, hepatoprotective, and immunomodulatory activities.	[23,37–39]
Leaves	Flavones glycosides (1–3%), quercetin, glycosides, kaempferol glycosides myricetin glycoside, betulorentic acid, caffeic acid, saponins, tannins, sesquiterpenes, chlorogenic acid, triterpene alcohol, malonyl esters of dimarene type, polymeric proanthocyanidins, macro- and micronutrients up to 38%	Oral health as preventive and therapeutic agent, anti-inflammatory antioxidant, bactericidal effect, natural surfactants.	[17,18,40–43]
Birch sap	Al, Ca, Mg, Zn, and Ni, ascorbic malic, citric, phosphoric, and succinic acids, botulin, betulic acid	Antiscorbutic, anticancer, bacteriostatic, anti-inflammatory.	[19–22,31,32,44,45]

Synthetic stoichiometric hydroxyapatite (HAP) may contain ionic substitutions like Mg^{2+}, Na^+, and CO_3^{2-}, making it well tolerated by living tissue [48]. Also, HAP is used in toothpastes or other medical applications substituted with physiological elements which enhance its bioactivity [49].

This study investigates the utilization of four novel nanomaterials in the formulation of toothpaste products. Specifically, these toothpastes were formulated by incorporating four types of different hydroxyapatites (simple, substituted, and multi-substituted HAPs)—HAP [theoretical formula: $Ca_{10}(PO_4)_6(OH)_2$], HAP-5%Zn [theoretical formula; $Ca_{9.22}Zn_{0.78}(PO_4)_6(OH)_2$], HAP-0.23%Mg-3.09%Zn-2%Si-10%Sr [theoretical formula: $Ca_{8.19}Mg_{0.10}Zn_{0.5}Sr_{1.21}(PO_4)_{5.25}(SiO_4)_{0.75}(OH)_{1.25}$], and HAP-2.5%Mg-2.9%Si-1.34%Zn [theoretical formula: $Ca_{8.80}Mg_{1.00}Zn_{0.20}(PO_4)_{5.00}(SiO_4)_{1.00}(OH)_{1.00}$]. The nanostructure of the HAPs was not altered by the replacement of the elements [10,50]. The underlying advantages for the incorporation of these substitutive elements in our toothpaste formulations stems from the known ability of substitution ions to engage with adjacent tissues, thereby enhancing biomineralization and facilitating the processes associated with the regeneration of biological structures [50,51].

Zinc oxide nanoparticles exhibit antimicrobial properties against both bacteria and fungi, along with documented abilities to stimulate mineralization, cell proliferation, and differentiation [52,53].

Magnesium ions have the capacity to substitute a portion of calcium ions Ca^{2+} within the hydroxyapatite lattice. This substitution affects the crystal structure and characteristics of HAP, influencing its chemical stability, including dissolution behavior and biocompatibility. Furthermore, these ions make a significant contribution to the inhibition of acid-producing bacteria, thereby diminishing their ability to induce dental caries. Moreover, they have the capacity to ameliorate tooth sensitivity and irritation by effectively sealing exposed dentinal tubules [54].

Strontium ions can serve as a suitable substitute for calcium ions within the hydroxyapatite (HAP) structure [55]. Notably, strontium has been observed to possess desensitizing properties, which are characterized by its ability to impede or slow nerve impulse transmission within dentin [56]. Moreover, it exhibits the capability to promote remineralization, thereby reinforcing enamel and addressing the initial stages of dental decay [57].

The integration of silicon into the hydroxyapatite structure leads to an enhanced remineralization process. Additionally, it augments acid resistance without inducing any deleterious effects or irritation in the teeth or gingival tissues [58,59].

The purpose of this paper is to select and optimize the chemical composition of toothpaste formulations that possess the dual attributes of remineralization and antibacterial efficacy. To this end, we conducted a comprehensive assessment of the effectiveness of eleven distinct toothpaste formulations, each comprised of varying combinations of both pure and substituted nano-hydroxyapatite, in conjunction with birch extract. It is noteworthy that contemporary scientific literature highlights an existing gap in the realm of toothpaste development, specifically in the creation of multifaceted toothpaste products capable of delivering both remineralizing and antibacterial agents concurrently, with the potential to enhance overall enamel health. Consequently, our study represents an extension of our previous work [10], wherein we made substantial advancements by formulating specialized multisubstituted hydroxyapatites (ms-HAPs) that offer adaptability in terms of structural modifications, crystallinity adjustments, nanoparticle morphology, and size modulation [50,51]. Moreover, our formulations incorporate antibacterial properties derived from birch extract. In order to comprehensively assess the potential of these toothpaste formulations in the treatment of compromised enamel and to lay the groundwork for future investigations into novel materials for oral disease management, we conducted a rigorous examination encompassing morpho-structural characteristics, surface quality, and in vitro antibacterial activity.

2. Materials and Methods

2.1. Materials

All chemicals and reagents employed in this research were of analytical grade (AR) with a purity level equal to or exceeding 99.7%. These materials were sourced from Sigma-Aldrich and included $Ca(NO_3)_2 \cdot 4H_2O$, $Mg(NO_3)_2 \cdot 6H_2O$, $Zn(NO_3)_2 \cdot 6H_2O$, and $Sr(NO_3)_2$. Additional chemicals, namely sorbitol, polyethylene glycol (PEG 400), silicon dioxide, H_3PO_4, $(NH_4)_2HPO_4$, ammonia solution (25%), and xanthan gum, were supplied by Chempur. Tetraethyl orthosilicate (TEOS) of 98% purity was acquired from Thermo Fischer Scientific (Waltham, MA, USA) for use in experimental procedures.

Hydroglycerin alcoholic extract (96% vol. ethyl alcohol obtained from cereals, glycerin, and purified water) of *Betula verrucosa* sap (10%), made from organically harvested plants, containing 18% vol. ethyl alcohol, was purchased from Plant Extrakt, Romania.

2.2. Synthesis of nHAPs

The 4 types of different hydroxyapatites, simple, substituted, and two multi-substituted, were synthesized following a method developed in our labs [50,51].

2.3. Formulation Design and Development of Toothpastes

The four synthesized nHAPs jointly with birch extract were added in the desired toothpaste formulations, as can be seen in the next table.

The experimental design proposed three groups representing the independent variable, with 11 levels. The P1-P4 group represents the basic formulation to which varied nHAPs were added; the P5-P8 group contained the basic formulation, nHAPs (3.40%), and 1.30% birch extract; and the P9-P11 group contained variants of toothpastes without nHAPs and with varying concentrations of birch extract. As toothpaste remineralization agents, variants P1 and P5 both contained HAP-5%Zn, variants P2 and P6 contained pure nHAPs, variants P3 and P7 contained HAP-0.23%Mg-3.09%Zn-2%Si-10%Sr, and variants P4 and P8 contained HAP-2.5%Mg-2.9%Si-1.34%Zn. The experiment's dependent variables include the toothpaste's remineralization capacity and antibacterial action. The temperature, working technique, and reagents utilized were the standardized experimental constants.

2.4. Preparation of Toothpastes

To create experimental toothpaste formulations, a complex procedure involving multiple technological steps was undertaken. These steps are integral to the production of an aqueous suspension, which necessitates precise blending of various components. The initial step (Step 1) involves the mixing of a specific quantity of silica dioxide with distilled water. Following a resting period of 25 min, the suspension underwent vigorous homogenization within a sealed container, followed by an additional half hour of resting. In the subsequent step (Step 2), an aqueous suspension was prepared by dispersing hydroxyapatite in distilled water, followed by continuous mixing for a duration of 50 min. The hydrated silica dioxide was then introduced into this mixture and blended until complete homogeneity was achieved. Moving on to Step 3, sorbitol was mixed with distilled water, and subsequently, PEG 400 and xanthan gum were incorporated into the mixture. The blending continued until a fine, white paste was formed. In the final step (Step 4), the paste generated in Step 3 was thoroughly mixed with the product from Step 2, and this combined mixture was stirred for approximately 10 min, after which sodium dodecyl sulfate was added. Notably, in this step, birch extract of varying concentrations was introduced in the P5-P11 toothpaste variants. The prepared toothpaste formulations were stored at a temperature of 4 °C and were employed twice daily for the treatment of enamel slices.

2.5. Procedure for Obtaining Enamel Specimens

The procedure for obtaining enamel specimens adhered to rigorous ethical standards and received approval from the Ethics Committee of University of Medicine and Pharmacy, Cluj-Napoca, under Approval Number 85 dated 19 July 2017. The enamel slices were obtained using the following experimental protocol: 21 healthy third molars extracted for orthodontic purposes with healthy enamel, and without abnormalities or dental restorations on the molar surfaces, were selected and ultrasonicated in distilled water for 5 min. The apical region of the tooth was securely sealed to prevent the ingress of liquids, and the root structures were enveloped within a polymer material to enhance the manageability of the samples. Subsequently, the teeth were encased within autopolymerizing acrylate prisms (Duracryl Plus, Spofadental Inc., Jin, Czech Republic) with the coronal region remaining exposed. Two molars were used as a control (Ctrl) and were maintained in deionized water without any treatment. Nineteen molars were treated for 60 s with 37.5% orthophosphoric acid and washed for 30 s with distilled water to remove contaminants. Utilizing a microtome, specifically the Microtome IsoMet®, longitudinal enamel specimens measuring 7 mm × 5 mm in size and possessing a thickness of 1.5 mm were meticulously sliced from the crowns of molars. This procedure resulted in the acquisition of a total of 84 samples, which were obtained from the buccal, lingual, mesial, and distal surfaces of the 21 molars utilized in the study. The NC-negative control group ($n = 6$) was selected from the artificially demineralized slices, and each slice was immersed in deionized water. The demineralized enamel surfaces of the molars were treated with a certain toothpaste

(P1–P11) according to the experimental design. The sample sizes were $n = 6$ for Ctrl, $n = 6$ for NC, and $n = 6$ for each of the eleven test groups treated with different toothpastes.

2.6. Enamel Treatment with Toothpaste

Over the course of ten consecutive days, a particular toothpaste formulation chosen from the array of tested formulations (designated as P1 to P11) was administered daily to a specific experimental group of enamel slices (corresponding to P1–P11). The 10-day duration of the treatment was determined according to the remineralizing effect of nHAPs [10]. The application of this treatment involved the utilization of circular brushing motions, facilitated by a brush applicator, specifically employing the 3M™ Applicator Brush, procured from Corona, CA, USA. The protocol entailed brushing the teeth for a duration of 3 min, twice a day, followed by a gentle rinse. Subsequently, the collected specimens were carefully stored in sterile containers, immersed in deionized water. Prior to conducting Atomic Force Microscopy (AFM) measurements, the specimens underwent meticulous cleaning and drying procedures.

2.7. AFM Investigations

Images were captured using a JEOL JSPM 4210 Scanning Probe Microscope manufactured by the Jeol Company, Tokyo, Japan in tapping mode with typical silicon nitride cantilevers [60–64]. After the treatment, the enamel was scanned at 5 μm × 5 μm areas. For each sample, at least five different areas were observed to acquire the Ra data (mean arithmetic surface roughness). Topographic images revealed surface morphology, while tridimensional profiles revealed Ra surface roughness [62,63]. Histograms were processed using Microcal Origin v6.0 (Microcal Software Inc., Northampton, MA, USA).

2.8. Evaluation of the Antibacterial Activity

The microorganisms subjected to examination within this research comprised the following: *Streptococcus mutans* ATCC 25175; *Porphyromonas gingivalis* ATCC 33277; *Enterococcus faecalis* ATCC-29212; *Escherichia coli* ATCC 25922; and *Staphylococcus aureus* ATCC 25923. The evaluation of antibacterial activity was conducted utilizing the Agar Disk Diffusion Test, a recognized method for standard antimicrobial susceptibility assessment, which entails the measurement of inhibitory zone diameters [65].

To prepare the bacterial cultures, overnight incubation in Nutrient Broth was carried out. Subsequently, suspensions were diluted to a concentration of 1% (v/v) within the culture medium. Volumes of 500 μL from these diluted suspensions were applied onto Petri plates employing sterile swabs to ensure coverage of the entire solid culture medium (Mueller–Hinton agar). In the case of *S. mutans*, an overnight culture grown in Brain Heart Infusion (BHI) at 37 °C was combined with 3.5 mL of soft Mueller–Hinton agar and uniformly poured over the plates, encircling the disks. Following incubation at 37 °C for a period of 48 h, the zones of inhibition were gauged employing a scale designed for measuring inhibition zones. All assessments were conducted in triplicate under aseptic conditions.

2.9. Statistical Analysis

GraphPad Prism v6.0 for Windows (GraphPad Software, Inc., La Jolla, CA, USA) was used to pursue statistical analysis following a 10-day period of enamel treatment with toothpaste formulations. All surface roughness data, denoted as Ra, represent the mean values ± standard deviation (SD) derived from a minimum of three independent experiments. To discern significant distinctions among various groups of enamel slices, statistical analysis involved the utilization of One-Way ANOVA. Also, a post-test Bonferroni's Multiple Comparison Test was applied, with a significance level set between 0.01 and 0.001.

For the statistical evaluation of bacterial growth inhibition, the GraphPad Prism v5.0 software program was employed, employing a Two-Way ANOVA analysis supplemented with a Bonferroni posttest.

3. Results

3.1. Nanostructure of the Tested Samples

Utilizing Atomic Force Microscopy (AFM), the dental slices, encompassing both natural specimens and those subjected to demineralization through phosphoric acid, as well as those treated with the recently formulated toothpaste, were meticulously examined. The results can be visualized in the following images (Figure 1).

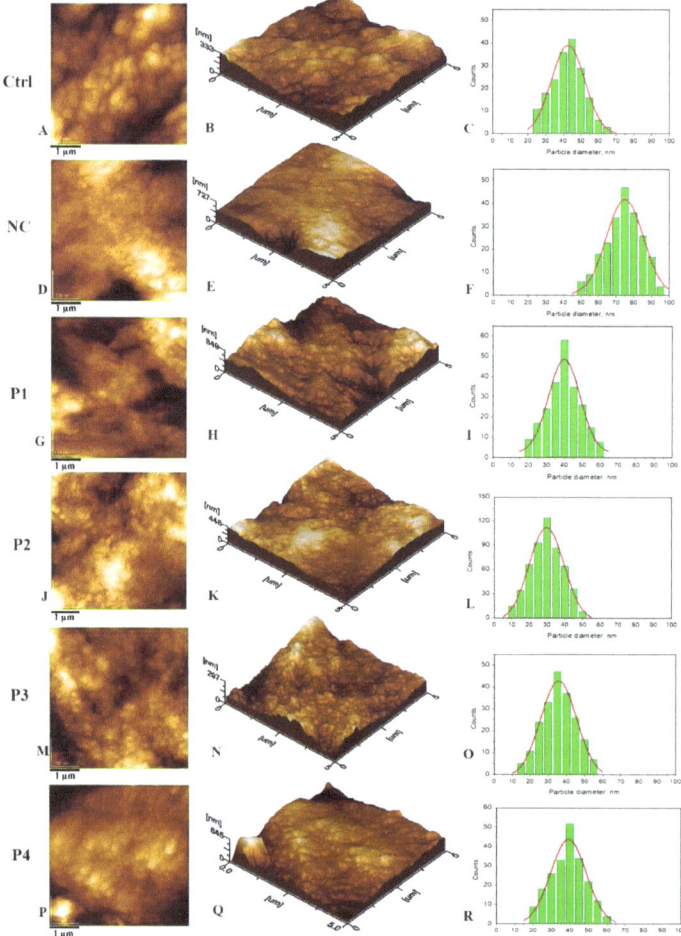

Figure 1. The 2D topography AFM images (**A,D,G,J,M,P**) and 3D topography (**B,E,H,K,N,Q**); scanned area of 5 μm × 5 μm. Histograms (**C,F,I,L,O,R**) on 2D images with the distribution of counts by particle diameter (nm) for untreated enamel (Ctrl), demineralized enamel (NC), and treated enamel with toothpastes: P1–P4.

By comparing the histograms of natural enamel (Ctrl) Figure 1C and artificial demineralized enamel (NC) obtained by treating samples with orthophosphoric acid (F), a significant increase in particle size was observed from values of approximately 41 nm to 75 nm.

Figure 1 also displays AFM images of HAP samples as follows: HAP-5%Zn used in toothpaste P1 (G–I), pure HAP used in P2 (J–L), HAP-0.23%Mg-3.09%Zn-2%Si-10%Sr used in toothpaste P3 (M–O), and HAP-2.5%Mg-2.9%Si-1.34%Zn used in P4 (P–R). It is important to highlight the particles observed within the hydroxyapatite (HAP) samples exhibit either spherical or oval morphology, characterized by dimensions that span from 30 nm in the case of unsubstituted HAP (as depicted in Figure 1J–L) to 40 nm for HAP containing 5% zinc (Figure 1G–I). Notably, these measurements closely resemble the size of particles found in natural enamel, which stands at 41 nm (as shown in Figure 1, labeled as Ctrl).

After a 10-day regimen of enamel treatment with toothpaste formulations, a thorough surface examination was conducted to gather data on the parameter Ra, representing surface roughness. The results unveiled substantial variations between artificially demineralized enamel (labeled as NC) and natural enamel (referred to as Ctrl).

Following the 10-day treatment period involving toothpaste formulations P1 to P4, it was observed that the toothpaste denoted as P2, containing nanostructured hydroxyapatite (HAP), exhibited the lowest Ra values. Notably, these Ra values were not statistically distinguishable from the Ctrl values in the conducted statistical analysis, suggesting a noteworthy level of remineralization efficacy relative to the Ra value corresponding to untreated enamel. It should be noted that the Ra values for toothpaste formulations P1 to P4 exhibited a descending order as follows: P1 > P4 > P3 > P2 > Ctrl (as illustrated in Figure 2A).

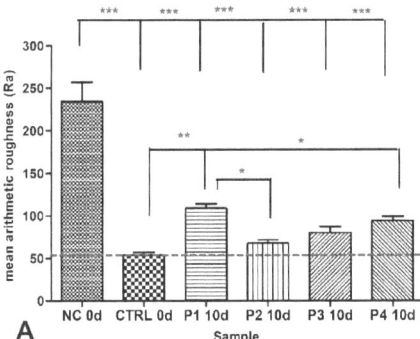
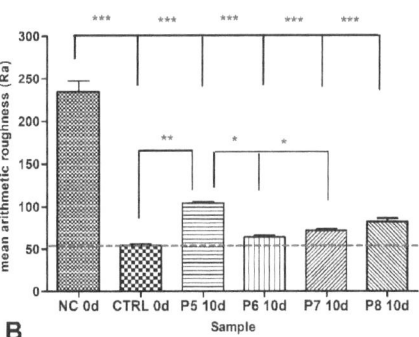

Figure 2. Statistical analysis of Ra values of enamel surfaces treated with toothpastes P1-P4 (**A**) compared to control (Ctrl) and demineralized enamel (NC); Ra values of enamel surfaces treated with toothpastes P5-P8 (**B**). The following degrees of statistical significance are denoted by stars: * $0.01 < p < 0.05$; ** $0.001 < p < 0.01$; *** $p < 0.001$. Scanned area: 5 µm × 5 µm.

The Ra values for toothpaste formulations P5–P8 exhibited the same trend of descending order: P5 > P8 > P7 > P6 > Ctrl as for toothpastes P1–P4 (Figure 2B).

3.2. Antibacterial Activity Evaluation

The toothpastes were inoculated in a volume of 80 µL of cultivation medium in Petri dishes. Most of the tested bacterial species are found in the oral cavity or accidentally arrive there and cause various diseases. Distilled water served as the control sample.

The results are presented in Figures 3 and 4 and Table 3.

The control sample recorded no inhibition for all strains tested in the study. *Streptococcus mutans*, a Gram-positive anaerobic coccus strain, showed resistance for samples 3 and 4 (Figure 3). P1 and P2 toothpaste samples exhibited the same growth inhibition value of 8.3 mm with a standard deviation of 0.57 mm, indicating that both toothpastes suppress the development of *Streptococcus mutans*. With a value of 22.0 mm, the P9 toothpaste sample had the maximum growth inhibition. Among all toothpastes examined, this toothpaste appears to be the most effective at suppressing the growth of *Streptococcus mutans*. With values of 21.6 mm and 20.3 mm, respectively, the P5 and P10 toothpaste samples showed considerable growth inhibition. Both toothpastes appear to be highly successful at inhibiting bacterial development, However, P9 appears to be slightly more effective (Table 3).

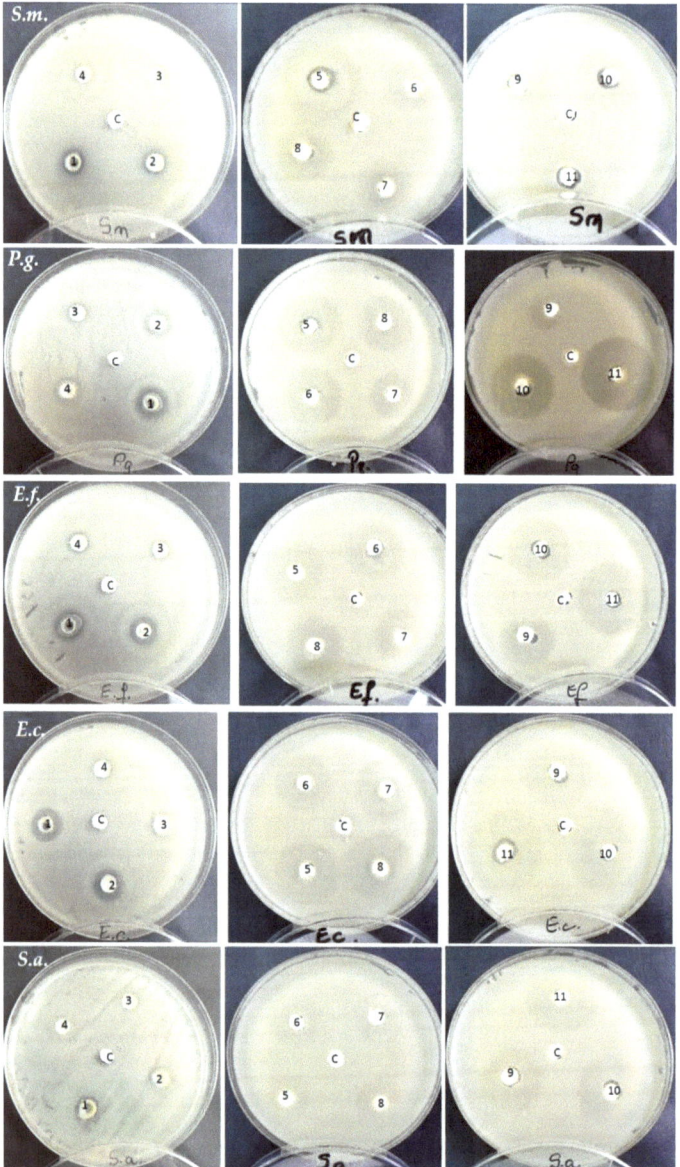

Figure 3. Agar disk diffusion susceptibility test of five bacterial strains *Streptococcus mutans* (S.m.); *Porphyromonas gingivalis* (P.g.); *Enterococcus faecalis* (E.f.); *Escherichia coli* (E.c.); and *Staphylococcus aureus* (S.a.) to the 11 toothpastes (P1–P11). The clear, circular zones around the disks indicate the growth inhibition of bacterial strains compared to control (C-distilled water).

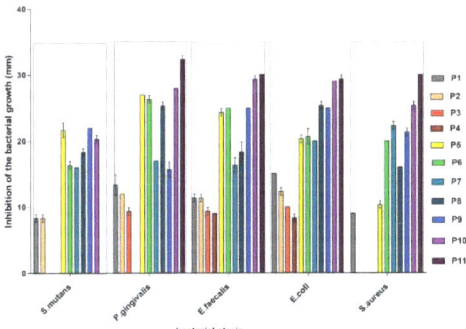

Figure 4. Inhibition of the bacterial growth induced by different toothpaste treatments.

The diameter of the inhibitory area in the Gram-negative bacillus *Porphyromonas gingivalis* was found to be larger for samples 11, 10, 5, and 6.

For all samples analyzed, a clear region was detected in the comensal Gram-positive and anaerobic bacteria *Enterococcus faecalis*. The diameters varied, with the greatest being recorded in samples 11 and 10.

In the Gram-negative, anaerobic strain *Escherichia coli*, inhibition areas were also observed for all tested samples. In this strain, the highest inhibition diameter was obtained for samples 11 and 10. The other samples recorded smaller inhibition areas. The existence of sensitivity in the Gram-positive bacterium *Staphylococcus aureus* was shown in variants P10, P11, P9, and P7. There was no distinct region around the disks in experimental variants P2–P4.

4. Discussion

This experiment on the remineralization effect of nHAPs suggests that simple HAP nanoparticles, which are smaller and uniformly arranged, have the best behavior in toothpaste due to their uniform adsorption. However, these nanoparticles must bond to the enamel structure via local epitaxial regeneration [66]. Larger nanoparticles fill deeper gaps and surround them, ensuring smoothness and optimal adsorption on uneven surfaces. This behavior can be observed in 3D imaging (Figure 1B,E,H,K,N,Q).

Figure 1A–C illustrate the fine microstructure of healthy enamel (Ctrl), which is characterized by excellent mineral material cohesiveness both inside and between the prisms. The nanoparticles are extensively welded together, resulting in a smooth enamel topography. Orthophosphoric acid etching, on the other hand, produces morphological modifications. The demineralized enamel (NC—negative control) exhibits severe surface disorganization after demineralization, as demonstrated by strongly individualizing the surrounding portions between two successive prisms and eroding the innermost layer of the prisms (Figure 1D,E). The histogram in Figure 1F (NC) shows a significant "increase" in HAP nanoparticle size from an average of 41 ± 5 nm for normal enamel (Figure 1C) to roughly 60–80 nm for etched enamel, with an average size of 75 ± 5 nm. A possible explanation for this fact can be that the demineralized nanostructural HAP unit diameter increases due to partial dissolution of the protein binder of hydroxyapatite crystallites, which tends to create some space between them [67]. The surface morphology of the treated samples indicated the presence of globular hydroxyapatite nanoparticles that exhibit uniform dispersion across the enamel surface. The average particle diameter for enamel treated with P1 was approximately 40 nm (Figure 1I), while it was around 30 nm for P2 (Figure 1L), approximately 37 nm for P3 (Figure 1O), and about 39 nm for P4 (Figure 1R).

In Figure 2, the roughness of the surfaces expressed by mean Ra values obtained from AFM imaging is statistically analyzed. Notably, significant differences were observed between the control group (Ctrl) and artificially demineralized enamel (NC), as well as between NC and all other experimental samples ($p < 0.001$, ***). Statistically significant differences were also noted when comparing Ctrl with individual values of P2, P3, and P4 (p values falling between 0.01 and 0.05, denoted as *), and between Ctrl and P1 (p values between 0.001 and 0.01, represented as **). The relative Ra values of remineralized enamel, treated with toothpaste, exhibited a descending order as follows: P1 > P4 > P3 > P2 > Ctrl, with close values noted between Ctrl and P2, as well as P3. It is pertinent to mention that the effectiveness of these toothpaste formulations in the process of remineralizing artificially demineralized enamel could be ranked in the following order: Ctrl = P2 = P3 > P4 > P1. These claims are supported by the fact that small-sized HAP nanoparticles are capable of penetrating the pores and cracks of the dental enamel and repairing the damaged microstructure of the tooth. During the restoration of the demineralized enamel, synergy among the substituted ions released from the ms-HAPs might be observed. From the literature, it is known that substituted ions can interact with protein units to enhance the enamel resistance [68,69].

In the context of enamel surface remineralization induced by the treatment with the toothpastes denoted as P5–P8, containing HAPs and birch extract (as given in Figure 2B), a similar trend was observed as in the case of toothpaste formulations (P1–P4), which exclusively comprised only HAPs. Consequently, it can be inferred that the incorporation of birch extract does not exert a discernible influence on the remineralization potential of HAPs (unpublished data).

After testing the antimicrobial activity of toothpastes, the following observation can be drawn: namely, all strains showed varying sensitivity for each tested sample. Analyzing the data within the P1–P4 group represented by toothpastes containing only nHAPs, it can be found that there is some antibacterial activity, including in the P2 toothpaste containing only pure nHAPs. Of the first group of tested toothpaste, P1 and P2 were more effective at stopping the growth of bacteria in the culture medium. Within this group, the most significant inhibition, manifested in most species of bacteria, was recorded in the experimental variant P1 consisting of nHAP-5%Zn. It is known from the literature that zinc has an antimicrobial effect [70,71].

In the group of P5–P8 toothpastes containing both nHAPs (3.4%) and 1.3% birch extract, there was a great variability in the inhibition reaction of bacterial strains depending on the species. In general, P5, represented by nHAP-5%Zn, induced the most pronounced inhibition within the group in all bacterial species except *Staphylococcus aureus* (Table 3). It should be noticed that the P7 variant, represented by HAP-0.23%Mg-3.09%Zn-2%Si-10%Sr, significantly inhibited this species.

Comparing the P1–P4 group that contained only nHAPs with the P5–P8 group where birch extract was added, significant differences were found in terms of inhibition of the growth of bacterial strains. This inhibition can be attributed to the secondary metabolites contained in the birch extract. A particular case is *Staphylococcus aureus*, which showed resistance to the P2–P4 variants of toothpaste but whose growth was inhibited in the presence of birch extract in P6–P8 toothpastes. Similarly, *Streptococcus mutans* was resistant to P3–P4 variants but was inhibited by the addition of birch extract in P5–P8 toothpastes.

In the next experimental group (P9–P11) without nHAPs, the concentration of birch extract added to toothpaste was reduced (Table 2). The analysis of the P9–P11 group reveals that there was significantly greater inhibition of bacterial growth compared to the previous toothpastes, especially at 1.3% birch extract concentration.

Among the examined bacterial species, *Enterococcus faecalis* and *Escherichia coli* had the greatest sensitivity, with *Porphyromonas gingivalis* close behind. *Streptococcus mutans* was classified in the center of the bacterial species tested. Among the examined species, *Staphylococcus aureus* had the lowest growth inhibition under the applied treatments.

Table 2. Chemical formulations of the toothpastes.

Variant	nHAP 3.40% for Each Formulation	Birch Extract (%)	Basic Chemical Composition of the Group (%)	
P1	HAP-5%Zn	-	Distilled water	58.58
P2	Pure HAP	-	Glycerol	25.18
			Sorbitol	2.99
P3	HAP-0.23%Mg-3.09%Zn-2%Si-10%Sr	-	Silicon dioxide	3.73
			Xanthan gum	0.17
P4	HAP-2.5%Mg-2.9%Si-1.34%Zn	-	Na lauryl sulphate	0.17
P5	HAP-5%Zn	1.30	Distilled water	58.49
P6	Pure HAP	1.30	Glycerol	25.15
			Sorbitol	2.99
			Silicon dioxide	3.73
P7	HAP-0.23%Mg-3.09%Zn-2%Si-10%Sr	1.30	HAP	3.42
			Xanthan gum	0.17
			Na lauryl sulphate	0.17
P8	HAP-2.5%Mg-2.9%Si-1.34%Zn	1.30	Ethyl alcohol	3.7
P9	-	0.25	Distilled water	83.32
			Glycerol	5.9
			Silicon dioxide	5.32
			Xanthan gum	0.25
			Na lauryl sulphate	0.25
			Sorbitol	4.27
			Ethyl alcohol	0.44
P10	-	0.70	Distilled water	79.41
			Glycerol	9.06
			Sorbitol	4.06
			Silicon dioxide	5.06
			Xanthan gum	0.23
			Na lauryl sulphate	0.23
			Ethyl alcohol	1.25
P11	-	1.30	Distilled water	74.2
			Glycerol	13.15
			Sorbitol	3.8
			Silicon dioxide	4.72
			Xanthan gum	0.21
			Na lauryl sulphate	0.21
			Ethyl alcohol	2.41

Overall, based on the results from the experiments performed under the same conditions, the toothpastes can be ranked in terms of growth inhibition effectiveness (Table 3) for each bacterial species (from the highest to the lowest) as follows:

For *Streptococcus mutans*: P9 > P5 > P10 > P8 ≈ P7 ≈ P6 > P1 ≈ P2 > P3 ≈ P4 ≈ P11.
For *Porphyromonas gingivalis*: P5 > P6 > P11 > P10 > P8 > P7 ≈ P9 > P1 > P2 > P3 > P4.
For *Enterococcus faecalis*: P11 > P10 > P9 = P6 ≈ P5 > P8 > P1 > P2 > P3 > P4.
For *Escherichia coli*: P11> P10 > P8 ≈ P9 > P5 = P6 ≈ P7 > P1 > P2 > P3 > P4.
For *Staphylococcus aureus*: P11 > P10 > P8 ≈ P9 > P5 = P6 ≈ P7 > P1 > P2 = P3 = P4.

The efficiency of toothpaste varies depending on the bacterial species. Toothpaste may be extremely efficient against one species while being ineffective against another. Toothpaste P11, consisting of a basic formulation with 1.3% birch extract, appears to be among the most effective at inhibiting growth in all studied bacterial species. Toothpaste P10 is frequently listed as one of the most effective, but its efficacy differs according to species. P5 and P6 toothpastes are effective against several species, most notably *Porphyromonas gingivalis*. Toothpastes P1–P4, while inhibiting in some cases, are generally less effective than others.

Table 3. Bacterial growth inhibition induced by toothpastes.

Sample	Diameter of the Inhibition Zone (mm)				
	Streptococcus mutans	Porphyromonas gingivalis	Enterococcus faecalis	Escherichia coli	Staphylococcus aureus
P1	8.3 ± 0.57	13.3 ± 1.52	11.3 ± 0.57	15.0 ± 0	9.0 ± 0
P2	8.3 ± 1.15	12.0 ± 0	11.3 ± 1.15	12.3 ± 0.57	-
P3	-	9.3 ± 0.57	9.3 ± 0.57	10.0 ± 0	-
P4	-	0	9.0 ± 0	8.3 ± 1.52	-
P5	21.6 ± 1.15	27.0 ± 0	24.3 ± 0.57	20.3 ± 0.57	10.3 ± 0.57
P6	16.3 ± 0.57	26.6 ± 1.15	25.0 ± 0	20.3 ± 1.15	20.0 ± 0
P7	16.0 ± 0	17.0 ± 0	15.3 ± 1.15	20.0 ± 0	22.3 ± 1.15
P8	18.3 ± 1.52	25.3 ± 0.57	18.3 ± 1.52	25.3 ± 1.15	16.0 ± 0
P9	22.0 ± 0	15.3 ± 1.15	25.0 ± 0	25.0 ± 0	21.3 ± 1.52
P10	20.3 ± 0.57	28.0 ± 0	29.3 ± 0.57	29.0 ± 0	25.3 ± 0.57
P11	-	32.3 ± 0.57	30.0 ± 0	29.3 ± 0.57	30.0 ± 0

According to these data, toothpaste P11 is the most effective against bacterial strains, ranking first in three of the five bacterial species studied. It consistently outperformed other bacterial inhibitors across a wide range of bacterial species, making it the clear choice for bacterial growth inhibition.

Considering both remineralization effectiveness, expressed by the ranking Ctrl ≈ P6 ≈ P2 > P7 ≈ P3 > P8 ≈ P4 > P5 ≈ P1, and antibacterial effectiveness, expressed by the ranking P11 > P10 > P9 > P5 > P6 > P8 > P7 > P1 > P2 > P3 > P4, it can be identified that toothpaste P5 is an appropriate option for both effective remineralization and antibacterial activity. This shows that toothpaste P5 may provide an efficient combination of remineralization and antibacterial properties.

As future developments of this experiment, time-course tests can be conducted to measure the lifetime of toothpaste's efficiency in preventing bacterial growth over different time intervals. In addition to growth inhibition trials, oral microbiome studies may shed light on the broader effects of toothpaste variants on the oral microflora. Exploring other oral health parameters, such as the anti-inflammatory or anti-adhesive properties of toothpastes and investigating the mechanisms by which specific toothpaste variants inhibit bacterial growth, could provide insights for developing targeted oral care products. By integrating these future discoveries, we can acquire a better understanding of toothpaste effectiveness and enhance oral health outcomes. These improvements can contribute to the development of more effective oral care products in addition to enhancing oral hygiene practices.

5. Conclusions

Oral healthcare holds considerable significance in the broader context of overall well-being and quality of life. There is an increasing trend toward the adoption of functional toothpaste formulations for routine oral health maintenance. The goal of this research paper is to formulate functional toothpaste products that possess the dual capabilities of enamel remineralization and antibacterial properties, achieved through the incorporation of nano-hydroxyapatite and birch extract.

When considering both remineralization and antibacterial effectiveness, toothpaste P5 emerged as a compelling option due to its moderate antibacterial activity and good remineralization potential.

Optimizing the chemical composition of a functional toothpaste by incorporating hydroxyapatite and birch extract is a challenging process. The substantial enhancement in remineralization (P1–P4) attributed to nano-hydroxyapatite is intricately regulated by the presence of substituted elements. It is worth noting that the simultaneous substitution of multiple ions imparts a superior influence compared to the substitution of a single ion, indicating a synergistic interaction among these ions. Furthermore, it is noteworthy that the inclusion of birch extract does not alter the remineralization potential of HAPs.

In terms of antimicrobial activity, the most robust effectiveness of toothpastes was observed in formulations (P9–P11) devoid of nHAPs, as the presence of nHAPs (P5–P8) mitigated the immediate impact of birch extract. It would be of scientific interest to elucidate the mechanism underlying this mitigation of birch extract's effect by the presence of nHAPs, which could involve a delay in the release of active molecules or a reduction in their efficacy.

Author Contributions: Conceptualization, A.-D.F., C.T.D. and M.T.-C.; methodology, A.-D.F., G.T. and A.M.; software, A.A. and L.C.P.; validation, C.T.D., M.T.-C. and A.-D.F.; formal analysis, A.A.; investigation, R.C. and L.C.P.; resources, M.T.-C., C.-P.R., C.T.D. and O.S.; writing—original draft preparation, A.-D.F., C.T.D., R.C., M.T.-C. and G.T.; writing—review and editing, C.T.D. and A.M.; visualization, R.C. and O.S.; supervision, M.T.-C.; project administration, M.T.-C.; funding acquisition, C.-P.R. and M.T.-C.; A.-D.F. and C.T.D. had equal contributions. All authors have read and agreed to the published version of the manuscript.

Funding: The Ministry of Research, Innovation, and Digitization financed this research within Project no. 186 of the PN-III-P4-ID-PCE-2020-1910 Program.

Institutional Review Board Statement: The study protocol and all the procedures were approved by the Ethics Committee of "Iuliu Hatieganu" University of Medicine and Pharmacy, Cluj-Napoca (Approval No. 85/19 July 2017).

Informed Consent Statement: Informed consent was obtained from all subjects involved in the study.

Data Availability Statement: Data are contained within the article.

Conflicts of Interest: The authors declare no conflict of interest.

References

1. Pedro, A.C.; Paniz, O.G.; Fernandes, I.d.A.A.; Bortolini, D.G.; Rubio, F.T.V.; Haminiuk, C.W.I.; Maciel, G.M.; Magalhães, W.L.E. The Importance of Antioxidant Biomaterials in Human Health and Technological Innovation: A Review. *Antioxidants* **2022**, *11*, 1644. [CrossRef]
2. Insuasti-Cruz, E.; Suárez-Jaramillo, V.; Mena, K.A.; Pila-Varela, K.O.; Fiallos-Ayala, X.; Dahoumane, S.A.; Alexis, F. Natural biomaterials from biodiversity for healthcare applications. *Adv. Healthc. Mater.* **2022**, *11*, 2101389. [CrossRef]
3. Davison-Kotler, E.; Marshall, W.S.; García-Gareta, E. Sources of collagen for biomaterials in skin wound healing. *Bioengineering* **2019**, *6*, 56. [CrossRef]
4. Nakahara, M.; Toyama, N.; Ekuni, D.; Takeuchi, N.; Maruyama, T.; Yokoi, A.; Morita, M. Trends in self-rated oral health and its associations with oral health status and oral health behaviors in Japanese university students: A cross-sectional study from 2011 to 2019. *Int. J. Environ. Res. Public Health* **2022**, *19*, 13580. [CrossRef]
5. Sun, L.; Chow, L.C. Preparation and properties of nano-sized calcium fluoride for dental applications. *Dent. Mater.* **2008**, *24*, 111–116. [CrossRef]
6. Prabhu, S.; Poulose, E.K. Silver nanoparticles: Mechanism of antimicrobial action, synthesis, medical applications, and toxicity effects. *Int. Nano Lett.* **2012**, *2*, 32. [CrossRef]
7. Degli Esposti, L.; Ionescu, A.C.; Brambilla, E.; Tampieri, A.; Iafisco, M. Characterization of a toothpaste containing bioactive hydroxyapatites and In Vitro evaluation of its efficacy to remineralize enamel and to occlude dentinal tubules. *Materials* **2020**, *13*, 2928. [CrossRef]
8. Ionescu, A.C.; Cazzaniga, G.; Ottobelli, M.; Garcia-Godoy, F.; Brambilla, E. Substituted nano-hydroxyapatite toothpastes reduce biofilm formation on enamel and resin-based composite surfaces. *J. Funct. Biomater.* **2020**, *11*, 36. [CrossRef]
9. Kranz, S.; Heyder, M.; Mueller, S.; Guellmar, A.; Krafft, C.; Nietzsche, S.; Tschirpke, C.; Herold, V.; Sigusch, B.; Reise, M. Remi-neralization of artificially demineralized human enamel and dentin samples by zinc-carbonate hydroxyapatite nanocrystals. *Materials* **2022**, *15*, 7273. [CrossRef]
10. Florea, A.-D.; Pop, L.C.; Benea, H.-R.-C.; Tomoaia, G.; Racz, C.-P.; Mocanu, A.; Dobrota, C.-T.; Balint, R.; Soritau, O.; Tomoaia-Cotisel, M. Remineralization Induced by Biomimetic Hydroxyapatite Toothpastes on Human Enamel. *Biomimetics* **2023**, *8*, 450. [CrossRef]
11. Silva, J.C.; Pereira, R.L.S.; de Freitas, T.S.; Rocha, J.E.; Macedo, N.S.; Nonato, C.d.F.A.; Linhares, M.L.; Tavares, D.S.A.; Cuhna, F.A.B.; Coutinho, H.D.M.; et al. Evaluation of antibacterial and toxicological activities of essential oil of *Ocimum gratissimum* L. and its major constituent eugenol. *Food Biosci.* **2022**, *50*, 102128. [CrossRef]
12. Noshad, M.; Behbahani, B.A.; Nikfarjam, Z. Chemical composition, antibacterial activity and antioxidant activity of citrus bergamia essential oil: Molecular docking simulations. *Food Biosci.* **2022**, *50*, 102123. [CrossRef]
13. Banday, J.A.; Rather, Z.U.; Yatoo, G.N.; Hajam, M.A.; Bhat, S.A.; Santhanakrishnan, V.P.; Farozi, A.; Rather, M.A.; Rasool, S. Gas chromatographic-mass spectrometric analysis, antioxidant, antiproliferative and antibacterial activities of the essential oil of prangos pabularia. *Microb. Pathog.* **2022**, *166*, 105540. [CrossRef] [PubMed]

14. Laszczyk, M.; Jäger, S.; Simon-Haarhaus, B.; Scheffler, A.; Schempp, C.M. Physical, chemical and pharmacological characterization of a new oleogel-forming triterpene extract from the outer bark of birch (*Betulae cortex*). *Planta Med.* **2006**, *72*, 1389–1395. [CrossRef] [PubMed]
15. Rastogi, S.; Pandey, M.M.; Kumar Singh Rawat, A. Medicinal plants of the genus Betula—Traditional uses and a phytochemical-pharmacological review. *J. Ethnopharmacol.* **2015**, *159*, 62–83. [CrossRef] [PubMed]
16. European Medicines Agency. *Evaluation of Medicines for Human Use*; 7 Westferry Circus, Canary Wharf, London, E14 4HB, UK, Doc. Ref. EMEA/HMPC/244569/2006; European Medicines Agency: London, UK, 2008.
17. Olmstead, M.J. Organic Toothpaste Containing Saponin. U.S. Patent 6,485,711, 26 November 2002. Available online: http://www.freepatentsonline.com/6485711.html (accessed on 30 March 2022).
18. Al-Ghutaimel, H.; Riba, H.; Al-Kahtani, S.; Al-Duhaimi, S. Common periodontal diseases of children and adolescents. *Int. J. Dent.* **2014**, *2014*, 850674. [CrossRef]
19. Nishida, N.; Grossi, S.G.; Dunford, R.G.; Ho, A.W.; Trevisan, M.; Genco, R.J. Dietary vitamin C and the risk for periodontal disease. *J. Periodontol.* **2000**, *71*, 1215–1223. [CrossRef]
20. Rao, P.; Rao, R.; Langade, D.; Rathod, V. Rare Case of Scorbutic Gingivitis. *Ind. Med. Gaz.* **2014**, *4*, 81–84.
21. Pussinen, P.J.; Laatikainen, T.; Alfthan, G.; Asikainen, S.; Jousilahti, P. Periodontitis is associated with a low concentration of vitamin C in plasma. *Clin. Diagn. Lab. Immunol.* **2013**, *10*, 897–902. [CrossRef]
22. Jäger, S.; Laszczyk, M.N.; Scheffler, A. A preliminary pharmacokinetic study of betulin, the main pentacyclic triterpene from extract of outer bark of birch (*Betulae alba* cortex). *Molecules* **2008**, *13*, 3224–3235. [CrossRef]
23. Zdzisińska, B.; Szuster-Ciesielska, A.; Rzeski, W.; Kanderfer-Szerszen, M. Therapeutic properties of betulin and betulinic acid, components of birch bark extract. *Farm. Prz. Nauk.* **2010**, *7*, 33–39.
24. Krasutsky, P.A. Birch bark research and development. *Nat. Prod. Rep.* **2006**, *23*, 919–942. [CrossRef] [PubMed]
25. Koca, I.; Tekgüler, B.; Türkyilmaz, B. Bioactive terpenic acids: Their properties, natural sources and effects on health. *Int. Congr. Med. Aromat. Plants* **2017**, *1*, 429–439.
26. Haque, S.; Nawrot, D.A.; Alakurtti, S.; Ghemtio, L.; Yli-Kauhaluoma, J.; Tammela, P. Screening and characterisation of antimicrobial properties of semisynthetic Betulin derivatives. *PLoS ONE* **2014**, *9*, e102696. [CrossRef]
27. Viszwapriya, D.; Subramenium, G.A.; Radhika, S.; Pandian, S.K. Betulin inhibits cariogenic properties of *Streptococcus mutans* by targeting *vicRK* and *gtf* genes. *Antonie Van Leeuwenhoek* **2017**, *110*, 153–165. [CrossRef]
28. Godugu, C.; Patel, A.R.; Doddapaneni, R.; Somagoni, J.; Singh, M. Approaches to improve the oral bioavailability and effects of novel anticancer drugs berberine and betulinic acid. *PLoS ONE* **2014**, *9*, e89919. [CrossRef]
29. Gallo, M.B.P.; Bullet, M.; Sarachine, J. Biological activities of Lupeol. *Int. J. Res. Pharm. Biomed. Sci.* **2009**, *3*, 46–66. [CrossRef]
30. Lee, T.K.; Poon, R.T.P.; Wo, J.Y.; Ma, S.; Guan, X.Y.; Myers, J.N.; Altevogt, P.; Yuen, A.P. Lupeol suppresses cisplatin-induced nuclear factor-B activation in head and neck squamous cell carcinoma and inhibits local invasion and nodal metastasis in osteophatic nude mouse model. *Cancer Res.* **2007**, *67*, 8800–8809. [CrossRef]
31. Sousa, J.L.C.; Freire, C.S.R.; Silvestre, A.J.D.; Silva, A.M.S. Recent developments in the functionalization of betulinic acid and its natural analogues: A route to new bioactive compounds. *Molecules* **2019**, *24*, 355. [CrossRef]
32. Florea, A.D.; Tomoaia-Cotisel, M.; Dobrota, C.T. Use of Betula species extracts in therapeutic and preventive oral health care. In *Betula: Ecology and Uses*, 1st ed.; Bertelsen, C.T., Ed.; Nova Science Publishers, Inc.: New York, NY, USA, 2020; pp. 137–162.
33. Blondeau, D.; St-Pierre, A.; Bourdeau, N.; Bley, J.; Lajeunesse, A.; Desgagné-Penix, I. Antimicrobial activity and chemical composition of white birch (*Betula papyrifera* Marshall) bark extracts. *Microbiol. Open* **2019**, *9*, e00944. [CrossRef]
34. Kocaçalişkan, I.; Talan, I.; Terzi, I. Antimicrobial activity of catechol and pyrogallol as allelochemicals. *Z. Für Naturforschung C* **2006**, *61*, 639–642. [CrossRef] [PubMed]
35. Jeong, E.-Y.; Jeon, J.-H.; Lee, C.-H.; Lee, H.-S. Antimicrobial activity of catechol isolated from *Diospyros kaki* Thunb. roots and its derivatives toward intestinal bacteria. *Food Chem.* **2009**, *115*, 1006–1010. [CrossRef]
36. Berberian, V.; Allen, C.C.R.; Sharma, N.D.; Boyd, D.R.; Hardacre, C. A Comparative Study of the Synthesis of 3-Substituted Catechols using an Enzymatic and a Chemoenzymatic Method. *Adv. Synth. Catal.* **2007**, *349*, 727–739. [CrossRef]
37. Demirci, B.; Paper, D.H.; Demirci, F.; Can Başer, K.H.; Franz, G. Essential oil of *Betula pendula* roth. Buds. *Evid. Based Complement. Altern. Med.* **2004**, *1*, 301–303. [CrossRef] [PubMed]
38. Vladimirov, M.S.; Nikolic, V.D.; Stanojevic, L.P.; Stanojevic, J.S.; Nikolic, L.B.; Danilovic, R.B.; Marinkovic, V.D. Chemical composition, antimicrobial and antioxidant activity of birch (*Betula pendula* Roth.) Buds essential oil. *J. Essent. Oil-Bear. Plants* **2019**, *22*, 120–130. [CrossRef]
39. Markert, B.; Steinbeck, R. Some aspects of element distribution in *Betula alba*, a contribution to representative sampling of terrestrial plants for multi-element analysis. *Fresenius' Z. Für Anal. Chem.* **1988**, *331*, 616–619. [CrossRef]
40. Raal, A.; Boikova, T.; Püssa, T. Content and dynamics of polyphenols in *Betula* spp. Leaves naturally growing in Estonia. *Rec. Nat. Prod.* **2015**, *9*, 41–48.
41. Yang, H.; Li, K.; Yan, H.; Liu, S.; Wang, Y.; Huang, C. High-performance therapeutic quercetin-doped adhesive for adhesive–dentin interfaces. *Sci. Rep.* **2017**, *7*, 8189. [CrossRef]
42. Nakamura, K.; Shirato, M.; Kanno, T.; Lingström, P.; Örtengren, U.; Niwano, Y. Photo-irradiated caffeic acid exhibits antimicrobial activity against *Streptococcus mutans* biofilms via hydroxyl radical formation. *Sci. Rep.* **2017**, *7*, 6353. Available online: https://www.nature.com/articles/s41598-017-07007-z (accessed on 30 March 2023). [CrossRef]

43. Jumanca, D.; Galuscan, A.; Podariu, A.C.; Borcan, F.; Earar, K. Anti-inflammatory action of toothpastes containing betulin nanocapsules. *Rev. Chim.* **2014**, *65*, 1472–1476.
44. Zyryanova, O.A.; Terazawa, M.; Takayoshi, K.; Zyryanov, V.I. White birch trees as resource species of Russia: Their distribution, ecophysiological features, multiple utilizations. *Eurasian J. For. Res.* **2010**, *13*, 25–40.
45. Shu, X.; Zhao, S.; Huo, W.; Tang, Y.; Zou, L.; Li, Z.; Li, L.; Wang, X. Clinical study of a spray containing birch juice for repairing sensitive skin. *Arch. Dermatol. Res.* **2023**, *315*, 2271–2281. [CrossRef]
46. Imran, E.; Cooper, P.R.; Ratnayake, J.; Ekambaram, M.; Mei, M.L. Potential Beneficial Effects of Hydroxyapatite Nanoparticles on Caries Lesions In Vitro—A Review of the Literature. *Dent. J.* **2023**, *11*, 40. [CrossRef] [PubMed]
47. Maha, D.; Habib, A.; Badawy, R. Occlusion of Dentinal Tubules Using a Novel Dentifrice with Fluoro-Hydroxyapatite Nanoparticles Derived from a Biologic Source. (an in vitro study). *Dent. Sci. Updates* **2022**, *3*, 39–44. [CrossRef]
48. Makshakova, O.N.; Gafurov, M.R.; Goldberg, M.A. The Mutual Incorporation of Mg^{2+} and CO_3^{2-} into Hydroxyapatite: A DFT Study. *Materials* **2022**, *15*, 9046. [CrossRef]
49. Yazdanian, M.; Rahmani, A.; Tahmasebi, E.; Tebyanian, H.; Yazdanian, A.; Mosaddad, S.A. Current and advanced nanomaterials in dentistry as regeneration agents: An update. *Mini Rev. Med. Chem.* **2021**, *21*, 899–918. [CrossRef]
50. Garbo, C.; Locs, J.; D'Este, M.; Demazeau, G.; Mocanu, A.; Roman, C.; Horovitz, O.; Tomoaia-Cotisel, M. Advanced Mg, Zn, Sr, Si multi-substituted hydroxyapatites for bone regeneration. *Int. J. Nanomed.* **2020**, *15*, 1037–1058. [CrossRef] [PubMed]
51. Oltean-Dan, D.; Dogaru, G.-B.; Tomoaia-Cotisel, M.; Apostu, D.; Mester, A.; Benea, H.R.C.; Paiusan, M.G.; Jianu, E.-M.; Mocanu, A.; Balint, R.; et al. Enhancement of bone consolidation using high-frequency pulsed electromagnetic short-waves and titanium implants coated with biomimetic composite embedded into PLA matrix: In vivo evaluation. *Int. J. Nanomed.* **2019**, *14*, 5799–5816. [CrossRef] [PubMed]
52. Pillai, A.M.; Sivasankarapillai, V.S.; Rahdar, A.; Joseph, J.; Sadeghfar, F.; Rajesh, K.; Kyzas, G.Z. Green synthesis and characterization of zinc oxide nanoparticles with antibacterial and antifungal activity. *J. Mol. Str.* **2020**, *1211*, 128107. [CrossRef]
53. Fiume, E.; Magnaterra, G.; Rahdar, A.; Verné, E.; Baino, F. Hydroxyapatite for biomedical applications: A short Overview. *Ceramics* **2021**, *4*, 542–563. [CrossRef]
54. Peng, X.; Han, S.; Wang, K.; Ding, L.; Liu, Z.; Zhang, L. The Amelogenin-Derived Peptide TVH-19 Promotes Dentinal Tubule Occlusion and Mineralization. *Polymers* **2021**, *13*, 2473. [CrossRef] [PubMed]
55. Frangopol, P.T.; Mocanu, A.; Almasan, V.; Garbo, C.; Balint, R.; Borodi, G.; Bratu, I.; Horovitz, O.; Tomoaia-Cotisel, M. Synthesis and structural characterization of strontium substituted hydroxyapatites. *Rev. Roum. Chim.* **2016**, *61*, 337–344.
56. Dotta, T.C.; Hayann, L.; de Padua Andrade Almeida, L.; Nogueira, L.F.B.; Arnez, M.M.; Castelo, R.; Cassiano, A.F.B.; Faria, G.; Martelli-Tosi, M.; Bottini, M.; et al. Strontium Carbonate and Strontium-Substituted Calcium Carbonate Nanoparticles Form Protective Deposits on Dentin Surface and Enhance Human Dental Pulp Stem Cells Mineralization. *J. Funct. Biomater.* **2022**, *13*, 250. [CrossRef] [PubMed]
57. Vilhena, F.V.; Lonni, A.A.S.G.; D'Alpino, P. Silicon-enriched hydroxyapatite formed induced by REFIX-based toothpaste on the enamel surface. *Braz. Dent. Sci.* **2021**, *24*, 4. [CrossRef]
58. Khonina, T.G.; Chupakhin, O.N.; Shur, V.Y.; Turygin, A.P.; Sadovsky, V.V.; Mandra, Y.V.; Sementsova, E.A.; Kotikova, A.Y.; Legkikh, A.V.; Nikitina, E.Y.; et al. Silicon-hydroxyapatite—Glycerohydrogel as a promising biomaterial for dental applications. *Colloids Surf. B* **2020**, *189*, 110851. [CrossRef] [PubMed]
59. Fernandes, N.L.S.; Silva, J.G.V.C.; de Sousa, E.B.G.; D'Alpino, P.H.P.; de Oliveira, A.F.B.; de Jong, E.D.J.; Sampaio, F.C. Effectiveness of fluoride-containing varnishes associated with different technologies to remineralize enamel after pH cycling: An in vitro study. *BMC Oral Health* **2022**, *22*, 1–9. [CrossRef]
60. Horovitz, O.; Tomoaia, G.; Mocanu, A.; Yupsanis, T.; Tomoaia-Cotisel, M. Protein binding to gold autoassembled films. *Gold Bull.* **2007**, *40*, 295–304. [CrossRef]
61. Zdrenghea, U.V.; Tomoaia, G.; Pop-Toader, D.-V.; Mocanu, A.; Horovitz, O.; Tomoaia-Cotisel, M. Procaine effect on human erythrocyte membrane explored by atomic force microscopy. *Comb. Chem. High Throughput Screen.* **2011**, *14*, 237–247. [CrossRef]
62. Machoy, M.; Wilczyński, S.; Szyszka-Sommerfeld, L.; Woźniak, K.; Deda, A.; Kulesza, S. Mapping of Nanomechanical Properties of Enamel Surfaces Due to Orthodontic Treatment by AFM Method. *Appl. Sci.* **2021**, *11*, 3918. [CrossRef]
63. Teutle-Coyotecatl, B.; Contreras-Bulnes, R.; Rodríguez-Vilchis, L.E.; Scougall-Vilchis, R.J.; Velazquez-Enriquez, U.; Almaguer-Flores, A.; Arenas-Alatorre, J.A. Effect of Surface Roughness of Deciduous and Permanent Tooth Enamel on Bacterial Adhesion. *Microorganisms* **2022**, *10*, 1701. [CrossRef]
64. Besnard, C.; Marie, A.; Sasidharan, S.; Harper, R.A.; Marathe, S.; Moffat, J.; Shelton, R.M.; Landini, G.; Korsunsky, A.M. Time-Lapse In Situ 3D Imaging Analysis of Human Enamel Demineralisation Using X-ray Synchrotron Tomography. *Dent. J.* **2023**, *11*, 130. [CrossRef] [PubMed]
65. EUCAST. *Antimicrobial Susceptibility Testing: EUCAST Disk Diffusion Method*; EUCAST: Basel, Switzerland, 2021; p. 16. Available online: www.eucast.org (accessed on 1 March 2023).
66. Wang, S.; Zhang, L.; Chen, W.; Jin, H.; Zhang, Y.; Wu, L.; Li, Q. Rapid regeneration of enamel-like-oriented inorganic crystals by using rotary evaporation. *Mater. Sci. Eng.* **2020**, *115*, 111141. [CrossRef] [PubMed]
67. Lee, W.H.; Loo, C.Y.; Rohanizadeh, R. A review of chemical surface modification of bioceramics: Effects on protein adsorption and cellular response. *Colloids Surf. B Biointerfaces* **2014**, *122*, 823–834. [CrossRef]

68. Zhang, X.; Ramirez, B.E.; Liao, S.; Diekwisch, T.G.H. Amelogenin supramolecular assembly in nanospheres defined by a complex helix-coil-PPII helix 3D-structure. *PLoS ONE* **2011**, *6*, e24952. [CrossRef] [PubMed]
69. Hu, J.C.-C.; Hu, Y.; Lu, Y.; Smith, C.E.; Lertlam, R.; Wright, J.T.; Suggs, C.; MacKee, M.D.; Beniah, E.; Kabir, M.E.; et al. Enamelin Is critical for ameloblast integrity and enamel ultrastructure formation. *PLoS ONE* **2014**, *9*, e89303. [CrossRef] [PubMed]
70. Predoi, D.; Iconaru, S.L.; Predoi, M.V.; Motelica-Heino, M.; Guegan, R.; Buton, N. Evaluation of Antibacterial Activity of Zinc-Doped Hydroxyapatite Colloids and Dispersion Stability Using Ultrasounds. *Nanomaterials* **2019**, *9*, 515. [CrossRef] [PubMed]
71. Stanic, V.; Dimitrijevic, S.; Stankovic, J.A.; Mitrić, M.; Jokic, B.; Plećaš, I.B.; Raičević, S. Synthesis, characterization and antimicrobial activity of copper and zinc-doped hydroxyapatite nanopowders. *Appl. Surf. Sci.* **2010**, *256*, 6083–6089. [CrossRef]

Disclaimer/Publisher's Note: The statements, opinions and data contained in all publications are solely those of the individual author(s) and contributor(s) and not of MDPI and/or the editor(s). MDPI and/or the editor(s) disclaim responsibility for any injury to people or property resulting from any ideas, methods, instructions or products referred to in the content.

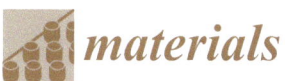

Article

Comparative Evaluation of Microleakage of Flowable Composite Resin Using Etch and Rinse, Self-Etch Adhesive Systems, and Self-Adhesive Flowable Composite Resin in Class V Cavities: Confocal Laser Microscopic Study

Ekta Varma Sengar [1], Sanjyot Mulay [1], Lotika Beri [1], Archana Gupta [2], Thamer Almohareb [3], Sultan Binalrimal [4], Ali Robaian [5], Maha A. Bahammam [6,7], Hammam Ahmed Bahammam [8], Sarah Ahmed Bahammam [9], Bassam Zidane [10], Nassreen H. Albar [11], Shilpa Bhandi [11,12], Deepti Shrivastava [13], Kumar Chandan Srivastava [14,*] and Shankargouda Patil [15,16,*]

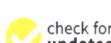

1. Department of Conservative Dentistry and Endodontics, Dr. D. Y. Patil Dental College & Hospital, Dr. D. Y. Patil Vidyapeeth, Pimpri, Pune 411018, India; ektavarma1993@gmail.com (E.V.S.); sanjyot.mulay@dpu.edu.in (S.M.); lotika.lb@gmail.com (L.B.)
2. Independent Researcher, Pune 411018, India; archanaanshumangupta@gmail.com
3. Restorative Dental Science Department, College of Dentistry, King Saud University, Riyadh 11451, Saudi Arabia; talmohareb@ksu.edu.sa
4. Restorative Department, College of Dentistry, Riyadh Elm University, Riyadh 13244, Saudi Arabia; sultan@riyadh.edu.sa
5. Conservative Dental Sciences Department, College of Dentistry, Prince Sattam Bin Abdulaziz University, Alkharj 16245, Saudi Arabia; ali.alqahtani@psau.edu.sa
6. Department of Periodontology, Faculty of Dentistry, King Abdulaziz University, Jeddah 21589, Saudi Arabia; mbahammam@kau.edu.sa
7. Executive Presidency of Academic Affairs, Saudi Commission for Health Specialties, Riyadh 11614, Saudi Arabia
8. Department of Pediatric Dentistry, College of Dentistry, King Abdulaziz University, Jeddah 21589, Saudi Arabia; habahammam@kau.edu.sa
9. Department of Pediatric Dentistry and Orthodontics, College of Dentistry, Taibah University, Medina 42353, Saudi Arabia; sbahammam@taibahu.edu.sa
10. Restorative Dentistry Department, Faculty of Dentistry, King Abdulaziz University, Jeddah 21589, Saudi Arabia; bzidane@kau.edu.sa
11. Department of Restorative Dental Sciences, Division of Operative Dentistry, College of Dentistry, Jazan University, Jazan 45412, Saudi Arabia; nalbar01@gmail.com (N.H.A.); shilpa.bhandi@gmail.com (S.B.)
12. Department of Cariology, Saveetha Dental College & Hospitals, Saveetha Institute of Medical and Technical Sciences, Saveetha University, Chennai 600077, India
13. Department of Preventive Dentistry, College of Dentistry, Jouf University, Sakaka 72345, Saudi Arabia; sdeepti20@gmail.com
14. Department of Oral & Maxillofacial Surgery & Diagnostic Sciences, College of Dentistry, Jouf University, Sakaka 72345, Saudi Arabia
15. Department of Maxillofacial Surgery and Diagnostic Sciences, Division of Oral Pathology, College of Dentistry, Jazan University, Jazan 45412, Saudi Arabia
16. Centre of Molecular Medicine and Diagnostics (COMMaND), Saveetha Dental College & Hospitals, Saveetha Institute of Medical and Technical Sciences, Saveetha University, Chennai 600077, India
* Correspondence: drkcs.omr@gmail.com (K.C.S.); dr.ravipatil@gmail.com (S.P.)

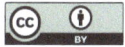

Abstract: The essential factor in determining the preservation of restoration is the marginal seal. Restoring cervical lesions with a resin composite has always been a challenge. Composite resins with various viscosities and different bonding systems are being researched to reduce the microleakage. Confocal laser scanning microscopy (CLSM) is the latest non-destructive technique for visualizing the microleakage. **Objectives:** To evaluate and compare the microleakage of Universal Flo composite resin (G-aenial) using etch and rinse adhesive system ER-2 steps (Adper Single Bond 2), self-etch adhesive system SE-1 step (G-Bond), and self-adhesive flowable composite resin (Constic) in Class V cavities using a confocal laser scanning microscope. **Materials and Method:** Class V cavities were prepared on 27 caries-free human extracted premolar teeth on the buccal and lingual surfaces with standardized dimensions of 2 mm height, width 4 mm, and a depth of 2 mm. After the cavity preparation, all teeth were randomly divided into three groups, namely Group-I: G-aenial Universal Flo with Single Bond 2 (n = 9 teeth); Group-II: G- aenial Universal Flo with G-Bond (n = 9 teeth), and Group-III: Constic (n = 9 teeth). The prepared and restored specimens were then subjected to thermocycling for 500 cycles in a water bath at 5 °C and 55 °C with a dwelling time of 30 s. The specimens were placed in 0.6% aqueous rhodamine dye for 48 h. Sectioning was carried out bucco-lingually and specimens were evaluated for microleakage under a confocal laser scanning microscope. **Results:** There was a significant difference (p = 0.009) in microleakage when comparing total etch and rinse, specifically between Adper Single Bond 2 ER-2 steps (fifth generation) and self-adhesive flowable composite resin, which is Constic. There was more microleakage in the self-etch bonding agent, particularly G-Bond, SE-1 step (seventh generation), when compared to ER-2 steps (fifth generation bonding agent); however, the results were not statistically significant (p = 0.468). The self-adhesive flowable composite resin showed more microleakage than SE-1 step and ER-2 steps. **Conclusions:** None of the adhesive systems tested were free from microleakage. However, less microleakage was observed in the total etch and rinse, especially Adper Single Bond 2 (ER-2 steps), than the self-etch adhesive system SE-1 step and self-adhesive flowable composite resin. **Clinical significance**: Constant research and technological advancements are taking place in dentin adhesives to improve the marginal seal. This has led to the evolution of total acid-etching dentin bonding agents termed as etch and rinse (ER)-2 steps (fifth generation dentin bonding agents) and self-etching (SE) 2 steps, and SE-1 step dentin bonding agents termed as the sixth and seventh generation bonding agents, respectively.

Keywords: restorative material; polymer; composite resin; flowable composite; dental leakage; dentin bonding agent

1. Introduction

Restorative dentistry has always thrived to obtain biocompatible restorations with superior aesthetic demand and a good marginal seal [1]. In today's clinical practice, composite resins have gained wide acceptance due to their high aesthetic quality [2].

Late 1996 led to the development of flowable composites. Their lower filler content, low viscosity and coefficient of thermal expansion being similar to that of the tooth structure made them widely used for restoring class V cavities [3]. Composite resins have progressed from macro-filled to micro-filled restoratives and from hybrids to micro-hybrids, and now the introduction of new nano-filled flowable composite and self-adhesive flowable resins has opened doors in dentistry. These are composed of nanocluster filler particle and nanomer, and thus have a better physical property and less marginal leakage [4].

Despite continuous development in the field of resin material, polymerization shrinkage still occurs. This is the crucial factor for determining the marginal integrity of the restoration [5]. The incidence of cervical lesions are on the rise [5,6]. Present literature states that the reason for the development of these lesions cannot be stated under one etiological factor, but is multifactorial in origin [7,8].

Abfraction is considered as a pathological loss of tooth structure in the cervical region of the tooth when eccentric and excessive occlusal forces act on the teeth [9,10]. Restoring cervical lesions with composite resins is always challenging, chiefly due to gingival margin lying in cementum, leaving no enamel margin for bonding. Isolation is difficult at gingival margins, which may lead to microleakage, and the outcome will be sensitivity, bacterial invasion and failure in the restoration. The longevity and success of such restorations can be assured by establishing a complete seal [11–13]. An adequate seal is a fundamental goal to obtain in either direct or in indirect adhesive restorations [14].

Despite continuous development in the field of resin material, polymerization shrinkage still occurs, which is the crucial factor for determining the marginal integrity of the restoration [15]. An increase in aesthetic demands and ease of operative procedures has also led to research and development in newer bonding systems [16]. Approximately 20 years ago, in 1960, Castan began an evolution regarding the concept of the self-etching approach that has reached a hallmark [17]. Recently, the new dentin bonding agents permit the use of acid, primer and bonding agents all together concomitantly [18]. Dentin demineralization followed by monomer penetration into the porosities are the mechanism of action [19]. Thus, these systems are considered to be simple and time- saving [20].

Although total etch adhesives are considered as the 'gold standard' for many years [21], studies have shown that total adhesives are incapable of preventing nanoleakage, and post-operative sensitivity has been reported [22]. The increase in the number of clinical steps is technique-sensitive and also time-consuming [23]. Therefore, the current trend is to transpose towards self-etch adhesives.

Currently, self-adhesive flowable composites are developed in order to overcome the time consumption by traditional materials. Bringing novel perception to restorative dentistry [24], they combine the merits of adhesive and restorative resin in a single technology, making new changes in the field of restorative dentistry and claiming to have less microleakage and a high bond strength [25].

Self-etch flowable composite resin requires no etching and bonding as a separate step. It claims that the material provides a good sealing ability, reduces the chair side time and is also less technique-sensitive [26].

Confocal laser scanning microscopy (CLSM) has been used for the three-dimensional evaluation of an object and obtaining a clear image. CLSM has powerful software that displays and analyzes 3D data, and images obtained have a greater sensitivity contrast and high resolution. In addition, optical sectioning giving three-dimensional reconstruction avoids the physical sectioning of specimen [27].

Hence, there is a need to study and evaluate the bonding efficacy of these newly developed self-etch adhesives and self-etch composites in comparison to etch and rinse adhesives in Class V cavities. The commercially available branded materials of a reputed company were selected for this purpose. Progress in the field of adhesive dentistry has given us a unique, less researched, all-in-one composite material called Constic.

This study aims to evaluate and compare the microleakage of Universal Flo composite resin (G-aenial) using an etch and rinse adhesive system, i.e., fifth generation ER-2steps (Adper Single Bond 2), self-etch adhesive system, i.e., seventh generation SE-1 step (G-Bond) and self-adhesive flowable composite resin (Constic) in Class V cavities using a confocal laser scanning microscope.

The null hypothesis states that there is no difference in the microleakage amongst the etch and rinse adhesive system ER-2steps (Adper Single Bond 2), self-etch adhesive system SE-1 step (G-Bond) and self-adhesive flowable composite resin (Constic) in Class V cavities.

2. Materials and Methods

This experimental in vitro research study was carried out in Dr. D.Y.Patil Dental College and Hospital, Pimpri, Pune. Prior approval from ethics committee was taken (DYPDCH/696/2016/20).

Twenty-seven human-extracted premolar teeth were selected for the study, and were extracted for orthodontic reasons. Maxillary and mandibular teeth were selected. After removal of residual tags, the specimens were cleaned with pumice, kept in normal saline and used in less than 2 months. Class V cavities were prepared on buccal and lingual surfaces of the teeth.

Cavities were prepared with uniform dimensions of height 2 mm, width 4 mm and depth of 2 mm using No. 329 fissure bur (Mani INC, Utsunomiya, Japan), and airotor handpiece (NSK, Shinagawa City, Japan), and diagnostic instruments such as single-end straight probe (GDC, Bangalore, India), William periodontal probe (GDC, Bangalore, India) and tweezer (GDC, Bangalore, India) were used.

After cavity preparation, all teeth were randomly divided into three groups with different adhesive systems to evaluate microleakage of each under flowable composite resin.

- Group I—G-aenial Universal Flo with Adper Single Bond2 (n = 9 teeth) (Etch and rinse adhesive system, ER-2 steps);
- Group-II—G-aenial Universal Flo with G-Bond (n = 9 teeth) (Self-etch adhesive system, SE-1 step);
- Group-III—Constic (Self-adhesive flowable composite resin) (n = 9 teeth).

In Group I, after preparation of Class V cavities, they were etched for 15 s using 37% phosphoric acid etching gel (3M ESPE, USA) and washed off for 10–15 s, and the cavities were dried until moist cavity surface was visible. Then, one coat of Adper Single Bond 2 (ER-2 steps-fifth generation bonding agent, 3M ESPE, Schiller Park, IL, USA) was applied on the inner surface of the cavity using an applicator brush (Denbur, Westmont, IL, USA) and air dried, followed by another coat, which was light cured using LED light curing unit (Confident, Bengaluru, India) for 10 s. The cavity was then restored with G-aenial universal Flo (GC Corp., Tokyo, Japan), and then again light cured for 20 s.

In Group II, after preparation of Class V cavities, two coats of G-Bond (SE-1 step-seventh generation bonding agent, GC Corp., Tokyo, Japan) was applied on the inner surface of the cavity using an applicator brush, air dried and cured for 10 s. The cavity was then restored with G-aenial universal Flo (GC Corp., Tokyo, Japan) and then cured for 20 s.

In Group III, after preparation of Class V cavities, it was restored with Constic (DMG, Davis, CA, USA). The resin composite surface was rubbed with the help of a brush and then cured for 20 s each.

The restored cavities were polished using composite polishing kit (Shofu, San Marcos, CA, USA). The prepared and restored specimens were then subjected to thermocycling for 500 cycles in water bath (Thermocycler 1100 SD, Mechatronik, Pleidelsheim, Germany) at 5° and 55 °C with a dwell time of 30 s. Nail varnish was applied, except on restorative material and 1 mm area around it. The specimens were placed in 0.6% aqueous rhodamine dye (HiMedia, Mumbai, India) for 48 h. The specimens were then rinsed with water and sectioned bucco-lingually through the center of restoration using slow-speed diamond disc (Shofu, San Marcos, CA, USA) on micromotor (Marathon-4, Seoul, Korea). A total of 36 sections were thus obtained in each group. Each cavity section was evaluated for microleakage by two observers using confocal laser scanning microscope (Zeiss LSM 710, Oberkochen, Germany) at 10× magnification.

The scores were given to the images according to the scoring criteria of Silveira de Araujo et al. [1].

- Score 0—No dye penetration.
- Score 1—Penetration involving half the occlusal and/or gingival wall.
- Score 2—Penetration involving more than half the occlusal and/or gingival wall.
- Score 3—Penetration involving up to the axial wall.

Statistical analysis was carried out using Kruskal–Wallis and Mann–Whitney U test. The p value was set at (0.025). The results were processed and analyzed using SPSS software version 19—SPSS Inc., Chicago, IL, USA.

3. Results

In statistical analysis, mean value/ score for microleakage was 46.65, 51.69 and 65.15 in Group I, II and III, respectively, with the highest microleakage observed in Group III compared to other groups (Figure 1).

Later pair-wise comparisons were carried out using the Mann–Whitney U test. Regarding the intergroup comparison, a higher (38.18 vs. 34.82) although non-significant (p = 0.468) microleakage score was found in Group II when compared with Group I (Figure 2). However, a significantly (p = 0.009) higher microleakage (42.67 vs. 30.33) was reported in Group

III in contrast to Group I (Figure 3). Lastly, a non-significant ($p = 0.058$) difference in microleakage was observed between Group II and Group III (Figure 4).

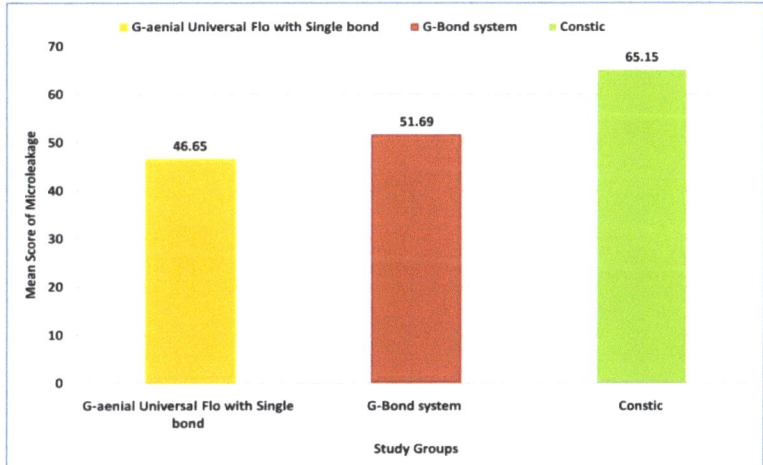

Figure 1. Comparison of mean values of microleakage in class V cavities with Single Bond and G-Bond system and Constic, using G-aenial Universal Flo.

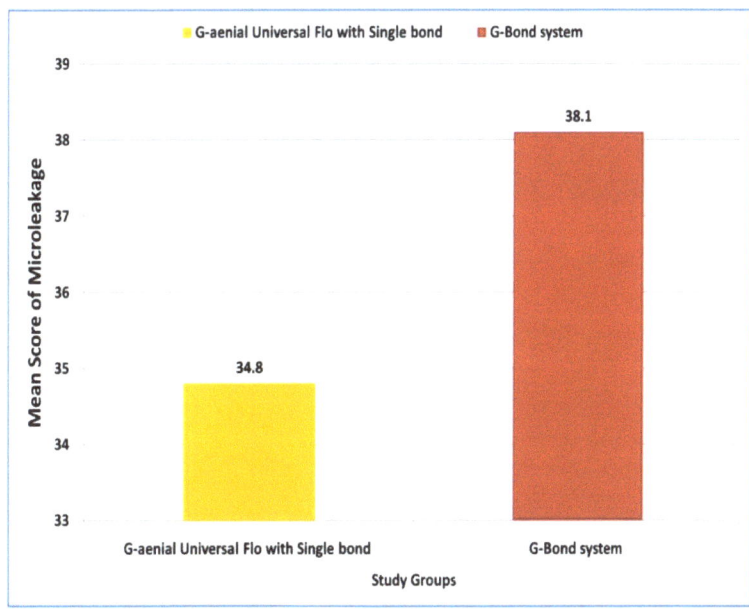

Figure 2. Comparison of mean values of microleakage in class V cavities with Single Bond and G-Bond system, using G-aenial Universal Flo.

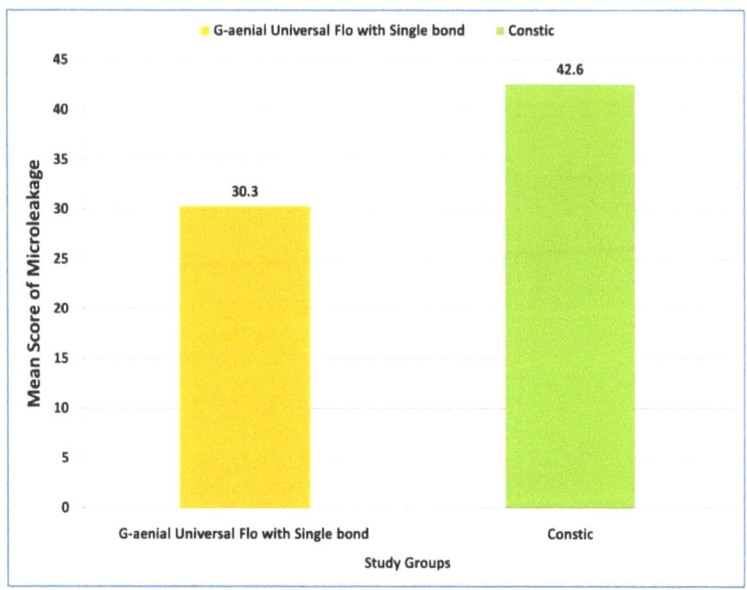

Figure 3. Comparison of mean values of microleakage in class V cavities with Single Bond and Constic, using G-aenial Universal Flo.

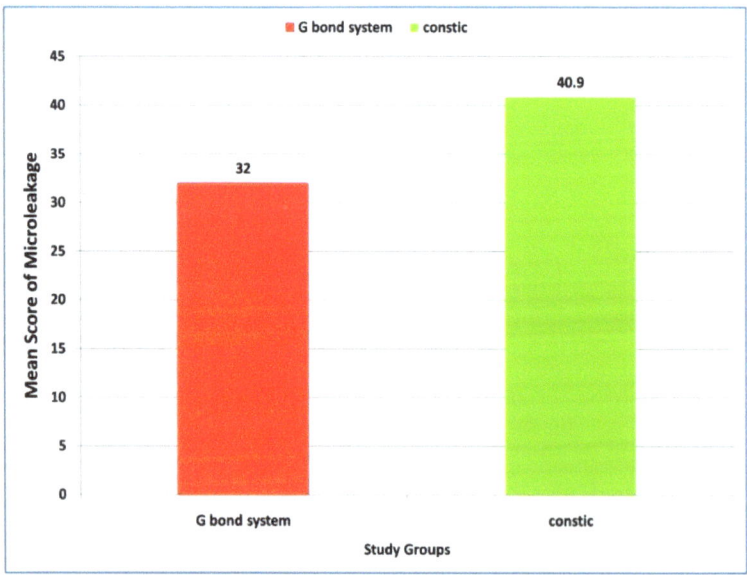

Figure 4. Comparison of mean values of microleakage in class V cavities with G-Bond system and Constic using G-aenial Universal Flo.

4. Discussion

Restorative dentistry endeavors to meet the aesthetic demands. Today, composite resins play a pivotal role in order to meet these demands. Other than aesthetics, composite resins have many more advantages, such as the conservation of the tooth structure, a low thermal conductivity and being repairable [2]. The longevity of composite resin restoration is, however, related to its marginal integrity. Marginal integrity is influenced by numerous factors, such as tooth preparation, type of restorative material used, restorative technique and also the finishing procedure [28,29].

However, as adhesion to enamel is a predictable entity, it is difficult for it to achieve an adequate bond to dentin. Various technological advancements of dentin adhesives have taken place over time to overcome this challenge. This has led to the evolution of fifth generation total acid-etching dentin bonding agents (ER-2 steps) and self-etching dentin bonding agents termed as the sixth (SE-2 steps) and seventh generation (SE-1step) bonding agents [30].

Adper Single Bond is ER-2 steps (fifth generation total acid etching dentin bonding agent). It consists of 2-hydroxyethyl methacrylate (HEMA), diurethanedimethacrylate, ethyl alcohol, glycerol 1,3-dimethacrylate Bis-GMA, silane-treated silica, itaconic acids and copolymers of acrylic acids [31]. Its composition involves the combination of the functions of a primer and components of an adhesive of a three-step conventional adhesive system, and its solvent consists of alcohol and water. The diffusion of the adhesive into the dentinal tubules is improved by the alcohol present in the solvent, which helps in enhancing the adhesion. The mechanism of action taking place is that the moisture present in the dentinal tubules draws the alcohol into and within the dentinal tubules along with the resin. From the substrate, the moisture content and alcohol vaporize, leaving the resin behind [32].

G-Bond is a SE-1 step (seventh generation) all-in-one self-etching adhesive system. It consists of 4-methacryloxethyl trimellitate anhydride, urethane dimethacrylate (UDMA), triethyleneglycoldimetacrylate, acetone and distilled water [11]. Vinay et al. studied the microleakage of G-Bond in class V cavities. The study showed that, when the samples were treated with this bonding agent, there was no exposure of the collagen fibers, and a slight decalcification was seen at dentin [29]. The functional monomers in the G-Bond react at the nano level with the hydroxyapatite crystals and form insoluble calcium. It has been shown that the G-bond is expected to be more durable and stronger. Five percent of the G-Bond consists of fillers, which seals the dentinal tubules and also decreases pulpal sensitivity [33]. A close marginal adaptation and less gap formation between the adhesive and dentin causes less microleakage and prevents microbial invasion, further leading to an increase in the longevity of restoration.

Constic, a self-adhesive flowable composite resin, was used for this study. Constic consists of 10-methacryloyloxydecyl dihydrogen phosphate. MDP, in a comparison with glycerol phosphate dimethacrylate (GPD), which a monomer used in other selfetch adhesive resins, is found to hold on to a greater number of hydrophobic spacer chains [34]. MDP has shown to form strong bonding with the hydroxyapatite crystals, forming stable 10-MDP-Ca salts.

The confocal microscopic evaluation of the samples in this study was carried out using the scoring system depicted in Figure 5. Microleakage was found in all of the materials tested. However, regarding the statistical analysis, the lowest amount of microleakage was seen in Adper Single Bond (ER-2 steps), which is a fifth generation bonding agent with a mean value (46.65), followed by G-Bond (SE-1 step), which is a seventh generation bonding agent with a mean value (51.69), and self-adhesive flowable composite resin (Constic), with a mean value (65.15). The difference in the microleakage of restorations carried out using the materials Single Bond and Constic was statistically significant.

The possible reasons for this result could be due to the fact that Single Bond is a fifth generation (ER-2 steps) bonding agent that comprises priming action and adhesive components of the conventional three-step adhesive system. It is composed of ethanol and water as a solvent. The presence of alcohol as a solvent has shown to increase the penetration into the dentinal tubules, thus aiding in adhesion. Moisture present in the dentinal tubules tends to draw the alcohol content into the dentinal tubules, which also takes resin along with it. Moisture and alcohol vaporize from the substrate and leave behind the resin content, thus providing a better bond strength [35].

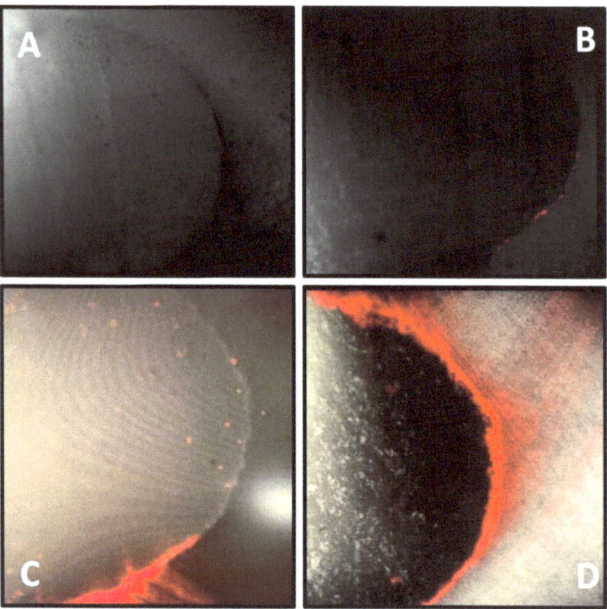

Figure 5. (**A**–**D**) Images of confocal laser microscopy showing scoring criteria with (**A**) Score 0; (**B**) Score 1; (**C**) Score 2; (**D**) Score 3.

The G-Bond showed a greater microleakage when compared with Single Bond, but this was not statistically significant. The possible reasons for this result could be due to G-Bond being the seventh generation (SE-1 step), and so working on a different mechanism of modifying the smear layer and not removing it; thus, the interface formed is different from the previously introduced adhesive systems. The decalcification of the dentin surface is less and there is almost no exposure of the collagen fibers. Hence, a very thin layer of the interface is formed, explaining the results obtained in this study. A nano level of insoluble calcium is formed due to the interaction between the functional monomers and the hydroxyapatite crystals. Thus, a strong bonding is expected from this bonding agent. This nano-level interaction is also termed the nano interaction zone or a "nano-level" interacted layer. These could be the reasons for better adaptation and microleakage values close to the gold standard etch and rinse system [33].

The current study results are in harmony with research carried out by Alfonso Sánchez-Ayala et al. to evaluate the microleakage in class V resin restorations bonded with six one-step self-etch systems and one etch and rinse adhesive. Seventy class V resin-based composite restorations were prepared on the buccal and lingual surfaces of 35 premolars by using: Clearfil S3 Bond, G-Bond, iBond, One Coat 7.0, OptiBond All-In-One or Xeno IV. The Adper Single Bond etch-and-rinse two-step adhesive was employed as a control. Specimens were thermocycled. None of the adhesives avoided microleakage at the dentin margins, and they displayed similar performances ($p = 0.76$). Their study showed that less microleakage was seen in Adper Single Bond compared to the G-Bond. They justified that Adper Single Bond 2 is able to wet and impregnate the etched enamel in an efficient manner comparable to those of three-step systems. However, its efficiency on dentin is lower because the adhesive incompletely diffuses under wet-bonding conditions, and a porous collagen network remains. Phase-separation also occurs in the interphase region between the hydrophilic primers and hydrophobic resins, resulting in water absorption. This effect may be justified by the incorporation of a high-molecular-weight polyalkenoic acid and the presence of HEMA. Nevertheless, the incorporation of alcohol as a cosolvent may help to explain its performance [11].

MitraTabari et al. conducted a study to evaluate the microleakage of composite resin restoration using a fifth generation bonding agent and two seventh generation bonding agents. This study was performed on 45 intact human-extracted primary teeth. Following class V cavity preparation, the samples were randomly divided into three groups, including 15 teeth based on the type of bonding agent: Single Bond 2, Clearfil S3 Bond, or G-Bond. There was no significant difference between incisal and gingival microleakage considering the different types of bonding [35].

In this study, Constic showed a greater amount of microleakage when compared with Single Bond and G-Bond. The possible reasons could be due to the incorporation of different monomers and compositions. A hard tissue interaction of self-adhesive flowable composites is found to be unlike the conventional composites [36]. The flowable composite tends to show a high water absorption. When the hydrophilic monomers are correlated to the conventional composites, they display a high tendency of water absorption. This, in turn, results in the breakdown of the polymer chains as the matrix swells due to water absorption because of the hydrophilic nature of the monomers in self-adhesive flowable composites. Such interactions might affect the bonding ability of the self-adhesives, which, in turn, cause a weak adhesion and failure [37].

Anshula Deshpande carried out an in vivo study to evaluate the retention rate, marginal integrity and marginal discoloration of two different sealants in which Constic and Conseal was used as a pit and fissure sealant. Constic showed a lower sealing ability when compared to Conseal. The Conseal-F sealant was better than the flowable composite as a sealant with respect to the marginal integrity and anatomical form. Both the materials showed similar results with respect to marginal discoloration [26].

However, a study carried out by Amey Panse compared the efficacy of the new material to the conventional sealant. Seventy-six noncarious primary molars were randomly assigned into two groups, Fissurit F (Group A) and Constic (Group B). Each group was further subdivided into four groups: G1—microleakage ($n = 18$), G2—fracture strength ($n = 18$), G3—tensile strength ($n = 20$), G4—shear strength ($n = 20$). The microleakage and fracture strength of Constic were found to be better, but the bond strength of Fissurit F (tensile strength—14.30 ± 4.49; shear bond strength—6.12 ± 2.84) was greater than that of Constic (tensile strength—6.33 ± 1.47; shear bond strength—2.06 ± 0.635). Their results showed Constic to be more fracture-resistant and presented less microleakage [38].

Hence, the null hypothesis for this study was rejected, as there was a difference in microleakage amongst the study groups, i.e., etch and rinse adhesive system ER-2steps (Adper Single Bond 2), self-etch adhesive system SE-1 step (G-Bond), and self-adhesive flowable composite resin (Constic) in Class V cavities.

The biocompatibility of these new products may be a matter of concern, but the dentin bonding agents and composite resins mentioned in this study are commercially available materials. Research by Pagano S et al. suggested that adhesives showed an effect on the functionality of fibroblasts, with a cytotoxic effect on time, that was concentration-dependent. The in-depth analysis of the effects of universal adhesives and possible functional effects represents important information for the clinician towards choosing the most suitable adhesive system [38].

Continued technological development in dental materials has led to the introduction of 'bioactive materials' that can activate dental tissue repair mechanisms, as well as elicit a positive response from the dental tissue. With characteristics similar to composites and glass ionomer cements, these can be especially useful in restorative dentistry. This could be future scope for scientific research in the ever-increasing clinical use of bioactive composites in the restoration of cervical lesions [39].

The limitation of this in vitro study is that the simulation of oral environment was not possible. There is a need for further in vivo research with regards to microleakage that compares the self-adhesive composite resin. Recently, different adhesive systems have been introduced in dentistry for better marginal adaptations and less microleakage. Their sealing ability should be assessed both in vitro and in vivo using different techniques.

5. Conclusions

None of the adhesive systems tested in the above study were free from microleakage. In the present study, the total etch adhesive ER-2 steps, i.e., fifth generation bonding agent (Adper Single Bond 2), showed the least microleakage values, followed by SE-1 step i.e., seventh generation bonding agent (G-Bond) and self-adhesive flowable composite (Constic). Constic showed the highest amount of microleakage.

The difference in microleakage between the self-adhesive flowable composite (Constic), etch and rinse (ER-2 steps) fifth generation (Adper Single Bond), and self-etch (SE-1 step) seventh generation bonding agent (G-Bond) was statistically significant. When etch and rinse (Adper Single Bond 2) and self-etch (G-Bond) were compared, more microleakage was seen in the G-Bond compared to Adper Single Bond 2, the difference not being statistically significant.

Author Contributions: Conceptualization, E.V.S. and S.M.; methodology, S.M., L.B. and A.G.; software, T.A. and S.B. (Shilpa Bhandi); validation, A.R. and M.A.B; formal analysis, H.A.B., S.A.B. and B.Z.; investigation, N.H.A., S.B. (Sultan Binalrimal), and S.P.; resources, A.G. and T.A.; data curation, L.B., A.G., T.A., D.S., K.C.S. and S.P.; writing—original draft preparation, E.V.S., S.M., L.B., A.G., T.A., S.B. (Sultan Binalrimal), A.R. and M.A.B.; writing—review and editing, E.V.S., S.M., L.B., A.G., T.A., S.B. (Sultan Binalrimal), A.R., M.A.B., H.A.B., S.A.B., B.Z., N.H.A., S.B. (Shilpa Bhandi), D.S., K.C.S. and S.P.; visualization, E.V.S. and S.M.; supervision, S.M., L.B., A.R. and M.A.B.; project administration, S.A.B., B.Z. and S.P. All authors have read and agreed to the published version of the manuscript.

Funding: This research received no external funding.

Institutional Review Board Statement: The study was conducted in accordance with the Declaration of Helsinki, and approved by the Institutional Review Board of Dr. DY. Patil Vidyapeeth, Pimpri, Pune, Maharashtra (Approval number: DPU/R &R(D)/971(27)/16).

Informed Consent Statement: Not applicable.

Data Availability Statement: Not applicable.

Conflicts of Interest: The authors declare no conflict of interest.

References

1. Sooraparaju, S.G.; Kanumuru, P.K.; Nujella, S.K.; Konda, K.R.; Reddy, K.B.K.; Penigalapati, S. A Comparative Evaluation of Microleakage in Class V Composite Restorations. *Int. J. Dent.* **2014**, *2014*, 1–4. [CrossRef] [PubMed]
2. Ferracane, J.L. Resin composite—State of the art. *Dent. Mater.* **2011**, *27*, 29–38. [CrossRef] [PubMed]
3. Yazici, A.R.; Baseren, M.; Dayangaç, B. The effect of flowable resin composite on microleakage in class V cavities. *Oper. Dent.* **2003**, *28*, 42–46. [PubMed]
4. Jain, A.; Deepti, D.; Tavane, P.N.; Singh, A.; Gupta, P.; Gupta, A.; Sonkusre, S. Evaluation of Microleakage of Recent Nano-hybrid Composites in Class V Restorations: An In Vitro Study. *Int. J. Adv. Health Sci.* **2015**, *2*, 8–12.
5. Lyttle, H.A.; Sidhu, N.; Smyth, B. A study of the classification and treatment of noncarious cervical lesions by general practitioners. *J. Prosthet. Dent.* **1998**, *79*, 342–346. [CrossRef]
6. Bader, J.D.; Levitch, L.C.; Shugars, D.A.; Heymann, H.O.; McClure, F. How Dentists Classified and Treated Non-Carious Cervical Lesions. *J. Am. Dent. Assoc.* **1993**, *124*, 46–54. [CrossRef]
7. Grippo, J.O.; Simring, M.; Schreiner, S. Attrition, abrasion, corrosion and abfraction revisited. *J. Am. Dent. Assoc.* **2004**, *135*, 1109–1118. [CrossRef]
8. Osborne-Smith, K.L.; Burke, F.J.T.; Wilson, N.H.F. The aetiology of the non-carious cervical lesion. *Int. Dent. J.* **1999**, *49*, 139–143. [CrossRef]
9. Grippo, J.O.; Simring, M.; Coleman, T.A. Abfraction, Abrasion, Biocorrosion, and the Enigma of Noncarious Cervical Lesions: A 20-Year Perspective. *J. Esthet. Restor. Dent.* **2012**, *24*, 10–23. [CrossRef]
10. Marcauteanu, C.; Bradu, A.; Sinescu, C.; Topala, F.I.; Negrutiu, M.L.; Podoleanu, A.G. Quantitative evaluation of dental abfraction and attrition using a swept-source optical coherence tomography system. *J. Biomed. Opt.* **2013**, *19*, 021108. [CrossRef]
11. Sánchez-Ayala, A.; Farias-Neto, A.; Vilanova, L.S.R.; Gomes, J.C.; Gomes, O.M.M. Marginal microleakage of class V resin-based composite restorations bonded with six one-step self-etch systems. *Braz. Oral Res.* **2013**, *27*, 225–230. [CrossRef] [PubMed]

12. Geerts, S.; Bolette, A.; Seidel, L.; Guéders, A. An In Vitro Evaluation of Leakage of Two Etch and Rinse and Two Self-Etch Adhesives after Thermocycling. *Int. J. Dent.* **2012**, *2012*, 1–7. [CrossRef] [PubMed]
13. Sadeghi, M. An in vitro microleakage study of class V cavities restored with a new self-adhesive flowable composite resin versus different flowable materials. *Dent. Res. J.* **2012**, *9*, 460–465.
14. Baldi, A.; Comba, A.; Michelotto Tempesta, R.; Carossa, M.; Pereira, G.K.R.; Valandro, L.F.; Paolone, G.; Vichi, A.; Goracci, C.; Scotti, N. External Marginal Gap Variation and Residual Fracture Resistance of Composite and Lithium-Silicate CAD/CAM Overlays after Cyclic Fatigue over Endodontically-Treated Molars. *Polymers* **2021**, *13*, 3002. [CrossRef]
15. Scotti, N.; Comba, A.; Gambino, A.; Paolino, D.S.; Alovisi, M.; Pasqualini, D.; Berutti, E. Microleakage at enamel and dentin margins with a bulk fills flowable resin. *Eur. J. Dent.* **2014**, *8*, 1–8. [CrossRef] [PubMed]
16. Atash, R.; van den Abbeele, A. Bond strengths of eight contemporary adhesives to enamel and to dentine: An in vitro study on bovine primary teeth. *Int. J. Paediatr. Dent.* **2005**, *15*, 264–273. [CrossRef] [PubMed]
17. Somani, R.; Jaidka, S.; Arora, S. Comparative evaluation of microleakage of newer generation dentin bonding agents: An in vitro study. *Indian J. Dent. Res.* **2016**, *27*, 86. [CrossRef]
18. Yaseen, S.; Subba Reddy, V. Comparative evaluation of shear bond strength of two self-etching adhesives (sixth and seventh generation) on dentin of primary and permanent teeth: An in vitro study. *J. Indian Soc. Pedod. Prev. Dent.* **2009**, *27*, 33. [CrossRef]
19. Agostini, F.G.; Kaaden, C.; Powers, J.M. Bond strength of self-etching primers to enamel and dentin of primary teeth. *Pediatr. Dent.* **2001**, *23*, 481–486.
20. Uekusa, S.; Yamaguchi, K.; Miyazaki, M.; Tsubota, K.; Kurokawa, H.; Hosoya, Y. Bonding Efficacy of Single-step Self-etch Systems to Sound Primary and Permanent Tooth Dentin. *Oper. Dent.* **2006**, *31*, 569–576. [CrossRef]
21. Giannini, M.; Makishi, P.; Ayres, A.P.A.; Vermelho, P.M.; Fronza, B.M.; Nikaido, T.; Tagami, J. Self-Etch Adhesive Systems: A Literature Review. *Braz. Dent. J.* **2015**, *26*, 3–10. [CrossRef]
22. Van Meerbeek, B. The "myth" of nanoleakage. *J. Adhes. Dent.* **2007**, *9*, 491–492. [PubMed]
23. Sundfeld, R.H.; Valentino, T.A.; Sversut de Alexandre, R.; Fraga Briso, A.L.; Marçal Mazza Sundefeld, M.L. Hybrid layer thickness and resin tag length of a self-etching adhesive bonded to sound dentin. *J. Dent.* **2005**, *33*, 675–681. [CrossRef] [PubMed]
24. Khalil Yousef, M.; Abo El Naga, A.; Ramadan, R.; Fayez, C.; Alshawwa, L. Does the use of a novel self-adhesive flowable composite reduce nanoleakage? *Clin. Cosmet. Investig. Dent.* **2015**, *7*, 55. [CrossRef] [PubMed]
25. Ozel Bektas, O.; Eren, D.; Akin, E.G.; Akin, H. Evaluation of a self-adhering flowable composite in terms of micro-shear bond strength and microleakage. *Acta Odontol. Scand.* **2013**, *71*, 541–546. [CrossRef]
26. Deshpande, A.; Sudani, U.; Bargale, S.; Poonacha, K.S.; Kadam, M.; Joshi, N. Six months clinical performance of self etch-self adhesive flowable composite and conventional pit-and-fissure sealants in 7 to 10 year old children. *J. Adv. Med. Dent. Sci. Res.* **2016**, *4*, 38–43.
27. Wright, S.J.; Wright, D.J. Introduction to confocal microscopy. *Methods Cell Biol.* **2002**, *72*, 85.
28. Jefferies, S.R. The art and science of abrasive finishing and polishing in restorative dentistry. *Dent. Clin. N. Am.* **1998**, *42*, 613–627. [CrossRef]
29. Hoelscher, D.C.; Neme, A.M.; Pink, F.E.; Hughes, P.J. The effect of three finishing systems on four esthetic restorative materials. *Oper. Dent.* **1998**, *23*, 36–42.
30. Langalia, A.; Buch, A.; Khamar, M.; Patel, P. Polymerization Shrinkage of Composite Resins: A Review. *J. Med. Dent. Sci. Res.* **2015**, *2*, 23–27.
31. Kidd, E.A. Microleakage in relation to amalgam and composite restorations. A laboratory study. *Br. Dent. J.* **1976**, *141*, 305–310. [CrossRef]
32. Migliau, G. Classification review of dental adhesive systems: From the IV generation to the universal type. *Ann. Stomatol.* **2017**, *8*, 1. [CrossRef] [PubMed]
33. Radovic, I.; Vulicevic, Z.R.; García-Godoy, F. Morphological Evaluation of 2- and 1-step Self-etching System Interfaces with Dentin. *Oper. Dent.* **2006**, *31*, 710–718. [CrossRef] [PubMed]
34. Wang, R.; Shi, Y.; Li, T.; Pan, Y.; Cui, Y.; Xia, W. Adhesive interfacial characteristics and the related bonding performance of four self-etching adhesives with different functional monomers applied to dentin. *J. Dent.* **2017**, *62*, 72–80. [CrossRef] [PubMed]
35. Amaral, C.M.; Hara, A.T.; Pimenta, L.A.; Rodrigues, A.L. Microleakage of hydrophilic adhesive systems in Class V composite restorations. *Am. J. Dent.* **2001**, *14*, 31–33. [PubMed]
36. Brueckner, C.; Schneider, H.; Haak, R. Shear Bond Strength and Tooth-Composite Interaction With Self-Adhering Flowable Composites. *Oper. Dent.* **2017**, *42*, 90–100. [CrossRef]
37. Peterson, J.; Rizk, M.; Hoch, M.; Wiegand, A. Bonding performance of self-adhesive flowable composites to enamel, dentin and a nano-hybrid composite. *Odontology* **2018**, *106*, 171–180. [CrossRef]
38. Panse, A.; Nair, M.; Patil, A.; Bahutule, S. Comparison of microleakage, bond strength, and fracture strength of no etch no bond novel flowable composite as a pit and fissure sealant in comparison to the conventional sealants: An In vitro Study. *Int. J. Pedod. Rehabil.* **2018**, *3*, 28. [CrossRef]
39. Bordea, I.R.; Sîrbu, A.; Lucaciu, O.; Ilea, A.; Câmpian, R.S.; Todea, D.A.; Alexescu, T.G.; Aluaș, M.; Budin, C.; Pop, A.S. Microleakage—The Main Culprit in Bracket Bond Failure? *J. Mind Med. Sci.* **2019**, *6*, 86–94. [CrossRef]

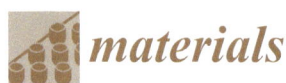

Article

Influence of Factors in the Photopolymerization Process on Dental Composites Microhardness

Jordan Maximov [1], Tsanka Dikova [2,*], Galya Duncheva [1] and Georgi Georgiev [2]

[1] Faculty of Mechanical Engineering, Technical University of Gabrovo, 4 Hadji Dimitar Str., 5300 Gabrovo, Bulgaria
[2] Faculty of Dental Medicine, Medical University of Varna, 84 Tsar Osvoboditel Blvd., 9000 Varna, Bulgaria
* Correspondence: tsanka_dikova@abv.bg

Abstract: The aim of the present paper is to investigate the influence of factors in photopolymerization process that govern microhardness of three types of dental composites—universal (UC), bulk-fill (BC), and flowable (FC). Cylindrical specimens with different thicknesses are made and light cured. The significance of light intensity, irradiation time, and layer thickness on Vickers microhardness is evaluated by experimental design, analysis of variance, and regression analysis. It is found that the main factor influencing the microhardness on the top surface of the three composites is light intensity. The second factor is layer thickness for the UC and FC, while for BC, it is curing time. The third factor is curing time for the first two composites and layer thickness for bulk-fill. The significance of factors' influence on the microhardness of the bottom surface is the same for the UC and FC, but different for BC. The main factor for the first two composites is layer thickness, followed by curing time and light intensity. For bulk-fill, curing time is main factor, light intensity is second, and layer thickness is last. Different significance of factors influencing the microhardness on top and bottom surfaces of investigated composites is revealed for the first time in the present study.

Keywords: light-cured dental composites; microhardness; light intensity; irradiation time; layer thickness

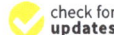

Citation: Maximov, J.; Dikova, T.; Duncheva, G.; Georgiev, G. Influence of Factors in the Photopolymerization Process on Dental Composites Microhardness. *Materials* **2022**, *15*, 6459. https://doi.org/10.3390/ma15186459

Academic Editors: Lavinia Cosmina Ardelean and Laura-Cristina Rusu

Received: 19 August 2022
Accepted: 13 September 2022
Published: 17 September 2022

Publisher's Note: MDPI stays neutral with regard to jurisdictional claims in published maps and institutional affiliations.

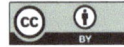

Copyright: © 2022 by the authors. Licensee MDPI, Basel, Switzerland. This article is an open access article distributed under the terms and conditions of the Creative Commons Attribution (CC BY) license (https://creativecommons.org/licenses/by/4.0/).

1. Introduction

Resin-based composites (RBCs), also known as dental composites, are widely used in restorative dentistry due to their many advantages, such as excellent esthetics, conservation of tooth structure, good longevity, affordable price, and possibility for repair [1]. They are used in dental practices as restorative materials, sealants, liners, veneers, crowns, cements, etc. [2]. The main components of RBC include organic matrix, inorganic filler, coupling agents, and initiators of the polymerization process [3–5]. The organic resin matrix phase is made from a mixture of multifunctional monomers (Bis-GMA, UDMA, TEGDMA, etc.), while the filler phase contains micro/nano-sized fillers, which are mainly used as a reinforcement [6,7].

Depending on their viscosity, composites can be divided into compactable and flowable. The latter have a reduced filler content (37–53 vol. %), which gives them a low viscosity with a flowable character, spreading uniformly, and adapting intimately to the prepared tooth surfaces. The main advantages of flowable over compactable composites are easier handling properties during manipulation, better adaptation to the tooth surface, and higher flexibility [8]. Of course, what makes flowable composites so effective for some restorations also limits their effectiveness in others. The lower filler content of these materials can lead to more polymerization shrinkage. Moreover, less filler leads to a reduction in the composite's mechanical properties [9]. However, not all flowables have the same composition. Newer materials have higher filler contents than their predecessors, which improves some of the well-known disadvantages and gives them higher strength and wear resistance. These improved materials can be used for Class I, II, III, IV, and V restorations, and with similar results to more viscous composites [10].

Conventional RBCs are applied using an incremental technique, which is a time-consuming process and contributes to greater inaccuracies. To simplify the procedure, the manufacturers create bulk-fill composites that allow light curing layers of up to 5 mm, while ensuring sufficient depth of cure. These materials can be divided into two groups: Base and full-body bulk-fill composites. Base bulk-fill composites have a low viscosity (they are flowable), which enables placement and adaptation in less accessible cavities. These composites have a lower filler content and, respectively, lower wear resistance, hence, capping with a conventional composite is required [11]. The full-body bulk-fill composites are highly viscous because of their higher filler loads and allow the whole restoration to be placed at once without requiring any coverage. The application of bulk fill composites in posterior restorations reduces cusp deflection [12–14] and polymerization stress [15], thus increasing the fracture resistance of the restoration and hard dental tissues [12].

The degree of conversion achieved within a composite is important because it controls several properties of the cured material, including mechanical strength, polymerization shrinkage, wear behavior, and monomer release [16]. The degree of conversion depends on many factors: Light intensity, curing time, layer thickness, distance and angulation of the light curing tip to the irradiated surface, color of the composite, type and amount of filler, and material temperature [17].

Many in vitro studies have been conducted over the years to show how different irradiation times and light intensities affect the mechanical properties of the restoration [18–20]. They all confirm that the amount of light energy needed for the proper polymerization of the restoration can be achieved by many combinations between light intensity and irradiation time, and the higher the intensity of the light curing unit, the shorter the duration of the polymerization. The abovementioned studies indicate that increasing the light curing time results in higher overall radiant exposure reaching the composite layer. Therefore, better polymerization can be obtained, especially with a thick composite layer or a light curing unit with low light intensity.

Another factor of fundamental importance for the proper polymerization of the RBC restoration is the layer thickness. Many authors in their studies have reported that for conventional composite, a layer thickness of 2 mm is optimal when the incremental technique is applied [13,21]. Placing increments thicker than 2–2.5 mm significantly reduces the mechanical and physical properties of the restoration and, respectively, its longevity [17,22]. The use of bulk-fill composites allows adequate polymerization for thicker layers up to 5 mm.

The successful polymerization of RBCs can be evaluated by their hardness. There is a positive correlation between the conversion ratio and hardness of dental composites [23,24]. It was found that an 80% bottom-to-top hardness ratio corresponds to a 90% conversion ratio [25]. On the other hand, the wear and fracture resistance, as well as the durability of the restoration, are defined by the composite hardness.

The present study aims to investigate the influence of factors in the photopolymerization process (light intensity, irradiation time, and layer thickness) on the microhardness of three types of dental composites (conventional, bulk-fill, and flowable). The evaluation of the factors is performed by dispersion and regression analyses. The combination of these methods gives the opportunity to study the influence of each factor on the hardness and also to determine the significance of the different factors. To the best of our knowledge, different significance of the factors influencing the microhardness on the top and bottom surfaces of the investigated composites is established for the first time in the present study.

2. Materials and Methods

2.1. Materials and Specimen Preparation

Three types of light-cured resin-based composites were used in the research: Universal nanohybrid composite (UC) (Evetric, Ivoclar Vivadent, Liechtenstein), nanohybrid bulk-fill composite (BC) for posterior restorations (Filtek One Bulk Fill Restorative, 3M, Saint Paul, MN, USA), and universal nanofilled flowable composite (FC) with high filler content (G-aenial Universal Flo, GC, Fuchu, Japan) with composition shown in Table 1. Round samples (5 mm diameter) were made of the three composites with the same A2 shade. The samples were manufactured in polyurethane molds with thicknesses of 2, 3, and 4 mm. The polymerization was carried out by a light-curing unit (LCU) (Curing Pen, Eighteeth, Changzhou Sifary Medical Technology Co., Ltd., Changzhou, China), varying the light intensity (600, 1000, and 1500 mW/cm^2) and irradiation time (20, 40, and 60 s). More detailed information about sample preparation was given in our previous works [26,27].

Table 1. Composition of the investigated dental composites [26].

No.	Composite	Composition		Matrix/Filler Ratio, wt %
		Component	Amount	
1	UC Evetric [28]	Matrix: UDMA (Urethane dimethacrylate) Bis-GMA (Bisphenol A glycydil dimethacrylate) Bis-EMA (Bisphenol A polyethethylene glycol dimethacrylate) Fillers: Barium glass, ytterbium fluoride (YbF$_3$), mixed oxides, and prepolymers 40 nm–3 µm.	10–25%; 3–10%; 3–10%	19–20/80–81
2	BC Filtek One Bulk Fill Restorative [29]	Matrix: AUDMA (Aromatic Urethane Dimethacrylate) DDDMA (1,12-Dodecane Dimethycrylate) UDMA (Urethane dimethacrylate) Fillers: Non-aglomerated/non-agregated 20 nm silica and 4–11 nm zirconia, aggregated zirconia/silica cluster (comprised of 20 nm silica and 4–11 nm zirconia particles), and ytterbium fluoride (agglomerated 100 nm particles).	10–20% <10% 1–10%	23.5/76.5
3	FC G-aenial Universal Flo [30,31]	Matrix: UDMA (Urethane dimethacrylate) Bis-EMA Dimethacrylate component (TEGDMA) Fillers: Silicon dioxide (16 nm), strontium glass (200 nm), pigments.	10–20% 5–10% 5–10%	31/69

Three specimens were manufactured for each combination of parameters. According to the experimental design, shown in Table 2, fourteen different combinations of parameters were used for each composite type. Therefore, the specimens were divided into 3 groups depending on the composite type—UC, BC, and FC. Each group was divided into 14 subgropus (3 samples in each) according to the photopolymerization parameters. Totally, 126 specimens were prepared for the research, or 42 for each composite. After sample polymerization, they were stored for 24 h at room temperature in a dry, dark container before hardness measurements were made.

Table 2. Experimental design [26].

No.	Composite Type			UC		BC		FC	
	Dimensionless Governing Factors			$\overline{Y}_1, HV$	$\overline{Y}_2, HV$	$\overline{Y}_1, HV$	$\overline{Y}_2, HV$	$\overline{Y}_1, HV$	$\overline{Y}_2, HV$
	x_1	x_2	x_3						
1	−1	−1	−1	42.0	33.5	59.1	55.8	42.4	37.9
2	1	−1	−1	52.4	42.9	61.7	60.2	50.0	46.3
3	−1	1	−1	45.9	41.1	61.8	61.1	47.5	45.5
4	1	1	−1	57.8	51.3	68.4	67.5	49.9	47.7
5	−1	−1	1	45.0	12.2	57.9	45.4	42.9	13.1
6	1	−1	1	58.9	26.1	61.7	55.3	45.0	27.0
7	−1	1	1	49.3	32.7	60.3	57.5	45.3	31.7
8	1	1	1	62.7	45.0	67.2	65.3	48.1	42.6
9	−0.1111	−1	−1	54.1	42.2	62.2	60.3	47.7	42.3
10	−0.1111	1	1	56.9	35.8	65.1	61.6	45.8	37.6
11	−1	0	−1	42.4	38.2	63.8	60.3	45.3	43.5
12	1	0	1	61.7	38.4	65.3	62.5	45.5	36.5
13	−1	−1	0	44.3	22.2	59.2	51.8	46.1	29.9
14	1	1	0	59.3	48.7	69.1	67.3	51.1	47.1

2.2. Microhardness Measurements

The surface microhardness measurements on Vickers method ($HV_{0.05}$) were made using a ZHVμ Zwick/Roell microhardness tester with computerized processing of the measurement results, using a 0.05 kgf load and a 10 s holding time. Five measurements were made for the top and bottom surface of each specimen. The final value of the top and bottom surface microhardness corresponded to the grouping center.

2.3. Experimental Design

The governing factors and their levels are shown in Table 3. Physical coordinates $\tilde{x}_i$, $i = 1, 2, 3$ are transformed into dimensionless coordinates x_i, $i = 1, 2, 3$ by the formula

$$x_i = (\tilde{x}_i - \tilde{x}_{0,i})/\lambda_i, \qquad (1)$$

where $\lambda_i = (\tilde{x}_{max,i} - \tilde{x}_{min,i})/2$, $\tilde{x}_{0,i}$, $\tilde{x}_{max,i}$ and $\tilde{x}_{min,i}$ are, respectively, average, upper and lower levels of the i_{th} physical factor. The objective functions are Y_1 and Y_2, surface microhardness respectively on the top and bottom surface of the composite layer. An optimal second-order composition plan was chosen (Table 2).

Table 3. Governing factors and their levels.

Light intensity I [mW/cm^2]	$\tilde{x}_1$	600	1000	1500
Irradiation time t [s]	$\tilde{x}_2$	20	40	60
Layer thickness d [mm]	$\tilde{x}_3$	2	3	4

Analysis of variance (ANOVA)—two-way variant and regression analysis were conducted in order to study the factor influence, using QstatLab software (V. 5.5, creators Vuchkov I. N. and Vuchkov I. I., Sofia, Bulgaria). The objective functions in the regression models were chosen to be polynomials from the second order, given the number of levels of the governing factors:

$$Y_i = b_0 + \sum_{j=1}^{3} b_j x_j + \sum_{j=1}^{2}\sum_{k=j-1}^{3} b_{jk} x_j x_k + \sum_{j=1}^{3} b_{jj} x_j^2, \ i = 1, 2 \qquad (2)$$

The absolute value of the coefficients in the objective functions (2) shows the significance of the respective factor.

3. Results

The results we obtained show that the highest microhardness was in a sample of BC Filtek One Bulk Fill Restorative: 57.9–69.1 HV on the top surface and 45.4–67.5 HV on the bottom, depending on the curing modes used (Table 3). It is followed by FC G-aenial Universal Flo with hardness 42.4–51.1 HV and 13.1–47.7 HV on the top and bottom surfaces, respectively. The lowest hardness was observed in UC Evetric, with values of hardness on the top surface of 42.0–62.7 HV and 12.2–51.3 HV on the bottom. Regardless of the curing modes used, the smallest differences between the hardness of the two surfaces were observed in BC Filtek One Bulk Fill Restorative, and the largest—in UC Evetric.

The polynomial coefficients of the objective functions are shown in Table 4.

Table 4. Polynomial coefficients of the objective functions.

Composite/Objective Function		b_0	b_1	b_2	b_3	b_{11}	b_{22}	b_{12}	b_{13}	b_{23}	b_{123}
UC	Y_1	56.266	6.4	1.53	2.002	−4.458	0	0	0	0	0
	Y_2	35.936	6.11	6.459	−6.991	0	0	0	1.189	3.083	0
BC	Y_1	64.55	2.327	2.25	−0.704	0	−1.866	1.003	0	0	0
	Y_2	59.11	3.59	4.17	−2.74	0	0	0	1.162	1.397	0
FC	Y_1	46.762	1.715	1.054	−1.326	0	0	0	−0.766	0	0.730
	Y_2	37.091	4.214	5.271	−7.769	0	0	0	1.994	3.185	0

3.1. UC Evetric

The most significant factor influencing the surface hardness Y_1 of UC Evetric is light intensity (x_1), followed by layer thickness (x_3) and irradiation time (x_2) (Figure 1a). The upper levels of the three factors (x_1, x_2, x_3) maximize the objective function Y_1, and the lower levels minimize it. The maximum/minimum of the objective function Y_1 is reached when the three factors are maintained at the upper/lower level. This shows that the maximum hardness on the top surface is obtained at maximum values of the three parameters intensity, time, and layer thickness (1500 mW/cm^2, 60 s and 4 mm), and the minimum hardness at minimum values of the parameters (600 mW/cm^2, 20 s and 2 mm).

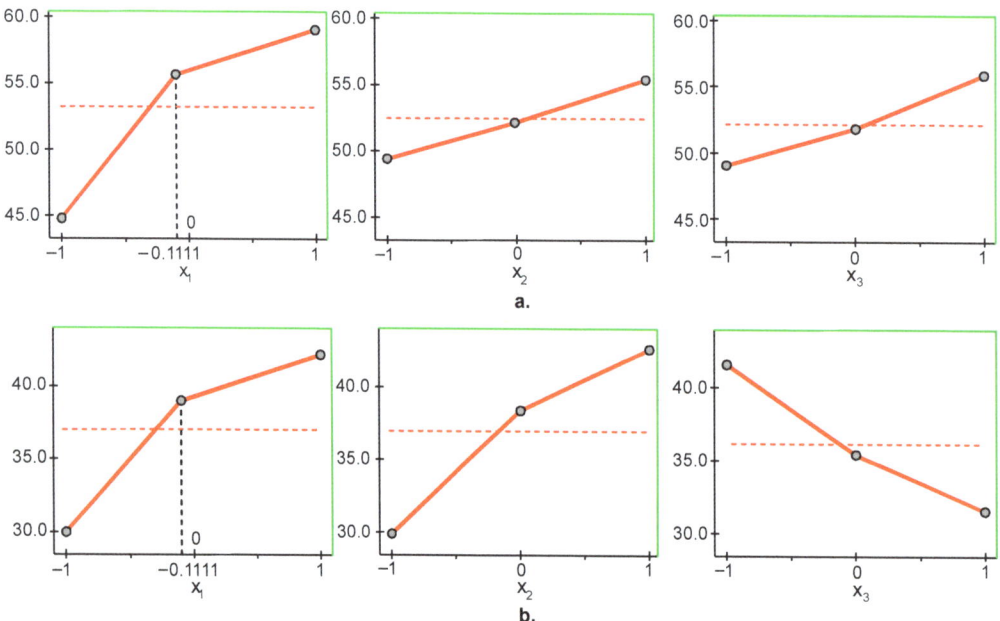

Figure 1. Influence of the different factors of photopolymerization on the microhardness on: (**a**) The top and (**b**) bottom surfaces of UC Evetric (x_1—light intensity, x_2—curing time, x_3—layer thickness). Red dashed line: average value of micro-hardness; black dashed line: the actual coded value of x_1.

The influence of the different factors on the hardness of the bottom surface Y_2 of UC Evetric is presented in Figure 1b. The graphs show that the most significant factor, in this case, is layer thickness (x_3), followed by irradiation time (x_2) and light intensity (x_1). The difference in the significance of the last two factors is very small, and a regression model in dimensionless coordinates is needed for a more accurate estimate. The maximum/minimum of the objective function Y_2 is achieved by maintaining the first two factors (x_1 and x_2) at the upper/lower level and the third factor (x_3) at the lower/upper level. Therefore, maximum/minimum hardness on the bottom surface is obtained at maximum/minimum values of the first two parameters, intensity and time (1500 mW/cm^2 and 60 s/600 mW/cm^2 and 20 s), and the values of the third parameter, layer thickness, are respectively minimum/maximum (2 mm/4 mm).

The coefficients in the objective functions (see Table 4) confirm the conclusions obtained via ANOVA (Figure 1). The visualization of the regression models for the hardness on the top surface (Y_1) of the composite layer and hardness on the bottom surface (Y_2) is presented in Figure 2. The coefficients in the regression model Y_1 confirm that light intensity (x_1) is the most significant factor, followed by layer thickness (x_3) and irradiation time (x_2). From the regression model Y_2 it is clear that the most significant factor is layer thickness (x_3), followed by irradiation time (x_2) and light intensity (x_1). Therefore, the intensity of the LCU has the greatest influence on the top surface hardness of the UC Evetric restoration, and as the intensity increases, so does the hardness. Layer thickness has the strongest effect on the hardness of the bottom surface, but here the dependence is reversed: Increasing the layer thickness leads to a decrease in hardness.

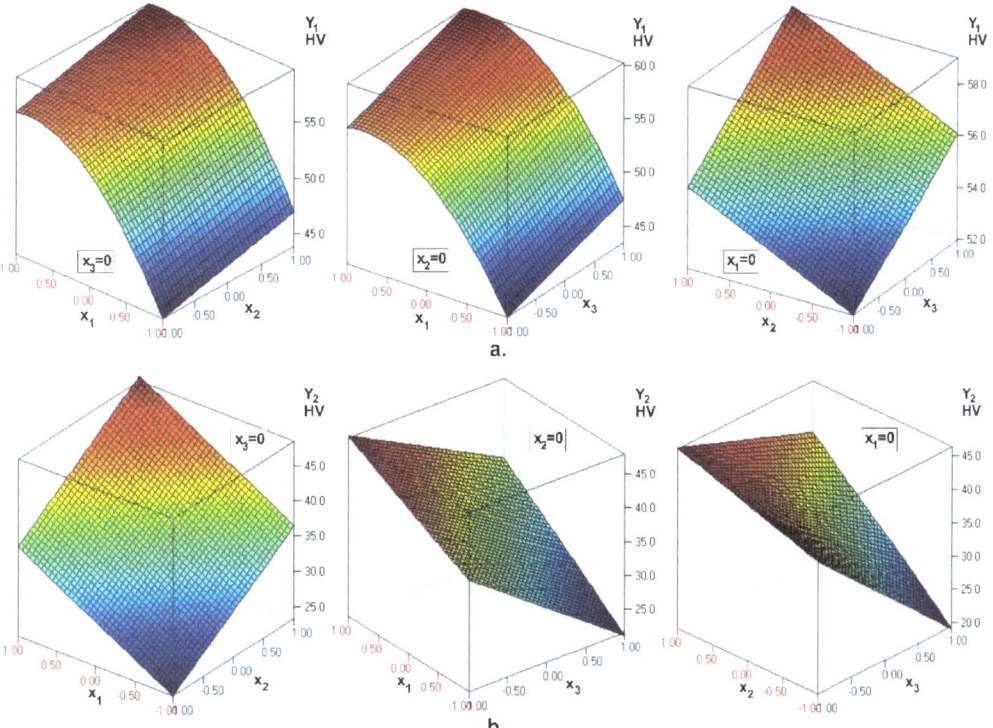

Figure 2. UC Evetric. Visualization of the regression models for: (**a**) Top surface microhardness and (**b**) bottom surface microhardness, Y_2 of the composite layer (x_1—light intensity, x_2—curing time, x_3—layer thickness). The dark blue color corresponds to the minimum micro-hardness values, and the deep red color corresponds to the maximum values.

3.2. BC Filtek One Bulk Fill Restorative

The graphs in Figure 3a show that the most significant factor influencing the hardness of the top surface Y_1 of BC Filtek One Bulk Fill Restorative is light intensity (x_1), followed by irradiation time (x_2) and layer thickness (x_3). The upper levels of the first two factors

(x_1 and x_2) and the medium level of the third factor (x_3) maximize Y_1, and the lower levels minimize the objective function. This means that the maximum hardness on the top surface is obtained when the light intensity and irradiation time have the highest values (1500 mW/cm^2 and 60 s) at a medium layer thickness of 3 mm, whereas working with the minimum values of the three factors (600 mW/cm^2, 20 s and 2 mm) ensures minimum hardness on the top surface.

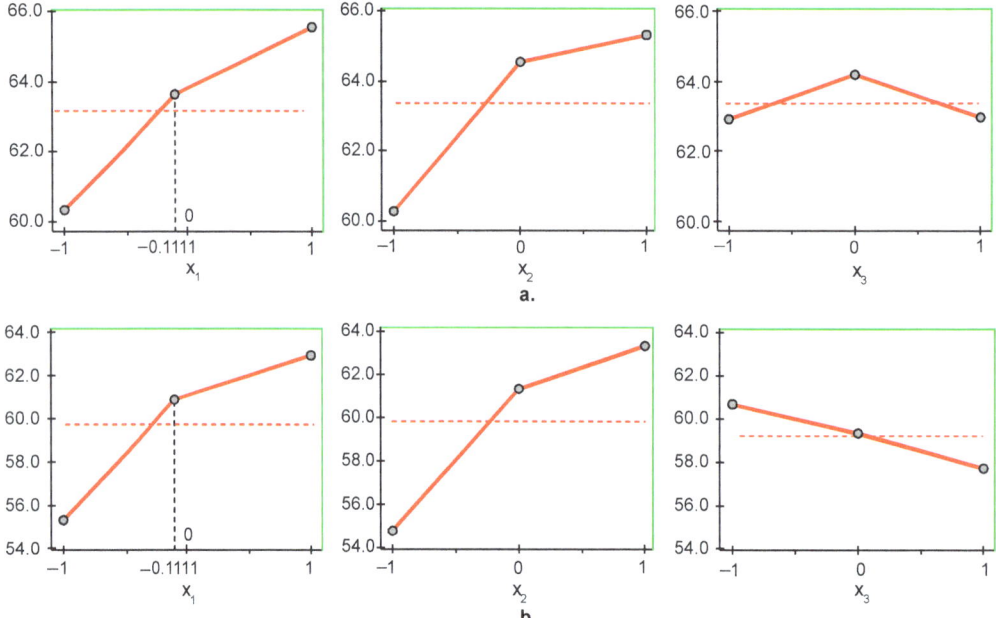

Figure 3. Influence of the different factors of photopolymerization on the microhardness on: (**a**) The top, and (**b**) bottom surfaces of BC Filtek One Bulk Fill Restorative (x_1—light intensity, x_2—curing time, x_3—layer thickness). Red dashed line: average value of micro-hardness; black dashed line: the actual coded value of x_1.

At the bottom surface hardness Y_2 (Figure 3b), however, the most significant factor is time (x_2), followed by intensity (x_1) and thickness (x_3). The maximum/minimum of Y_2 is achieved by maintaining the first two factors (x_1 and x_2) at the upper/lower level and the third factor (x_3) at the lower/upper level. Therefore, maximum/minimum hardness on the bottom surface is obtained at maximum/minimum values of intensity and time (1500 mW/cm^2 and 60 s/600 mW/cm^2 and 20 s) and at minimum/maximum layer thickness, respectively, 2 mm/4 mm.

Similar to UC Evetric, the coefficients (see Table 4) in front of the dimensionless coordinates confirm the conclusions of ANOVA. The visualization of the regression models for hardness on the top surface Y_1 of the composite layer and hardness on the bottom surface Y_2 is shown in Figure 4. The regression model Y_1 for surface hardness of BC Filtek One Bulk Fill Restorative confirms that the most significant factor is light intensity (x_1), followed by irradiation time (x_2) and layer thickness (x_3). For the bottom surface hardness Y_2, the most significant factor is time (x_2), followed by intensity (x_1) and thickness (x_3). Therefore, for BC Filtek One Bulk Fill Restorative, the intensity of the LCU has the greatest influence on the hardness of the top surface Y_1, and the irradiation time on the hardness of the bottom surface Y_2. Here, too, intensity and time have a positive effect: With their increase, the hardness on both surfaces increases. The layer thickness has a negative effect on the hardness of the bottom surface: Thicker composite layers have lower bottom surface hardness.

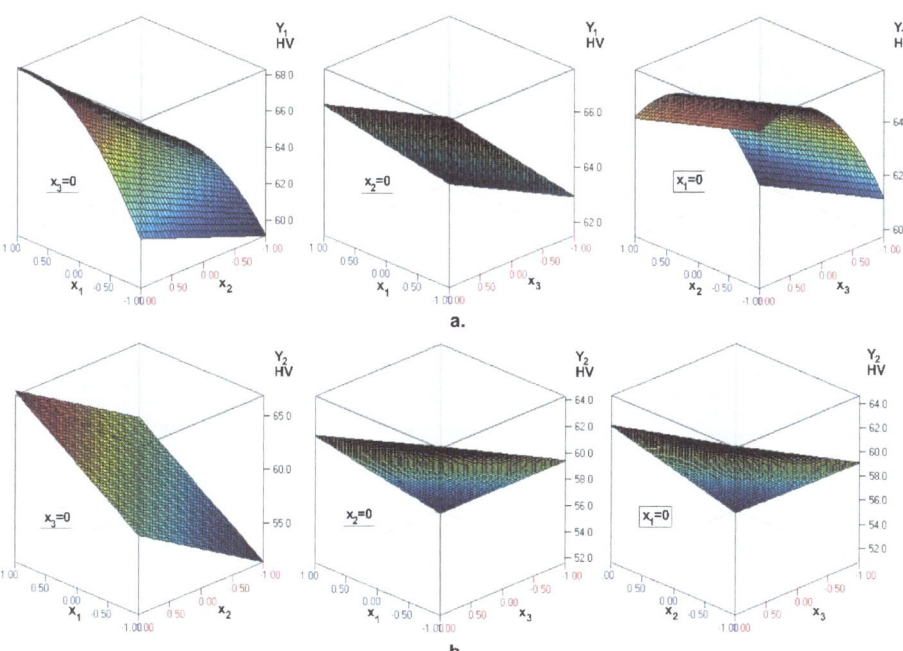

Figure 4. BC Filtek One Bulk Fill Restorative. Visualization of the regression models for: (**a**) Top surface microhardness Y_1 and (**b**) bottom surface microhardness Y_2, of the composite layer (x_1—light intensity, x_2—curing time, x_3—layer thickness). The dark blue color corresponds to the minimum micro-hardness values, and the deep red color corresponds to the maximum values.

3.3. FC G-aenial Universal Flo

The graphs in Figure 5a for FC G-aenial Universal Flo, similar to UC Evetric, show that the most significant factor for top surface hardness Y_1 is intensity (x_1), followed by layer thickness (x_3) and time (x_2). In contrast, different factors have different effects on the objective function. The upper levels of the first two factors (x_1 and x_2) and the middle level of the third factor (x_3) maximize Y_1. The lower level of the first factor (x_1), the middle level of the second factor (x_2) and the upper level of the third factor (x_3) minimize the objective function Y_1. Therefore, the maximum hardness on the top surface is obtained at maximum values of the intensity and irradiation time (1500 mW/cm^2 and 60 s) and at middle values of the layer thickness of 3 mm. The minimum hardness is obtained by working with a minimum intensity of 600 mW/cm^2, an irradiation time of 40 s, and a maximum layer thickness of 4 mm.

In Figure 5b it is shown that for the hardness on the bottom surface Y_2 the most important factor is layer thickness (x_3), followed by irradiation time (x_2) and light intensity (x_1). The difference in the significance is very small, and a regression model in dimensionless coordinates was used for a more accurate estimate. The maximum/minimum of Y_2 is achieved by maintaining the first two factors (x_1 and x_2) at the upper/lower level and the third factor (x_3) at the lower/upper level. Here, as with UC Evetric, maximum/minimum hardness on the bottom surface is obtained at maximum/minimum values of the first two parameters, intensity and time (1500 mW/cm^2 and 60 s/600 mW/cm^2 and 20 s), while the values of the third parameter, layer thickness, are minimum/maximum (2 mm/4 mm).

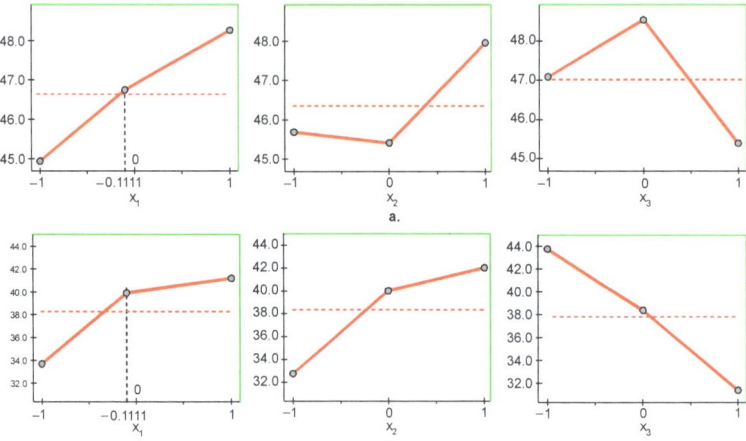

Figure 5. Influence of the different factors of photopolymerization on the microhardness on: (**a**) The top, and (**b**) bottom surfaces of FC G-aenial Universal Flo (x_1—light intensity, x_2—curing time, x_3—layer thickness). Red dashed line: average value of micro-hardness; black dashed line: the actual coded value of x_1.

Similar to the previous two composites, the coefficients (see Table 4) of the dimensionless coordinates confirm the conclusions of ANOVA. The visualization of the regression models for top surface hardness Y_1 of the composite layer and bottom surface hardness Y_2 is shown in Figure 6. The regression model for the objective function Y_1 (hardness on the top surface) confirms that the most significant factor is the intensity (x_1), followed by the thickness (x_3) and time (x_2).

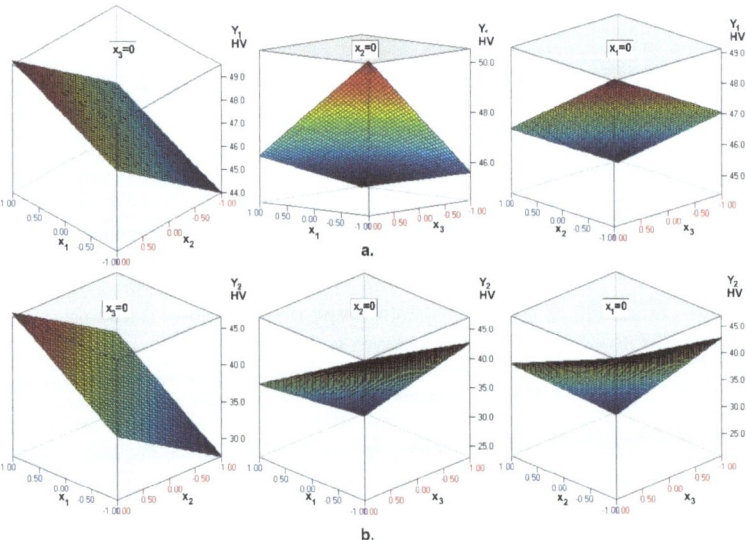

Figure 6. FC G-aenial Universal Flo. Visualization of the regression models for: (**a**) Top surface microhardness Y_1 and (**b**) bottom surface microhardness Y_2, of the composite layer (x_1—light intensity, x_2—curing time, x_3—layer thickness). The dark blue color corresponds to the minimum microhardness values, and the deep red color corresponds to the maximum values.

The regression model for the objective function Y_2 (hardness on the bottom surface) shows that the most important factor is layer thickness (x_3), followed by irradiation time (x_2) and light intensity (x_1). Therefore, similar to UC Evetric, in FC G-aenial Universal Flo the intensity of the LCU has the greatest influence on the hardness on the top surface Y_1, and the layer thickness has the strongest effect on the hardness on the bottom surface Y_2.

4. Discussion

Many factors influence the photopolymerization process of resin-based composites. They can be divided into two main groups: (1) External factors relating to the light-curing parameters and (2) internal ones, including the RBC compositions. The light-curing unit used, light intensity and spectrum, light tip position and distance from the composite surface, curing depth, and irradiation time belong to the first group. The co-monomer composition and ratio, photoinitiator type, type of fillers, and volume fraction, as well as their shapes and sizes, are part of the second group [32–36]. Among them, the composition of the RBC: Its monomer system, filler amount, and the filler-matrix interface, are the most important factors influencing the mechanical properties and microhardness [28,32,34,35,37]. The strength characteristics and hardness increase mainly with an increase in the filler quantity [4,38,39]. The composition of the fillers, their shapes, and sizes have an indirect influence, raising the filler volume fraction by varying shape, size, and distribution of the fille particles [34].

In our study, the highest microhardness on both surfaces is established for the BC Filtek One Bulk Fill Restorative, followed by the flowable composite G-aenial Universal Flo and the universal nano-hybrid Evetric. Their filler content is as follows: 76.5%, 69% and 80–81% (Table 1). According to the previous comments, the hybrid composite with the highest filler content should possess the highest microhardness, i.e., UC Evetric. However, in our study, this composite is characterized by having the lowest microhardness due to particles with lower hardness in its composition: Prepolymers and mixed oxides. The fillers of the BC Filtek One Bulk Fill Restorative and FC G-aenial Universal Flo consist mainly of particles with high hardness (ceramic, silica, zirconia, and strontium glass) that define their higher microhardness.

The depth to which the composite hardens in the light-curing process is referred to as the depth of cure [33]. If the bottom-to-top hardness ratio is equal to 0.80 or higher, the depth of cure is considered adequate [35,39]. The depth of cure depends on the fillers' composition, shade, and translucency as well as the light intensity and distance from the curing tip [33]. On the other hand, the depth of cure is defined by the degree of conversion of the composite matrix. Hence, the microhardness can also be considered as an indicator of the degree of conversion [37].

The degree of conversion depends mainly on the light penetration in the composite material, which is influenced by the filler organic matrix system [36]. The translucency of resin-based composites can be increased by reduction of the filler amount, usage of filler with larger sizes, and investigation of the refractive index of the fillers-organic matrix system [39]. The use of fillers with larger sizes decreases the total filler-matrix interface, thus reducing the scattered light and enhancing the transmission of the curing light [35,36].

Light transmission is characterized by the light attenuation coefficient and refractive index. The light attenuation through the composite thickness is a result of the complex process of scattering and absorption of light by the composite's components: Monomers, pigments, and fillers [40]. In RBCs, the light intensity scattering depends on the fillers' volume fraction, filler size, and refractive index of the monomers and fillers. There is a positive linear correlation between the attenuation coefficient and the filler volume: decreasing the volume fraction leads to low light attenuation. The refractive index is a measure of the speed of light in the material [40]. As RBCs are mixtures of different monomers and fillers, characterized by their own refractive indexes, it is highly difficult to define the resultant refractive index of the composite. It is found that the refractive index on the top surface is high due to the higher condensation due to high light intensity, while that on the bottom surface is lower with 0.17–0.55% for different composites due to the lower condensation with decreased light intensity [40]. The bulk-fill composites are characterized by a low attenuation coefficient compared to conventional RBCs, defining high light transmission through the material. Changes in refractive index and microhardness on the bottom surface of bulk-fill composites are low because of the low light attenuation.

In the nanofilled composites, the sizes of the particles vary between 0.005 and 0.01 μm [33,41]. The particles in this nano-range cannot react with visible light, and there is no scattering. As a result, significant absorption of the light occurs through the thickness of the composite, leading to a higher depth of cure and modulus of elasticity.

The viscosity of the monomers and the flexibility of their structure are other factors influencing the degree of conversion [42]. The established hybrid degree of conversion of the various monomers used in resin-based composites is in the following order: Bis-GMA < Bis-EMA < UDMA < TEGDMA [43]. Due to the lower viscosity of UDMA compared to Bis-GMA, the bulk-fill composites containing UDMA and TEGMA are characterized by having the highest degree of conversion [44].

With the use of dispersion and regression analyses, the present study establishes the influence of light intensity, irradiation time, and layer thickness on the hardness of three types of dental composites. These methods, on the one hand, show the influence of each factor on the hardness. On the other hand, they make it possible to determine the significance of the different factors.

Our study has shown that the main factor influencing the microhardness on the top surface of the three composites is the light intensity (Table 5). As the composites with the same A2 shade are used, and the distance between the top surface and the LCU tip is the same, the significance of this factor is defined by the high intensity of the curing light [40]. The second factor affecting the top surface microhardness is the layer thickness for the UC Evetric and FC G-aenial Universal Flo, while for the BC Filtek One Bulk Fill Restorative it is curing time. The third factor is the curing time for the first two composites and layer thickness for the bulk-fill.

Table 5. Factors influencing the photopolymerization process of resin-based dental composites.

Composite	Factors		
	Priority	Top Surface	Bottom Surface
UC Evetric	1 high 2 medium 3 low	x_1—light intensity x_3—layer thickness x_2—curing time	x_3—layer thickness x_2—curing time x_1—light intensity
BC Filtek One Bulk Fill Restorative	1 high 2 medium 3 low	x_1—light intensity x_2—curing time x_3—layer thickness	x_2—curing time x_1—light intensity x_3—layer thickness
FC G-aenial Universal Flo	1 high 2 medium 3 low	x_1—light intensity x_3—layer thickness x_2—curing time	x_3—layer thickness x_2—curing time x_1—light intensity

The significance of the factors' influence on the microhardness of the bottom surface is the same for the UC Evetric and FC G-aenial Universal Flo, but different for the BC Filtek One Bulk Fill Restorative. The main factor for the first two composites is layer thickness, followed by curing time and light intensity (Table 5). For the BC Filtek One Bulk Fill Restorative, the main factor is the curing time. The second is light intensity, and layer thickness is last.

The difference in the significance of the factors influencing the microhardness on the top and bottom surfaces of the investigated composites is defined mainly by their composition: The monomers of the resin matrix, filler type, amount, and sizes.

The UC Evetric is a typical representative of nano-hybrid universal composites with a high filler content of 80–81% and filler sizes ranging from 40 nm to 3 μm (Table 1). Its organic matrix consists mainly of UDMA, but also of 3–10% Bis-GMA and 3–10% Bis-

EMA. The last two monomers are characterized by a lower degree of conversion [43]. The highest volume fraction of the filler and the particle sizes, larger than the wavelength of the visible light, will cause scattering of the curing light and high attenuation coefficient. These circumstances will make it difficult to harden a thick layer of UC Evetric as the lower degree of conversion of Bis-GMA and Bis-EMA will have additional negative effects. That is the reason the layer thickness has a decisive role in the microhardness on the bottom surface of this composite (Table 3) and is the second-most significant factor affecting the microhardness on the top surface.

The organic matrix of the BC Filtek One Bulk Fill Restorative consists mainly of UDMA and AUDMA (Table 1), characterized by having the highest degrees of conversion [44]. The nanometer size of the fillers (from 4–20 nm of the particles up to 100 nm of the agglomerates) defines a low attenuation coefficient and high light transmission [33,40], resulting in a minimal difference between the microhardness of the top and bottom surfaces. Due to the high penetration of light through the material, the layer thickness has the lowest impact on the microhardness on the top and bottom surfaces of the bulk-fill composite (Table 3), and the curing time is the decisive factor for the microhardness on the bottom surface.

The presence of the low viscosity monomers UDMA, TEGDMA, and 5–10% Bis-EMA in the composition, the lower volume fraction of filler of 69%, and filler particles with sizes between 16 and 200 nm (Table 1) define the low viscosity of the flowable composite G-aenial Universal Flo. According to the producer [30], new glass particles are adopted as filler: Ultra-fine strontium glass that possesses superior translucency and low refractive index. The filler particles are treated by a new silane surface treatment and are homogeneously distributed in the organic matrix, thus providing the high strength of the composite. Similar to UC Evetric, the FC G-aenial Universal Flo has monomer Bis-EMA with a lower degree of conversion in its organic matrix. The filler particle sizes are larger than those of the BC Filtek One Bulk Fill Restorative, but smaller than the UC Evetric. Therefore, the characteristics of light penetration in this composite would occupy an intermediate place between those of the two other investigated materials. Taking into account the presence of a monomer with a lower degree of conversion and particles with larger sizes, higher scattering of light could be expected compared to the bulk-fill composite. This means the layer thickness is the most significant factor influencing the microhardness on the bottom surface of the FC G-aenial Universal Flo.

In the present study, three types of dental composites are polymerized by 14 different modes varying with three parameters (light intensity, curing time, and layer thickness). They are chosen on principle of investigating one typical representative of each group (conventional, bulk-fill, and flowable). Taking into account that there is a great variety of dental composites and light curing units on the market nowadays, the limitations of this study are that only three composites are used that are polymerized with one light curing unit.

5. Conclusions

The influence of light intensity, irradiation time, and layer thickness on the microhardness of three types of dental composites (conventional, bulk-fill, and flowable) has been established in the present work. The impact and significance of the factors are evaluated by dispersion and regression analyses.

It is found that the main factor influencing the microhardness on the top surface of the three composites is the light intensity. The second factor affecting the top surface microhardness is the layer thickness for the conventional and flowable composites, while for the bulk-fill, it is curing time. The third factor is the curing time for the first two composites and layer thickness for the bulk-fill.

Our study has shown that the significance of the factors influencing the microhardness on the bottom surface are the same for the conventional and flowable composites but different for the bulk-fill. The main factor for the first two composites is the layer thickness, followed by curing time and light intensity. For the bulk-fill, curing time is the main factor, light intensity is the second, and layer thickness is the last.

The different significance of the factors influencing the microhardness on the top and bottom surfaces of the investigated composites is defined mainly by their composition: The monomers of the resin matrix, filler type, amount, and sizes.

Author Contributions: Conceptualization, T.D. and J.M.; methodology, J.M., T.D. and G.D.; software, J.M.; experiment, G.G. and T.D.; data analysis, T.D. and J.M.; writing—original draft preparation, T.D. and G.G.; writing—review and editing, J.M.; visualization, J.M. and G.D.; supervision, J.M.; project administration, G.D.; funding acquisition, G.D. and J.M. All authors have read and agreed to the published version of the manuscript.

Funding: This research and APC were funded by the European Regional Development Fund within the OP "Science and Education for Smart Growth 2014–2020", Project CoC "Smart Mechatronics, Eco- and Energy Saving Systems and Technologies", No.BG05M2OP001-1.002-0023.

Institutional Review Board Statement: Not applicable.

Informed Consent Statement: Not applicable.

Conflicts of Interest: The authors declare no conflict of interest.

Nomenclature

b_{jk}	Polynomial coefficients
x_i	Variable in coded form
$\tilde{x}_i$	Variable in natural form
$\overline{Y}_i$	Measured microhardness: $i = 1$—top; $i = 2$—bottom
Y_i	Objective function

Abbreviations

ANOVA	Analysis of variance
BC	Bulk composite
FC	Flowable composite
LCU	Light curing unit
RBCs	Resin based composites
UC	Universal composite

References

1. Milosevic, M. Polymerization mechanics of dental composites–advantages and disadvantages. *Procedia Eng.* **2016**, *149*, 313–320. [CrossRef]
2. Aminoroaya, A.; Neisiany, R.E.; Khorasani, S.N.; Panahi, P.; Das, O.; Madry, H.; Cucchiarini, M.; Ramakrishna, S. A review of dental composites: Challenges, chemistry aspects, filler influences, and future insights. *Compos. Part B Eng.* **2021**, *216*, 108852. [CrossRef]
3. Sensi, L.G.; Strassler, H.E.; Webley, W. Direct composite resins. *Inside Dent.* **2007**, *3*, 76.
4. Anusavice, K.J.; Shen, C.; Rawls, H.R. *Phillips' Science of Dental Materials*; Elsevier Health Sciences: Amsterdam, The Netherlands, 2012; pp. 291–293.
5. Van Noort, R.; Barbour, R. *Introduction to Dental Materials-E-Book*; Elsevier Health Sciences: Amsterdam, The Netherlands, 2014; pp. 96–123.
6. Cho, K.; Sul, J.H.; Stenzel, M.H.; Farrar, P.; Prusty, B.G. Experimental cum computational investigation on interfacial and mechanical behavior of short glass fiber reinforced dental composites. *Compos. Part B Eng.* **2020**, *200*, 108294. [CrossRef]
7. Taheri, M.M.; Kadir, M.R.A.; Shokuhfar, T.; Hamlekhan, A.; Shirdar, M.R.; Naghizadeh, F. Fluoridated hydroxyapatite nanorods as novel fillers for improving mechanical properties of dental composite: Synthesis and application. *Mater. Des.* **2015**, *82*, 119–125. [CrossRef]
8. Mirică, I.C.; Furtos, G.; Bâldea, B.; Lucaciu, O.; Ilea, A.; Moldovan, M.; Câmpian, R.S. Influence of filler loading on the mechanical properties of flowable resin composites. *Materials* **2020**, *13*, 1477. [CrossRef]
9. Baroudi, K.; Rodrigues, J.C. Flowable resin composites: A systematic review and clinical considerations. *J. Clin. Diagn. Res. JCDR* **2015**, *9*, ZE18. [CrossRef]

10. Shaalan, O.O.; Abou-Auf, E.; El Zoghby, A.F. Clinical evaluation of flowable resin composite versus conventional resin composite in carious and noncarious lesions: Systematic review and meta-analysis. *J. Conserv. Dent. JCD* **2017**, *20*, 380. [CrossRef]
11. Van Ende, A.; De Munck, J.; Lise, D.P.; Van Meerbeek, B. Bulk-fill composites: A review of the current literature. *J. Adhes. Dent.* **2017**, *19*, 95–109.
12. Rosatto, C.M.P.; Bicalho, A.A.; Veríssimo, C.; Bragança, G.F.; Rodrigues, M.P.; Tantbirojn, D.; Soares, C.J. Mechanical properties, shrinkage stress, cuspal strain and fracture resistance of molars restored with bulk-fill composites and incremental filling technique. *J. Dent.* **2015**, *43*, 1519–1528. [CrossRef]
13. Van Ende, A.; De Munck, J.; Van Landuyt, K.L.; Poitevin, A.; Peumans, M.; Van Meerbeek, B. Bulk-filling of high C-factor posterior cavities: Effect on adhesion to cavity-bottom dentin. *Dent. Mater.* **2013**, *29*, 269–277. [CrossRef]
14. Van Ende, A.; Lise, D.P.; De Munck, J.; Vanhulst, J.; Wevers, M.; Van Meerbeek, B. Strain development in bulk-filled cavities of different depths characterized using a non-destructive acoustic emission approach. *Dent. Mater.* **2017**, *33*, e165–e177. [CrossRef]
15. Fronza, B.M.; Rueggeberg, F.A.; Braga, R.R.; Mogilevych, B.; Soares, L.E.S.; Martin, A.A.; Giannini, M. Monomer conversion, microhardness, internal marginal adaptation, and shrinkage stress of bulk-fill resin composites. *Dent. Mater.* **2015**, *31*, 1542–1551. [CrossRef]
16. Borges, A.F.S.; Chase, M.A.; Guggiari, A.L.; Gonzalez, M.J.; de Souza Ribeiro, A.R.; Pascon, F.M.; Zanatta, A.R. A critical review on the conversion degree of resin monomers by direct analyses. *Braz. Dent. Sci.* **2013**, *16*, 18–26. [CrossRef]
17. Rueggeberg, F.A.; Caughman, W.F.; Curtis, J.W., Jr.; Davis, H.C. Factors affecting cure at depths within light-activated resin composites. *Am. J. Dent.* **1993**, *6*, 91–95.
18. Ceballos, L.; Fuentes, M.; Tafalla Pastor, H.; Martínez, Á.; Flores, J.; Rodríguez, J. Curing effectiveness of resin composites at different exposure times using LED and halogen units. *Med. Oral Patol. Oral Cir. Bucal* **2009**, *1*, e8–e13.
19. Zorzin, J.; Maier, E.; Harre, S.; Fey, T.; Belli, R.; Lohbauer, U.; Petschelt, A.; Taschner, M. Bulk-fill resin composites: Polymerization properties and extended light curing. *Dent. Mater.* **2015**, *31*, 293–301. [CrossRef]
20. Selig, D.; Haenel, T.; Hausnerová, B.; Moeginger, B.; Labrie, D.; Sullivan, B.; Price, R.B. Examining exposure reciprocity in a resin based composite using high irradiance levels and real-time degree of conversion values. *Dent. Mater.* **2015**, *31*, 583–593. [CrossRef]
21. Park, J.; Chang, J.; Ferracane, J.; Lee, I.B. How should composite be layered to reduce shrinkage stress: Incremental or bulk filling? *Dent. Mater.* **2008**, *24*, 1501–1505. [CrossRef]
22. Flury, S.; Peutzfeldt, A.; Lussi, A. Influence of increment thickness on microhardness and dentin bond strength of bulk fill resin composites. *Dent. Mater.* **2014**, *30*, 1104–1112. [CrossRef]
23. Santini, A.; Miletic, V.; Swift, M.D.; Bradley, M. Degree of conversion and microhardness of TPO-containing resin-based composites cured by polywave and monowave LED units. *J. Dent.* **2012**, *40*, 577–584. [CrossRef]
24. Bouschlicher, M.R.; Rueggeberg, F.A.; Wilson, B.M. Correlation of bottom-to-top surface microhardness and conversion ratios for a variety of resin composite compositions. *Oper. Dent.* **2004**, *29*, 698–704.
25. Price, R.B.; Felix, C.A.; Andreou, P. Evaluation of a second-generation LED curing light. *J. Can. Dent. Assoc.* **2003**, *69*, 666.
26. Dikova, T.; Maximov, J.; Todorov, V.; Georgiev, G.; Panov, V. Optimization of photopolymerization process of dental composites. *Processes* **2021**, *9*, 779. [CrossRef]
27. Georgiev, G.; Dikova, T. Hardness investigation of conventional, bulk fill and flowable dental composites. *J. Achiev. Mater. Manuf. Eng.* **2021**, *109*, 68–77. [CrossRef]
28. Objelean, A.C.; Silaghi-Dimitrescu, L.; Furtos, G.; Badea, M.A.; Moldovan, M. The influence of organic-inorganic phase mixures on degradation behavior of some resin composites used in conservative dentistry. *J. Optoelectron. Adv. Mater.* **2016**, *18*, 567–575.
29. 3M Filtek One Bulk Fill Restorative, Technical Product Profile. 3m.com: St. Paul, MN, USA. Available online: https://multimedia.3m.com/mws/media/1317671O/3m-filtek-one-bulk-fill-restorative-technical-product-profile.pdf (accessed on 24 February 2022).
30. G-Aenial Universal Flo, Technical Manual. GC: Leuven, Belgium. Available online: www.gceurope.com; https://cdn.gceurope.com/v1/PID/gaenialuniversalflo/manual/MAN_Gaenial_Universal_Flo_Technical_Manual_en.pdf (accessed on 24 February 2022).
31. *Safety Data Sheet, G-Aenial Universal Flo. SDS_G-aenial Universal Flo.pdf*; GC America: Alsip, IL, USA, 2015.
32. Siagian, J.S.; Ikhsan, T.; Abidin, T. Effect of different LED light-curing units on degree of conversion and microhardness of bulk-fill composite resin. *J. Contemp. Dent. Pract.* **2020**, *21*, 615–620.
33. El-Nawawy, M.; Koraitim, L.; Abouelatta, O.; Hegazi, H. Depth of cure and microhardness of nanofilled, packable and hybrid dental composite resins. *Am. J. Biomed. Eng.* **2012**, *2*, 241–250. [CrossRef]
34. Masouras, K.; Silikas, N.; Watts, D.C. Correlation of filler content and elastic properties of resin-composites. *Dent. Mater.* **2008**, *24*, 932–939. [CrossRef]
35. Jang, J.H.; Park, S.H.; Hwang, I.N. Polymerization shrinkage and depth of cure of bulk-fill resin composites and highly filled flowable resin. *Oper. Dent.* **2015**, *40*, 172–180. [CrossRef]
36. AlShaafi, M.M. Factors affecting polymerization of resin-based composites: A literature review. *Saudi Dent. J.* **2017**, *29*, 48–58. [CrossRef]
37. Al Sunbul, H.; Silikas, N.; Watts, D.C. Surface and bulk properties of dental resin-composites after solvent storage. *Dent. Mater.* **2016**, *32*, 987–997. [CrossRef]
38. Dikova, T. *Dental Materials Science. Lectures and Laboratory Classes Notes Part II*; MU-Varna: Varna, Bulgaria, 2014; p. 150.

39. Rizzante, F.A.P.; Duque, J.A.; Duarte, M.A.H.; Mondelli, R.F.L.; Mendonca, G.; Ishikiriama, S.K. Polymerization shrinkage, microhardness and depth of cure of bulk fill resin composites. *Dent. Mater. J.* **2019**, *38*, 403–410. [CrossRef]
40. Son, S.; Park, J.K.; Seo, D.G.; Ko, C.C.; Kwon, Y.H. How light attenuation and filler content affect the microhardness and polymerization shrinkage and translucency of bulk-fill composites? *Clin. Oral Investig.* **2017**, *21*, 559–565. [CrossRef]
41. Dikova, T.; Milkov, M. Nanomaterials in dental medicine. In Proceedings of the 10th Workshops "Nanoscience & Nanotechnology", Sofia, Bulgaria, 27–28 November 2008; pp. 203–209.
42. Dickens, S.H.; Stansbury, J.W.; Choi, K.M.; Floyd, C.J.E. Photopolymerization kinetics of methacrylate dental resins. *Macromolecules* **2003**, *36*, 6043–6053. [CrossRef]
43. Sideridou, I.; Tserki, V.; Papanastasiou, G. Effect of chemical structure on degree of conversion in light-cured dimethacrylate-based dental resins. *Biomaterials* **2002**, *23*, 1819–1829. [CrossRef]
44. Papadogiannis, D.; Tolidis, K.; Gerasimou, P.; Lakes, R.; Papadogiannis, Y. Viscoelastic properties, creep behavior and degree of conversion of bulk fill composite resins. *Dent. Mater.* **2015**, *31*, 1533–1541. [CrossRef]

Article

An Evaluation of the Mechanical Properties of a Hybrid Composite Containing Hydroxyapatite

Leszek Klimek [1], Karolina Kopacz [2], Beata Śmielak [3,*] and Zofia Kula [4]

[1] Institute of Materials Science and Engineering, Faculty of Mechanical Engineering, Lodz University of Technology, ul. B. Stefanowskiego 1/15, 90-924 Lodz, Poland; leszek.klimek@p.lodz.pl
[2] "Dynamo Lab" Academic Laboratory of Movement and Human Physical Performance, Medical University of Lodz, ul. Pomorska 251, 92-213 Lodz, Poland; karolina.kopacz@umed.lodz.pl
[3] Department of Dental Prosthodontics, Medical University of Lodz, ul. Pomorska 251, 92-213 Lodz, Poland
[4] Department of Dental Technology, Medical University of Lodz, ul. Pomorska 251, 92-213 Lodz, Poland; zofia.kula@umed.lodz.pl
* Correspondence: beata.smielak@umed.lodz.pl; Tel.: +0048-603-691-851

Abstract: There is currently a lack of scientific reports on the use of composites based on UDMA resin containing HAp in conservative dentistry. The aim of this study was therefore to determine the effect of hydroxyapatite content on the properties of a hybrid composite used in conservative dentistry. This paper compares a commercial hybrid composite with experimental composites treated with 2% by weight (b/w), 5% b/w, and 8% b/w hydroxyapatite. The composites were subjected to bending strength, compression, and diametrical compression tests, as well as those for impact strength, hardness, and tribological wear. The obtained results were subjected to statistical analysis. Increased hydroxyapatite was found to weaken the mechanical properties; however, 2% b/w and 5% b/w hydroxyapatite powder was found to achieve acceptable results. The statistical analysis showed no significant differences. HAp is an effective treatment for composites when applied at a low concentration. Further research is needed to identify an appropriate size of HAp particles that can be introduced into a composite to adequately activate the surface and modification its composition.

Keywords: composite mechanical properties; composite tribological properties; dental composites; hydroxyapatite

1. Introduction

In dental practice, the ideal material for the reconstruction of hard tooth tissues is still being sought. The most used are composite materials based on polymers [1]. These materials consist of a polymer matrix (UDMA, Bis-GMA TEGDMA), a binding agent (vinyl silane), compounds regulating the polymerization process (initiators, inhibitors), substances conditioning aesthetic effects (dyes, UV absorbers and others), and filler particles (silicon oxide, quartz, colloidal silica, boron glass, alumina-lithium) [2–5]. The filler is one of the basic components of composites which constitutes 35 to 70% of the mass of the material [6]. Fillers are added to improve mechanical properties such as bending strength, fracture toughness, and abrasion resistance [7,8]. Fillers can be divided into macro-fillers and micro-fillers based on the size of the filler particles in the polymer matrix. There are also hybrid composites which contain different sizes of filler particles; these are characterized by favorable mechanical properties [9]. Indeed, the best properties are characterized by hybrid materials with filler particles below 0.1 μm (microhybrid and nanohybrid) [7–9]. Hydroxyapatite (HAp) has certain biological properties that make it a suitable filler. HAp, i.e., $Ca_3(PO_4)_2$, is part of the hard tissues of teeth and bones [10,11]. It is characterized by high biocompatibility and bioactivity [12–15]. It does not cause inflammation; it is not an irritant nor does it demonstrate toxic or carcinogenic effects [16–18]. Hydroxyapatite is used to fill bone defects, coat implants, and as an active agent against tooth hypersensitivity in toothpastes [10–12,19]. The addition of hydroxyapatite as a filler affects the mechanical properties of the dental filling [19–21]. Depending on the amount and form of the introduced filler, it may improve or deteriorate the mechanical properties. Santos et al. [19] showed an improvement in strength properties after adding 3% hydroxyapatite in the form of nanofibers to a TEGDMA/Bis-GMA polymer matrix. Domingo et al. [20] found a 30% improvement in mechanical properties after adding HAp in the form of powder. In turn, Elkassas and Arafa [21] and Priyadarsini et al. [22] confirmed that the addition of HAp on the nanometric scale improved to better understand the properties of composite materials containing hydroxyapatite fillers, and studies have examined the effect of hydroxyapatite treatment on selected mechanical properties [23–25]. One such property is hardness, which is easy to measure and comparable with other findings. It determines the ability of the material to resist deformation. However, to fully characterize the material, it is necessary to analyze the loads it will be subjected to and perform appropriate strength tests. During the chewing process, the teeth are exposed to various types of mechanical loads (bending, compression). Sometimes, the loads may have a shock character. The basic strength test is the static tensile test, which provides an insight into a number of important parameters characterizing both strength and plastic properties, as well as material constants. It is often used in studies on the mechanisms of deformation and fracture of materials. It is not generally used for materials used for dental fillings because it requires relatively large samples, and hence has a higher cost, and also entails various technical problems. Therefore, it is typically replaced by a diametrical compression test.

While existing studies on doping with hydroxyapatite have been based on composites based on TEGDMA, Bis-GMA, HEMA resins, and resin-modified glass ionomer cements [23–29], the present paper examines the hydroxyapatite modification of a UDMA resin dental composite, which is used in restorative dentistry. This type of composite enables direct reconstruction of all cavities according to Black's classification. Furthermore, the present work uses micro-scale hydroxyapatite, while previous studies have examined nano-sized hydroxyapatite [28–30], using hydroxyapatite in powder form. In addition to the typical mechanical loads, teeth are subject to wear processes, e.g., abrasion, when chewing and grinding food. Wear resistance determines the service life of the dental filling.

The aim of this paper is to study compare the hardness, static strength properties (compression and bending), dynamic properties (impact strength and fracture toughness), and wear resistance of three experimental composites with different HAp contents with those of a commercial filler. The null hypothesis assumes that the use of hydroxyapatite as a filler in dental composites affects its mechanical properties.

2. Materials and Methods

Samples were prepared for testing as rectangular ($n = 120$) and cylindrical ($n = 120$) beams of appropriate sizes in accordance with ISO standards [20–22,31]. The samples consisted of a commercial composite material based on urethane dimethacrylate (UDMA) (Gradia Direct, GC Tokyo, Japan) ($n = 60$) as a reference, and three test substances with self-sintered hydroxyapatite (HAp): 2% b/w HAp (administered as 30 μm grain size) ($n = 60$), 5% b/w ($n = 60$) and 8% b/w ($n = 60$). Experimental material was prepared in accordance with ISO standards [31–35]. Table 1 shows the content and size of the filler in individual samples.

Table 1. Filler content and size in individual samples.

Sample Symbol	Composite Type	Resin Type	Filler Content HAp [%] wag.	Filler Size HAp [μm]
HAp 0	light-curing	UDMA	0	-
HAp 2	light-curing	UDMA	2	30
HAp 5	light-curing	UDMA	5	30
HAp 8	light-curing	UDMA	8	30

Hydroxyapatite was synthesized by the wet method. The dried HAp grains obtained were fractionated using an LPzE-3e laboratory shaker (MULTISERW-Morek, Brzeźnica, Poland) and passed through a set of three sieves: 0.1 mm, 0.05 mm, and 0.025 mm. The filler was then introduced into the composite material using a Roti-Speed stirrer (Carl Roth GmbH + Co., KG, Karlsruhe, Germany). This stirrer is used to mix very small samples in micro tubes at 5000 rpm. for about 5 min. The process of mixing was carried out in a darkened room under standardized conditions of temperature and humidity. The resulting material was stored in polypropylene syringes with a plunger. The samples were prepared for the strength by placing the composite in a silicone mold between basic laboratory slides to protect the surface against oxygen inhibition. Then, each layer of material, with a thickness of 1 mm, was irradiated for 20 s using a diode polymerization lamp (Elipar S10, 3M ESPE, St. Paul, MS, USA) with a real power of 1400 mW/cm^2, emitting light radiation in the range of 450–490 nm. Before the mechanical tests, the samples were artificially aged by incubation at 37 °C in distilled water for 24 h. Then, tests of bending strength, compression, diametrical compression, impact tests, hardness measurements, and tribological wear resistance tests were carried out (Table 2).

Table 2. Test methods, devices, and the shape and size of the samples used in the tests.

Research Method	Devices	Dimensions and Shape of Samples
Bending Strength Test	UMT TriboLab Bruker multifunctional device (Bruker, Karlsruhe, Germany).	Rectangular beam with dimensions of 2 mm × 2 mm × 25 mm
Compression Strength Test	Walter + Bai testing machine (Walter + Bai AG, Lohningen, Switzerland).	A cylinder with a diameter of 4 mm and a height of 6 mm
Diametral Compression Strength Test (DTS)	Universal testing machine (Zwick/Roell, Ulm, Germany)	A disc with a diameter of 4 mm and a thickness of 2 mm
Impact Strength Test	HIT 5.5p Zwick/Roeler impact hammer (Zwick/Roell, Ulm, Germany)	A cuboid with dimensions of 5 mm × 10 mm × 20 mm
Hardness Measurements	Shore type D hardness tester (Elcometer Inc, Warren, MI, USA)	A cuboid with dimensions of 10 mm × 20 mm × 5 mm
Tribological Wear Resistance Test	CSM Instruments Tribometer device (CSM Instruments, Freiburg, Germany) with the Tribox program installed, the Hommel Waveline 200 profilometer (ITA, Skórzewo, Poland).	A disc with a diameter of 21 mm and a thickness of 2

2.1. Bending Strength Test

Ten rectangular beam-shaped samples (2 mm × 2 mm × 25 mm) from each series were prepared for the three-point bending strength test. The tests were performed with a UMT TriboLab Bruker multifunctional device (Bruker, Karlsruhe, Germany). The travel speed of the traverse was 0.5 mm/min while maintaining the support spacing of 20 mm. The radii of the supports and the mandrel implementing the excitation were 1 mm. Figure 1 shows a photo of a sample placed in the device during the test. For comparative purposes, the strength was calculated according to the following formula:

$$\delta = 3FL/2bh^2$$

where
　　δ—flexural strength [MPa];
　　F—destructive force [N];
　　L—spacing of supports [mm];
　　b—sample width [mm];
　　h—sample thickness [mm].

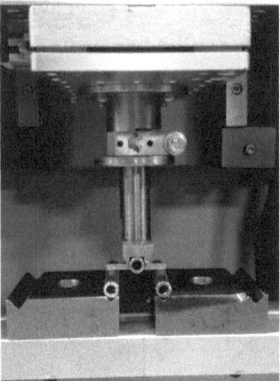

Figure 1. Photo showing the sample placed in the device during the bending test.

2.2. Compression Strength Test

For the compression strength test, 10 cylindrical samples were created from each material series with a diameter of 4 mm and a height of 6 mm. This test was carried out on a Walter + Bai testing machine (Walter + Bai AG, Lohningen, Switzerland). The compressive strength was calculated according to the formula:

$$\delta = F/\pi r^2$$

where
    δ—compressive strength [MPa];
    F—destructive force [N];
    r—sample radius [mm].

Figure 2 shows a photo of a sample placed in the device during the test.

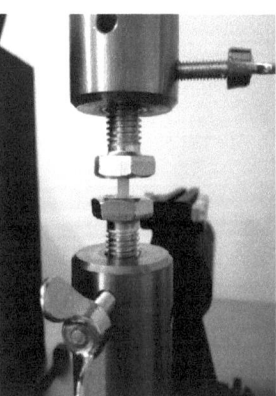

Figure 2. The sample placed in the device during the compression test.

2.3. Diametral Compression Strength Test (DTS)

For the diametrical compressive strength test, 10 cylindrical samples were created from each material series with a diameter of 4 mm and a height of 6 mm. The DTS test was performed on a Zwick/Roell Z020 universal testing machine (Zwick/Roell, Ulm, Germany) at a traverse speed of 1 mm/min. The strength value was calculated according to the following formula:

$$DTS = 2P/\pi DT$$

where
P—compressive force that caused the destruction of the material structure and surface [N];
D—sample diameter [mm];
T—sample thickness [mm].
Figure 3 shows a photo of a sample placed in the device during the test.

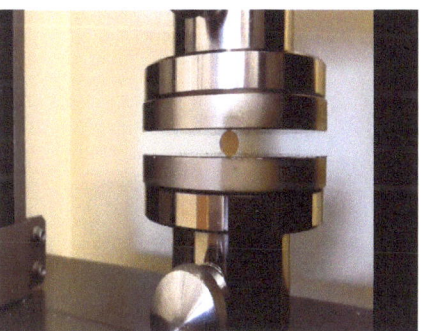

Figure 3. The sample placed in the device during the diametrical compressive strength.

2.4. Impact Strength Test

For impact strength measurements, 10 cuboid samples (5 mm × 10 mm × 20 mm) were made from each material series. The tests were performed using a HIT 5.5p Zwick/Roeler impact hammer (Zwick/Roell, Ulm, Germany) at a hammer energy of 5.5 J. The impact strength of the material was calculated according to the formula:

$$U = A/(b \cdot h)$$

where
U—the impact strength of the sample [J/m^2];
A—breaking work (hammer energy) [J];
b—sample width [cm];
h—sample thickness [cm].
Figure 4 shows a photo of a sample placed in the device during the test.

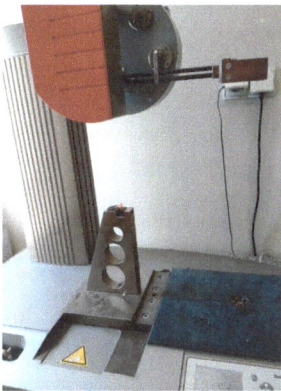

Figure 4. The sample placed in the device during the strength test.

2.5. Hardness Measurements

Hardness measurements were carried out on the surface of 10 cuboid samples (10 mm × 20 mm × 5 mm), with 5 measurements taken in randomly selected places. A

Shore type D hardness tester (Elcometer Inc., Warren, MI, USA) was used. Shor hardness indicates the resistance of the tested material penetrated by the needle. The value was read on the Shor durometer scale. Figure 5 shows a photo of a sample placed in the device during the test.

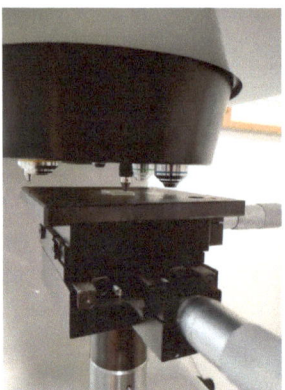

Figure 5. The sample placed in the device during hardness measurements.

2.6. Tribological Wear Resistance Test

The wear test was performed using a CSM Instruments Tribometer device (CSM Instruments, Freiburg, Germany) with the Tribox program installed, using the following parameters: friction radius 6.75 mm, speed 0.05 m/s, load 1 N, friction distance 100 m. The test was performed at a temperature of 25 °C in an artificial environment according to Fusayama Mayer (2 dm^3 of distilled water, 0.8 g NaCl, 0.8 g KCl, 1.59 g $CaCl_2 \bullet 2H_2O$, 1.56 g $NaH_2PO_4 \bullet 2H_2O$, 0.01 g $Na_2S \bullet 9H_2O$ and 2 g urea) [36]. The test was performed on disc-shaped samples with a diameter of 21 mm and a thickness of 2 mm, in a special Teflon holder. Artificial saliva was then added. The friction counter-sample was a 1/8-inch diameter zirconia ball. The wear of the materials was determined by measuring the linear wear in a friction trace based on the surface roughness measurement using the Hommel Waveline 200 profilometer (ITA, Skórzewo, Poland). The wear of the tested composites was calculated as the volume loss of the material, related to the friction path [37,38].

After the friction processes was completed, five abrasion marks were created on each sample and the mean cross-sectional area of the marks was calculated. The volume loss of the material was obtained by multiplying this value by the perimeter of the wear trace. The wear factor was calculated from the following formula:

$$k_v = V/(F \cdot L)$$

where:
  k—material consumption factor [m^3/(N·m)];
  V—volume of material used [m^3];
  F—pressing force [N];
  L—total friction path [m].
  Figure 6: A sample placed in the device during the test.

The obtained test results were subjected to statistical analysis using Excel (Microsoft Office 2010) and Statistica v. 13. The Shapiro–Wilk test of normality was used to evaluate the distribution of individual parameters. In the case of a non-normal distribution, the Kruskall–Wallis test was then used. In the case of a normal distribution, the equality of variances was assessed using Levene's test. For equal variances, ANOVA with the Scheffe Post Hoc test was used. The adopted significance level was $\alpha = 0.05$.

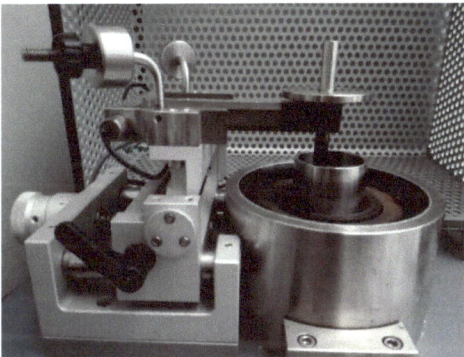

Figure 6. A sample placed in the device during the tribological test.

3. Results

3.1. Bending Strength Test

According to the ANOVA test, a statistically significant difference was demonstrated in the bending strength [MPa] ($p = 0.0000$). The results of the Scheffe post hoc test indicated statistically significant differences between 0% HAp and 2% HAp ($p = 0.0000$), 0% HAp and 5% HAp ($p = 0.0000$) and 0% Hap and 8% HAp ($p = 0.0000$) in all comparisons with larger values in the 0% wt. HAp samples. Moreover, statistically significant difference was demonstrated between 2% HAp and. 8% HAp ($p = 0.0000$) and 5% HAp and 8% HAp ($p = 0.0000$) with smaller values in 8% HAp (Figure 7).

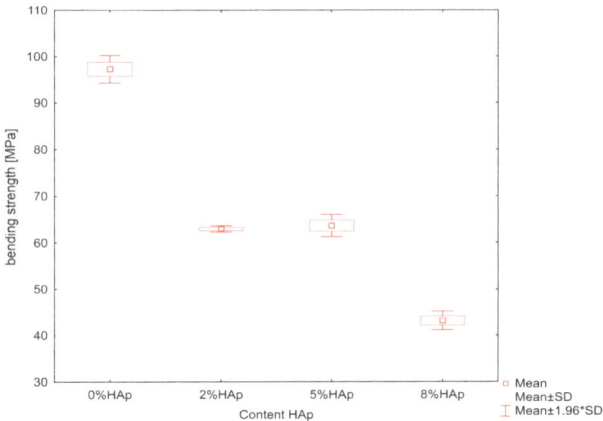

Figure 7. Statistically significant differences between the examined groups for bending strength.

In all cases, the addition of hydroxyapatite caused a decrease in flexural strength. Samples containing 2% and 5% hydroxyapatite filler yielded similar values.

3.2. Compression Strength Test

According to the ANOVA test, a statistically significant difference was demonstrated in the compression [MPa] ($p = 0.0000$). The results of the Scheffe post hoc test indicated statistically significant differences between 0% HAp and 5% HAp ($p = 0.0004$) and 0% HAp and 8% HAp with larger values in 0% HAp. Furthermore, a statistically significant difference was demonstrated between 2% HAp and 5% HAp ($p = 0.0062$) and 2% HAp and 8% HAp ($p = 0.0037$) with larger values in 2% HAp (Figure 8).

In all cases, the addition of hydroxyapatite caused a decrease in compressive strength. Samples containing 5% and 8% hydroxyapatite filler yielded similar strength values.

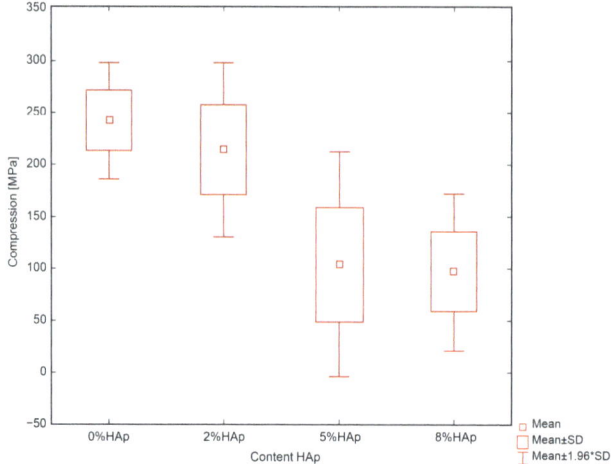

Figure 8. Statistically significant differences between the examined groups for compression.

3.3. Diametral Compression Strength Test (DTS)

According to the ANOVA test, a statistically significant difference was demonstrated in the DTS ($p = 0.0000$). The results of the Scheffe post hoc test indicated statistically significant differences between 0% HAp and 2% HAp ($p = 0.0000$), 0% HAp and 5% Hap ($p = 0.0000$), and 0% HAp and 8% HAp ($p = 0.0000$), with larger values in 0% HAp (Figure 9).

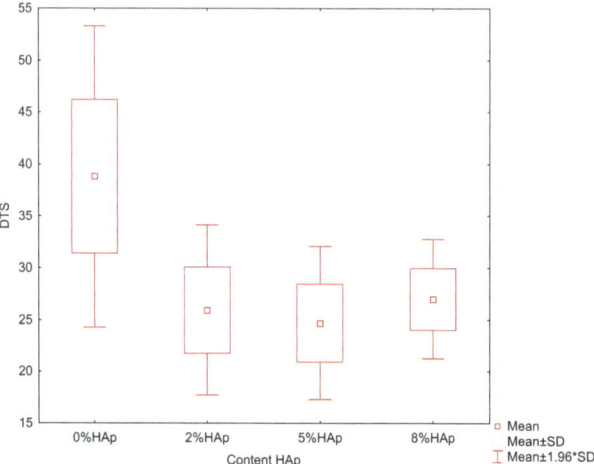

Figure 9. Statistically significant differences between the examined groups for DTS.

In all cases, the addition of hydroxyapatite caused a decrease in compressive strength. Samples containing 5% and 8% hydroxyapatite filler yielded similar strength values.

3.4. Impact Strength Tests

According to the ANOVA test, no statistically significant difference was found in the impact resistance [J/cm^2] ($p = 0.8304$) (Figure 10).

Impact tests indicate that the composites containing hydroxyapatite yield slightly lower values compared to the unmodified material.

3.5. Hardness Measurements

The Kruskal–Wallis test indicated significant differences in the hardness [ShoreŚ] ($p = 0.0021$). The post hoc test of multiple comparisons of mean ranks for all trials identified statistically significant differences between 0% HAp and 8% HAp ($p = 0.0005$), with larger values in 0% HAp (Figure 11).

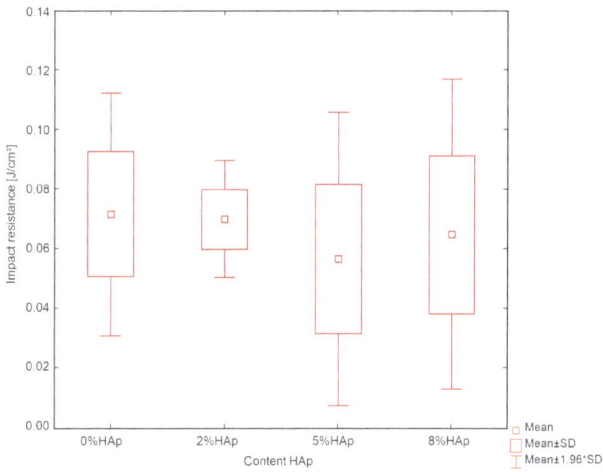

Figure 10. Insignificant differences between the examined groups for impact resistance.

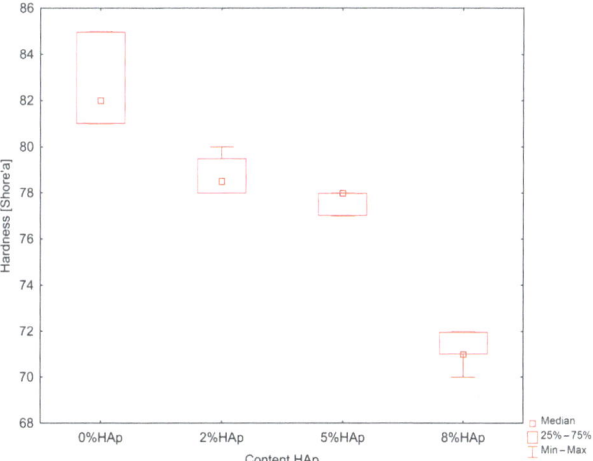

Figure 11. Statistically significant differences in examined groups in hardness.

Lower hardness was observed with increased hydroxyapatite content.

3.6. Impact Strength Tests Tribological Wear Resistance Test

The Kruskal–Wallis test revealed significant differences in the tribological wear ($p = 0.0074$). The post hoc test of multiple comparisons of mean ranks for all trials found significant differences between 5% HAp and 8% HAp ($p = 0.0467$), with larger values in 8% HAp (Figure 12).

Our findings suggest that the addition of 8% filler significantly reduces the wear resistance of the composite material. Composites that contain a larger amount of hydroxyapatite filler obtain a rougher and less even surface, which may reduce their wear rate.

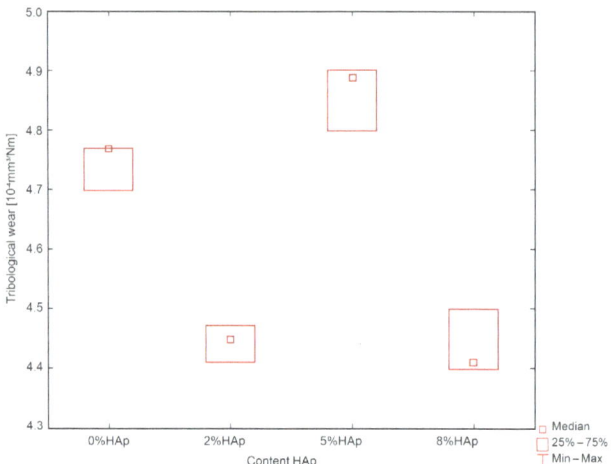

Figure 12. Significant differences between the examined groups for tribological wear.

4. Discussion

The study hypothesis was confirmed—the use of hydroxyapatite as a filler affects the mechanical properties of dental composites.

4.1. Bending Strength Test

In all cases, the addition of hydroxyapatite caused a significant decrease in flexural strength compared to the reference material. However, no significant differences were found between the materials treated with 2% or 5% HAp by weight. The 8% b/w group demonstrated more than double the strength of the untreated reference material; however, it did not achieve a flexural strength of 50 MPa, as specified by the ISO 4049 Dentistry-Polymer-based restorative materials 2009 standard [18] for fillings based on polymers rebuilding hard dental tissues. However, the 2% b/w and 5% b/w HAp had a flexural strength of 60 MPa, and hence are suitable for dental fillings.

4.2. Compression Strength

A key property of materials used for fillings is compression strength. Teeth are largely subject to compressive forces while chewing, with a mean force of about 100–150 N [39,40]. The addition of hydroxyapatite caused a decrease in compressive strength from about 230 MPa to about 100 MPa for the higher substitution values; however, no significant difference was observed for 2% b/w HAp. As there are no standards defining the minimum value of compressive strength of this type of material, all treated materials can be considered acceptable, particularly the samples with 2% b/w HAp. Hybrid composites are characterized by high resistance to compressive stresses [41,42]. This is probably due to the higher packing density of the fillers in the polymer matrix.

4.3. Diametral Compression Strength

Tensile strength is the basic mechanical test. However, in the case of brittle materials, it is difficult and sometimes even impossible to determine. Therefore, in order to determine the ability of brittle materials for dental fillings to resist tensile stresses that may occur during masticatory processes, a diametrical compression strength test is used [19]. This test can also be performed on small sample sizes, which is important in the case of expensive materials. However, it should be borne in mind that the obtained values are not identical with those obtained in the classic tensile test. In addition, the test provides useful information regarding the tensile strength of materials in FEM modeling of the behavior of teeth with fillings under load. Although there are no guidelines specifying the minimum strength of materials used in fillings for the reconstruction of hard tooth tissues, the minimum DTS value set by the American Dental Association is 24 MPa, as indicated by standard No. 27 "Resin-based fillings" [31]. In each case, the addition of hydroxyapatite reduced the diametrical compressive strength from about 38 MPa for the starting material to about 25–26 MPa for the remaining groups. Significant differences in strength were found between the initial and modified materials. Similar values were published by Okulus and Voelkel [43]. However, there were no differences between the modified groups. All obtained results appear to satisfy standard No. 27 (above).

4.4. Impact Strength

In the case of impact tests, no statistically significant differences were found between the groups. The obtained results approximated 0.07 J/cm^2, which is lower than those observed for flow composites [44].

4.5. Hardness

Hardness is an important value for materials as it determines their ability to resist deformation. Despite this, it is only an auxiliary parameter used to determine mechanical and operational values; it is difficult to clearly translate its value into other properties. Even so, due to its ease and speed of measurement, it is often used in research. In this case, an increase in HAp was associated with a decrease in the hardness of the tested samples, falling from 82 ShD for commercial samples to 72 ShD (8% b/w) or 78 ShD (2% b/w and 5% b/w). A significant difference was found between unmodified and 8% b/w HAp, but not for the other groups. Despite the observed slight decreases in hardness, the treated materials appear suitable for use in the reconstruction of hard dental tissues.

4.6. Wear Resistance Test

A very important property of dental filling materials is their wear resistance. It should be remembered that the chewing process is associated with friction processes and thus wear, which is especially intensified when grinding harder foods. Wear resistance largely determines the lifetime of the restoration, with high values leading to rapid wear of the filling [19,20]. The addition of hydroxyapatite to the tested composite reduces wear resistance. In addition, greater HAp content is associated with higher consumption. While the wear resistance values for 2% b/w and 5% b/w HAp were acceptable, it was significantly lower for 8% b/w.

Our findings do not fully agree with those of other authors. Akhtar et al. suggest that hydroxyapatite may be a promising filler material in dental filling materials [45]. Another study attempted to improve the mechanical properties of glass ionomers with the addition of HAp, with 10% b/w NHA being found to increase the abrasion resistance of Fuji II LC RMGI material [46]. However, excessive amounts of hydroxyaptite may lead to faster wear of the composite [21,22]. Indeed, the addition of hydroxyapatite to composites in an amount above 5% causes the surface to become rougher and heterogeneous, which may significantly reduce wear resistance [4,5]. Hongquan Zhang [47] and Bartoszewicz [48] indicate that the tribological and mechanical properties of a nanocomposite based on acrylic resin are strongly influenced by the morphology of the particles and their size. As such, it is probable that the differences in wear resistance observed between studies result from differences in the morphology of the hydroxyapatite used. It seems that the use of greater than 5% b/w HAp is pointless.

Our findings clearly show that hydroxyapatite affects the strength properties of the hybrid dental composite. It seems reasonable to introduce HAp at 2% b/w and 5% b/w. Despite the reduction in most strength parameters, the obtained values are within the requirements of the relevant standards. Increasing the amount of filler to 8% b/w disqualifies this material for use.

However, this should not be taken as a final conclusion. It is known that the properties of composite materials largely depend on the size of the filler particles and its surface properties, which allow for better bonding with the matrix. Filler grains of different sizes can mutually fill empty spaces, which can result in composite reinforcement [42]. Hydroxyapatite can be properly fractionated and added to the composite in such a diverse fraction, which should improve its properties. The addition of an additional filler, HAp, to a commercial dental composite resulted in a change in the ratio of the amount of filler to the amount of polymer matrix (matrix), and the overall increase in the total amount of fillers resulted in a relative decrease in the silanizing agent. This influences the quality of the connection of the filler with the matrix: an insufficient amount results in the deterioration of the connection of the polymer matrix and inorganic filler particles, as confirmed previously [49–51]. In addition to the amount of hydroxyapatite filler, its morphology can also influence the final result: its fragmentation and irregular surface significantly increases the surface area requiring silanization. Hence, in order to ensure proper silanization when adding HAp, it is necessary to consider its amount and morphology, as well as to increase the amount of pre-adhesive (silanizing) agents modifying the surface, as demonstrated previously [52]. Another solution that may improve the mechanical properties is to introduce additives that block the propagation of composite matrix cracking (e.g., graphene), which should also improve the properties of dental composites [53].

When trying to improve resistance to tribological wear, it must be considered that adding more than 5% HAp to composites causes the surface to become rougher and inhomogeneous, which may significantly reduce wear resistance [54,55].

The development of a dental filling containing hydroxyapatite is also clinically relevant. The current literature indicates that such materials have antibacterial properties [23,24] and such compounds inhibit the formation of secondary caries located under the dental filling, caused by bacterial microleakage.

5. Conclusions

Conclusions were reached as follows:

1. The content of hydroxyapatite (30 μm particle size) has a significant impact on the mechanical properties of a dental composite.
2. The mechanical properties of the composite decreased as the amount of hydroxyapatite filler increased.
3. Of the tested combinations, the best tribological properties were obtained by the composite containing 2% wt. hydroxyapatite.
4. Research shows unequivocally that the addition of hydroxyapatite in the amount of up to 5% by weight is legitimate.
5. HAp is an effective treatment for composites when applied at a low concentration. Further research is needed to identify an appropriate size of HAp particles that can be introduced into a composite, to adequately activate the surface and modification its composition.

Author Contributions: Conceptualization, Z.K. and L.K.; Methodology, L.K.; Software, B.Ś.; Validation, B.Ś., L.K. and K.K.; Formal Analysis, K.K.; Investigation, L.K.; Resources, B.Ś.; Data Curation, L.K.; Writing—Original Draft Preparation, Z.K.; Writing—Review and Editing, Z.K., L.K. and B.Ś.; Visualization, B.Ś.; Supervision, L.K.; Project Administration, L.K. and K.K.; Funding Acquisition, Z.K. and K.K. All authors have read and agreed to the published version of the manuscript.

Funding: This research received no external funding.

Institutional Review Board Statement: Not applicable.

Informed Consent Statement: Not applicable.

Data Availability Statement: Not applicable.

Conflicts of Interest: The authors declare no conflict of interest.

References

1. Rueggeberg, F.A.; Giannini, M.; Arriais, C.A.G.; Price, R.B.T. Light curing in dentistry and clinical implications: A literature review. *Braz. Oral Res.* **2017**, *31*, 64–91. [CrossRef] [PubMed]
2. Aminoroaya, A.; Esmaeely, N.R.; Nouri, K.S.; Panahi, P.; Das, O.; Ramakrishna, S. A Review of Dental Composites: Methods of Characterizations. *ACS Biomater. Sci. Eng.* **2020**, *13*, 3713–3744. [CrossRef] [PubMed]
3. Rachmia, R.Y.; Rahman, F.S. Dental composite resin: A review. *AIP Conf. Proc.* **2019**, *2193*, 020011. [CrossRef]
4. Bociong, K.; Szczesio, A.; Krasowski, M.; Sokołowski, J. The influence of filler amount on selected properties of new experimental resin dental composite. *Open Chem.* **2018**, *16*, 905–911. [CrossRef]
5. Oivanen, M.; Keulemans, F.; Garoushi, S.; Vallittu, P.K.; Lassila, V.L. The effect of refractive index of fillers and polymer matrix on translucency and color matching of dental resin composite. *Biomater. Investig. Dent.* **2021**, *8*, 48–53. [CrossRef]
6. Floyd, C.J.; Dickens, S.H. Network structure of Bis-GMA- and UDMA-based resin systems. *Dent. Mater.* **2006**, *22*, 1143–1149. [CrossRef]
7. Pratap, B.; Kant, R.; Bhardwaj, B.; Nag, M. Resin based restorative dental materials: Characteristics and future perspectives. *Jpn. Dent. Sci. Rev.* **2019**, *55*, 126–138. [CrossRef]
8. Domarecka, M.; Szczesio-Włodarczyk, A.; Krasowski, M.; Fronczek, M.; Gozdek, T.; Sokołowski, J.; Bociong, K.A. Comparative Study of the Mechanical Properties of Selected Dental Composites with a Dual-Curing System with Light-Curing Composites. *Coatings* **2021**, *11*, 1255. [CrossRef]
9. Jung, M.; Sehr, K.; Klimek, J. Surface Texture of Four Nanofilled and One Hybrid Composite After Finishing. Laboratory research. *Oper. Dent.* **2007**, *32*, 45–52. [CrossRef]
10. Bohner, M. Calcium orthophosphates in medicine: From ceramics to calcium phosphate cements. *Int. J. Care Inj.* **2000**, *31*, 37–47. [CrossRef]
11. Szcześ, A.; Hołysz, L.; Chibowski, E. Synthesis of hydroxyapatite for biomedical applications. *Adv. Colloid Interface Sci.* **2017**, *249*, 321–330. [CrossRef]
12. Lett, J.A.; Sundareswari, M.; Ravichandran, K. Porous hydroxyapatite scaffolds for orthopedic and dental applications—The role of binders. *Mater. Today Proc.* **2016**, *3*, 1672–1677.
13. Liu, Z.; Liang, H.; Shi, T.; Xie, D.; Chen, R.; Han, X.; Shen, L.; Wang, C.; Tian, Z. Additive manufacturing of hydroxyapatite bone scaffolds via digital light processing and in vitro compatibility. *Ceram. Int.* **2019**, *45*, 11079–11086. [CrossRef]
14. Sousa, A.C.; Biscaia, S.; Alvites, R.; Branquinho, M.; Lopes, B.; Sousa, P.; Valente, J.; Franco, M.; Santos, J.D.; Mendonça, C.; et al. Assessment of 3D-Printed Polycaprolactone, Hydroxyapatite Nanoparticles and Diacrylate Poly(ethylene glycol) Scaffolds for Bone Regeneration. *Pharmaceutics* **2022**, *14*, 2643. [CrossRef] [PubMed]
15. Kenry; Liu, B. Recent Advances in Biodegradable Conducting Polymers and Their Biomedical Applications. *Biomacromolecules* **2018**, *19*, 1783–1803. [CrossRef] [PubMed]
16. Bordea, I.; Candrea, S.; Alexescu, G.; Bran, S.; Baciut, M.; Baciut, G.; Lacaciu, O.; Dinu, C.; Todea, D. Nano-hydroxyapatite use in dentistry: A systematic review. *Drug Metab. Rev.* **2020**, *52*, 319–332. [CrossRef] [PubMed]
17. Dorozhkin, S.V. Calcium orthophosphates in dentistry. *Sci. Mater. Med.* **2013**, *24*, 1335–1363. [CrossRef] [PubMed]
18. Lopes, B.; Sousa, P.; Alvites, R.; Branquinho, M.; Sousa, A.C.; Mendonça, C.; Atayde, L.M.; Luís, A.L.; Varejão, A.S.P.; Maurício, A.C. Peripheral Nerve Injury Treatments and Advances: One Health Perspective. *Int. J. Mol. Sci.* **2022**, *23*, 918. [CrossRef]
19. Santos, C.; Luklinska, Z.B.; Clarke, R.L.; Davy, K.W. Hydroxyapatite as a filler for dental composite materials: Mechanical pro-perties and in vitro bioactivity of composites. *J. Mater. Sci. Mater. Med.* **2001**, *12*, 565–573. [CrossRef]
20. Domingo, C.; Arcıs, R.W.; Lopez-Macipe, A.; Osorio, R.; Rodrıguez-Clemente, R.; Murtra, J.; Fanovich, M.A.; Toledano, M. Dental composites reinforced with hydroxyapatite: Mechanical behavior and absorption/elution characteristics. *J. Biomed. Mater. Res.* **2001**, *56*, 297–305. [CrossRef]
21. Elkassas, D.; Arafa, A. The innovative applications of therapeutic nanostructures in dentistry. *Nanomedicine* **2017**, *13*, 1543–1562. [CrossRef]
22. Priyadarsini, S.; Mukherjee, S.; Mishra, M. Nanoparticles used in dentistry: A review. *J. Oral Biol. Craniofac. Res.* **2018**, *8*, 58–67. [CrossRef]
23. Li, Y.; Zhang, D.; Wan, Z.; Yang, X.; Cai, Q. Dental resin composites with improved antibacterial and mineralization properties via incorporating zinc/strontium-doped hydroxyapatite as functional fillers. *Biomed. Mater.* **2022**, *17*, 045002. [CrossRef] [PubMed]

24. Zhao, Y.; Zhang, H.; Hong, L.; Zou, X.; Song, J.; Han, R.; Chen, J.; Yu, Y.; Liu, X.; Zhao, H.; et al. A Multifunctional Dental Resin Composite with Sr-N-Doped TiO$_2$ and n-HA Fillers for Antibacterial and Mineralization Effects. *Int. J. Mol. Sci.* **2023**, *24*, 1274. [CrossRef]
25. Ulian, G.; Moro, D.; Valdrè, G. Hydroxylapatite and Related Minerals in Bone and Dental Tissues: Structural, Spectroscopic and Mechanical Properties from a Computational Perspective. *Biomolecules* **2021**, *11*, 72. [CrossRef]
26. Jardim, R.N.; Rocha, A.A.; Rossi, A.M.; de Almeida Neves, A.; Portela, M.B.; Lopes, R.T.; Moreira da Silva, E. Fabrication and characterization of remineralizing dental composites containing hydroxyapatite nanoparticles. *J. Mech. Behav. Biomed. Mater.* **2020**, *109*, 103817. [CrossRef] [PubMed]
27. Du, M.; Chen, J.; Liu, K.; Xing, H.; Song, C. Recent advances in biomedical engineering of nano-hydroxyapatite including dentistry, cancer treatment and bone repair. *Compos. Part B Eng.* **2021**, *215*, 108790. [CrossRef]
28. Alatawi, R.A.S.; Elsayed, N.H.; Mohamed, W.S. Influence of hydroxyapatite nanoparticles on the properties of glass ionomer cement. *J. Mater. Res. Technol.* **2019**, *8*, 344–349. [CrossRef]
29. Pagano, S.; Chieruzzi, M.; Balloni, S.; Lombardo, G.; Torre, L.; Bodo, M.; Cianetti, S.; Marinucci, L. Biological, thermal and mechanical characterization of modified glass ionomer cements: The role of nanohydroxyapatite, ciprofloxacin and zinc l-carnosine. *Mater. Sci. Eng. C Mater. Biol. Appl.* **2019**, *94*, 76–85. [CrossRef]
30. Balhuc, S.; Campian, R.; Labunet, A.; Negucioiu, M.; Buduru, S.; Kui, A. Dental Applications of Systems Based on Hydroxyapatite Nanoparticles—An Evidence-Based Update. *Crystals* **2021**, *11*, 674. [CrossRef]
31. EN ISO 4049;2009; Dentistry–Polymer-Based Restorative Materials. ISO: Geneva, Switzerland, 2009.
32. ASTM G133-05(2010); Standard Test Method for Linearly Reciprocating Ball-on-Flat Sliding Wear. ISO: Geneva, Switzerland, 2010.
33. PN-EN ISO 868:2003; Plastics and Ebonite—Determination of Indentation Hardness by Means of a Durometer (Shore Hardness). ISO: Geneva, Switzerland, 2003.
34. PN-EN ISO 604; Plastics—Determination of Compressive Properties 2002. ISO: Geneva, Switzerland, 2002.
35. PN-EN ISO 179-2:2020-12; Plastics—Determination of Charpy Impact Properties. ISO: Geneva, Switzerland, 2020.
36. ASTM D2240; Standard Test Method for Rubber Property—Durometer Hardness. ISO: Geneva, Switzerland, 2017.
37. Banaszek, K.; Klimek, L. Ti(C, N) as Barrier Coatings. *Coatings* **2019**, *9*, 432. [CrossRef]
38. Dziedzic, K.; Zubrzycka-Wróbel, J. Research on tribological properties of dental composite materials. *Adv. Sci. Technol. Res. J.* **2016**, *10*, 144–149. [CrossRef]
39. Sajewicz, E. On evaluation of wear resistance of tooth enamel and dental materials. *Wear* **2006**, *260*, 1256–1261. [CrossRef]
40. Chen, L.; Yu, Q.; Wang, Y.; Li, H. BisGMA/TEGDMA dental composite containing high aspect-ratio hydroxyapatite nanofibers. *Dent. Mater.* **2012**, *27*, 1187–1195. [CrossRef] [PubMed]
41. Chadda, H.; Satapathy, B.K.; Patnaik, A.; Ray, A.R. Mechanistic interpretations of fracture toughness and correlations to wear behavior of hydroxyapatite and silica/hydroxyapatite filled bis-GMA/TEGDMA micro/hybrid dental restorative composites. *Compos. Part B Eng.* **2017**, *130*, 132–146. [CrossRef]
42. Şahin, S.; Çehreli, M.C.; Yalçin, E. The influence of functional forces on the biomechanics of implant-supported prostheses—A review. *J. Dent.* **2002**, *30*, 271–282. [CrossRef] [PubMed]
43. Okulus, Z.; Voelkel, A. Mechanical properties of experimental composites with different calcium phosphates fillers. *Mater. Sci. Eng.* **2017**, *78*, 1101–1108. [CrossRef] [PubMed]
44. Kula, Z.; Klimek, L.; Kopacz, K.; Śmielak, B. Evaluation of the effect of the addition of hydroxyapatite on selected mechanical and tribological properties of a Flow type composite. *Materials* **2022**, *15*, 9016. [CrossRef]
45. Akhtar, K.; Pervez, C.; Zubair, N.; Khalid, H. Calcium hydroxyapatite nanoparticles as a reinforcement filler in dental resin nanocomposite. *J. Mater. Sci. Mater. Med.* **2021**, *32*, 129. [CrossRef]
46. Poorzandpoush, K.; Omrani, L.R.; Jafarnia, S.H.; Golkar, P.; Atai, M. Effect of addition of Nano hydroxyapatite particles on wear of resin modified glass ionomer by tooth brushing simulation. *J. Clin. Exp. Dent.* **2017**, *9*, 372–376. [CrossRef] [PubMed]
47. Zhang, H.; Darvell, B.W. Mechanical properties of hydroxyapatite whisker-reinforced bis-GMA-based resin composites. *Dent. Mater.* **2012**, *28*, 824–830. [CrossRef]
48. Bartoszewicz, M.; Rygiel, A.; Krzemiński, M.; Przondo-Mordarska, A. Penetration of a selected antibiotic and antiseptic into a biofilm formed on orthopedic steel implants. *Ortop. Traumatol. Rehabil.* **2007**, *9*, 310–318. [PubMed]
49. Meena, A.; Singh Mali, H.; Patnaik, A.; Ranjan Kumar, S. Comparative investigation of physical, mechanical and thermomechanical characterization of dental composite filled with nanohydroxyapatite and mineral trioxide aggregate. *e-Polymers* **2017**, *17*, 311–319. [CrossRef]
50. Lie, N.; Hilton, T.J.; Heintze, S.D.; Hickel, R.; Watts, D.C.; Silikas, N.; Stansbury, J.W.; Cadenaro, M.; Ferracane, J.L. Academy of Dental Materials Guidance-Resin Composites: Part I-Mechanical Properties. *Dent. Mater.* **2017**, *33*, 880–894.
51. Skapska, A.; Komorek, Z.; Cierech, M.; Mierzwinska-Nastalska, E. Comparison of Mechanical Properties of a Self-Adhesive Composite Cement and a Heated Composite Material. *Polymers* **2022**, *14*, 2686. [CrossRef] [PubMed]
52. Orczykowski, W.; Bieliński, D.M.; Anyszka, R.; Gozdek, T.; Klajn, K.; Celichowski, G.; Pędzich, Z.; Wojteczko, A. Fly Ash from Lignite Combustion as a Filler for Rubber Mixes—Part II: Chemical Valorisation of Fly Ash. *Materials* **2022**, *15*, 5979. [CrossRef]
53. Jaroniek, M.; Czechowski, L.; Kaczmarek, Ł.; Warga, T.; Kubiak, T. A New Approach of Mathematical Analysis of Structure of Graphene as a Potential Material for Composites. *Materials* **2019**, *12*, 3918. [CrossRef]

54. Vouvoudi, E.C.; Sideridou, I.D. Dynamic mechanical properties of dental nanofilled light-cured resin composites: Effect of food-simulating liquids. *J. Mech. Behav. Biomed. Mater.* **2012**, *10*, 87–96. [CrossRef]
55. Mansour, S.F.; El-Dek, S.I.; Ahmed, M.K. Physico-mechanical and morphological features of zirconia substituted hydroxyapatite nanocrystals. *Sci. Rep.* **2017**, *7*, 43202. [CrossRef]

Disclaimer/Publisher's Note: The statements, opinions and data contained in all publications are solely those of the individual author(s) and contributor(s) and not of MDPI and/or the editor(s). MDPI and/or the editor(s) disclaim responsibility for any injury to people or property resulting from any ideas, methods, instructions or products referred to in the content.

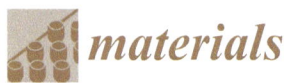

Article

Comparison of Shear Bond Strength of Three Types of Adhesive Materials Used in the Restoration of Permanent Molars after Treatment with Silver Diamine Fluoride: An In Vitro Study

Mannaa K. Aldowsari [1,*], Fatimah Alfawzan [2], Alanoud Alhaidari [2], Nada Alhogail [2], Reema Alshargi [2], Saad Bin Saleh [1], Ayman M. Sulimany [1] and Mohammed Alturki [3]

[1] Department of Pediatric Dentistry and Orthodontics, College of Dentistry, King Saud University, Riyadh 12372, Saudi Arabia
[2] College of Dentistry, King Saud University, Riyadh 12372, Saudi Arabia
[3] Department of Restorative Dental Science, College of Dentistry, King Saud University, Riyadh 12372, Saudi Arabia; mohaalturki@ksu.edu.sa
* Correspondence: maldowsari@ksu.edu.sa

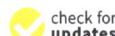

Citation: Aldowsari, M.K.; Alfawzan, F.; Alhaidari, A.; Alhogail, N.; Alshargi, R.; Bin Saleh, S.; Sulimany, A.M.; Alturki, M. Comparison of Shear Bond Strength of Three Types of Adhesive Materials Used in the Restoration of Permanent Molars after Treatment with Silver Diamine Fluoride: An In Vitro Study. *Materials* 2023, 16, 6831. https://doi.org/10.3390/ma16216831

Academic Editors: Lavinia Cosmina Ardelean and Laura-Cristina Rusu

Received: 12 September 2023
Revised: 6 October 2023
Accepted: 11 October 2023
Published: 24 October 2023

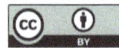

Copyright: © 2023 by the authors. Licensee MDPI, Basel, Switzerland. This article is an open access article distributed under the terms and conditions of the Creative Commons Attribution (CC BY) license (https://creativecommons.org/licenses/by/4.0/).

Abstract: Background: Permanent blackish discoloration of the tooth structure post application of silver diamine fluoride (SDF) is one of its drawbacks. Several restorative materials have been used to restore and mask the blackish discoloration of SDF-treated teeth. Recently, a new self-adhesive material has been introduced and is marketed as an all-in-one etchant, adhesive, and restorative material indicated for use in all clinical situations. This study aimed to assess the shear bond strength of the new self-adhesive restorative material and compare it with adhesive restorative materials-resin-based composite and resin-modified glass ionomer cement to dentin of extracted permanent teeth treated with 38% SDF. Methods: Thirty-nine caries-free extracted teeth (n = 39) were grouped into three groups. Following 38% SDF application, the specimens were loaded with resin-based (Group I), the new self-adhesive restorative material (SDR) Surefil (Group II), and resin-modified glass ionomer cement (RMGIC) (Group III). Shear bond strength (SBS) was calculated, and failure modes were evaluated using the universal testing device (3) Results: The composite showed the highest bond strength, followed by Group II while Group III had the lowest bond strength of all tested materials. Regarding failure type, the composite showed 100% adhesive failure, while Group III and Group II showed mostly adhesive failure with some combination. (4) Conclusions: RBC had a significantly stronger SBS to demineralized dentin surfaces of permanent molar teeth treated with SDF when compared to SDR Surefil and RMGIC.

Keywords: caries; composite; dental; SDF

1. Introduction

Dental caries is a dynamic, biofilm-mediated disease that causes phasic demineralization and remineralization of dental hard tissues. It results from complex interactions between acid-producing cariogenic bacteria, substrates like carbohydrates, and other host factors such as saliva and teeth [1]. Permanent and primary dentitions are susceptible to caries throughout life, which can affect the tooth's crown and, in the long term, exposed root surfaces [2].

Dental caries affecting children under six years of age are called early childhood caries (ECC). ECC spreads quickly and can cause children to experience extreme pain, abscesses, swelling, fever, and psychological disorders [3]. Two practical approaches for ECC prevention before the onset of cavitation are the use of fluoride varnishes containing 5% sodium fluoride (NaF) and fluoridated toothpaste [4]. In cases of cavity formation in ECC, removal of the infected tooth tissue and restoration are recommended.

SDF, a combination of silver nitrate and fluoride- in a 38% concentration has recently been used (off-label) as a caries-arresting agent [5]. Silver nitrate and fluoride work together to create SDF, thereby acting as both an anti-microbial as well as a remineralizing agent [6]. Silver phosphate and calcium fluoride are the products of the SDF's reaction with hydroxyapatite, and they operate as a reservoir for fluoride and phosphate ions that encourage remineralization. The silver ions enter the lesions (up to 30 microns into the enamel, up to 300 microns into the dentin, and up to 2 mm in a deep carious lesion) and exert their anti-bacterial effect [5,6].

The treatment's simplicity makes it suitable for treating caries in young children who may have intense dental fear, uncooperative patients with special needs, or elderly patients who have difficulty adapting to traditional dental care. Its straightforward application procedures do not require injection or drilling [6]. However, due to the presence of silver compounds like silver oxide and silver phosphate, the carious lesions stain black permanently. This influences the patient's and the parents' acceptability of the treatment. In efforts to mask the black staining, many clinicians place adhesive white or tooth-colored restorative materials as direct restorations in the cavitated lesions after SDF application [7].

Recently, a new self-adhesive material restorative material (SDR) Surefil, Dentsply Sirona, Konstanz, Germany) has been introduced as an all-in-one etchant, adhesive, and restorative material for restoring primary and permanent teeth. It offers the glass ionomer's simplicity and speed and a composite materials' restorative longevity and stability. The main component of Surefil One is MOPOS, a modified polyacid, which has a unique structure to allow new opportunities for creating self-adhesive restorative materials. MOPOS enables the material to adhere to tooth structure and form networks, which increases the material's mechanical strength. The addition of polymerizable groups to the polyacid base polymer, which is hydrolytically stable, is what distinguishes MOPOS from other technologies [8]. As the material is applied in one layer without needing adhesive or special retentive preparations, it makes it the ideal restorative material in clinical cases where time or cooperation aspects must be considered, as is the case with plenty of pediatric patients.

The number of clinical and in-vitro studies to test the biological, mechanical, and optical properties of this material is currently limited. In a clinical study by Rathke et al., the newly introduced material has shown acceptable clinical results over the follow-up period of one year. The study concluded that the restorations were in clinically acceptable condition with an annual failure rate of 2%. However, color stability showed the most significant change over time [9]. The mechanical properties of SDR in comparison with three direct composite resins and two GIC materials as evaluated by Lohbauer and Belli were found to be in a range similar to the resin composites [10]. Francois et al., on studying the share bond strength (SBS) of SDR One found the highest bond strength values among the tested materials in samples without any pre-treatment with a universal adhesive followed by etching [11]. Similar results were also found by Sadeghyar et al. in an animal study measuring the SBS values of different materials with and without pre-treatment [12]. However, data regarding the effect of SDF on the bond strength of this new self-adhesive material is inconclusive.

Therefore, the aim of this study was to assess the SBS of three different types of adhesive restorative materials, including resin-based composite (RBC), a new Self-adhesive restorative material (SDR) Surefil, and resin-modified glass ionomer cement (RMGIC) of dentin of extracted permanent teeth treated with 38% SDF. The null hypothesis was that there was no difference between the SBS of the three different materials with the dentin treated with 38% SDF.

2. Materials and Methods

An in vitro study was conducted to assess the SBS of three different types of adhesive restorative materials. The three materials included a resin-based composite (Neo Spectra ST LV, Dentsply Sirona, Charlotte, NC, USA) (RBC), a new self-adhesive restorative material (Dentsply Sirona, Konstanz, Germany) (SDR) Surefil and resin-modified glass ionomer cement (RMGIC, Fuji IX, GC Corporation, Tokyo, Japan) (RMGIC). The chemical composition of the investigated materials is presented in Table 1.

Table 1. Materials used in this study and their composition and application mode.

Material, Manufacturer	Composition	Application Mode
Advantage arrest, silver diamine fluoride 38%, Elevate Oral Care, West Palm Beach, FL, USA)	Silver fluoride, ammonia, and deionized water	-Dry the surface -Apply the material using a micro brush to the tooth surface -Dry with a gentle flow of compressed air for one minute.
Best-Etch, Vista Dental designs, New York, NY, USA	Phosphoric acid 37%	-Apply to the surface of the bonding for 15 s. -Rinse with water for 5 s and dry.
Prime & Bond NT, Dentsply Sirona)	MDP Phosphate Monomer, dimethacrylate, HEMA, Vitrebond copolymer, fillers, ethanol, water, initiator, and saline	-Apply for 20 s using a microbrush. -Air dry gently for 5 s. -Cure for 10 s
Neo Spectra ST LV, Dentsply Sirona	A blend of spherical, pre-polymerized Sphere fillers (d3,50 ≈ 15 μm), non-agglomerated barium glass and ytterbium fluoride. Highly dispersed, methacrylic polysiloxane nano-particles	-Apply 2 mm thickness and light cure for 20 s
Surefil One, Dentsply Sirona, Konstanz, Germany	Aluminum-phosphor-strontium-sodium-fluoro-silicate glass, water, silicon dioxide, acrylic acid, polycarboxylic acid, ytterbium fluoride, bifunctional acrylate, self-cure initiator, pigments, camphorquinone, and stabilizer	-Activate capsule, and place in a mixer for 10 s -Apply 2 mm and light cure for 20 s.
Fuji IX, GC Corporation, Tokyo, Japan (RMGIC)	Powder: Fluro alumino silicate glass, Polyacrylic acid powder. Liquid: Polyacrylic acid Polybasic carboxylic acid	-Activate capsule, -Place in a mixer for 10 s, -Apply 2 mm then let it set for 3 min.

Abbreviations: HEMA—Hydroxyethyl methacrylate; MDP: 10-methacryloyloxydecyl dihydrogen phosphate.

2.1. Specimens and Sampling Technique

A power analysis was conducted to calculate the sample size. Based on previously available literature, using a package (pwr) in R software (R package version 1.3-0.) with a 95% confidence interval and 80% power of the study, the sample size was determined. Ethical clearance was obtained from the Institutional Review Board of the university. 39 permanent sound teeth indicated for orthodontic extraction were collected from dental clinics in Riyadh, Saudi Arabia after a written informed consent from the patients. The inclusion criterion was sound teeth. The exclusion criteria were teeth with restoration or caries. To remove debris and calculus, blood, and plaque, the teeth were thoroughly cleaned with an ultrasonic scaler and then placed in freshly prepared 0.5% chloramine-T solution and stored at 4–7 °C until further use. The sample was randomly split into three groups (n = 13) using a simple random sampling technique as follows: the first group (I) was loaded with RBC, the second group (II) was loaded with SDR Surefil and the third group (III) was loaded with RMGIC.

2.2. Specimens Preparation

The teeth were mounted in round metal molds in cold-cure clear acrylic. A slow-speed cutting machine (IsoMet, Buehler, Plymouth, MN, USA) was used to remove the occlusal enamel of the teeth specimens. The complete removal of the enamel was ensured by examining the dentin surfaces of the specimens under a stereomicroscope (SM80, Swift microscope, Carlsbad, CA, USA). The specimens were demineralized for seven days to simulate caries with pH adjusted to 5.0 (acidic) at 37 °C.

2.3. SDF Treatments

The occlusal surface of the demineralized dentin specimens was treated uniformly with one drop of 38% SDF (Advantage Arrest, Elevate Oral Care, West Palm Beach, FL, USA) using a micro brush applicator tip without a pre-etching step. After the SDF application had dried using a gentle flow of compressed air for one minute without rinsing, the dentin specimens were stored at 37 °C in distilled water for two weeks. After two weeks, the dentin specimens were loaded with assigned adhesive restorative materials as per the manufacturers' recommendations for each adhesive material (Table 1).

After loading the specimens with assigned restorative materials, the specimens were then loaded in a thermocycling machine (Huber, SD-Mechatronik-Thermocyclerr, Berching, Germany) and subjected to 5000 cycles of thermocycling between 5 °C and 55 °C to mimic 6 months of physiological use. The dwell time in each bath was set to 30 s.

2.4. SBS Measurements and Failure Modes

The universal testing device evaluated the SBS (Instron 5965, Norwood, MA, USA). The specimens were mounted in a metal mold 3 mm in diameter, serving as a drive surface for a metal plunger. This plunger touched the cylindrical test material at the contact point with the dentin at right angles. The testing device moved with a defined 1 mm/min speed toward the plunger. The shear bond strength was calculated with a special software program (Blue Heal 3). Failure modes were evaluated utilizing a stereomicroscope (SM80, Swift microscope, Carlsbad, CA, USA) and classified as adhesive, cohesive, and mixed failures.

2.5. Statistical Analysis

The statistical analysis used was the Statistical Package for the Social Sciences (SPSS) 19.0 (v.19.0, IBM, Chicago, IL, USA). Mean and standard deviation from the recorded shear bond strength values were calculated. Analysis of variance (ANOVA) with the Tukey Post hoc test was done to compare the bond strength between the three groups.

3. Results

The SBS of the three materials was tested, and the mean and standard deviation were calculated. The intergroup comparison was done using one-way ANOVA followed by Tukey HSD post hoc test (Table 2).

Table 2. Comparison of the mean shear bond strength of the test materials using one-way ANOVA and between group comparison using Tukey HSD post hoc test.

Study Group	n	Mean in (Mpa)	Std. Dev.	p Value
RBS	13	21.83	2.49	
RMGIC	13	15.70	2.06	<0.0001
SDR Surefil	13	17.71	1.79	
Between group comparison	Difference between means	95% Confidence Limits		p value
RBC vs. SDR Surefil	4.1204	2.0764	6.1645	<0.0001
RBC vs. RMGIC	6.1313	4.0872	8.1753	<0.0001
SDR Surefil vs. RMGIC	2.0108	−0.0332	4.0549	0.055

RBC showed the highest bond strength, followed by SDR Surefil, while RMGIC had the lowest bond strength of all tested materials. Statistically significant results were found between the RMGIC and RBC groups and between SDR Surefil and RBC groups when SBS was calculated after pretreatment of dentin with 38% SDF. However, no statistically significant difference was found between SDR Surefil and RMGIC (Table 2). Regarding the type of adhesive failure, RBC showed 100% adhesive failure, while RMGIC and SDR Surefil showed mostly adhesive failure with some combination. No cohesive failures were noted in any of the groups (Table 3) (Figure 1).

Table 3. Types of failure for the study groups.

Restorative Material	Adhesive n (%)	Cohesive n (%)	Combination n (%)	Total n (%)
RBC	13 (100%)	0 (0%)	0 (0%)	13 (100%)
SDR Surefil	9 (69.23%)	0 (0%)	4 (30.76)	13 (100%)
RMGIC	10 (76.92%)	0 (0%)	3 (23.07)	13 (100%)

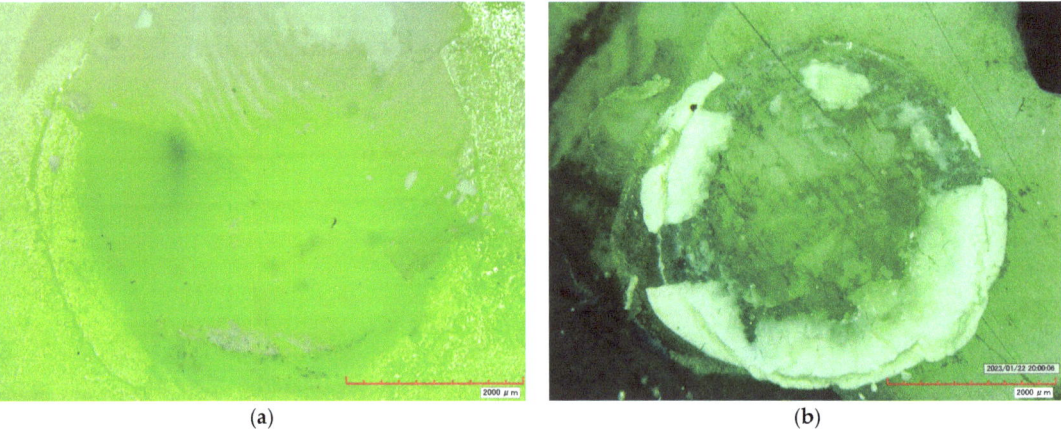

Figure 1. Stereomicroscope images at (×40) show the mode of failure of different experimental groups. (**a**) representative sample showing the adhesive type of failure of RBC specimen (**b**) representative sample showing the mixed type of failure of SDR surefil specimen.

4. Discussion

The aim of this in-vitro study was to evaluate the effect of pre-treatment of dentin with 38% SDF on the bond strength of three different restorative materials. In-vitro studies are often used to test the different variables of newly introduced materials and their interactions with other biomaterials in common clinical scenarios. SBS reveals the adhesive strength of the material at the restoration-tooth interface. It is at this interface that the forces of mastication, which are analogous to the shearing phenomenon, result in a complicated stress distribution during clinical weight-loading situations [13].

In this study, the maximum SBS was noted with the RBC, followed by SDR Surefil, and the least values were noted with RMGIC. Statistically significant results were found between the RMGIC and RBC groups and between SDR Surefil and RBC groups when SBS was calculated after pretreatment of dentin with 38% SDF.

SDF has become a popular alternative in managing dental caries, which was approved by the US Food and Drug Administration (FDA) in 2014 as a commercial product for dental use. However, concerns have been raised about its impact on the bond strength of restorative materials to dentin [14]. Multiple in-vitro studies have been conducted to investigate SDF's effects on the bond strength of restorative materials. Zhao et al. showed that pre-treatment with SDF did not negatively affect the adhesion of GIC to caries-affected dentine [15]. Similarly, Wu et al. showed that the bond strengths of composite to sound primary molars were not affected using 38% SDF on primary dentin [16]. In contrast, pre-treatment of sound primary dentin with SDF significantly increased the SBS between RMGIC and primary dentin as studied by Sa'ada et al. [17]. In addition, the light curing of RMGIC for 20 s may increase the SBS between SDF pre-treated primary dentin and RMGIC [18]. Fröhlich et al. in their systematic review stated that the effect of SDF on dentin bonding was material-dependent, no effect was noted on adhesion of GIC, but a significant decrease in bond strength with adhesive systems was observed [19]. In an updated systematic review published by the same authors, it was found that SDF application, followed by rinsing, does not jeopardize adhesive bond strength, and could improve the adhesion of the restorative material to caries-affected dentin [20]. The mean SBS in the present study was lower than the universal adhesive values. This could be due to the effect of pre-treatment of SDF as shown previously in a recent systematic review, which showed a significant decrease in bond strength with adhesive systems [19].

An ideal restorative material should have optimal biocompatibility, chemical adhesion, adequate strength, and be usable in all clinical situations. SDR Surefil was introduced by the manufacturer as a one-step bulk-fill material, eliminating the need for etching and bonding procedures, and was indicated for use in all clinical situations. It has initiators to enable both photo and chemo polymerization and a high molecular weight polymer called MOPOS by the manufacturer. This polymer is claimed to promote bonding to the tooth and create a strong composite-like structure [20]. Abuljadayel and co-workers in an invitro study, studied the effect of SDF and Chlorhexidine on the SBS of various bio-active restorative materials, including SDR Surefil [8]. Higher values were noted with the SDF-treated specimens as compared to the chlorhexidine group. However, the results of this study must be treated with caution as this study assessed immediate SBS values without any artificial aging. This is not in line with the recent recommendations which recommend placement of a restorative material two weeks after treatment with SDF to minimize black discoloration [21].

The RMGIC, evaluated in this study, is a commonly used material in posterior restorations and ART (atraumatic restorative treatment). There are numerous studies comparing the bonding of GIC with and without surface treatment of SDF. No solid conclusion was drawn in a systematic review by Jiang et al. based on this topic [14]. A high degree of variation of data comparing the effect of SDF application on the bond strength of dentine to adhesives and to GICs was the reason behind their findings. Ng et al. found no difference in the bond strength of glass ionomer cement to dentin lesions after SDF treatment. They noted improved retention by allowing the SDF solution to be set for one week prior to GIC placement [22]. Abdullah et al. in an in vitro study involving primary molars, have noted lower SBS for GIC, composite resin, and resin-modified bioactive resin for SDF-treated dentin as compared to the control group (sound dentine without SDF) [23].

Of the three restorative materials tested in this study, Neo Spectra ST is a nano-hybrid composite with a patented SphereTEC technology as claimed by the manufacturer. The fillers have a micro-granulated structure, thereby allowing them to bind more free resin than conventional fillers [24]. Our results showed that RBC exhibited the highest SBS after SDF treatment. This was probably because the etching and bonding step was performed only for this material group. It is well known that the bonding of adhesives is based on micromechanical retention and hybrid layer formation. SDF is a highly alkaline fluid that reacts with hydroxyapatite forming a silver phosphate layer, resulting in an impermeable layer and dentinal tubule obstruction, making it both a physical and chemical barrier to adhesion [25–27]. This interferes with resin impregnation, thereby affecting the SBS of composite resin. The application of phosphoric acid has been suggested by Koizumi et al. to remove some precipitate SDF and thereby increase the bond strength [28]. Using an etchant and delaying restoration placement positively affects the SBS of the composite.

Similarly, there is no consensus on the effect of immediate rinsing of SDF with water on the bond strength of the adhesive materials. While some authors have noted increased bond strength values after rinsing SDF-applied specimens with water [15,29], others have reported no significant changes in the same [30,31]. There was no rinsing of the specimens with water in this study, which could have possibly influenced the final results. Francois et al., had compared the differences in SBS of SDR Surefil, with or without the use of an adhesive system, and recorded higher values for specimens where an adhesive was used [11]. In the same study, when different materials SDR Surefil and Activa BioActive Restorative) were compared without the use of an adhesive, SDR Surefil demonstrated the highest SBS. They attributed this high adhesion value to the structural composition of Surefil. The functionalized polyacrylic acid of high molecular weight facilitates hybridization of the smear layer, interactions between calcium contained in dentin and carboxyl groups of MOPOS have been shown to promote adhesion between the material and the tooth structure [32]. In another study by Latta et al., similar SBS values were found between light-cured and self-cured SDR Surefil specimens [33]. However, no adhesives were used in this case. They concluded that on dentin surfaces, the self-adhesive materials including SDR Surefil generated lower SBS values than a composite resin and a universal adhesive. The results of this study are on similar lines as our study where the values of SDR Surefil were similar to RMGIC but lesser than RBC.

In terms of failure, RBC showed 100% adhesive failure. This is supported by Aldosari et al. and Atalay et al., who found adhesive failure to be the more frequent mode [34,35]. Most RMGIC and SDR Surefil samples had an adhesive failure, with some samples showing combination failure. This contrasts with Poorzandpoush K. et al., which found RMGIC to have 100% adhesive failure [36]. There were no cohesive failures with any of the samples. Instead of indicating the bonding properties, cohesive failures often indicate different mechanical properties of the materials involved or some other problems like errors in alignment of the testing assembly, or microcracks in the specimens. Scherrer et al. in their literature review have suggested avoiding cohesive failure specimens and analyzing data from specimens with adhesive failure or mixed failure with small region (<10%) only, to get more accurate results [37]. Ignoring any data may however lead to bias in the final results and should be treated with caution.

The main limitation of this study is that it is an in vitro study; it cannot mimic the in vivo conditions. However, Thermocycling was used in this study to simulate some aspects of the oral environment to overcome this limitation. Moreover, SDF is mainly used in primary teeth. However, in this study, permanent molars were used instead of primary teeth. The differences in the dentinal tubules' structures may also be a factor affecting the action of SDF on the natural tooth and the subsequent restorative material. Another limitation could be that the bond strength of teeth affected by clinical caries may be different from artificial caries. However, in spite of these limitations, the present study's findings can contribute to the ongoing studies that investigate the effect of pre-treatment of SDF on the physical properties of the dental materials.

The interface between the restoration and the SDF-treated tooth is exposed to diverse forces that act simultaneously in the oral cavity. Therefore, long-lasting clinical trials remain necessary to validate the laboratory observations. Only the shear bond strength was calculated in this study. Further scope of the research includes the assessment of other mechanical and optical properties of the new self-adhesive material, SDR Surefil, in SDF-treated teeth and correlating its clinical survival and success rates. Also, further studies using different restorative materials might be considered.

5. Conclusions

Within the limitations of this in vitro study, the following conclusions were made:

1. RBC had a significantly stronger SBS to demineralized dentin surfaces of permanent molar teeth treated with SDF when compared to SDR Surefil and RMGIC.
2. SDR Surefil showed better properties of SBS compared with RMGIC, making it a good alternative choice to conventional restorative materials.
3. The bond strength between SDF-treated tooth and SDR Surefil found to be within the clinical acceptable limits, makes the material a good alternative choice to be used to mask the discoloration caused by SDF application. This is particularly helpful in young and un-cooperative patients since the material is marketed by the manufacturer as a self- adhesive material without the requirement of any tooth preparation procedures.

Author Contributions: Conceptualization, M.K.A.; methodology, M.K.A. and M.A.; validation, A.M.S., M.A. and M.K.A.; formal analysis, A.M.S.; investigation, M.K.A.; resources data curation, writing—original draft preparation, M.K.A., F.A., A.A., N.A., R.A. and S.B.S.; writing—review and editing, M.K.A.; visualization, M.K.A., F.A., A.A., N.A., R.A. and S.B.S.; supervision, M.K.A., A.M.S., S.B.S. and M.A. All authors have read and agreed to the published version of the manuscript.

Funding: This research received no external funding.

Institutional Review Board Statement: This study was conducted according to the guidelines of the Declaration of Helsinki and approved by the Ethics Committee Institutional Review Board of King Saud University (E-22-7136, approval date 10 September 2022).

Informed Consent Statement: Informed consent was obtained from all subjects involved in the study.

Data Availability Statement: The database is available upon request from the corresponding author).

Acknowledgments: The authors would like to thank the College of Dentistry Research Center and the Deanship of Scientific Research at King Saud University, Saudi Arabia, for funding this research project.

Conflicts of Interest: The authors declare no conflict of interest.

References

1. Selwitz, R.H.; Ismail, A.I.; Pitts, N.B. Dental caries. *Lancet* **2007**, *369*, 51–59. [CrossRef]
2. Pitts, N.B.; Zero, D.T.; Marsh, P.D.; Ekstrand, K.; Weintraub, J.A.; Ramos-Gomez, F.; Ismail, A. Dental caries. *Nat. Rev. Dis. Primers* **2017**, *25*, 17030. [CrossRef] [PubMed]
3. Mathur, V.P.; Dhillon, J.K. Dental Caries: A Disease Which Needs Attention. *Indian J. Pediatr.* **2018**, *85*, 202–206. [CrossRef]
4. Duangthip, D.; Chen, K.J.; Gao, S.S.; Lo, E.C.M.; Chu, C.H. Managing Early Childhood Caries with Atraumatic Restorative Treatment and Topical Silver and Fluoride Agents. *Int. J. Environ. Res. Public Health* **2017**, *14*, 1204. [CrossRef]
5. Janakiram, C.; Ramanarayanan, V.; Devan, I. Effectiveness of Silver Diammine Fluoride Applications for Dental Caries Cessation in Tribal Preschool Children in India: Study Protocol for a Randomized Controlled Trial. *Methods Protoc.* **2021**, *4*, 30. [CrossRef]
6. Nuvvula, S.; Mallineni, S.K. Silver diamine fluoride in pediatric dentistry. *J. South Asian Assoc. Pediatr. Dent.* **2019**, *2*, 73–80. [CrossRef]
7. Horst, J.A.; Ellenikiotis, H.; Milgrom, P.M. UCSF Protocol for Caries Arrest Using Silver Diamine Fluoride: Rationale, Indications and Consent. *Pa. Dent. Assoc.* **2017**, *44*, 16–28. [CrossRef]
8. Abuljadayel, R.; Aljadani, N.; Almutairi, H.; Turkistani, A. Effect of Antibacterial Agents on Dentin Bond Strength of Bioactive Restorative Materials. *Polymers* **2023**, *15*, 2612. [CrossRef] [PubMed]
9. Rathke, A.; Pfefferkorn, F.; McGuire, M.K.; Heard, R.H.; Seemann, R. One-year clinical results of restorations using a novel self-adhesive resin-based bulk-fill restorative. *Sci. Rep.* **2022**, *12*, 3934. [CrossRef]
10. Lohbauer, U.; Belli, R. The Mechanical Performance of a Novel Self-Adhesive Restorative Material. *J. Adhes. Dent.* **2020**, *22*, 47–58. [PubMed]
11. François, P.; Remadi, A.; Le Goff, S.; Abdel-Gawad, S.; Attal, J.-P.; Dursun, E. Flexural properties and dentin adhesion in recently developed self-adhesive bulk-fill materials. *J. Oral Sci.* **2021**, *63*, 139–144. [CrossRef]

12. Sadeghyar, A.; Lettner, S.; Watts, D.C.; Schedle, A. Alternatives to amalgam: Is pretreatment necessary for effective bonding to dentin? *Dent. Mater.* **2022**, *38*, 1703–1709. [CrossRef]
13. Nujella, B.S.; Choudary, M.T.; Reddy, S.P.; Kumar, M.K.; Gopal, T. Comparison of shear bond strength of aesthetic restorative materials. *Contemp. Clin. Dent.* **2012**, *3*, 22–26. [CrossRef]
14. Jiang, M.; Mei, M.L.; Wong, M.C.M.; Chu, C.H.; Lo, E.C.M. Effect of silver diamine fluoride solution application on the bond strength of dentine to adhesives and to glass ionomer cements: A systematic review. *BMC Oral Health* **2020**, *20*, 40. [CrossRef]
15. Zhao, I.S.; Chu, S.; Yu, O.Y.; Mei, M.L.; Chu, C.H.; Lo, E.C.M. Effect of silver diamine fluoride and potassium iodide on shear bond strength of glass ionomer cements to caries-affected dentine. *Int. Dent. J.* **2019**, *69*, 341–347. [CrossRef]
16. Wu, D.I.; Velamakanni, S.; Denisson, J.; Yaman, P.; Boynton, J.R.; Papagerakis, P. Effect of Silver Diamine Fluoride (SDF) Application on Microtensile Bonding Strength of Dentin in Primary Teeth. *Pediatr. Dent.* **2016**, *38*, 148–153.
17. Sa'ada, M.M.; Khattab, N.M.; Amer, M.I. Effect of Silver Diamine Fluoride Pretreatment on Shear Bond Strength of Resin Modified Glass Ionomer Cement to Primary Dentin. *Open Access Maced. J. Med Sci.* **2021**, *9*, 243–247. [CrossRef]
18. Wang, A.S.; Botelho, M.G.; Tsoi, J.K.; Matinlinna, J.P. Effects of silver diammine fluoride on microtensile bond strength of GIC to dentine. *Int. J. Adhes. Adhes.* **2016**, *70*, 196–203. [CrossRef]
19. Fröhlich, T.T.; Rocha, R.O.; Botton, G. Does previous application of silver diammine fluoride influence the bond strength of glass ionomer cement and adhesive systems to dentin? Systematic review and meta-analysis. *Int. J. Paediatr. Dent.* **2020**, *30*, 85–95. [CrossRef]
20. Fröhlich, T.T.; Botton, G.; Rocha, R.O. Bonding of Glass-Ionomer Cement and Adhesives to Silver Diamine Fluoride-treated Dentin: An Updated Systematic Review and Meta-Analysis. *J. Adhes. Dent.* **2022**, *24*, 29–38.
21. Cryst Young, D.A.; Quock, R.L.; Horst, J.; Kaur, R.; MacLean, J.K.; Frachella, J.C.; Duffin, S.; Semprum-Clavier, A.; Ferreira Zandona, A.G. Clinical Instructions for Using Silver Diamine Fluoride (SDF) in Dental Caries Management. *Compend. Contin. Educ. Dent.* **2021**, *42*, e5–e9.
22. Ng, E.; Saini, S.; A Schulze, K.; Horst, J.; Le, T.; Habelitz, S. Shear Bond Strength of Glass Ionomer Cement to Silver Diamine Fluoride-Treated Artificial Dentinal Caries. *Pediatr. Dent.* **2020**, *42*, 221–225. [PubMed]
23. Abdullah, A.; Finkelman, M.; Kang, Y.; Loo, C.Y. Shear Bond Strength of Different Restorative Materials to Primary Tooth Dentin Treated with Silver Diamine Fluoride. *J. Dent. Child.* **2022**, *89*, 68–74.
24. Joshi, C.; Patel, D.; Shah, M.; Patel, A.; Khunt, A.; Kanabar, A.K. Comparative Evaluation of The Effects of Different Alcoholic Beverages and Sports/Energy Drinks on the Surface Roughness of a Recently Marketed Universal Nanohybrid with a Nano-Filled Composite Resin. *J. Pharm. Negat. Results* **2022**, *13*, 2423–2429.
25. Li, Y.; Liu, Y.; Psoter, W.J.; Nguyen, O.M.; Bromage, T.G.; Walters, M.A.; Hu, B.; Rabieh, S.; Kumararaja, F.C. Assessment of the Silver Penetration and Distribution in Carious Lesions of Deciduous Teeth Treated with Silver Diamine Fluoride. *Caries Res.* **2019**, *53*, 431–440. [CrossRef] [PubMed]
26. Sayed, M.; Matsui, N.; Hiraishi, N.; Inoue, G.; Nikaido, T.; Burrow, M.F.; Tagami, J. Evaluation of discoloration of sound/demineralized root dentin with silver diamine fluoride: In-vitro study. *Dent. Mater. J.* **2019**, *38*, 143–149. [CrossRef]
27. Lutgen, P.; Chan, D.; Sadr, A. Effects of silver diammine fluoride on bond strength of adhesives to sound dentin. *Dent. Mater. J.* **2018**, *37*, 1003–1009. [CrossRef]
28. Koizumi, H.; Hamama, H.H.; Burrow, M.F. Effect of a Silver Diamine Fluoride and Potassium Iodide-Based Desensitizing and Cavity Cleaning Agent on Bond Strength to Dentine. *Int. J. Adhes. Adhes.* **2016**, *68*, 54–61. [CrossRef]
29. Thomas, M.S.; Gupta, J.; Radhakrishna, M.; Srikant, N.; Ginjupalli, K. The effect of silver fluoride and potassium iodide on the bond strength of auto cure glass ionomer cement to dentine. *Aust. Dent. J.* **2006**, *51*, 42–45.
30. Francois, P.; Fouquet, V.; Attal, J.-P.; Dursun, E. Effect of silver diamine fluoride and potassium iodide on bonding to demineralized dentin. *Am. J. Dent.* **2019**, *32*, 143–146.
31. Thomas, M.S.; Gupta, J.; Radhakrishna, M.; Srikant, N.; Ginjupalli, K. Effect of silver diamine fluoride-potassium iodide and 2% chlorhexidine gluconate cavity cleansers on the bond strength and microleakage of resin-modified glass ionomer cement. *J. Conserv. Dent.* **2019**, *22*, 201–206. [CrossRef] [PubMed]
32. Francois, P.; Fouquet, V.; Attal, J.-P.; Dursun, E. Commercially available fluoride-releasing restorative materials: A review and a proposal for classification. *Materials* **2020**, *13*, 2313. [CrossRef]
33. Latta, M.A.; Tsujimoto, A.; Takamizawa, T.; Barkmeier, W.W. Enamel and Dentin Bond Durability of Self-Adhesive Restorative Materials. *J. Adhes. Dent.* **2020**, *22*, 99–105.
34. Aldosari, M.M.; Al-Sehaibany, F.S. Evaluation of the Effect of the Loading Time on the Microtensile Bond Strength of Various Restorative Materials Bonded to Silver Diamine Fluoride-Treated Demineralized Dentin. *Materials* **2022**, *15*, 4424. [CrossRef] [PubMed]
35. Atalay, C.; Vural, U.K.; Tugay, B.; Miletić, I.; Gurgan, S. Surface Gloss, Radiopacity and Shear Bond Strength of Contemporary Universal Composite Resins. *Appl. Sci.* **2023**, *13*, 1902. [CrossRef]

36. Poorzandpoush, K.; Shahrabi, M.; Heidari, A.; Hosseinipour, Z.S. Shear Bond Strength of Self-Adhesive Flowable Composite, Conventional Flowable Composite and Resin-Modified Glass Ionomer Cement to Primary Dentin. *Front. Dent.* **2019**, *16*, 62–68. [CrossRef] [PubMed]
37. Scherrer, S.S.; Cesar, P.F.; Swain, M.V. Direct comparison of the bond strength results of the different test methods: A critical literature review. *Dent. Mater.* **2010**, *26*, e78–e93. [CrossRef]

Disclaimer/Publisher's Note: The statements, opinions and data contained in all publications are solely those of the individual author(s) and contributor(s) and not of MDPI and/or the editor(s). MDPI and/or the editor(s) disclaim responsibility for any injury to people or property resulting from any ideas, methods, instructions or products referred to in the content.

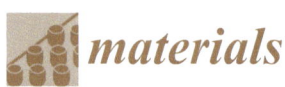 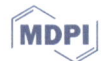

Article

In Vitro Evaluation of *Candida albicans* Adhesion on Heat-Cured Resin-Based Dental Composites

Francesco De Angelis [1,†], Simonetta D'Ercole [1,*,†], Mara Di Giulio [2], Mirco Vadini [1], Virginia Biferi [1], Matteo Buonvivere [1], Lorenzo Vanini [3], Luigina Cellini [2], Silvia Di Lodovico [2,†] and Camillo D'Arcangelo [1,†]

1. Department of Medical, Oral and Biotechnological Sciences, "G. d'Annunzio" University of Chieti–Pescara, 66100 Chieti, Italy; fda580@gmail.com (F.D.A.); m.vadini@unich.it (M.V.); virg.bif@gmail.com (V.B.); matteo.buonvivere@unich.it (M.B.); camillo.darcangelo@unich.it (C.D.)
2. Department of Pharmacy, "G. d'Annunzio" University of Chieti–Pescara, 66100 Chieti, Italy; mara.digiulio@unich.it (M.D.G.); l.cellini@unich.it (L.C.); silvia.dilodovico@unich.it (S.D.L.)
3. Corso S. Gottardo 25, 6830 Chiasso, Switzerland; vaniniodonto@gmail.com
* Correspondence: simonetta.dercole@unich.it
† These authors contributed equally to this work.

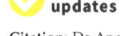

Citation: De Angelis, F.; D'Ercole, S.; Di Giulio, M.; Vadini, M.; Biferi, V.; Buonvivere, M.; Vanini, L.; Cellini, L.; Di Lodovico, S.; D'Arcangelo, C. In Vitro Evaluation of *Candida albicans* Adhesion on Heat-Cured Resin-Based Dental Composites. *Materials* 2023, *16*, 5818. https://Doi.org/10.3390/ma16175818

Academic Editors: Lavinia Cosmina Ardelean and Laura-Cristina Rusu

Received: 28 July 2023
Revised: 18 August 2023
Accepted: 22 August 2023
Published: 25 August 2023

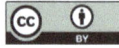

Copyright: © 2023 by the authors. Licensee MDPI, Basel, Switzerland. This article is an open access article distributed under the terms and conditions of the Creative Commons Attribution (CC BY) license (https://creativecommons.org/licenses/by/4.0/).

Abstract: Microbial adhesion on dental restorative materials may jeopardize the restorative treatment long-term outcome. The goal of this in vitro study was to assess *Candida albicans* capability to adhere and form a biofilm on the surface of heat-cured dental composites having different formulations but subjected to identical surface treatments and polymerization protocols. Three commercially available composites were evaluated: GrandioSO (GR), Venus Diamond (VD) and Enamel Plus HRi Biofunction (BF). Cylindrical specimens were prepared for quantitative determination of *C. albicans* S5 planktonic CFU count, sessile cells CFU count and biomass optical density ($OD_{570\,nm}$). Qualitative Concanavalin-A assays (for extracellular polymeric substances of a biofilm matrix) and Scanning Electron Microscope (SEM) analyses (for the morphology of sessile colonies) were also performed. Focusing on planktonic CFU count, a slight but not significant reduction was observed with VD as compared to GR. Regarding sessile cells CFU count and biomass $OD_{570\,nm}$, a significant increase was observed for VD compared to GR and BF. Concanavalin-A assays and SEM analyses confirmed the quantitative results. Different formulations of commercially available resin composites may differently interact with *C. albicans*. The present results showed a relatively more pronounced antiadhesive effect for BF and GR, with a reduction in sessile cells CFU count and biomass quantification.

Keywords: microbial adhesion; resin composites; heat-cured; *Candida albicans*; dental biofilm; dental caries

1. Introduction

Due to their current improvements in mechanical properties and aesthetic performance, dental resin composites (DRCs) have become the most preferred filling material in direct dental restorations. [1–5]. DRCs are typically made out of an organic matrix, inorganic fillers and a silane coupling agent, which connects the two components [6]. The organic matrix consists of several monomers, such as BisGMA (2,2-bis [p-(2′-hidroxy-3′-methacryloxypropoxy) phenyl]- propane), UDMA (urethane dimethacrylate), TEGDMA (trietylenglycol di-methacrylate), DMAEMA (dimethylaminoethyl methacrylate) and various additives (photoinitiators-camphoroquinone, inhibitors, stabilizers). The organic matrix, in the form of a three-dimensional cross-linked network, is created during the polymerization reaction of the monomer mixture of resin composites [7]. The most used technique for starting the polymerization reaction of resin composites is photo-activation [7]. However, monomer conversion is never complete during the polymerization of light-cured resin composites [8] and, according to data from the literature, up to 45% of monomer and double bonds may go unreacted as methacrylate pendant groups [9]. The degree of conversion of double carbon bonds to single carbon bonds achieved during polymerization directly affects the final characteristics of photo-cured composites [10]. When resin composites are used for indirect restorations, before final restoration delivery, they can be further processed in the dental laboratory; here, they are typically subjected to additional heat curing protocols that, according to several studies, allow for enhanced material's microhardness, flexural strength, fracture toughness, wear resistance, tensile strength and color stability [11–14]. The conversion of monomers into durable polymer chains is increased as a result of such a heat curing [15,16]. As stated in the literature, in fact, without a post-curing heat treatment process, the polymer matrix is not strong enough, and failure of composites under loading is typically caused by the crushing of the polymer matrix [17]. Many different heat-curing protocols are described in the literature, in which an additional material photopolymerization is performed for a prolonged time (ranging from 10 min to a maximum of 6 h) at an increased temperature (even up to 120 °C) [18–20].

Dental materials have been widely investigated in terms of their mechanical performances [21–24]. At the same time, their biological properties should also be considered of paramount clinical relevance. Oral microorganisms are found in highly structured and ordered microbial communities called biofilms, where microbial cells are embedded in a self-produced extracellular polymeric substance [25–28]. In this environment, several interactions between species occur, so that the presence of one microorganism is able to create a niche for others, which helps to promote colonization and retention [29,30]. The ability of *Streptococcus mutans* to create very large amounts of glucans, release acid and survive in an acidic environment, combined with its strong binding to teeth, ultimately leads to the disintegration of hydroxyapatite in tooth enamel and dentin [31–35]. Cariogenic bacteria, such as *S. mutans*, can cause degradation of resin composites through bacterial production of acidic derivatives [36–39], mainly acting at the adhesive tooth-restoration interface, which can limit the functional and esthetic longevity of a composite restoration [40–42] resulting in interfacial gaps [43].

Although *S. mutans* has traditionally been seen as the primary cariogenic species, current research appears to suggest that *Candida albicans*, through interactions with *S. mutans*, may also play a significant cariogenic role [44–47]. Alike *S. mutans*, *C. albicans* is a natural commensal colonizer of the oral cavity [30,48]. However, this opportunistic organism can quickly turn into a pathogen that causes oral candidiasis under conditions of immune suppression or changes in the host environment [49–51]. It is well known that *C. albicans* and *S. mutans* interact in the oral cavity in a synergistic way [52–58] and both physical connections and metabolic interactions have been shown. For example, *S. mutans* uses lactic acid to supply a carbon source for *C. albicans* growth, which in turn causes the oxygen tension to drop to levels favorable to facultative streptococci [59]. *C. albicans* has been described on mineralized tooth surfaces, has shown the ability to adapt in dental biofilms and to possess virulence attributes associated with caries pathogenesis, such as the ability to produce acids, to grow under low pH conditions, combined with a high proteolytic activity [60]. The results of a recent study have clearly shown how the different chemical composition of different light-cured composites subjected to identical surface treatments can determine significant differences in terms of adhesion for *S. mutans* [61]. Similarly, it would be of definite clinical interest to further investigate on the potential of *C. albicans* to adhere and proliferate on the surface of different DRCs, particularly on the surface of composite materials subjected to additional heat-curing protocols aimed at improving their mechanical properties.

Thus, the aim of the present in vitro study was to analyze the ability of *C. albicans* to adhere and form biofilms on the surface of three commercially available heat cured dental composite resins having different chemical formulations but subjected to identical surface treatment and polymerization protocols.

2. Materials and Methods

Table 1 shows the experimental groups and composite resins used in the current study design and provides details on the material composition.

Table 1. Composite resins included in this study.

Experimental Group	Material	Manufacturer	Batch	Composition
GR	GrandioSO - Shade A2 - (Nanohybrid)	Voco GmbH (Cuxhaven, Germany)	2028459	89% (w/w) fillers (1 µm glass ceramic filler, 20 nm–40 nm silicon dioxide fillers), Bis-GMA, Bis-EMA, TEGDMA.
VD	Venus Diamond - Shade A2 - (Nanohybrid)	Kulzer GmbH (Hanau, Germany)	E8292	71% (w/w) fillers (0.2 µm Si-Zr fillers), Bis-GMA, TEGDMA.
BF	Enamel Plus HRi Biofunction - Shade BF2 - (Nanohybrid)	Micerium (Avegno, Genova, Italy)	2021006247	74% in weight (60% in volume) fillers (0.005 µm–0.05 µm silicon dioxide fillers), (0.2–3.0 µm glass fillers), Urethane dimethacrylate, Tricyclodecane dimethanol dimethacrylate.

2.1. Realization of Composite Discs

Disc-shaped specimens were manufactured by placing the gel material in polyvinylsiloxane molds, 2 mm high and having a 4 mm inner hole. To extrude the surplus material, filled molds were positioned between two glass slides held in place with a paper clip. A light-emitting diode curing unit (Celalux 3, VOCO, Cuxhaven, Germany) with an 8 mm tip diameter and an output power of 1300 mW/cm^2 was used to light-cure the material for 20 s. Each final composite disc had a total surface area of 50.27 mm^2. An ultrasonic bath was used to clean every disc, which were then subjected to an additional cycle of heat curing in a composite oven at 70 °C for 10 min (Bulb PlusT, Micerium, Avegno, Genova, Italy).

2.2. Saliva Collection

Human saliva samples were collected according to D'Ercole et al. (2022) and the Ethics Committee of "G. d'Annunzio" University, Chieti–Pescara, Italy (approval code SALI, N. 19 of the 10 September 2020) [61]. Healthy volunteers were enrolled who had not brushed or flossed their teeth for two hours, without active oral caries, periodontitis, dental care in progress or antibiotic therapy for at least three months before the study start. Saliva was collected, combined, centrifuged (16.000× g for 1 h at 4 °C) and filtered through filters with pores of 0.8, 0.45 and 0.2 mm to remove microorganisms. After being incubated for 24–48 h at 37 °C, saliva samples were deemed to be sterile if no growth could be seen in either an aerobic or anaerobic environment [61]. To perform the investigation, sterile saliva was collected into sterile tubes and stored in the freezer. Saliva was used to allow the saliva-acquired pellicle formation on the disks to reproduce a human-like environment.

2.3. Microbial Strain

Candida albicans S5 clinical strain, isolated from the oral cavity of patients who gave their informed consent for this study (reference number: BONEISTO N. 22-10.07.2021, G. d'Annunzio University, Chieti–Pescara, 10 July 2021), was used for the experiments. *C. albicans* S5, grown on Sabouraud dextrose agar (SAB, Oxoid, Milan, Italy) was cultured in RPMI 1640 (Sigma-Aldrich, Milan, Italy) plus 2% glucose and standardized to Optical Density (OD$_{600}$) = 0.15 corresponding to ≈10^6 CFU/mL [62]. *C. albicans* S5 was characterized for its capability to form a biofilm on a polystyrene surface, and it was a good biofilm producer.

2.4. Experimental Design

All disks, previously sterilized with ultraviolet UV light for 40 min, were placed on 96-well polystyrene microtiter plates and inoculated for 2 h in saliva at 37 °C in a shaking incubator with slight agitation to form the protein pellicle layer on the surface and to provide microbial adhesion. Subsequently, 200 µL of standardized *C. albicans* S5 suspension was added in each well with disk and incubated at 37 °C for 48 h in aerobic atmosphere.

For negative control, each composite disk was inoculated with only medium without the microbial culture and incubated as described above. For each test, a negative control was evaluated. After incubation, the evaluations were performed following the experimental plan (Figure 1).

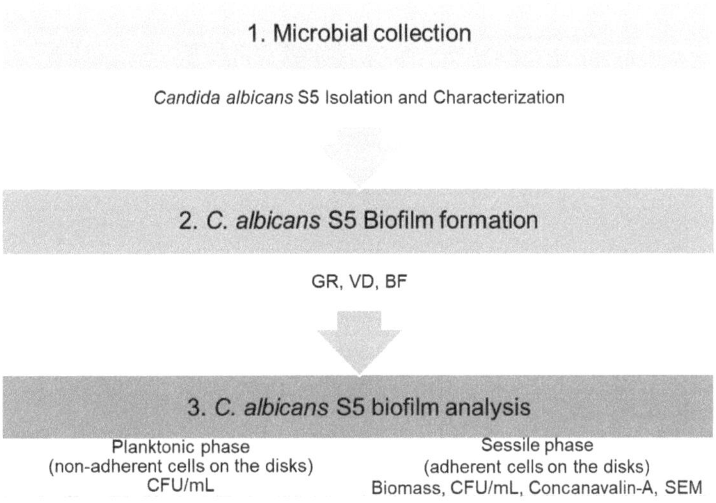

Figure 1. Schematic summary of the study design.

The planktonic phase was carefully removed from each well, diluted, spread on SAB and incubated at 37 °C for 48 h for the planktonic CFU count (CFU/mL), according to previous studies [55,57]. For the planktonic evaluation, 39 disks (10 tests and 3 negative controls for each different material), in triplicate, for a total of 117 disks were used.

The amount of *C. albicans* S5 adhered to each disk was evaluated for the following:
(i) Sessile CFU count (CFU/mL);
(ii) Biofilm biomass production;
(iii) Extracellular polymeric substances (EPS) of the biofilm matrix;
(iv) Morphology of the sessile colonies by Scanning Electron Microscopy (SEM).

The experimental planning was developed according to D'Ercole et al. [61].

Briefly, for sessile CFU/mL detection, after incubation for 48 h, the adherent viable cells were washed with PBS, detached by ultrasonication and vortexing, spread on SAB plates, incubated for 48 h at 37 °C and counted. The *C. albicans* S5 biomass was determined by Crystal violet (CV) staining at $OD_{570\,nm}$. A Concanavalin-A assay was carried out to evaluate the EPS of the biofilm's matrix. SEM evaluation was performed to morphologically analyze the sessile colonies. After 48 h of in vitro biofilm formation, 5 specimens from each group were fixed for 1 h in 2.5% glutaraldehyde, dehydrated in six ethanol washes (10%, 25%, 50%, 75% and 90% for 20 min and 100% for 1 h) and then dried overnight in a bacteriological incubator at 37 °C. Then, they were coated with gold (Emitech K550, Emitech Ltd., Ashford, Kent, UK) and observed carefully under a SEM (EVO 50 XVP LaB6, Carl Zeiss SMT Ltd., Cambridge, UK) at 15 kV, under 1000× and 5000× magnifications.

For the sessile phase, a total of 294 specimens (10 tests and 3 negative controls for each different material; 117 disks for sessile CFU/mL count and 117 disks for biofilm biomass quantification; 5 disks from each group for Concanavalin A assay and SEM evaluation) were used.

2.5. Statistical Analysis

In each group, means and standard deviations were calculated from raw data related to quantitative tests (planktonic CFU count, sessile cells CFU count and biomass quantification by $OD_{570\,nm}$). Statistical analysis was carried out according to the analysis of variance (ANOVA) and the Tukey's test for post hoc intergroup comparisons, using the SPSS for Windows version 21 (IBM SPSS Inc, Chicago, IL, USA). Levene's and Kolmogorov–Smirnov tests were used to validate the homogeneity of the variances and the normality of data, respectively. The level of α was set at 0.05 for all tests.

3. Results

Table 2 summarizes the results achieved from the quantitative tests carried out.

Table 2. C. albicans S5 detection on the three resin composites investigated.

	Experimental Group		
	GR	VD	BF
Planktonic CFU count ($\times 10^5$ CFU/mL) (SD)	29.80 [a] (3.16)	27.40 [a] (2.07)	31.00 [a] (2.49)
Sessile Cells CFU count ($\times 10^3$ CFU/mL) (SD)	2.65 [b] (0.47)	3.44 [a] (0.56)	2.90 [b] (0.17)
Biomass quantification $OD_{570\,nm}$ (SD)	0.6637 [b] (0.0427)	1.0327 [a] (0.1642)	0.5641 [c] (0.0752)

Different superscript letters indicate statistically significant differences.

3.1. Planktonic CFU/mL Count

Figure 2 shows the C. albicans S5 CFU/mL count in planktonic phase. Not statistically significant differences were detected among all groups ($p > 0.05$). A slight, but not significant, C. albicans S5 CFU/mL reduction was obtained with heat-cured VD ($27.40 \times 10^5 \pm 2.07 \times 10^5$ CFU/mL) as compared to heat-cured GR ($29.80 \times 10^5 \pm 3.16 \times 10^5$ CFU/mL) and BF ($31.00 \times 10^5 \pm 2.49 \times 10^5$ CFU/mL).

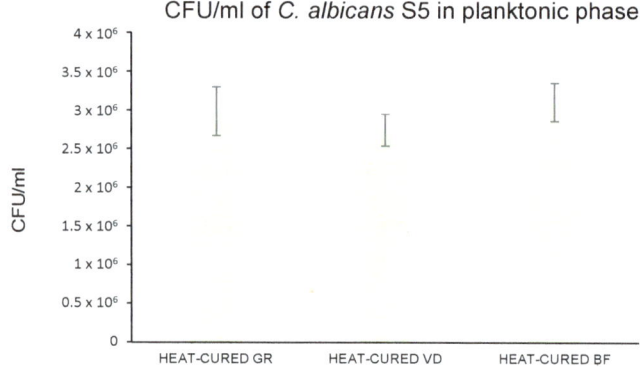

Figure 2. Planktonic C. albicans S5 CFU/mL count ($\times 10^5$ CFU/mL).

3.2. Sessile Cells CFU/mL Count

The CFU/mL of *C. albicans* S5 adherent to each tested disk are showed in Figure 3. In detail, the least fungal growth was observed on GR heat-cured ($2.65 \times 10^5 \pm 0.47 \times 10^5$ CFU/mL), with no statistically significant difference ($p < 0.05$) compared to BF heat-cured ($2.90 \times 10^5 \pm 0.17 \times 10^5$ CFU/mLt). A significantly increased number of CFU/mL was observed for VD ($3.44 \times 10^5 \pm 0.56 \times 10^5$) ($p < 0.05$).

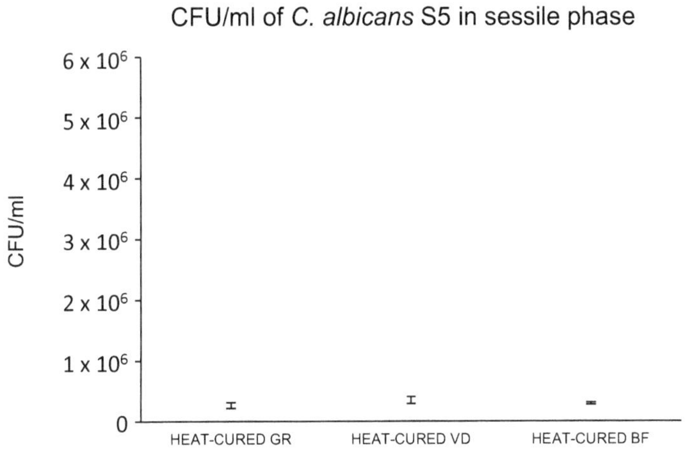

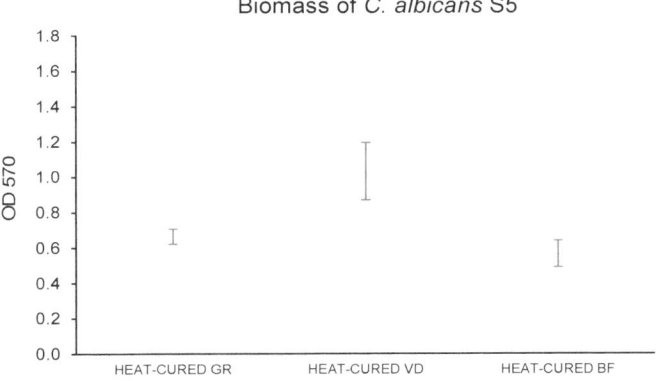

Figure 3. Sessile *C. albicans* S5 CFU/mL count ($\times 10^3$ CFU/mL).

3.3. Biofilm Biomass Quantification by Optical Density ($OD_{570\,nm}$)

The biomass production of *C. albicans* S5 adherent to each tested disk (Figure 4) showed a trend similar to that observed for the sessile cells CFU/mL count. The best results were displayed by heat-cured BF, with an $OD_{570\,nm}$ of the produced biofilm biomass equal to 0.564 ± 0.0752, significantly reduced as compared to both heat-cured GR (0.6637 ± 0.0427) ($p < 0.05$) and VD (1.0327 ± 0.1642) ($p < 0.05$). The biofilm biomass quantification on GR was significantly lower than VD ($p < 0.05$).

Figure 4. Biomass quantification by optical density ($OD_{570\,nm}$).

3.4. Concanavalin Assay

Figure 5 shows the polysaccharide matrix (EPS) production by *C. albicans* S5 biofilms on different composites disks. The images confirmed the biofilm biomass results with a major production of carbohydrates displayed on a heat-cured VD disk as compared to the other composites. A slight EPS reduction was also observed when comparing heat-cured BF to heat-cured GR.

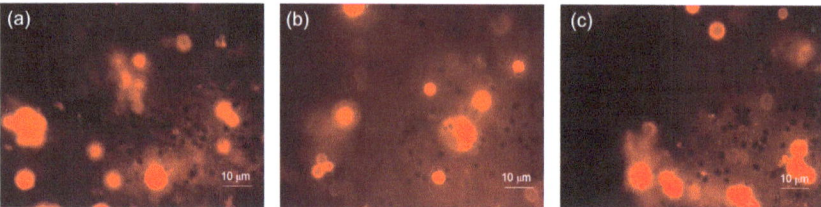

Figure 5. Representative images (original magnification 100×) of polysaccharide matrix (EPS) production by *C. albicans* S5 biofilms observed using Concanavalin-A on heat-cured GR (**a**), heat-cured VD (**b**) and heat-cured BF specimens (**c**).

3.5. SEM Analysis

Figure 6 shows representative SEM microphotographs of the *C. albicans* S5 biofilm formation on the composite disks. The VD group, which contained the greatest amount of fungal cells on its surface, showed relatively large adherent aggregates after 48 h of in vitro biofilm development (Figure 6b), while GR and BF showed smaller aggregates and an apparent reduced biofilm formation.

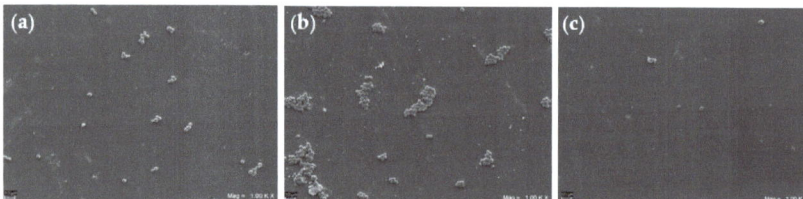

Figure 6. Representative SEM images (original magnification 10,000×) of *C. albicans* S5 biofilm formed on disk-shaped specimens from heat-cured GR (**a**), heat-cured VD (**b**) and heat-cured BF (**c**) groups.

4. Discussion

In the present investigation, the behavior of *C. albicans* S5 in the presence of three commercially available, nanohybrid DCRs, coated with human saliva, was evaluated by assessing the planktonic and sessile growth modes, the biofilm biomass quantification and the qualitative analysis of the extracellular polymeric substances (EPS) of the biofilm matrix by the Concanavalin-A assay and SEM observation. All samples were polymerized using the same standardized heat-curing protocol and received the same surface treatment. This made it possible to exclude the impact of possible confounding factors and allowed us to properly assess the effect of the only one variable under investigation (i.e., the unique chemical formulation of each different resin) on the biofilm formation [63,64]. Focusing on planktonic CFU assay, a not statistically significant difference among the tested groups emerged. A slight, but not significant, *C. albicans* S5 planktonic CFU/mL reduction was observed with VD as compared to GR. Regarding the sessile cells CFU count, a significant increase was observed for VD compared to GR and BF. The current findings demonstrated a relevant antiadhesive effect for GR and BF, with a significant decrease in the number of sessile CFUs, in the biomass quantification and in the presence of EPS matrix. BF had the most promising behavior when compared to the other composite, both in terms of antiadhesive activity and due to a general decrease in the biofilm biomass quantification. The *C. albicans* capability to adhere to disk is affected by the nature of the surface, the molecules involved in quorum sensing and the production of adhesin [65]. In particular, Park et al. demonstrated that the *C. albicans* adhesion on resin was reduced by the electrostatic repulsion force created and hydrophobic interactions between the surface and yeast [66]. Probably, even in the present study, a decreased yeast cells growth might be related to an increased surface hydrophilicity. As already reported by Kim et al., cells grown under bis-GMA showed significantly increased surface hydrophobicity, which could potentially enhance the ability of *C. albicans* S5 to adhere to hydrophobic surfaces [67]. As a result, in the current investigation, both bis-GMA-based composites (GR and VD), when compared to a bis-GMA free material (BF), showed a slight rise in the sessile CFU count.

Of course, antiadhesive and antibacterial qualities need to be carefully considered together with any potential cytotoxicity brought on by the monomers present in (and released from) dental materials [68,69]. Numerous in vitro investigations have shown that the free methacrylate monomer residues left over after the polymerization phase, which may cause the production of prostaglandin E2 (PGE2), the expression of cyclooxygenase 2 and an activation of the proinflammatory response via an increase in interleukin-1 (IL-1), IL-6 and nitric oxide (NO), are primarily responsible for the potential cytotoxicity of the CR organic components [70,71]. It has also been observed that resin monomers can affect cellular physiology and adaptive cell responses by boosting ROS generation [72,73]. In a recent study, De Angelis et al. investigated the biological effect of different resin-based composites on human gingival fibroblast by means of flow cytometry analysis and immunofluorescence. Interestingly, based on their results, GrandioSo (Voco GmbH) and Enamel Plus HRi Biofunction (Micerium) seemed the least cytotoxic among the materials they tested, leading to reduced oxidative stress and fewer genotoxic effects [74]. Therefore, for the abovementioned resins (GR and BF), the antiadhesive action and the general reduction in biomass quantification herein observed seems even more promising and clinically relevant, if combined with the reduced cytotoxicity shown in previous studies [70–73]. Furthermore, as far as GrandioSo (Voco GmbH) is concerned, in a recent study on light-cured materials, D'Ercole et al. found a stronger capability to reduce *S. mutans* growth (in terms of sessile CFU count, biofilm biomass, metabolic activity and polysaccharide production) compared to that of Venus Diamond (Kulzer GmbH), somehow strengthening the clinical relevance of the present findings [61]. In fact, several studies provided striking evidence that *S. mutans* and *C. albicans* develop a symbiotic relationship that enhances the virulence of cospecies plaque biofilms formed on tooth surfaces, ultimately amplifying the severity of disease [53,56,57]. Such an association between *C. albicans* and *S. mutans* appears to be largely mediated by a physical interaction that relies on the production of glucans, which are produced by bacterial exoenzymes (Gtfs), on yeast and hyphal cell surfaces. These interactions are essential for the assembly of an EPS-rich matrix, the formation of enlarged microcolonies containing densely packed *S. mutans* cells and the development of cospecies biofilms [45]. For these reasons, it should be underlined how the ability suggested for GR to limit the proliferation of both *C. albicans* and *S. mutans* might definitely be promising.

A lower amount of biofilm matrix, with a reduced biofilm thickness and less carbohydrate amount accumulation, may be clinically advantageous, as a biofilm with a reduced biomass is supposed to be less resistant to the salivary buffering effect, antibacterial agents and to the action of fluoride ions [61]. The presence of a thick and stable plaque biofilm, on the contrary, makes those defense mechanisms less effective, compromising the long-term outcome of composite resin restorations [43] and potentially increasing the risk for secondary caries. Thus, from a clinical point of view, it would be advisable to select a material that impairs adhesion, proliferation or even just extracellular matrix production of pathogenic microorganisms, in particular (based on the results of the present study) when dealing with indirect composites subjected to post-polymerization thermal cycles.

Among the limitations of the present study, it should be underlined that only the heat-curing protocol was herein evaluated, without taking into account the simple light-curing procedure. Photoactivation is the most prevalent method used to activate and promote the polymerization of resin based dental composites. The irradiance emitted by different models/brands of light-curing devices is variable, usually ranging between 400 and 1200 mW/cm^2 [75]. However, as already mentioned, monomer conversion is never complete during the polymerization of light-cured resin composites. This is the reasons why, when dealing with indirect restorations, resin composites are conveniently subjected to further heat curing. Such an additional heat treatment leads to an increase in the degree of conversion and improved mechanical properties such as microhardness, flexural strength, fracture toughness, wear resistance, tensile strength, color stability and a reduction of wear [11–14]. Thus, it seemed of greater clinical interest to investigate the antimicrobial activity of materials when they are used in their best performing modes.

As already mentioned, several studies have reported high prevalence for *S. mutans* in dental biofilms where *C. albicans* resides, suggesting that such a fungal–bacterial interaction can potentially contribute to dental caries [25,26,44,45]. Considering this association between *C. albicans* S5 and *S. mutans*, further studies seem necessary to better investigate the combined susceptibility of both microorganisms to resin-based material formulation in terms of adhesion and proliferation.

In brief, based on the present results, it can be concluded that different formulations of commercially available heat-cured resin composites may interact differently with *C. albicans*. In comparison to VD, GR and BF led to a decreased biofilm growth in terms of sessile CFU count, biofilm biomass and polysaccharide synthesis. Despite the fact that they also permitted *C. albicans* development to a certain level, these characteristics would suggest that GR and BF as more suitable restorative materials. Understanding that heat-cured composites may show a different affinity with *Candida albicans*, depending on their intrinsic chemical composition and despite the surface treatment, may be of great clinical relevance. In fact, an informed clinician could wisely select those materials that are able to limit the formation of biofilms by potentially cariogenic species, which might lead to secondary caries over time. Moreover, a better understanding about the affinity between restorative materials and cariogenic species would also encourage manufacturers of the dental industry towards the production and commercialization of resin composites that are less prone to allow an intense microbial proliferation.

Author Contributions: Conceptualization, F.D.A., S.D., M.V., L.V. and C.D.; methodology, F.D.A., S.D., M.V., L.V., S.D.L. and C.D.; software, F.D.A.; validation, F.D.A., S.D.L., M.D.G. and S.D.; formal analysis, F.D.A., S.D. and C.D.; investigation, F.D.A., V.B., M.V., M.B., S.D.L. and S.D.; resources, L.V. and C.D.; data curation, F.D.A., V.B., M.B. and S.D.; writing—original draft preparation, F.D.A., V.B., S.D.L. and S.D.; writing—review and editing, F.D.A., V.B., M.V., C.D. and L.C.; visualization, F.D.A., M.B. and M.D.G.; supervision, F.D.A., C.D., L.C. and S.D.; project administration, C.D. and L.C.; funding acquisition, C.D. All authors have read and agreed to the published version of the manuscript.

Funding: This research received no external funding.

Institutional Review Board Statement: This study was conducted according to the guidelines of the Declaration of Helsinki and approved by the Ethics Committee of "G. d'Annunzio" University, Chieti–Pescara, Italy (approval code SALI, N. 19 of 10 September 2020).

Informed Consent Statement: Informed consent was obtained from all subjects involved in this study.

Data Availability Statement: The data presented in this study are available on request from the corresponding author.

Conflicts of Interest: The authors declare no conflict of interest.

References

1. Van Landuyt, K.L.; Yoshida, Y.; Hirata, I.; Snauwaert, J.; De Munck, J.; Okazaki, M.; Suzuki, K.; Lambrechts, P.; Van Meerbeek, B. Influence of the chemical structure of functional monomers on their adhesive performance. *J. Dent. Res.* **2008**, *87*, 757–761. [CrossRef] [PubMed]

2. De Angelis, F.; D'Arcangelo, C.; Maliskova, N.; Vanini, L.; Vadini, M. Wear properties of different additive restorative materials used for onlay/overlay posterior restorations. *Oper. Dent.* **2020**, *45*, E156–E166. [CrossRef]
3. D'Arcangelo, C.; Vanini, L.; Rondoni, G.D.; Vadini, M.; De Angelis, F. Wear evaluation of prosthetic materials opposing themselves. *Oper. Dent.* **2018**, *43*, 38–50. [CrossRef]
4. D'Arcangelo, C.; Vanini, L.; Rondoni, G.D.; Pirani, M.; Vadini, M.; Gattone, M.; De Angelis, F. Wear properties of a novel resin composite compared to human enamel and other restorative materials. *Oper. Dent.* **2014**, *39*, 612–618. [CrossRef]
5. D'Arcangelo, C.; Vadini, M.; Buonvivere, M.; De Angelis, F. Safe clinical technique for increasing the occlusal vertical dimension in case of erosive wear and missing teeth. *Clin. Case Rep.* **2021**, *9*, e04697. [CrossRef] [PubMed]
6. Ferracane, J.L. Current trends in dental composites. *Crit. Rev. Oral Biol. Med.* **1995**, *6*, 302–318. [CrossRef] [PubMed]
7. Obici, A.C.; Sinhoreti, M.A.C.; Frollini, E.; Correr Sobrinho, L.; Consani, S. Degree of conversion of z250 composite determined by fourier transform infrared spectroscopy: Comparison of techniques, storage periods and photo-activation methods. *Mater. Res.* **2004**, *7*, 605–610. [CrossRef]
8. Peutzfeldt, A. Resin composites in dentistry: The monomer systems. *Eur. J. Oral Sci.* **1997**, *105*, 97–116. [CrossRef]
9. Amirouche-Korichi, A.; Mouzali, M.; Watts, D.C. Effects of monomer ratios and highly radiopaque fillers on degree of conversion and shrinkage-strain of dental resin composites. *Dent. Mater.* **2009**, *25*, 1411–1418. [CrossRef]
10. Daronch, M.; Rueggeberg, F.; De Goes, M. Monomer conversion of pre-heated composite. *J. Dent. Res.* **2005**, *84*, 663–667. [CrossRef]
11. Grazioli, G.; Francia, A.; Cuevas-Suárez, C.E.; Zanchi, C.H.; Moraes, R.R.D. Simple and low-cost thermal treatments on direct resin composites for indirect use. *Braz. Dent. J.* **2019**, *30*, 279–284. [CrossRef]
12. Lapesqueur, M.; Surriaga, P.; Masache, M.E.; Vásquez, B.; Peña, M.; Gómes, O.M.M.; Domínguez, J.A. Efectos sobre microdureza y grado de conversión de dos tipos de resinas sometidas a tratamientos de pospolimerización. *Rev. Nac. Odontol.* **2015**, *11*, 49–56. [CrossRef]
13. Cruz, F.L.; Carvalho, R.F.; Batista, C.H.T.; Siqueira-Júnior, H.M.; Queiroz, J.R.C.; Leite, F.P. Efecto del tratamiento térmico y de fibras de polietileno en la resistencia a la flexión de resinas compuestas. *Acta Odontol. Venez.* **2014**, *52*, 3–4.
14. Zamalloa-Quintana, M.; López-Gurreonero, C.; Santander-Rengifo, F.M.; Ladera-Castañeda, M.; Castro-Pérez Vargas, A.; Cornejo-Pinto, A.; Cervantes-Ganoza, L.; Cayo-Rojas, C. Effect of additional dry heat curing on microflexural strength in three types of resin composite: An in vitro study. *Crystals* **2022**, *12*, 1045. [CrossRef]
15. Al-Zain, A.O.; Platt, J.A. Effect of light-curing distance and curing time on composite microflexural strength. *Dent. Mater. J.* **2021**, *40*, 202–208. [CrossRef] [PubMed]
16. Al-Zain, A.O.; Marghalani, H.Y. Influence of light-curing distances on microflexural strength of two resin-based composites. *Oper. Dent.* **2020**, *45*, 297–305. [CrossRef]
17. Kumar, D.; Shukla, M.; Mahato, K.; Rathore, D.; Prusty, R.; Ray, B. Effect of Post-Curing on Thermal and Mechanical Behavior of gfrp Composites. *IOP Conf. Ser. Mater. Sci. Eng.* **2015**, *75*, 012012. [CrossRef]
18. Lucena-Martin, C.; Gonzalez-Lopez, S.; Navajas-Rodriguez de Mondelo, J.M. The effect of various surface treatments and bonding agents on the repaired strength of heat-treated composites. *J. Prosthet. Dent.* **2001**, *86*, 481–488. [CrossRef] [PubMed]
19. Uzay, C.; Boztepe, M.H.; Bayramoğlu, M.; Geren, N. Effect of post-curing heat treatment on mechanical properties of fiber reinforced polymer (frp) composites. *Mater. Test.* **2017**, *59*, 366–372. [CrossRef]
20. Takeshige, F.; Kinomoto, Y.; Torii, M. Additional heat-curing of light-cured composite resin for inlay restoration. *J. Osaka Univ. Dent. Sch.* **1995**, *35*, 59–66.
21. De Angelis, F.; Minnoni, A.; Vitalone, L.M.; Carluccio, F.; Vadini, M.; Paolantonio, M.; D'Arcangelo, C. Bond strength evaluation of three self-adhesive luting systems used for cementing composite and porcelain. *Oper. Dent.* **2011**, *36*, 626–634. [CrossRef] [PubMed]
22. De Angelis, F.; Vadini, M.; Buonvivere, M.; Valerio, A.; Di Cosola, M.; Piattelli, A.; Biferi, V.; D'Arcangelo, C. In vitro mechanical properties of a novel graphene-reinforced pmma-based dental restorative material. *Polymers* **2023**, *15*, 622. [CrossRef]
23. Re, D.; De Angelis, F.; Augusti, G.; Augusti, D.; Caputi, S.; D'Amario, M.; D'Arcangelo, C. Mechanical properties of elastomeric impression materials: An in vitro comparison. *Int. J. Dent.* **2015**, *2015*, 428286. [CrossRef] [PubMed]
24. D'Amario, M.; De Angelis, F.; Mancino, M.; Frascaria, M.; Capogreco, M.; D'Arcangelo, C. Canal shaping of different single-file systems in curved root canals. *J. Dent. Sci.* **2017**, *12*, 328–332. [CrossRef] [PubMed]
25. Jenkinson, H.F.; Lala, H.C.; Shepherd, M.G. Coaggregation of *Streptococcus sanguis* and other streptococci with *Candida albicans*. *Infect. Immun.* **1990**, *58*, 1429–1436. [CrossRef]
26. Kolenbrander, P.E.; Andersen, R.N.; Blehert, D.S.; Egland, P.G.; Foster, J.S.; Palmer, R.J., Jr. Communication among oral bacteria. *Microbiol. Mol. Biol. Rev.* **2002**, *66*, 486–505. [CrossRef]
27. Rickard, A.H.; Gilbert, P.; High, N.J.; Kolenbrander, P.E.; Handley, P.S. Bacterial coaggregation: An integral process in the development of multi-species biofilms. *Trends. Microbiol.* **2003**, *11*, 94–100. [CrossRef] [PubMed]
28. Vu, B.; Chen, M.; Crawford, R.J.; Ivanova, E.P. Bacterial extracellular polysaccharides involved in biofilm formation. *Molecules* **2009**, *14*, 2535–2554. [CrossRef]
29. Xiao, J.; Klein, M.I.; Falsetta, M.L.; Lu, B.; Delahunty, C.M.; Yates, J.R., III; Heydorn, A.; Koo, H. The exopolysaccharide matrix modulates the interaction between 3d architecture and virulence of a mixed-species oral biofilm. *PLoS Pathog.* **2012**, *8*, e1002623. [CrossRef]

30. Sultan, A.S.; Kong, E.F.; Rizk, A.M.; Jabra-Rizk, M.A. The oral microbiome: A lesson in coexistence. *PLoS Pathog.* **2018**, *14*, e1006719. [CrossRef]
31. Islam, B.; Khan, S.N.; Khan, A.U. Dental caries: From infection to prevention. *Med. Sci. Monit.* **2007**, *13*, RA196-203.
32. Koo, H.; Falsetta, M.L.; Klein, M.I. The exopolysaccharide matrix: A virulence determinant of cariogenic biofilm. *J. Dent. Res.* **2013**, *92*, 1065–1073. [CrossRef] [PubMed]
33. Lemos, J.A.; Quivey, R.G.; Koo, H.; Abranches, J. *Streptococcus mutans*: A new Gram-positive paradigm? *Microbiology* **2013**, *159*, 436–445. [CrossRef]
34. Klein, M.I.; Hwang, G.; Santos, P.H.; Campanella, O.H.; Koo, H. *Streptococcus mutans*-derived extracellular matrix in cariogenic oral biofilms. *Front. Cell. Infect. Microbiol.* **2015**, *5*, 10. [CrossRef] [PubMed]
35. Valm, A.M. The structure of dental plaque microbial communities in the transition from health to dental caries and periodontal disease. *J. Mol. Biol.* **2019**, *431*, 2957–2969. [CrossRef] [PubMed]
36. Bourbia, M.; Ma, D.; Cvitkovitch, D.G.; Santerre, J.P.; Finer, Y. Cariogenic bacteria degrade dental resin composites and adhesives. *J. Dent. Res.* **2013**, *92*, 989–994. [CrossRef]
37. Huang, B.; Siqueira, W.L.; Cvitkovitch, D.G.; Finer, Y. Esterase from a cariogenic bacterium hydrolyzes dental resins. *Acta Biomater.* **2018**, *71*, 330–338. [CrossRef]
38. Kruger, J.; Maletz, R.; Ottl, P.; Warkentin, M. In vitro aging behavior of dental composites considering the influence of filler content, storage media and incubation time. *PLoS ONE* **2018**, *13*, e0195160. [CrossRef]
39. Marashdeh, M.Q.; Gitalis, R.; Levesque, C.; Finer, Y. *Enterococcus faecalis* hydrolyzes dental resin composites and adhesives. *J. Endod.* **2018**, *44*, 609–613. [CrossRef]
40. Delaviz, Y.; Finer, Y.; Santerre, J.P. Biodegradation of resin composites and adhesives by oral bacteria and saliva: A rationale for new material designs that consider the clinical environment and treatment challenges. *Dent. Mater.* **2014**, *30*, 16–32. [CrossRef]
41. Opdam, N.J.; van de Sande, F.H.; Bronkhorst, E.; Cenci, M.S.; Bottenberg, P.; Pallesen, U.; Gaengler, P.; Lindberg, A.; Huysmans, M.C.; van Dijken, J.W. Longevity of posterior composite restorations: A systematic review and meta-analysis. *J. Dent. Res.* **2014**, *93*, 943–949. [CrossRef] [PubMed]
42. Demarco, F.F.; Collares, K.; Coelho-de-Souza, F.H.; Correa, M.B.; Cenci, M.S.; Moraes, R.R.; Opdam, N.J. Anterior composite restorations: A systematic review on long-term survival and reasons for failure. *Dent. Mater.* **2015**, *31*, 1214–1224. [CrossRef] [PubMed]
43. Kusuma Yulianto, H.D.; Rinastiti, M.; Cune, M.S.; de Haan-Visser, W.; Atema-Smit, J.; Busscher, H.J.; van der Mei, H.C. Biofilm composition and composite degradation during intra-oral wear. *Dent. Mater.* **2019**, *35*, 740–750. [CrossRef]
44. Metwalli, K.H.; Khan, S.A.; Krom, B.P.; Jabra-Rizk, M.A. *Streptococcus mutans*, *Candida albicans*, and the human mouth: A sticky situation. *PLoS Pathog.* **2013**, *9*, e1003616. [CrossRef] [PubMed]
45. Falsetta, M.L.; Klein, M.I.; Colonne, P.M.; Scott-Anne, K.; Gregoire, S.; Pai, C.-H.; Gonzalez-Begne, M.; Watson, G.; Krysan, D.J.; Bowen, W.H. Symbiotic relationship between *Streptococcus mutans* and *Candida albicans* synergizes virulence of plaque biofilms in vivo. *Infect. Immun.* **2014**, *82*, 1968–1981. [CrossRef]
46. Pereira, D.F.A.; Seneviratne, C.J.; Koga-Ito, C.Y.; Samaranayake, L.P. Is the oral fungal pathogen *Candida albicans* a cariogen? *Oral Dis.* **2018**, *24*, 518–526. [CrossRef] [PubMed]
47. Xiao, J.; Huang, X.; Alkhers, N.; Alzamil, H.; Alzoubi, S.; Wu, T.T.; Castillo, D.A.; Campbell, F.; Davis, J.; Herzog, K.; et al. Candida albicans and early childhood caries: A systematic review and meta-analysis. *Caries Res.* **2018**, *52*, 102–112. [CrossRef]
48. Krom, B.P.; Kidwai, S.; Ten Cate, J.M. Candida and other fungal species: Forgotten players of healthy oral microbiota. *J. Dent. Res.* **2014**, *93*, 445–451. [CrossRef]
49. Fidel, P.L., Jr. Candida-host interactions in hiv disease: Implications for oropharyngeal candidiasis. *Adv. Dent. Res.* **2011**, *23*, 45–49. [CrossRef]
50. Williams, D.; Lewis, M. Pathogenesis and treatment of oral candidosis. *J. Oral Microbiol.* **2011**, *3*, 5771. [CrossRef]
51. Jabra-Rizk, M.A.; Kong, E.F.; Tsui, C.; Nguyen, M.H.; Clancy, C.J.; Fidel, P.L., Jr.; Noverr, M. *Candida albicans* pathogenesis: Fitting within the host-microbe damage response framework. *Infect. Immun.* **2016**, *84*, 2724–2739. [CrossRef] [PubMed]
52. Jenkinson, H.; Barbour, M.; Jagger, D.; Miles, M.; Bamford, C.; Nobbs, A.; Dutton, L.; Silverman, R.; McNally, L.; Vickerman, M. *Candida albicans*-bacteria interactions in biofilms and disease. *Univ. Bristol. Dent. Sch.* **2008**, *16*. [CrossRef]
53. Diaz, P.I.; Xie, Z.; Sobue, T.; Thompson, A.; Biyikoglu, B.; Ricker, A.; Ikonomou, L.; Dongari-Bagtzoglou, A. Synergistic interaction between *Candida albicans* and commensal oral streptococci in a novel in vitro mucosal model. *Infect. Immun.* **2012**, *80*, 620–632. [CrossRef] [PubMed]
54. Xu, H.; Dongari-Bagtzoglou, A. Shaping the oral mycobiota: Interactions of opportunistic fungi with oral bacteria and the host. *Curr. Opin. Microbiol.* **2015**, *26*, 65–70. [CrossRef]
55. Ellepola, K.; Liu, Y.; Cao, T.; Koo, H.; Seneviratne, C.J. Bacterial gtfb augments *Candida albicans* accumulation in cross-kingdom biofilms. *J. Dent. Res.* **2017**, *96*, 1129–1135. [CrossRef] [PubMed]
56. Koo, H.; Andes, D.R.; Krysan, D.J. Candida-streptococcal interactions in biofilm-associated oral diseases. *PLoS Pathog.* **2018**, *14*, e1007342. [CrossRef]
57. Montelongo-Jauregui, D.; Lopez-Ribot, J.L. Candida interactions with the oral bacterial microbiota. *J. Fungi* **2018**, *4*, 122. [CrossRef]
58. Montelongo-Jauregui, D.; Saville, S.P.; Lopez-Ribot, J.L. Contributions of *Candida albicans* dimorphism, adhesive interactions, and extracellular matrix to the formation of dual-species biofilms with *Streptococcus gordonii*. *mBio* **2019**, *10*, e01179-19. [CrossRef]

59. Jenkinson, H.F.; Lamont, R.J. Oral microbial communities in sickness and in health. *Trends Microbiol.* **2005**, *13*, 589–595. [CrossRef] [PubMed]
60. Xiang, Z.; Wakade, R.S.; Ribeiro, A.A.; Hu, W.; Bittinger, K.; Simon-Soro, A.; Kim, D.; Li, J.; Krysan, D.J.; Liu, Y.; et al. Human tooth as a fungal niche: *Candida albicans* traits in dental plaque isolates. *mBio* **2023**, *14*, e0276922. [CrossRef]
61. D'Ercole, S.; De Angelis, F.; Biferi, V.; Noviello, C.; Tripodi, D.; Di Lodovico, S.; Cellini, L.; D'Arcangelo, C. Antibacterial and antibiofilm properties of three resin-based dental composites against *Streptococcus mutans*. *Materials* **2022**, *15*, 6933. [CrossRef]
62. Di Lodovico, S.; Dotta, T.C.; Cellini, L.; Iezzi, G.; D'Ercole, S.; Petrini, M. The antibacterial and antifungal capacity of eight commercially available types of mouthwash against oral microorganisms: An in vitro study. *Antibiotics* **2023**, *12*, 675. [CrossRef] [PubMed]
63. Mena Silva, P.A.; Garcia, I.M.; Nunes, J.; Visioli, F.; Castelo Branco Leitune, V.; Melo, M.A.; Collares, F.M. Myristyltrimethylammonium bromide (mytab) as a cationic surface agent to inhibit *Streptococcus mutans* grown over dental resins: An in vitro study. *J. Funct. Biomater.* **2020**, *11*, 9. [CrossRef] [PubMed]
64. Cazzaniga, G.; Ottobelli, M.; Ionescu, A.; Garcia-Godoy, F.; Brambilla, E. Surface properties of resin-based composite materials and biofilm formation: A review of the current literature. *Am. J. Dent.* **2015**, *28*, 311–320.
65. Gad, M.M.; Fouda, S.M. Current perspectives and the future of *Candida albicans*-associated denture stomatitis treatment. *Dent. Med. Probl.* **2020**, *57*, 95–102. [CrossRef]
66. Park, S.E.; Blissett, R.; Susarla, S.M.; Weber, H.P. *Candida albicans* adherence to surface-modified denture resin surfaces. *J. Prosthodont.* **2008**, *17*, 365–369. [CrossRef]
67. Masuoka, J.; Hazen, K.C. Cell wall protein mannosylation determines *Candida albicans* cell surface hydrophobicity. *Microbiology* **1997**, *143*, 3015–3021. [CrossRef] [PubMed]
68. Trubiani, O.; Caputi, S.; Di Iorio, D.D.; Amario, M.; Paludi, M.; Giancola, R.; Di Nardo Di Maio, F.; De Angelis, F.; D'Arcangelo, C. The cytotoxic effects of resin-based sealers on dental pulp stem cells. *Int. Endod. J.* **2010**, *43*, 646–653. [CrossRef]
69. Trubiani, O.; Cataldi, A.; De Angelis, F.; D'Arcangelo, C.; Caputi, S. Overexpression of interleukin-6 and -8, cell growth inhibition and morphological changes in 2-hydroxyethyl methacrylate-treated human dental pulp mesenchymal stem cells. *Int. Endod. J.* **2012**, *45*, 19–25. [CrossRef] [PubMed]
70. Kuan, Y.H.; Huang, F.M.; Lee, S.S.; Li, Y.C.; Chang, Y.C. Bisgma stimulates prostaglandin e2 production in macrophages via cyclooxygenase-2, cytosolic phospholipase a2, and mitogen-activated protein kinases family. *PLoS ONE* **2013**, *8*, e82942. [CrossRef] [PubMed]
71. Huang, F.M.; Chang, Y.C.; Lee, S.S.; Yeh, C.H.; Lee, K.G.; Huang, Y.C.; Chen, C.J.; Chen, W.Y.; Pan, P.H.; Kuan, Y.H. Bisgma-induced cytotoxicity and genotoxicity in macrophages are attenuated by wogonin via reduction of intrinsic caspase pathway activation. *Environ. Toxicol.* **2016**, *31*, 176–184. [CrossRef] [PubMed]
72. Lottner, S.; Shehata, M.; Hickel, R.; Reichl, F.X.; Durner, J. Effects of antioxidants on DNA-double strand breaks in human gingival fibroblasts exposed to methacrylate based monomers. *Dent. Mater.* **2013**, *29*, 991–998. [CrossRef]
73. Gallorini, M.; Petzel, C.; Bolay, C.; Hiller, K.A.; Cataldi, A.; Buchalla, W.; Krifka, S.; Schweikl, H. Activation of the nrf2-regulated antioxidant cell response inhibits hema-induced oxidative stress and supports cell viability. *Biomaterials* **2015**, *56*, 114–128. [CrossRef] [PubMed]
74. De Angelis, F.; Mandatori, D.; Schiavone, V.; Melito, F.P.; Valentinuzzi, S.; Vadini, M.; Di Tomo, P.; Vanini, L.; Pelusi, L.; Pipino, C.; et al. Cytotoxic and genotoxic effects of composite resins on cultured human gingival fibroblasts. *Materials* **2021**, *14*, 5225. [CrossRef] [PubMed]
75. Rueggeberg, F.A.; Giannini, M.; Arrais, C.A.G.; Price, R.B.T. Light curing in dentistry and clinical implications: A literature review. *Braz. Oral Res.* **2017**, *31*, e61. [CrossRef]

Disclaimer/Publisher's Note: The statements, opinions and data contained in all publications are solely those of the individual author(s) and contributor(s) and not of MDPI and/or the editor(s). MDPI and/or the editor(s) disclaim responsibility for any injury to people or property resulting from any ideas, methods, instructions or products referred to in the content.

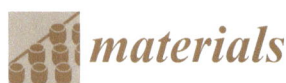 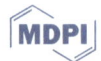

Article

Effectiveness of a Single Chair Side Application of NovaMin® [Calcium Sodium Phosphosilicate] in the Treatment of Dentine Hypersensitivity Following Ultrasonic Scaling—A Randomized Controlled Trial

Jeeth Janardhan Rai [1], Saurabh Chaturvedi [2,*], Shankar T. Gokhale [3], Raghavendra Reddy Nagate [3], Saad M. Al-Qahtani [3], Mohammad Al. Magbol [3], Shashit Shetty Bavabeedu [4], Mohamed Fadul A. Elagib [3], Vatsala Venkataram [5] and Mudita Chaturvedi [6]

[1] Department of Periodontology, Bharati Vidyapeeth Dental College and Hospital, Sangli 416406, Maharastra, India
[2] Department of Prosthetic Dentistry, College of Dentistry, King Khalid University, Abha 61421, Saudi Arabia
[3] Department of Periodontics and Community Dental Sciences, College of Dentistry, King Khalid University, Abha 61421, Saudi Arabia
[4] Restorative Dental Sciences, College of Dentistry, King Khalid University, Abha 61421, Saudi Arabia
[5] Department of Pedodontics & Preventive Dentistry, KVG Dental College & Hospital, Sullia 574327, Karnataka, India
[6] Independent Researcher, Bhopal 462008, Madhya Pradesh, India
* Correspondence: survedi@kku.edu.sa; Tel.: +966-580697248

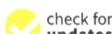

Citation: Rai, J.J.; Chaturvedi, S.; Gokhale, S.T.; Nagate, R.R.; Al-Qahtani, S.M.; Magbol, M.A.; Bavabeedu, S.S.; Elagib, M.F.A.; Venkataram, V.; Chaturvedi, M. Effectiveness of a Single Chair Side Application of NovaMin® [Calcium Sodium Phosphosilicate] in the Treatment of Dentine Hypersensitivity Following Ultrasonic Scaling—A Randomized Controlled Trial. *Materials* 2023, *16*, 1329. https://doi.org/10.3390/ma16041329

Academic Editors: Lavinia Cosmina Ardelean and Laura-Cristina Rusu

Received: 31 October 2022
Revised: 8 January 2023
Accepted: 1 February 2023
Published: 4 February 2023

Copyright: © 2023 by the authors. Licensee MDPI, Basel, Switzerland. This article is an open access article distributed under the terms and conditions of the Creative Commons Attribution (CC BY) license (https:// creativecommons.org/licenses/by/ 4.0/).

Abstract: Dentinal hypersensitivity or cervical dentinal sensitivity is one of the commonest clinical problems. The aim of this randomized controlled trial was to evaluate the effectiveness of a single chair side application of 100% pure calcium sodium phosphosilicate (NovaMin®) in reducing dentin hypersensitivity following ultrasonic scaling as evaluated on a visual analogue scale (VAS). The study included 50 subjects who were selected based on an evaluation of dentinal hypersensitivity on a VAS carried out using a metered air blast from a three-way syringe and divided into two groups (n = 25/group); i.e., the test group (Group A) received the NovaMin® paste and the control group (Group B) received a placebo paste made from pumice. All the 50 subjects included in the study were had VAS scores of 3 or more. The NovaMin® powder mixed with distilled water was applied. Dentinal hypersensitivity was reassessed immediately and after 1, 2 and 4 weeks after the procedure. Results showed that the percentage reduction of dentinal hypersensitivity following a single application of NovaMin® in powder form was about 76.38% immediately, 67.72% one week postoperatively, 52.76% two weeks postoperatively and 26.78% four weeks postoperatively. It can be concluded from the results of the current clinical study demonstrated that a single chair side application of NovaMin® in powder form has a significant and immediate reduction in dentinal hypersensitivity, which lasted nearly for four weeks.

Keywords: NovaMin®; bioactive glass; dentinal hypersensitivity; calcium sodium phosphosilicate

1. Introduction

The hypersensitivity arising from the tooth as a whole or especially from the cervical part of the tooth is one of the commonest clinical problems. It is characterized by acute, non-spontaneous, short or long-lasting pain arising from exposed dentine in response to stimuli typically thermal, evaporative, tactile, osmotic or chemical, and which cannot be corelated to pathology arising from a dental defect of any other origin form [1–3]. Hypersensitivity is attributed to the general increase in exposed dentine over the root surfaces of the teeth resulting from periodontal disease, toothbrush abrasion or a pointed load of repetitive stress at the thin enamel near the cementoenamel junction [4,5].

The age for occurrence of dentinal hypersensitivity generally ranges from early teenagers up to 70-year-old individuals [6]. However, the increased incidence is generally reported to be between the range of 20 to 40 years old, and it is more prevalent in females [6–8]. The buccal cervical area has the highest predilection for dentinal hypersensitivity [7]. Several studies have shown that the prevalence rate of dentinal hypersensitivity varies from 2 to 85% [9,10]. Dentinal hypersensitivity has also been shown to have a negative effect on psychological and emotional wellbeing. The causes of dentine hypersensitivity are basically from three factors, viz.: (i) recession leading to root exposure, (ii) formation of porosities at the surface followed by exposure of nascent dentinal tubules and (iii) susceptibility of pulp nerves to alteration of movement of the fluid in the dentine. Overall, it appears that it is the combination of more than one of the above-mentioned factors that might lead to dentinal hypersensitivity, rather than just the one factor responsible for it. Irrespective of etiologies for exposure to dentine, the apparent cause and effect is the open dentinal tubules which provide a direct link between the oral environment and the pulp chamber. The occurrence of hypersensitivity will be very unlikely when the dentinal tubules are fully covered by overlying enamel and cementum. The apertures of the dentinal tubules around the sensitive teeth are patent, and this causes the availability of stimuli close to the nerves. The hydrodynamic theory put forth by Brannstrom and colleagues [11,12] is by far the most widely accepted explanation for dentinal hypersensitivity. According to this theory's postulates, temperature, physical, or osmotic changes can upset the fluids in the dentinal tubules, and these fluid movements can activate a baroreceptor and cause a neural discharge.

Periodontal therapy including surgical and non-surgical therapies are routinely carried out by dentists. Patients often report an immediate increase in dentinal sensitivity during the procedure or post-procedure once the anesthetic effect wears off. Studies have shown that routine periodontal therapies like ultrasonic scaling have been shown to cause an increase in dentinal sensitivity [13–17]. The duration required for the dentinal sensitivity to slowly subside would be around two weeks [14]. Sensitivity following ultrasonic scaling may be attributed to the inadvertent damage occurring to the tooth structure exposing the dentine to the oral cavity. It is also linked to the presence of calculus which occludes the tubules and can lead to the exposure of dentinal tubules following its removal from that area.

There are various treatment modalities presently in vogue towards managing and preventing dentinal hypersensitivity, including nerve desensitization, anti-inflammatory agents, plugging dentinal tubules, dentinal sealers, periodontal soft tissue grafting, crown placement/restorative materials and LASERS (light amplification by the stimulated emission of radiation) [18,19].

Out of all of these methods, the one most frequently used to treat dentinal hypersensitivity is plugging the exposed dentinal tubules with a substance that forms a deposition layer and mechanically occludes dentinal tubules. This method lessens sensitivity by putting a barrier between the flow of pulpal fluid and dentine. The different substances used in this route include potassium oxalate, sodium monofluorophosphate, calcium hydroxide, ferrous oxide, potassium oxalate, sodium monofluorophosphate, sodium fluoride, sodium fluoride/stannous fluoride combination, stannous fluoride, strontium chloride, formaldehyde, glutaraldehyde, silver nitrate, strontium chloride, hexahydrate, casein phosphopeptides, burnishing fluoride and iontophoresis [8,20–27].

Numerous studies have been conducted on the use of NovaMin®, a type of bioactive glass that contains calcium sodium phosphosilicate, to alleviate dentinal sensitivity [28–37]. The brand name NovaMin® refers to a particulate bioactive glass that was created and patented by NovaMin® Technology, Inc. and is used in dental care products to remineralize teeth (Alachua, FL, USA). NovaMin® is made up of 45% SiO_2, 24.5% Na_2O, 24.5% CaO, and 6% P_2O_5 in aqueous solutions. Calcium, phosphorus, silica, and sodium, which are essential for the mineralization of bones and teeth, are provided by NovaMin® in an ionic form. When these substances are exposed to bodily fluids, they react strongly and deposit hydroxyapatite, a mineral that is chemically similar to the minerals found in bone, enamel, and dentin.

When NovaMin® is exposed to an aqueous environment, the physical occlusion of NovaMin® particles begins. The particles' sodium ions start exchanging with hydrogen cations rapidly. This quick release of ions enables the release of phosphate and calcium ions from the structure of the NovaMin® particle. As soon as the particles are exposed, a number of early reactions start to take place. As long as the particles are exposed to an aqueous environment, the calcium and phosphate ions continue to be released. When NovaMin® is first exposed, the release of sodium causes a localized, brief rise in pH. By precipitating the calcium and phosphate ions from the NovaMin® particle, as well as the calcium and phosphorus present in saliva, this rise in pH aids in the formation of a calcium phosphate layer. The layer crystallizes into hydroxycarbonate apatite, which is chemically and structurally identical to biological apatite, as the particle reactions and calcium and phosphorus complex deposition proceed. The physical blockage of dentinal tubules caused by the interaction of the remaining NovaMin® particles and the hydroxycarbonate apatite layer will reduce hypersensitivity [28,29].

Clinical trials have shown the efficacy of NovaMin®-containing toothpaste in significantly reducing dentinal hypersensitivity over an eight-week period with follow-up interviews up to twelve weeks after cessation of product use [33]. Another study comparing NovaMin®-containing toothpaste with other desensitizing toothpastes showed that NovaMin®-containing toothpaste performs as well as or better than the positive control with respect to rapidly relieving tooth hypersensitivity after two weeks and six weeks of daily use [34]. There are a few studies showing the efficacy of the NovaMin® powder applied after ultrasonic scaling followed by using the NovaMin® toothpaste at home later [36,37]. A literature search shows no study mentioning the effects of a single use of NovaMin® following ultrasonic scaling on dentinal sensitivity.

The aim of the current randomized clinical trial was to evaluate the efficacy of single chair-side application of NovaMin® in powder form to reduce dentin hypersensitivity as evaluated on a visual analogue scale (VAS) [38] over a four-week period.

2. Materials and Methods

2.1. Study Design

A double-blind parallel arm randomized controlled study was planned to evaluate the effectiveness of single chair-side application of NovaMin® in powder form and to compare with pumice as a negative control to reduce dentin hypersensitivity as evaluated on a visual analogue scale (VAS) following ultrasonic scaling. The study was conducted in accordance with the Declaration of Helsinki, and the protocol was approved by the Ethics Committee of the Institute, College of Dentistry, King Khalid University, Abha, KSA. (IRB/KKUCOD/ETH/2019-20/012). Before taking part in the study, all subjects provided their informed consent for inclusion and the study protocol was created.

2.2. Study Subjects and Sample Size

Sample size (n) was calculated by using formula

$$n = \frac{2(\text{Standard deviation})^2}{(\text{Effect size})^2}(Z_{\alpha/2} + Z_{1-\beta})^2$$

where $Z_{\alpha/2}$ = 1.96 and $Z_{1-\beta}$ = 0.842, respectively, represent the 95% confidence intervals based on the usual normal distribution with an 80% study power. To identify a significant difference in dentin hypersensitivity following intervention with NovaMin®, with an effect size of 0.50 and a standard deviation of 0.45 from the pilot trial utilizing ten patients, at least seventeen subjects were required. To reach the final sample size, 10% of n is added to account for dropouts. As a result, we kept n = 25 patients in each group even though the minimal sample size needed for each group was n = 20.

The study was conducted on 50 subjects (aged between 25 to 40 years) having mild to moderate localized dentinal hypersensitivity in the Department of Periodontology. The patients were divided randomly into two groups i.e., the test group (Group A) receiving NovaMin® paste and the control group (Group B) receiving a placebo paste made from pumice. Dentin hypersensitivity was measured in each selected subject. Each group was subdivided again based on the time from T0 to T5. T0 was before the start of the treatment, T1 was immediately after ultrasonic scaling, T2 was post-treatment, T3 was one week after treatment, T4 was 2 weeks after treatment and T5 was 4 weeks after treatment.

2.3. Preparation of NovaMin® Paste and Pumice Paste

The NovaMin® paste was prepared by using pure NovaMin® powder (Denshield; NovaMin® Technology, Alachua, FL, USA, Shield Starter) (Figure 1) and mixing it with distilled water to form a mono-structured paste. Pumice paste was prepared by using a fine pumice powder and mixing it with distilled water to give a similar paste.

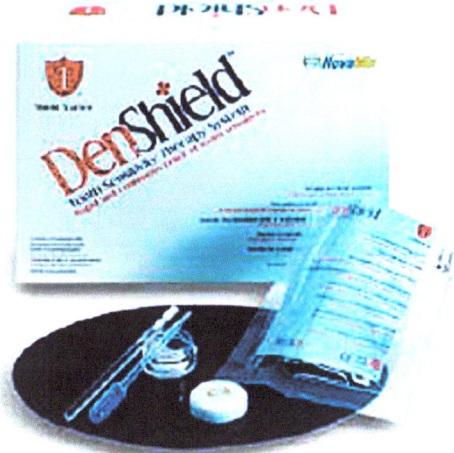

Figure 1. NovaMin® paste prepared by mixing pure novamin powder (Denshield; Shield Starter) and with distilled water.

2.4. Assessment of Dentin Hypersensitivity

Sensitivity was measured using a metered air blast of a five-second duration on a visual analogue scale (VAS) with a rating of 0 to 10 [38] (Figure 2). Subjects having at least one tooth sensitive to air stimulation with a VAS rating of 3 or more were included in the study (T1). All 50 subjects included in the study had a VAS rating of 3 or more. The most sensitive tooth in the oral cavity was selected (Figure 3). Exclusion criteria included patients already using desensitizing toothpaste or mouthwashes which may alter the study, severe wasting disease of teeth, restorations in the quadrant of the study and extreme dentinal hypersensitivity which may require restorative or endodontic treatment. Before the start of the treatment, both groups received a thorough ultrasonic scaling. Sensitivity was re-assessed after ultrasonic scaling again (T1).

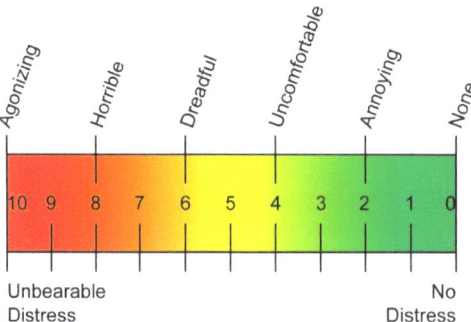

Figure 2. Visual analogue scale (VAS).

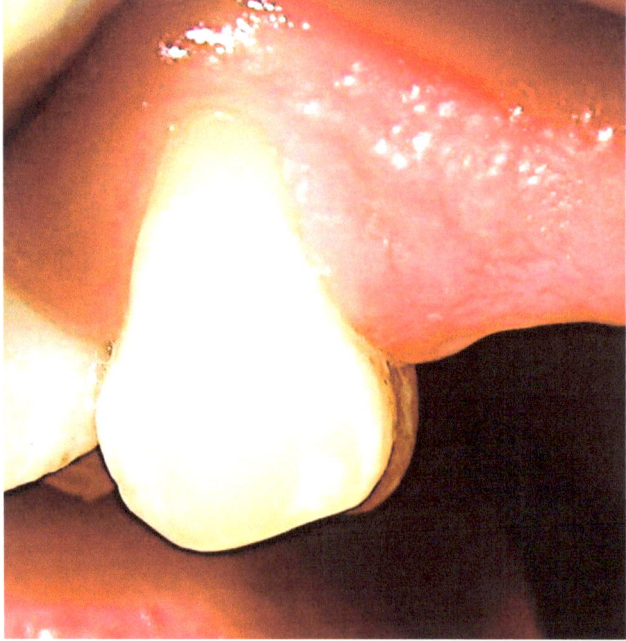

Figure 3. Selection of the most sensitive tooth in the oral cavity.

2.5. Study Procedure

A total of fifty subjects were randomly divided into two equal intervention groups using a lottery approach, with Group A subjects receiving NovaMin® as the intervention (n = 25) and Group B receiving Pumice (n = 25). The intervention groups were only known to one researcher, and the subjects were given identifying codes. For the subsequent follow-up visits, the VAS assessment was carried out by the same researcher.

The NovaMin® powder was mixed with distilled water to get a smooth paste-like consistency. The identified tooth in the test group was isolated using cotton rolls and dried using a blast of air for 5 s leaving the tooth moist but not wet. The NovaMin® paste was gently applied on the tooth surface and left for 2 min which allows mineralization to take place (Figure 4). Then the tooth was irrigated lightly with water from a three-way syringe for 15 to 20 s until all the NovaMin® paste was removed. Dentinal hypersensitivity was re-evaluated (T2). Similarly, the control group received a placebo made from mixing pumice and distilled water with a similar consistency as the NovaMin® paste and the prepared paste was applied to the isolated sensitive tooth, left for 2 min, and irrigated lightly to remove the pumice mixture. Sensitivity was re-evaluated again (T2).

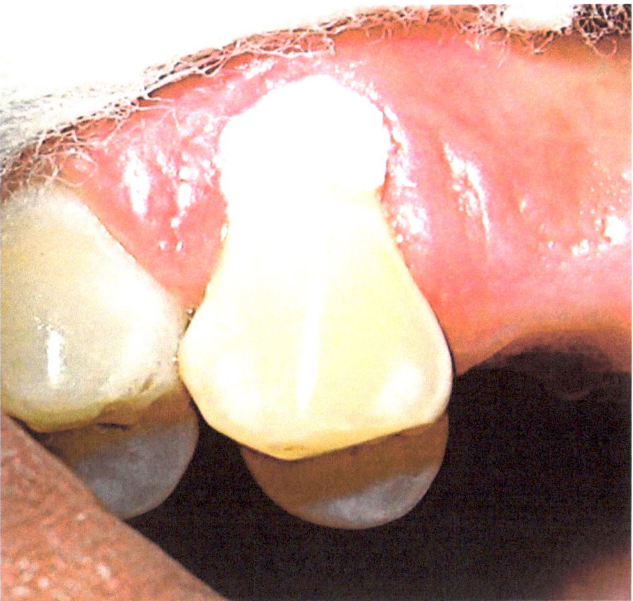

Figure 4. Application of the NovaMin® paste on the most sensitive tooth.

The subjects were advised not to eat or drink anything for the next 30 min. Patients were given oral hygiene instructions and recalled after 1, 2 and 4 weeks to reassess the sensitivity (T3, T4 and T5).

Every participant finished the research, and no one experienced any problems at the follow-up sessions. Desensitizing agents were prescribed to patients who felt the need for their use at the completion of the research.

2.6. Statistical Analysis

First, the data collected was entered into an MS-Excel spreadsheet, and then was subjected to analysis using SPSS for Windows, Version 16.0. USA, Chicago, Illinois: SPSS Inc. Frequency, mean, and standard deviation were used to show the results in a descriptive manner. The study used Freidman's test, the Mann—Whitney test, and the Wilcoxon signed-rank post hoc test for statistical analysis in order to compare the mean VAS scores between the two groups, between time intervals, the mean difference between the two groups' mean VAS scores, and the mean percentage increase between the test and control groups' mean VAS scores.

3. Results

The results show that ultrasonic scaling increases the amount of dentinal sensitivity from an average VAS score of 3.46 to a score of 4.96. The average VAS score in the test group fell from 5.04 to 0.96 immediately following the NovaMin® application and increased slightly to 1.76 one week postoperatively, 2.04 two weeks postoperatively and 1.92 four weeks postoperatively. The control group also showed a slight fall in VAS scores, from an average VAS score of 4.88 to an average VAS score of 3.76 with the follow-up VAS scores being 3.84 one week postoperatively, 3.6 two weeks postoperatively and 3.08 four weeks postoperatively (Table 1).

Table 1. VAS reading at different time intervals in two groups. (T0–Before Scaling; T1–After Scaling; T2–Post Procedure, T3–Post 1 Week, T4–Post 2 weeks and T5–Post 4 weeks).

Time Interval	Test Group						Control Group					
	T0	T1	T2	T3	T4	T5	T0	T1	T2	T3	T4	T5
Patient-1	2	3	0	1	1	1	2	4	3	3	3	2
Patient-2	2	4	2	3	3	2	2	4	3	2	2	2
Patient-3	2	4	1	1	2	2	5	6	4	5	5	4
Patient-4	4	6	2	3	3	4	3	4	3	3	3	3
Patient-5	4	5	1	2	2	3	2	5	3	3	2	2
Patient-6	4	4	0	1	2	2	2	3	2	2	3	3
Patient-7	2	3	0	1	1	2	4	6	5	4	4	4
Patient-8	4	4	0	1	1	2	6	7	5	5	4	5
Patient-9	5	6	2	3	3	2	5	5	5	5	5	4
Patient-10	3	5	1	2	2	2	2	4	4	4	4	3
Patient-11	3	7	3	2	2	1	4	5	3	4	4	4
Patient-12	3	4	0	1	1	2	5	6	4	4	4	3
Patient-13	5	7	2	2	3	2	5	7	5	5	4	4
Patient-14	4	7	1	2	2	2	3	3	2	3	2	1
Patient-15	4	4	0	2	2	2	4	5	5	5	4	3
Patient-16	4	5	1	2	2	2	2	3	3	3	3	3
Patient-17	4	6	0	3	3	2	2	4	3	3	3	2
Patient-18	3	6	2	1	2	2	3	3	3	2	2	2
Patient-19	5	7	1	2	2	1	4	7	5	5	4	3
Patient-20	2	4	0	1	1	1	3	6	4	5	5	4
Patient-21	3	4	0	1	2	1	3	5	5	4	5	3
Patient-22	4	5	1	2	3	2	2	3	2	3	3	2
Patient-23	5	6	2	3	3	2	2	4	3	3	2	2
Patient-24	5	7	2	1	2	3	5	7	5	6	5	5
Patient-25	3	3	0	1	1	2	4	6	5	5	5	4
Mean	3.56	5.04	0.96	1.76	2.04	1.96	3.36	4.88	3.76	3.84	3.6	3.08
SD	1.04	1.367	0.935	0.78	0.73	0.68	1.29	1.39	1.09	1.143	1.080	1.039
% Change	41.57	0	80.95	65.08	59.52	61.11	31.15	0	22.95	21.311	26.23	36.88

The percentage of reduction of dentinal hypersensitivity in the test group was about 80.95% immediately, 65.08% one week postoperatively, 59.52% two weeks postoperatively and 61.1% four weeks postoperatively. The percentage of reduction of dentinal hypersensitivity in the control group was about 22.95% immediately, 21.31% one week postoperatively, 26.23% two weeks postoperatively and 36.88% four weeks postoperatively (Table 1).

The Mann—Whitney test, performed for different time intervals, showed that there was no significant difference in the mean VAS scores between Test and Control group at T0 & T1 time intervals, at $p = 0.48$ & 0.68, respectively. However, at the T2 to T5 time intervals, the test group showed a significant decrease in the mean VAS scores as compared to the control group, and the mean difference in the VAS scores was statistically significant at $p < 0.001$ (Figure 5).

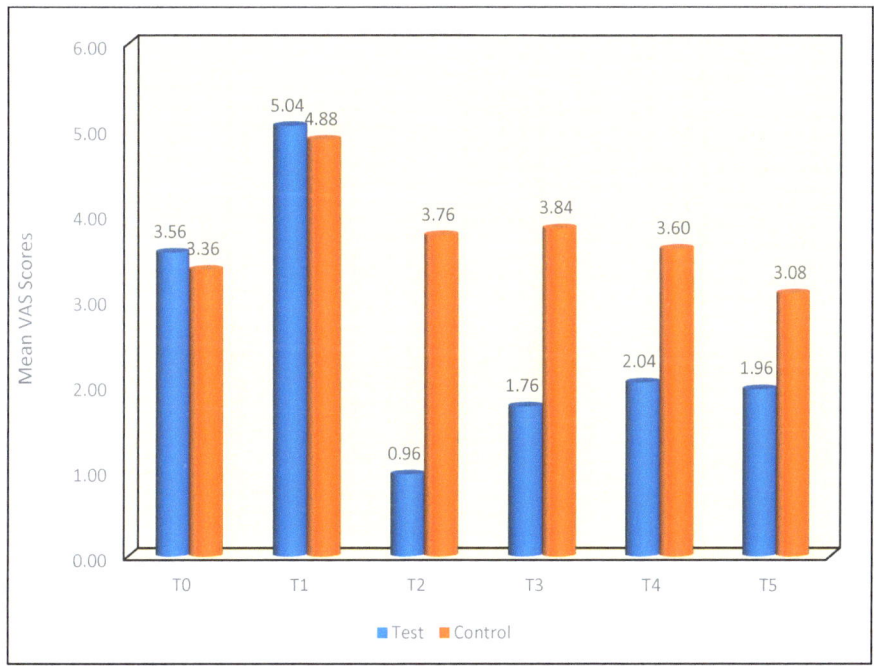

Figure 5. Mean VAS scores between two groups at different time intervals.

A comparison of the mean VAS scores between various time intervals using Freidman's test also gave a statistically significant result at $p < 0.001$ between different time frames. (Table 2).

Table 2. Comparison of mean VAS scores between time intervals in the test group using Friedman's test.

Time	N	Mean	SD	Min	Max	p-Value
T0	25	3.56	1.04	2	5	
T1	25	5.04	1.37	3	7	
T2	25	0.96	0.94	0	3	<0.001 *
T3	25	1.76	0.78	1	3	
T4	25	2.04	0.74	1	3	
T5	25	1.96	0.68	1	4	

*—Statistically significant.

Multiple comparisons of the mean difference in VAS scores in the test group between different time intervals using the Wilcoxon signed-rank post hoc test demonstrated that the mean VAS scores showed a significant increase from the T0 to T1 time interval at $p < 0.001$. Furthermore, there was a significant reduction noted from the T2 to T5 time intervals at $p < 0.001$. This was next followed by the T2 to T5 time intervals showing significantly lower mean VAS scores as compared to T1 at $p < 0.001$. Similarly, the T2 time interval showed significantly lower mean VAS scores as compared to the T3 to T5 time intervals at $p \leq 0.001$. This was followed with the T3 time interval which showed significantly lower mean VAS scores as compared to the T4 time interval at $p = 0.008$. However, no significant difference was noted between T3 and T5 [$p = 0.25$] or between the T4 and T5 time intervals [$p = 0.62$]. (Table 3).

Table 3. Multiple comparisons of mean difference in VAS scores b/w time intervals in test group using Wilcoxon signed-rank post hoc test.

(I) Time	(J) Time	Mean Diff. (I − J)	95% CI for the Diff.		p-Value
			Lower	Upper	
T0	T1	−1.48	−2.14	−0.83	<0.001 *
	T2	2.60	1.85	3.35	<0.001 *
	T3	1.80	1.15	2.45	<0.001 *
	T4	1.52	0.92	2.12	<0.001 *
	T5	1.60	0.92	2.28	<0.001 *
T1	T2	4.08	3.46	4.70	<0.001 *
	T3	3.28	2.49	4.07	<0.001 *
	T4	3.00	2.27	3.73	<0.001 *
	T5	3.08	2.16	4.00	<0.001 *
T2	T3	−0.80	−1.36	−0.24	<0.001 *
	T4	−1.08	−1.58	−0.59	<0.001 *
	T5	−1.00	−1.65	−0.35	0.001 *
T3	T4	−0.28	−0.58	0.02	0.008 *
	T5	−0.20	−0.76	0.36	0.25
T4	T5	0.08	−0.45	0.61	0.62

*—Statistically significant.

A comparison of mean VAS scores between time intervals in the control group using Friedman's test showed that there was a significant difference in the mean VAS scores between different time intervals in the control group at $p < 0.001$. (Table 4).

Table 4. Comparison of mean VAS scores between time intervals in the control group using Friedman's test.

Time	N	Mean	SD	Min	Max	p-Value
T0	25	3.36	1.29	2	6	
T1	25	4.88	1.39	3	7	
T2	25	3.76	1.09	2	5	<0.001 *
T3	25	3.84	1.14	2	6	
T4	25	3.60	1.08	2	5	
T5	25	3.08	1.04	1	5	

*—Statistically significant.

Multiple comparisons of the mean difference in VAS scores between time intervals in the control group using the Wilcoxon signed-rank post hoc test demonstrated that the mean VAS scores showed a significant increase from the T0 to T1 time interval at $p < 0.001$. Furthermore, a significant reduction was noted from the T2 to T3 time intervals at $p = 0.04$ & $p = 0.01$, respectively. This was next followed by the T2 to T5 time intervals showing significantly lower mean VAS scores as compared to T1 at $p < 0.001$. Similarly, the T2 time interval showed significantly lower mean VAS scores as compared to the T5 time interval at $p = 0.001$. This was followed with the T5 time interval showing significantly lower mean VAS scores as compared to the T3 & T4 time intervals at $p < 0.001$ and $p = 0.002$. However, no significant difference was noted between T0 and the T4 and T5 time intervals [$p = 0.24$ and $p = 0.11$, respectively] or between the T2 and T3 and T4 time intervals [$p = 0.53$ and $p = 0.29$, respectively] and between the T3 & T4 time interval at $p = 0.06$. (Table 5).

Table 5. Multiple comparison of mean difference in VAS scores b/w time intervals in the control group using the Wilcoxon signed-rank post hoc test.

(I) Time	(J) Time	Mean Diff. (I − J)	95% CI for the Diff.		p-Value
			Lower	Upper	
T0	T1	−1.52	−2.09	−0.95	<0.001 *
	T2	−0.40	−1.00	0.20	0.04 *
	T3	−0.48	−1.02	0.06	0.01 *
	T4	−0.24	−0.90	0.42	0.24
	T5	0.28	−0.27	0.83	0.11
T1	T2	1.12	0.61	1.63	<0.001 *
	T3	1.04	0.56	1.52	<0.001 *
	T4	1.28	0.61	1.95	<0.001 *
	T5	1.80	1.21	2.40	<0.001 *
T2	T3	−0.08	−0.50	0.34	0.53
	T4	0.16	−0.33	0.65	0.29
	T5	0.68	0.16	1.20	0.001 *
T3	T4	0.24	−0.15	0.63	0.06
	T5	0.76	0.29	1.23	<0.001 *
T4	T5	0.52	0.09	0.95	0.002 *

*—Statistically significant.

A comparison of the mean percentage increase in VAS between the two groups at the T1 Time Interval was carried out using Mann—Whitney Test. The mean percentage increase in the VAS scores from the T0 to T1 time interval showed that the test group showed a relatively lower mean increase in VAS scores as compared to the control group. However, the difference in the mean percentage increase in VAS scores between the two groups was not statistically significant at $p = 0.53$. (Figure 6).

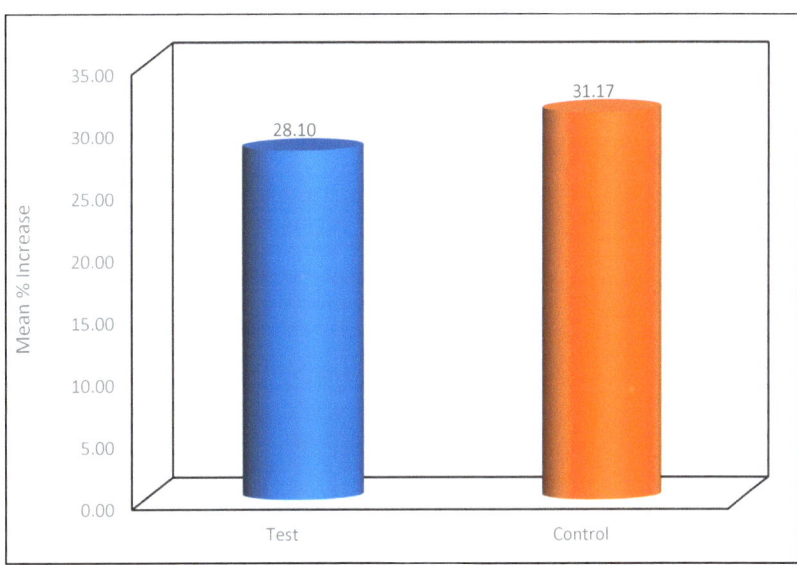

Figure 6. Mean percentage increase in VAS between the two groups at the T1 Time Interval.

A comparison of the mean percentage decrease in VAS between the two groups at the T2 to T5 Time Intervals using the Mann—Whitney Test revealed that the test group demonstrated a significantly higher mean percentage reduction in VAS scores as compared to the control group and the difference between the two groups at the T2 to T5 time intervals was statistically significant at $p < 0.001$. (Figure 7).

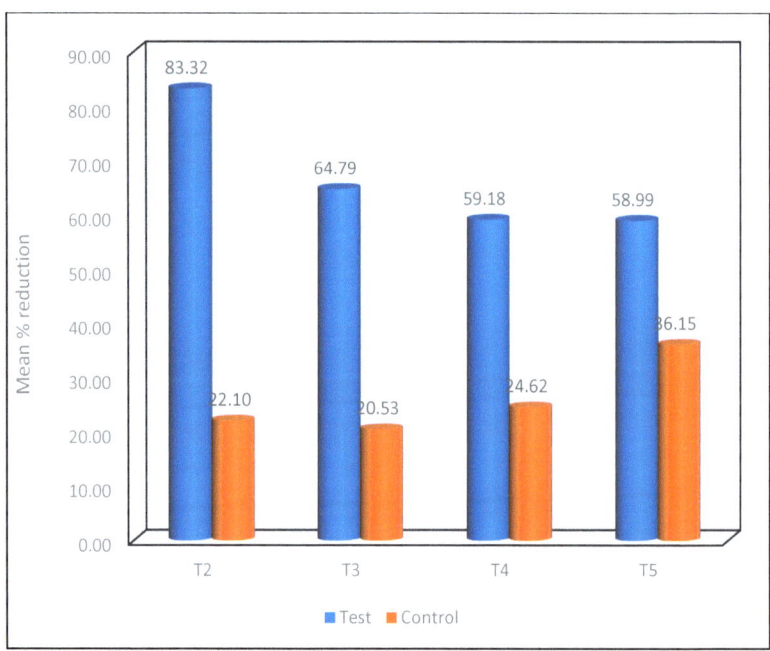

Figure 7. Mean percentage reduction in VAS between the two groups at the T2 to T5 Time Intervals.

The results show that a single chair-side application of NovaMin® in powder form significantly reduced dentinal hypersensitivity immediately after application and the effect lasted until the 4-week post-operative follow-up.

4. Discussion

Dentin sensitivity is a chronic condition and may be one of the most common painful conditions of the oral cavity; yet it is one of the least satisfactorily treated. The prevalence of dentin sensitivity is likely to increase as the adult population lives longer and retains their teeth later in life, and as populations of all age groups engage in lifestyles and behaviors that promote dentin exposure through gingival recession or erosion of protective tooth surfaces. A survey among oral care professionals reports that dental care providers feel confident about diagnosing dentin hypersensitivity but not about treating it [2]. Studies show that the incidence of dentinal sensitivity increases after supra or sub-gingival scaling. Different theories have been proposed to explain the concept of dentin hypersensitivity. The Brannstrom theory which deals with the flow of fluid inside the dentinal tubules is currently accepted as a valid theory [11,12]. Dentine sensitivity is generally measured using visual analogue scales (VAS) in many clinical situations. VAS have proved to be a good tool for the measurement of dentinal sensitivity as pain is subjective and can vary greatly among different individuals.

Clinicians dealing with dentin hypersensitivity would benefit greatly from the development of a therapy that offers both rapid relief following expert administration and a long-lasting desensitizing impact. Increased patient compliance with professional oral care

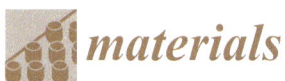

Article

The Effects of a Novel Nanohydroxyapatite Gel and Er: YAG Laser Treatment on Dentin Hypersensitivity

Demet Sahin [1,*], Ceren Deger [2], Burcu Oglakci [2], Metehan Demirkol [3], Bedri Onur Kucukyildirim [3], Mehtikar Gursel [1] and Evrim Eliguzeloglu Dalkilic [2]

1. Department of Periodontology, Faculty of Dentistry, Bezmialem Vakif University, 34093 Istanbul, Turkey; mihtikar@gmail.com or mgursel@bezmialem.edu.tr
2. Department of Restorative Dentistry, Faculty of Dentistry, Bezmialem Vakif University, 34093 Istanbul, Turkey; crndgr1@gmail.com or cdeger@bezmialem.edu.tr (C.D.); burcu923@hotmail.com or boglakci@bezmialem.edu.tr (B.O.); eeliguzeloglu@hotmail.com or edalkilic@bezmialem.edu.tr (E.E.D.)
3. Department of Mechanical Engineering, Yildiz Technical University, 34349 Istanbul, Turkey; demirkol@yildiz.edu.tr (M.D.); kucukyil@gmail.com or kucukyil@yildiz.edu.tr (B.O.K.)
* Correspondence: demetsahin_87@hotmail.com or dsahin1@bezmialem.edu.tr; Tel.: +90-212-453-18-50 or +90-212-523-22-88; Fax: +90-212-523-22-88

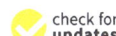

Citation: Sahin, D.; Deger, C.; Oglakci, B.; Demirkol, M.; Kucukyildirim, B.O.; Gursel, M.; Eliguzeloglu Dalkilic, E. The Effects of a Novel Nanohydroxyapatite Gel and Er: YAG Laser Treatment on Dentin Hypersensitivity. *Materials* 2023, 16, 6522. https://doi.org/10.3390/ma16196522

Academic Editors: Laura-Cristina Rusu, Lavinia Cosmina Ardelean and Nikolaos Silikas

Received: 12 August 2023
Revised: 1 September 2023
Accepted: 29 September 2023
Published: 30 September 2023

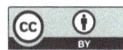

Copyright: © 2023 by the authors. Licensee MDPI, Basel, Switzerland. This article is an open access article distributed under the terms and conditions of the Creative Commons Attribution (CC BY) license (https://creativecommons.org/licenses/by/4.0/).

Abstract: Purpose: This study evaluates the effects of a novel nanohydroxyapatite gel and Er: YAG laser on the surface roughness, surface morphology, and elemental content after dentin hypersensitivity treatments. Methods: Dentin discs (2 × 3 × 3 mm^3) were prepared from 75 human molars. Out of 75 human molars, 50 were used to evaluate surface roughness and randomly divided into five groups: Group ID (intact dentin), Group DD (demineralized dentin), Group BF (fluoride varnish/Bifluorid 10), Group Lsr (Er: YAG laser-50 mJ, 0.50 W, 10 Hz), and Group NHA (nanohydroxyapatite-containing gel). Dentin hypersensitivity was stimulated by 35% phosphoric acid for 1 min (except Group ID). The surface roughness (Ra, µm) was measured via contact profilometry (n = 10). Out of the 75 sound human molars, 25 were used to evaluate the surface morphology and elemental content using scanning electron microscopy and energy-dispersive X-ray spectroscopy (n = 5). The data were statistically analyzed using Welsch ANOVA, Games–Howell, Kruskal–Wallis, and Dunn tests ($p < 0.05$). Results: Group Lsr showed significantly lower surface roughness than Group NHA and Group BF ($p < 0.05$). The SEM analysis indicated that most of the dentinal tubules were obliterated for Group NHA. Precipitant plugs with partially occluded dentinal tubules were observed for Group BF, while partially or completely occluded tubules with a melting appearance were detected for Group Lsr. The EDS analysis revealed that Group NHA and Group Lsr presented similar calcium and phosphorus amounts to Group ID. All dentin hypersensitivity treatment methods could provide promising results in terms of tubular occlusion efficiency. However, laser treatment resulted in smoother surfaces, which could help prevent dental plaque accumulation.

Keywords: nanohydroxyapatite; fluoride varnish; laser; dentin hypersensitivity; surface roughness

1. Introduction

Dentin hypersensitivity is a frequent clinical condition, and it has multifactorial etiology [1]. Dentin hypersensitivity is the pain that derives from exposed dentin in response to chemical, thermal tactile, or osmotic stimuli which cannot be explained by other dental problems [2]. If a patient experiences dentin hypersensitivity, brushing the affected teeth or consuming cold food and beverages could cause pain, and the individual may therefore avoid those practices [3]. Dentin hypersensitivity prevalence is reported to affect between 4% and 69% of the adult population [4], with an average prevalence of 57%. It mostly affects individuals aged between 20 and 40 years [5] and more commonly afflicts women [6]. Dentin hypersensitivity is more prevalent among periodontally compromised patients (60–98%). Buccal surfaces clearly show the highest prevalence rates [6]. The number, size, and diameter of the patent dentinal tubules determine the level of sensitivity that individuals experience [7]. The activated nerve endings generate a severe, sharp, and sudden pain [2] that derives from the exposed cervical pulp–dentine complex. Ultimately, this pain may discourage the individual from consuming food and beverages, brushing their teeth, or even breathing [8].

Hypersensitive dentin can be treated with various procedures. Together with the elimination of nociceptive stimuli, two major treatment approaches stand out: (1) altering the nervous response by inhibiting or decreasing neuronal transmission and (2) occluding the permeable dentinal tubules [9]. Regarding potassium salts applications, potassium nitrate is the most preferred for use as a nervous modifier [10]. With regard to managing tubular occlusion, various methods are employed, including chemical interventions using fluorides [11], oxalates [12], or arginine [13,14] and physical interventions using adhesives [15] or laser therapies [16]. Low-power lasers (GaAlAs diode laser) have effects on neural transmission and medium-power lasers (Nd: YAG, CO and Er: YAG laser) reduce the diameter of dentinal tubules and cause occlusion. Because of this, these two approaches are preferred for eliminating dentin hypersensitivity [16,17]. Compared with conventional desensitizing topical agents, laser treatment methods lead to rapid results with less application time and less time spent for the patient [18]. However, laser treatments have certain disadvantages, such as their high cost and complexity of use [19]. Thus, recent studies have focused on identifying new materials and new treatment methods [20].

Nanohydroxyapatite resembles an inorganic bone structure, and it is biocompatible; therefore, it can be used for various dental purposes. Recently, interest in nanotechnology has produced promising applications in dentistry for nanohydroxyapatite, which offers crystals ranging in size from 50 to 1000 nm. The ability of nanohydroxyapatite to bind to proteins is due to the size of the nanoparticles, which noticeably extend the surface area to which proteins can bind. In addition, nanohydroxyapatite fills the small gaps and depressions on the enamel surface. It also has impressive remineralizing effects on initial enamel lesions and is more effective than fluorides in this regard [21]. Since it is a bioactive material and can enhance the mineralization process, this material has the potential to inhibit dentine hypersensitivity [22]. Several types of treatments for dentin hypersensitivity involve using products or laser applications directly on the affected dentin tissue. In this way, such treatments are likely to change the surface roughness of the dentin [23]. Bacterial adhesion and plaque retention on tooth structures might be accelerated due to an increase in surface roughness, and this can make the surface prone to caries and periodontal disease [24]. Existing research has limited data regarding the selection of reliable treatment modalities for dentin hypersensitivity [25]. Hence, this study aims to investigate the effects of a novel nanohydroxyapatite gel and Er:YAG laser on the surface roughness, surface morphology, and elemental content after dentin hypersensitivity treatments.

The null hypothesis of this study was as follows:

There will be no differences in surface roughness, dentinal tubule morphology, or elemental content after different dentin hypersensitivity treatments.

2. Materials and Methods

This in vitro study was approved by the local ethics committee (Bezmialem Vakif University Ethics Committee for Non-Invasive Studies, Process no: 2022/323). The specimen size was determined on the basis of the estimated effect size between groups, in accordance with the literature [26,27]. In this study, 10 specimens for surface roughness measurement and 5 specimens for elemental content analysis were necessary for each group to obtain a medium effect size (d = 0.50) using 95% power and a 5% type 1 error rate.

A total of 75 extracted sound human molars were used. Out of the 75 sound human molars, 50 were used to evaluate surface roughness and 25 out of the 75 sound human molars were used to evaluate surface morphology and elemental content. Teeth with caries, root resorption, cracks, fractures, or restorations were excluded. The teeth were cleaned with curettes and stored in distilled water until the experiment. Dentin specimens ($2 \times 3 \times 3$ mm^3 area) were obtained using a model trimmer and high-speed diamond saw

(MT3 Wet trimmer, Renfert GmbH, Hilzingen, Germany) under water irrigation. Enamel was cut up to 2 mm below the central fossa to expose the dentin parallel to the occlusal surface. A stereomicroscope (SMZ 1000, Nikon, Japan) was used to control the dentin specimens for lack of enamel. Additionally, the thickness of the specimen was verified with a digital caliper (Insize/China). The surfaces were polished using 400-, 600-, and 800-grit silicon carbide papers on a polishing device (Minitech 233, Presi, Grenoble, France) under water cooling (B.0.) [28].

Table 1 summarizes the materials used in this study and their compositions. The specimens were randomly divided into five groups according to different dentin hypersensitivity treatment methods:

Group ID (Intact Dentin/positive control): The specimen received no dentin exposure application and no dentin hypersensitivity treatment.

Group DD (Demineralized Dentin/negative control): The specimen received no dentin hypersensitivity treatment.

Group BF (Bifluorid 10): The fluoride varnish (Bifluorid 10, Voco GmbH, Cuxhoven, Germany) was applied to the specimen with a microbrush under dry conditions. It was allowed to be absorbed for 10–20 s and was then air-dried according to the manufacturers' instructions.

Group Lsr (Er:YAG laser): The Er: YAG laser (Fotona AT Fidelis, Ljubljana, Slovenia) was applied to the specimen under the sets of parameters (50 mJ, 0.50 W, 10 Hz) with a wavelength of 2940 nm at 1 cm distance for 30 s [29]. A non-contact hand piece (H02) was applied perpendicular to the surfaces with a cylindrical sapphire optical fiber tip (1.3 mm in diameter, 8 mm in length). The tip was moved mesiodistally at a speed of approximately 1 mm/s.

Group NHA (nanohydroxyapatite): A novel nanohydroxyapatite-containing gel (Biodent Medical, Istanbul, Turkey) was applied to the specimen for 1 min at 500 rpm with a slow hand piece using a rubber cap under dry conditions according to the manufacturers' instructions.

Table 1. The materials used in this study and their compositions.

Materials	Trade	Composition
Bifluorid 10	Voco GmBh, Cuxhoven, Germany	5% NaF, 5% CaF, (22.600 ppm)
Nanohydroxiapatite containing gel	Biodent Medical, Istanbul, Turkey	Nanohydroxyapatite particles with typical particle size below 50 nm in a rod-like shape (typically 30–40 nm length and 5–10 nm width).

To expose the dentinal tubules and simulate dentin hypersensitivity, 35% phosphoric acid (Scotchbond Universal Etchant, 3M ESPE, St. Paul, MN, USA) was applied to the surfaces for 1 min for all tested groups except Group ID. After that, etched specimens were rinsed with distilled water for 20 s. Then, all the etched and rinsed specimens were air-dried. All dentin hypersensitivity treatments were performed with a single operator for standardization (D.S.).

Next, 10 specimens from each group were assessed using a contact profilometer (Mahr GmbH, Marsurf PS1, Göttingen, Germany) for surface roughness (Ra, mm). The measurements were obtained from three different parts of the surface for each specimen with a stylus tip radius of 5 μm and a stylus driving speed of 0.5 mm/s, in accordance with EN ISO 4288.21. The arithmetic mean of these measurements was calculated. After measuring every five specimens, the tool was calibrated for reliable findings. A second operator (M.D.), who was blind to the dentin hypersensitivity treatment method, performed this surface roughness procedure [30,31].

Five specimens from each group were chosen, and the surface morphology and elemental content was evaluated via SEM (Thermo Fisher Scientific, Phenom XL, Waltham, MA, USA). These specimens were gold-sputter-coated to obtain the electrical conductivity necessary for SEM imaging. A CeB6 thermionic source using 5, 10, or 15 kV acceleration voltages provided illumination during SEM imaging, which achieved a resolution below 20 nm. The morphology was evaluated using a secondary electron detector, which monitored the geometrical differences on the surface in three dimensions. The micromorphology of the surfaces was completed at 5000× magnification. Then, the surface content was evaluated using the backscattered electron detector (BSD), which demonstrates chemical composition based on the density variances of different elemental contents.

For the chemical characterization of the dentin specimens, a semiquantitative chemical microanalysis method, namely energy-dispersive X-ray spectroscopy (EDS), was utilized. The EDS module of the scanning electron microscope (Phenom XL, Thermo Fisher Scientific) was selected, since this module has the ability to identify elements from boron (B) to americium (Am) by virtue of the ultrathin silicon nitride X-ray window. A thermoelectrically cooled (LN2-free) silicon drift detector was utilized, and an energy resolution below 137 eV at Mn Kα was achieved with a 10 eV/ch processing capability, with 2048 channels and 300,000 counts/second. Thus, an elemental analysis with high certainty was performed for the basic elements (C, O, F, P, Ca, Mg). A researcher who was blind to the dentin hypersensitivity treatment method performed all the SEM and EDS analyses.

Statistical Analysis

Statistical analysis was performed using SPSS 23.0 for Windows (SPSS Inc., Chicago, IL, USA). The Shapiro–Wilk test was first used to indicate the normality of variables, and the data were then analyzed with Levene's test for homogeneity of variances. The surface roughness data were normally distributed. Welch ANOVA was used to show differences between groups. Pairwise comparisons were performed via Games Howell test. Since EDS data did not satisfy parametric test assumptions, the data were analyzed with non-parametric tests. The Kruskal–Wallis test was performed to compare between-group differences in terms of EDS. Pairwise comparisons were developed via Dunn test. Statistical significance was determined at a confidence level of 0.05 in all analyses.

3. Results

3.1. Surface Roughness Evaluation

Mean surface roughness values and standard deviations are presented in Table 2. Group Lsr exhibited significantly lower surface roughness than group NHA and group BF ($p < 0.05$). Moreover, no significant differences in surface roughness were found between the other tested groups ($p > 0.05$).

Table 2. Mean surface roughness values and standard deviations (±) of all tested groups (Ra, μm).

Group	Surface Roughness (±)	p
Group ID	0.865 ± 0.289 [ab]	0.015
Group DD	1.121 ± 0.355 [ab]	0.015
Group BF	1.262 ± 0.419 [a]	0.015
Grup Lsr	0.856 ± 0.094 [b]	0.015
Group NHA	1.155 ± 0.319 [a]	0.015

The lowercase letters indicate significant differences between groups.

3.2. Surface Morphology and Elemental Content Analysis

Representative SEM images of all tested groups are given in Figure 1. The SEM analysis indicated that most of the dentinal tubules with deposit formations (red arrows) were obliterated for Group NHA. Additionally, precipitant plugs (blue arrows) with partially occluded dentinal tubules were observed in Group BF, while either partially or completely occluded tubules with a melting appearance (blue circle) were detected in Group Lsr.

The representative semiquantitative chemical analyses and distribution of elements for all tested groups are provided in Figure 2 and Table 3 (%). The EDS analysis revealed that phosphorus (P) and calcium (Ca) were the predominant elements. Significantly lower Ca and P amounts were found for Group DD compared with Group ID. Group NHA and Group Lsr yielded similar amounts of all tested elements to Group ID. Significant differences in the P and F amounts were detected among the treated groups. F amounts were found to be significantly higher in Group BF compared with Group Lsr, but similar to those in Group NHA. Significantly higher F amounts were found for Group BF compared with Group ID. The amount of Mg in Group NHA and Group Lsr was significantly higher than in Group DD. All treated groups showed a similar Mg amount to Group ID.

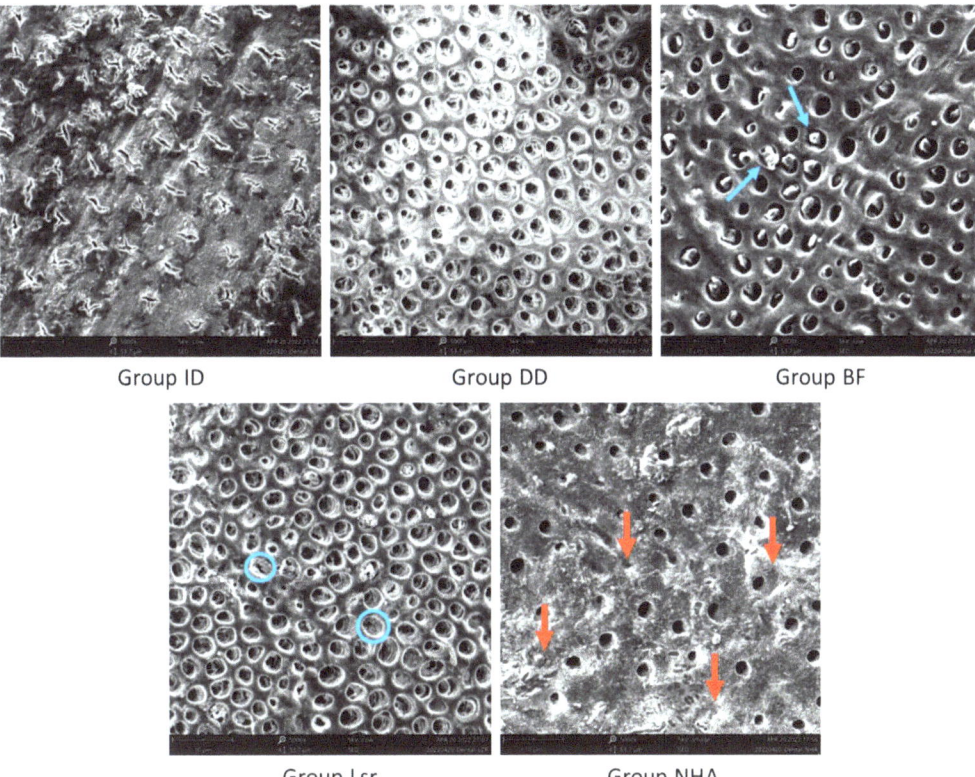

Figure 1. Representative SEM images of all tested groups. (Red arrows: deposit formation, blue arrows: precipant plugs, blue circles: occluded tubules with melting appearance).

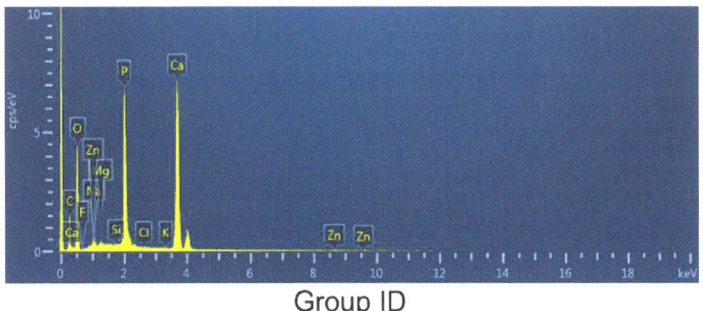

Figure 2. *Cont.*

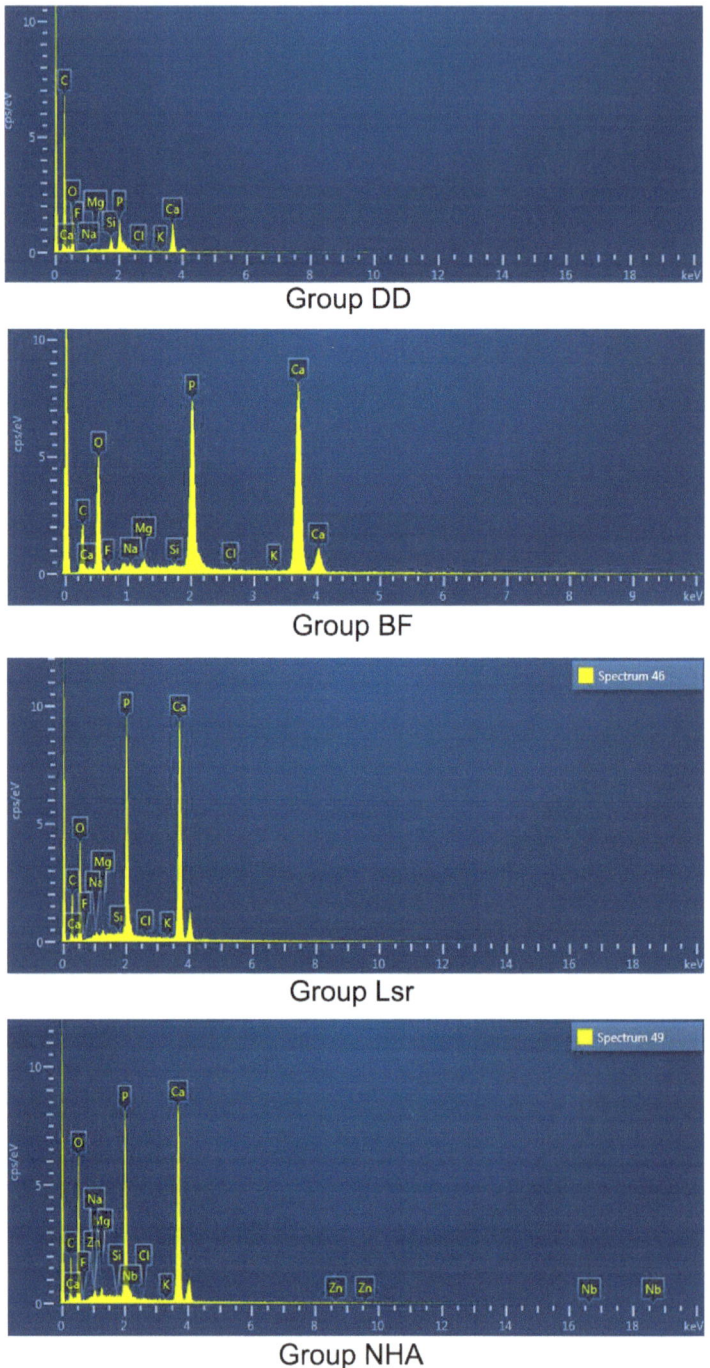

Figure 2. Representative semi-quantitative chemical analysis and distribution of elements of all tested groups.

Table 3. The chemical distribution of elements for all tested groups (%).

	O	P	Ca	F	C	Mg
Group ID	52.59 ± 1 [b]	12.06 ± 0.81 [b]	23.43 ± 1.3 [b]	0.04 ± 0.07 [a]	10.16 ± 0.95 [b]	0.26 ± 0.1 [ab]
Group DD	68.46 ± 0.72 [a]	2.41 ± 0.52 [ac]	4.83 ± 0.94 [a]	0.02 ± 0.04 [a]	23.6 ± 0.61 [a]	0.06 ± 0.02 [a]
Group BF	55.41 ± 2.53 [ab]	1.16 ± 0.17 [a]	19.02 ± 3.15 [ab]	1.07 ± 0.36 [b]	13.2 ± 2.01 [ab]	0.43 ± 0.04 [b]
Group Lsr	57.28 ± 2.41 [ab]	9.25 ± 1.43 [bc]	18.74 ± 3.02 [ab]	0.03 ± 0.08 [a]	14.1 ± 2.03 [ab]	0.23 ± 0.03 [ab]
Group NHA	55.95 ± 2.86 [ab]	9.76 ± 1.51 [bc]	19.39 ± 3.48 [ab]	0.26 ± 0.17 [ab]	13.13 ± 2.34 [ab]	0.4 ± 0.05 [b]
p	<0.001	<0.001	<0.001	<0.001	<0.001	<0.001

The lowercase letters indicate significant differences between groups.

4. Discussion

In this study, the effects of a novel nanohydroxyapatite-containing gel and Er: YAG laser on surface roughness, surface morphology, and elemental content after dentin hypersensitivity treatments were evaluated. The null hypothesis that proposed that there would be no differences in surface roughness, dentinal tubule morphology, or elemental content after different dentin hypersensitivity treatments was rejected because the treated groups exhibited partial or complete occlusion of the dentinal tubules and because significant differences in P and F amounts were detected among treated groups. In addition, the laser-treated groups exhibited significantly lower surface roughness values compared with the other tested groups.

Rough surfaces favor plaque accumulation and maturation [32]. The influence of surface roughness on supragingival plaque supports the need for smooth surfaces with a low surface free energy to eliminate plaque accumulation, thereby decreasing the number of teeth with caries and periodontitis [33]. The contact profilometry method has advantages, since it is an easily accessible and cost-effective measurement of surface roughness [34].

Thus, in this study, surface roughness was analyzed with this method. The laser-treated group revealed the most favorable surface roughness values. The Er: YAG laser is one of the most preferred types of lasers to treat dental hard tissues because its wavelength (2940 nm) is in harmony with the main absorption peak of water, which is absorbed well in all biological tissues, including enamel and dentin. Absorption of water was 15 and 10,000 times higher with Er: YAG lasers than with CO_2 and Nd: YAG lasers, respectively. Thus, as a result of the high water absorption peak in comparison with other commercially available lasers, Er: YAG lasers have often been preferred for treating dental and oral conditions [29]. Zhuang et al., who investigated the effects of Er: YAG lasers used at various power- and wavelength levels (0.5 W/50 mJ/10 Hz, 1 W/50 mJ/20 Hz, 2 W/100 mJ/20 Hz and 4 W/200 mJ/20 Hz) on dentinal tubule occlusion, intrapulpal heat, and pulpal tissue structure, reported that the parameters 0.5 W/50 mJ were suitable for proper tubule occlusion. Furthermore, they indicated that the accumulation of energy from laser treatments might damage pulp [35]. Thus, in this study, the Er: YAG laser parameters 0.5 W/50 mJ/10 Hz were used to treat dentin hypersensitivity.

This expansion process results in the ablation of the surrounding material [36]. Therefore, the surface roughness findings of laser-treated specimens could be attributable to the ablation of dentin tissue. In addition, differences in surface roughness were found to be insignificant between other tested groups.

In the present study, SEM and EDS analysis were chosen to examine the dentin tubule morphology and elemental content of the dentin surfaces. It has been well documented that the level of dentin hypersensitivity is dependent on the magnitude and potency of the dentinal tubules [5]. Furthermore, according to hydrodynamic theory, as the dentinal fluid movement diminishes, dentine hypersensitivity also decreases. Fluoride is used often in clinical settings and studies to decrease dentin hypersensitivity. The action mechanism of fluoride accounts for its efficiency, as fluoride is able to form precipitates and occlude the tubules [1]. It has been reported that bifluorid varnish containing sodium fluoride and calcium fluoride provided the occlusion of open tubules and precipitation of calcium fluoride or proteins [37]. This fact is consistent with the SEM images of the current experiment, which indicated that Bifluorid 10 caused precipitant plugs with partially occluded dentinal tubules. EDS analysis showed that the Biflorid 10-treated group had higher F levels than the laser-treated groups, but similar to those of the NHA-treated groups.

Roughly, 97% of tooth enamel and 70% of dentin consists of hydroxyapatite (HA) [38]. NHA can act as a template for mineral crystal nucleation and growth to form a dentin-like structure during the remineralization process. Calcium and phosphate ions from the oral environment may attach to the dentin surface during the precipitation and will fill the empty places in the crystal complex [39]. In this study, SEM analysis revealed that most of the tubules were occluded for the NHA-treated specimens. The sizes of NHA particles allowed the material to penetrate through microcracks to reach the dentinal tubules [40]. The increase in surface area associated with the reduction in NHA particle size may have resulted in increased penetration and deposition of these molecules into the dentinal tubules, resulting in large tubular occlusion [41]. The findings of this study are consistent with Vano et al. [42], who concluded that NHA-containing toothpaste was effective in treating dentin hypersensitivity. According to the SEM images of this study, the application of NHA was effective for the occlusion of the dentinal tubules. The application of an Er: YAG laser would be expected to reduce these fluid movements by evaporating the superficial parts of dentinal fluid [43]. These ablation and evaporation facilities of the laser could have enabled the obliteration and occlusion effects. Kurt et al. [44], who evaluated the efficacy of the Er: YAG laser and different dentin desensitizers on dentin permeability reduction, reported that the laser-treated groups performed best and that nanohydroxyapatite toothpaste can be considered an alternative therapeutic product. This finding is in line with the SEM images of the present study, which display partially or completely occluded tubules with a melting appearance for the laser-treated specimens.

The occlusion effect and crystalline deposits result from the presence of calcium phosphate in the form of hydroxyapatite. In this study, for the laser- and NHA-treated groups, the EDS analysis indicated that the dentin surface deposits had similar levels of calcium and phosphorous to intact dentin. These findings could have contributed to the promising tubule occlusion of these groups' SEM images. Moreover, P amounts for these groups were significantly higher than the amount of Biflorid 10. This finding is in line with Contrera-Arriaga et al. [45], who reported similar P amounts after Er:YAG laser irradiation. Mg concentration is 1% (wt) in dentin tissue. Mg^{2+} is involved in the biomineralization of teeth and directly affects crystallization and pattern generation of the inorganic mineral phase [46]. EDS analysis highlighted that all treated groups showed similar Mg amounts to Group ID. The discovered Mg^{2+} could contribute to the positive effect on the remineralization potentials of those desensitizing agents.

Regarding the limitations of the current in vitro study, only the early-term effects of BF, Lsr, and NHA were evaluated via SEM EDS and contact profilometry analysis, and the long-term effects were not examined. In addition, the erosion–abrasion cycle step was not used in our study. Further damage and different occlusion rates on dentinal tubules could be expected with such an approach. What is more, future studies could focus on combination therapies for dentinal tubule occlusion. Different specimen groups treated with dentin hypersensitivity agents such as NHA and subsequent Lsr application and other combination approaches might provide promising results.

5. Conclusions

Within the limitations of this study, it can be concluded that all dentin hypersensitivity treatment methods could provide promising results in terms of tubular occlusion efficiency. However, laser treatment resulted in smoother surfaces, which could help to prevent dental plaque accumulation.

Author Contributions: Conceptualization and design: B.O., E.E.D., D.S., M.G. and C.D.; Literature review: B.O., C.D., E.E.D., D.S. and M.G.; Formal analysis: B.O., D.S., C.D., B.O.K., M.D., E.E.D. and M.G.; Investigation and data collection: B.O., D.S., C.D., B.O.K., M.D., E.E.D. and M.G.; Data analysis and interpretation: B.O., D.S., C.D., B.O.K., M.D., E.E.D. and M.G.; Writing: B.O., D.S., C.D.,

B.O.K., M.D., E.E.D. and M.G.; Review and editing: B.O., D.S., C.D., B.O.K., M.D., E.E.D. and M.G. All authors have read and agreed to the published version of the manuscript.

Funding: The authors do not have any financial interests in the companies whose materials are included in this article.

Institutional Review Board Statement: Not applicable.

Informed Consent Statement: Not applicable.

Data Availability Statement: Not applicable.

Acknowledgments: This study was co-funded by Voco GmbH (Cuxhoven, Germany) and Biodent Medical, (Istanbul, Turkey). The funders had no role in the design, conduct, evaluation or interpretation of the study, or in writing the manuscript. The authors do not have any financial interests in the companies whose materials are included in this article.

Conflicts of Interest: The authors declare no conflict of interest.

References

1. Davari, A.; Ataei, E.; Assarzadeh, H. Dentin hypersensitivity: Etiology, diagnosis and treatment: A literature review. *J. Dent.* **2013**, *14*, 136–145.
2. Canadian Advisory Board on Dentin Hypersensitivit. Consensus-based recommendations for the diagnosis and management of dentin hypersensitivity. *J. Can. Dent. Assoc.* **2003**, *69*, 221–226.
3. Arua, S.O.; Fadare, A.S.; Adamu, V.E. The etiology and management of dentinal hypersensitivity. *Orapuh J.* **2021**, *2*, e815.
4. Gillam, D.G.; Orchardson, R. Advances in the treatment of root sensitivity: Mechanisms and treatment principles. *Endod. Topics* **2006**, *13*, 13–33. [CrossRef]
5. Favaro Zeola, L.; Soares, P.V.; Cunha-Cruz, J. Prevalence of dentin hypersensitivity: Systematic review and meta-analysis. *J. Dent. Feb.* **2019**, *81*, 1–6. [CrossRef] [PubMed]
6. Splieth, C.H.; Tachou, A. Epidemiology of dentin hypersensitivity. *Clin. Oral Investig.* **2013**, *17* (Suppl. S1), 3–22. [CrossRef] [PubMed]
7. West, N.X.; Lussi, A.; Seong, J.; Hellwig, E. Dentin hypersensitivity: Pain mechanisms and aetiology of exposed cervical dentin. *Clin. Oral Investig.* **2013**, *17* (Suppl. S1), S9–S19. [CrossRef] [PubMed]
8. Bartold, P. Dentinal hypersensitivity: A review. *Aust. Dent. J.* **2006**, *51*, 212–218. [CrossRef]
9. Shiau, H. Dentin hypersensitivity. *J. Evid. Based Dent. Pract.* **2012**, *12* (Suppl. S3), 220–228. [CrossRef] [PubMed]
10. Hong, J.Y.; Lim, H.C.; Herr, Y. Effects of a mouthwash containing potassium nitrate, sodium fluoride, and cetylpyridinium chloride on dentin hypersensitivity: A randomized, double-blind, placebo-controlled study. *J. Periodontal Implant Sci.* **2016**, *46*, 46–56. [CrossRef]
11. Petersson, L.G. The role of fluoride in the preventive management of dentin hypersensitivity and root caries. *Clin. Oral Investig.* **2013**, *17*, 63–71. [CrossRef] [PubMed]
12. Arnold, W.H.; Prange, M.; Naumova, E.A. Effectiveness of various tooth-pastes on dentine tubule occlusion. *J. Dent.* **2015**, *43*, 440–449. [CrossRef] [PubMed]
13. Petrou, I.; Heu, R.; Stranick, M.; Lavender, S.; Zaidel, L.; Cummins, D.; Sullivan, R.J.; Hsueh, C.; Gimzewski, J.K. A breakthrough therapy for dentin hypersensitivity: How dental products containing 8% arginine and calcium carbonate work to deliver effective relief of sensitive teeth. *J. Clin. Dent.* **2009**, *20*, 23–31.
14. Yang, Z.Y.; Wang, F.; Lu, K.; Li, Y.H.; Zhou, Z. Arginine-containing desensitizing toothpaste for the treatment of dentin hypersensitivity: A meta-analysis. *Clin. Cosmet. Investig. Dent.* **2016**, *8*, 1–14. [PubMed]
15. Kathariya, R. Dental hypersensitivity: A common cold in dentistry. *J. Dent. Res. Rev.* **2016**, *3*, 49. [CrossRef]
16. Kimura, Y.; Wilder-Smith, P.; Yonaga, K.; Matsumoto, K. Treatment of dentine hypersensitivity by lasers: A review. *J. Clin. Periodontol.* **2000**, *27*, 715–721. [CrossRef]
17. Asnaashari, M.; Moeini, M. Effectiveness of lasers in the treatment of dentin hypersensitivity. *J. Lasers Med. Sci.* **2013**, *4*, 1.
18. Biagi, R.; Cossellu, G.; Sarcina, M.; Pizzamiglio, I.T.; Farronato, G. Laser-assisted treatment of dentinal hypersensitivity: A literature review. *Ann. Stomatol.* **2016**, *6*, 75–80. [CrossRef] [PubMed]
19. Orchardson, R.; Gillam, D.G. The efficacy of potassium salts as agents for treating dentin hypersensitivity. *J. Orofac. Pain* **2000**, *14*, 9–19. [PubMed]
20. Jones, J.A. Dentin hypersensitivity: Etiology, risk factors, and prevention strategies. *Dent. Today* **2011**, *30*, 112–113.
21. Pepla, E.; Besharat, L.K.; Palaia, G.; Tenore, G.; Migliau, G. Nano-hydroxyapatite and its applications in preventive, restorative and regenerative dentistry: A review of literature. *Ann. Stomatol.* **2014**, *5*, 108–114. [CrossRef]
22. Roxana Bordea, I.; Candrea, S.; Teodora Alexescu, G.; Bran, S.; Băciuț, M.; Băciuț, G.; Lucaciu, O.; Mihail Dinu, C.; Adina Todea, D. Nano-hydroxyapatite use in dentistry: A systematic review. *Drug. Metab. Rev.* **2020**, *52*, 319–332. [CrossRef] [PubMed]
23. Tawakoli, P.N.; Sener, B.; Attin, T. Mechanical effects of different Swiss market-leading dentifrices on dentin. *Swiss. Dent. J.* **2015**, *125*, 1210–1219. [PubMed]

24. Solis Moreno, C.; Santos, A.; Nart, J.; Levi, P.; Velasquez, A.; Sanz Moliner, J. Evaluation of root surface microtopography following the use of four instrumentation systems by confocal microscopy and scanning electron microscopy: An in vitro study. *J. Periodontal Res.* **2012**, *47*, 608–615. [CrossRef]
25. Liu, X.X.; Tenenbaum, H.C.; Wilder, R.S.; Quock, R.; Hewlett, E.R.; Ren, Y.F. Pathogenesis, diagnosis and management of dentin hypersensitivity: An evidence-based overview for dental practitioners. *BMC Oral Health* **2020**, *20*, 220. [CrossRef]
26. Küçükkaya Eren, S.; Uzunoğlu, E.; Sezer, B.; Yılmaz, Z.; Boyacı, İ.H. Mineral content analysis of root canal dentin using laser-induced breakdown spectroscopy. *Restor. Dent. Endod.* **2018**, *43*, e11. [CrossRef]
27. Oglakci, B.; Kucukyildirim, B.O.; Özduman, Z.C.; Eliguzeloglu Dalkilic, E. The Effect of Different Polishing Systems on the Surface Roughness of Nanocomposites: Contact Profilometry and SEM Analyses. *Oper. Dent.* **2021**, *46*, 173–187. [CrossRef]
28. Reis, B.O.; Prakki, A.; Stavroullakis, A.T.; Souza, M.T.; Siqueira, R.L.; Zanotto, E.D.; Briso, A.L.F.; Tavares Ângelo Cintra, L.; Henrique Dos Santos, P. Analysis of permeability and biological properties of dentin treated with experimental bioactive glasses. *J. Dent.* **2021**, *111*, 103719. [CrossRef]
29. Mahmoud, B.; Abdulaziz, Y. A comparative evaluation of CO2 and erbium-doped yttrium aluminium garnet laser therapy in the management of dentin hypersensitivity and assessment of mineral content. *J. Periodontal Implant Sci.* **2014**, *44*, 227–234. [CrossRef]
30. *ISO 4288*; Geometrical Product Specifications (GPS)–Surface Texture: Profile Method–Rules and Procedures for the Assessment of Surface Texture. ISO-Standards: Geneva, Switzerland, 1996.
31. *ISO 16610-21*; Geometrical Product Specifications (GPS)–Filtration—Part 21: Linear Profile Filters: Gaussian Filters. ISO-Standards: Geneva, Switzerland, 2011.
32. Gharechahi, M.; Moosavi, H.; Forghani, M. Effect of Surface Roughness and Materials Composition. *J. Biomater. Nanobiotechnol.* **2012**, *3*, 541–546. [CrossRef]
33. Yildirim, T.T.; Oztekin, F.; Keklik, E.; Tozum, M.D. Surface roughness of enamel and root surface after scaling, root planning and polishing procedures: An in-vitro study. *J. Oral Biol. Craniofac. Res.* **2021**, *11*, 287–290. [CrossRef]
34. Senawongse, P.; Pongprueksa, P. Surface roughness of nanofill and nanohybrid resin composites after polishing and brushing. *J. Esthet. Restor. Dent.* **2007**, *19*, 265–273. [CrossRef]
35. Zhuang, H.; Liang, Y.; Xiang, S.; Li, H.; Dai, X.; Zhao, W. Dentinal tubule occlusion using Er: YAG Laser: An in vitro study. *J. Appl. Oral Sci.* **2021**, *29*, e20200266. [CrossRef] [PubMed]
36. Eguro, T.; Maeda, T.; Tanabe, M.; Otsuki, M.; Tanaka, H. Adhesion of composite resins to enamel irradiated by the Er:YAG laser: Application of the ultrasonic scaler on irradiated surface. *Lasers Surg. Med.* **2001**, *28*, 365–370. [CrossRef] [PubMed]
37. Betke, H.; Kahler, E.; Reitz, A.; Hartmann, G.; Lennon, A.; Attin, T. Influence of bleaching agents and desensitizing varnishes on the water content of dentin. *Oper. Dent.* **2006**, *31*, 536–542. [CrossRef] [PubMed]
38. Ohta, K.; Kawamata, H.; Ishizaki, T.; Hayman, R. Occlusion of dentinal tubules by nano-hydroxyapatite. *J. Dent. Res.* **2007**, *86*. Available online: https://www.aclaim.co.in/wp-content/uploads/2018/09/occlusion-of-dentinal-tubules-by-nano-hydroxyapatite-min.pdf (accessed on 28 September 2023).
39. Zhang, M.; He, L.B.; Exterkate, R.A.M.; Cheng, L.; Li, J.Y.; Ten Cate, J.M.; Crielaard, W.; Deng, D.M. Biofilm Layers Affect the Treatment Outcomes of NaF and Nano-hydroxyapatite. *J. Dent. Res.* **2015**, *94*, 602–607. [CrossRef] [PubMed]
40. Gümüştaş, B.; Dikmen, B. Effectiveness of remineralization agents on the prevention of dental bleaching induced sensitivity: A randomized clinical trial. *Int. J. Dent. Hyg.* **2022**, *20*, 650–657. [CrossRef] [PubMed]
41. Netalkar, P.P.; Ym, K.; Natarajan, S.; Gadipelly, T.; Bhat, P.D.; Dasgupta, A.; Lewis, A. Effect of nano-hydroxyapatite incorporation on fluoride-releasing ability, penetration, and adaptation of a pit and fissure sealant. *Int. J. Paediatr. Dent.* **2022**, *32*, 344–351. [CrossRef]
42. Vano, M.; Derchi, G.; Barone, A.; Covani, U. Effectiveness of nano-hydroxyapatite toothpaste in reducing dentin hypersensitivity: A double-blind randomized controlled trial. *Quintessence Int.* **2014**, *45*, 703–711. [CrossRef] [PubMed]
43. Schwarz, F.; Arweiler, N.; Georg, T.; Reich, E. Desensitizing effects of an Er:YAG laser on hypersensitive dentine. *J. Clin. Periodontol.* **2022**, *29*, 211–215. [CrossRef] [PubMed]
44. Kurt, S.; Kırtıloğlu, T.; Yılmaz, N.A.; Ertaş, E.; Oruçoğlu, H. Evaluation of the effects of Er:YAG laser, Nd:YAG laser, and two different desensitizers on dentin permeability: In vitro study. *Lasers Med. Sci.* **2018**, *33*, 1883–1890. [CrossRef] [PubMed]
45. Contreras-Arriaga, B.; Rodríguez-Vilchis, L.E.; Contreras-Bulnes, R.; Olea-Mejia, O.F.; Scougall-Vilchis, R.J.; Centeno-Pedraza, C. Chemical and morphological changes in human dentin after Er:YAGlaser irradiation: EDS and SEM analysis. *Microsc. Res. Tech.* **2015**, *78*, 1019–1025. [CrossRef] [PubMed]
46. Todorovic, T.; Vujanovic, D. The influence of magnesium on the activity of some enzymes (AST, ALT, ALP) and lead content in some tissues. *Magnes. Res.* **2002**, *15*, 173–177. [PubMed]

Disclaimer/Publisher's Note: The statements, opinions and data contained in all publications are solely those of the individual author(s) and contributor(s) and not of MDPI and/or the editor(s). MDPI and/or the editor(s) disclaim responsibility for any injury to people or property resulting from any ideas, methods, instructions or products referred to in the content.

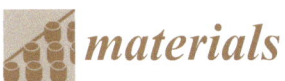

Article

Comparative Study Assessing the Canal Cleanliness Using Automated Device and Conventional Syringe Needle for Root Canal Irrigation—An Ex-Vivo Study

Keerthika Rajamanickam [1], Kavalipurapu Venkata Teja [1], Sindhu Ramesh [1,*], Abdulaziz S. AbuMelha [2], Mazen F. Alkahtany [3], Khalid H. Almadi [3], Sarah Ahmed Bahammam [4], Krishnamachari Janani [5], Sahil Choudhari [1], Jerry Jose [6], Kumar Chandan Srivastava [7,*], Deepti Shrivastava [8] and Shankargouda Patil [9,10]

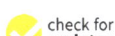

Citation: Rajamanickam, K.; Teja, K.V.; Ramesh, S.; AbuMelha, A.S.; Alkahtany, M.F.; Almadi, K.H.; Bahammam, S.A.; Janani, K.; Choudhari, S.; Jose, J.; et al. Comparative Study Assessing the Canal Cleanliness Using Automated Device and Conventional Syringe Needle for Root Canal Irrigation—An Ex-Vivo Study. *Materials* 2022, 15, 6184. https://doi.org/10.3390/ma15186184

Academic Editor: Abdelwahab Omri

Received: 21 July 2022
Accepted: 4 September 2022
Published: 6 September 2022

Publisher's Note: MDPI stays neutral with regard to jurisdictional claims in published maps and institutional affiliations.

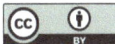

Copyright: © 2022 by the authors. Licensee MDPI, Basel, Switzerland. This article is an open access article distributed under the terms and conditions of the Creative Commons Attribution (CC BY) license (https:// creativecommons.org/licenses/by/ 4.0/).

[1] Department of Conservative Dentistry and Endodontics, Saveetha Dental College and Hospitals, Saveetha Institute of Medical and Technical Sciences, Chennai 600077, Tamil Nadu, India
[2] Restorative Dental Science Department, College of Dentistry, King Khalid University, Abha 62529, Saudi Arabia
[3] Department of RDS, Division of Endodontics, College of Dentistry, King Saud University, Riyadh 11545, Saudi Arabia
[4] Department of Pediatric Dentistry and Orthodontics, College of Dentistry, Taibah University, P.O. Box 344, Medina 42353, Saudi Arabia
[5] Department of Conservative Dentistry and Endodontics, SRM Dental College, SRM Institute of Science & Technology, Chennai 600089, Tamil Nadu, India
[6] Private Practice, Aluva, Ernakulam District, Kochi 683106, Kerala, India
[7] Department of Oral & Maxillofacial Surgery & Diagnostic Sciences, College of Dentistry, Jouf University, Sakaka 72388, Saudi Arabia
[8] Department of Preventive Dentistry, College of Dentistry, Jouf University, Sakaka 72388, Saudi Arabia
[9] Department of Maxillofacial Surgery and Diagnostic Sciences, Division of Oral Pathology, College of Dentistry, Jazan University, Jazan 45142, Saudi Arabia
[10] Centre of Molecular Medicine and Diagnostics (COMManD), Saveetha Dental College & Hospitals, Saveetha Institute of Medical and Technical Sciences, Saveetha University, Chennai 600077, Tamil Nadu, India
* Correspondence: drsinsushil@gmail.com (S.R.); drkcs.omr@gmail.com (K.C.S.)

Abstract: The success of endodontic treatment relies on both apical and coronal sealing. To achieve a good three-dimensional seal, the removal of the smear layer becomes mandatory. This study aims to assess the difference in debris accumulation and smear layer formation while using automated root canal irrigation and conventional syringe needle irrigation. Single-rooted human mandibular premolar teeth ($n = 30$) which were indicated for orthodontic extractions were selected. An endodontic access cavity was prepared, and a glide path was created. Based on the irrigation protocol decided upon for the study, the teeth were randomly allocated into three study groups, namely Group 1, where the manual syringe needle irrigation method was adopted; Group 2, in which automated root canal irrigation was undertaken; and Group 3, in which teeth remained un-instrumented as it was considered the Control group. The teeth were decoronated at the cement-enamel junction (CEJ) and were subjected for scanning electron microscopy (SEM) examination. Debris and smear layers were viewed in $1000\times$ magnification and scored. A statistically significant ($p < 0.05$) lower mean debris and smear layer score ($p < 0.05$) was observed in both study groups when compared with the control group. However, no significant difference ($p > 0.05$) in the debris and smear layer was observed between the manual syringe needle irrigation and automated irrigation, although automated irrigation devices can be a potential alternative. The present study concluded that the efficacy of smear layer removal remained the same with both automated irrigation and manual syringe irrigation.

Keywords: endodontic materials; automated root canal irrigation; manual syringe needle irrigation; root canal treatment; smear layer

1. Introduction

Biomechanical preparation is a crucial intermediate phase in root canal therapy, as it helps the irrigant to thoroughly disinfect the root canal system [1,2]. Evidence states that root canal preparation forms a smear layer which covers the root canal walls randomly up to 2–5 μm thickness [3,4]. Primarily, the smear layer is a crystalline structure containing remnants of pulp, dentinal debris, microorganisms, and their products [5]. It is usually contaminated and retains bacteria in the dentinal tubules, thereby limiting the optimal penetration of disinfecting agents such as irrigants and intracanal medicaments [6–8]. The smear layer contributes to increased coronal and apical microleakage by interfering with the penetration of root canal sealer [9,10]. Therefore, eliminating the tenacious smear layer is essential in order to achieve adequate disinfection [6] and to enhance the fluid-tight closure of the root canal system [11].

The preparation of the apical one-third segment of the root canal is a challenging task as the canals here are more constricted and curved with ramification [12]. Studies have proven that smear formation is more significant at the apical one third of the root canal, and it is quite challenging to clean and disinfect, due to the inherent anatomical complexities [13]. A recent study demonstrated that irrespective of the technique employed and the subjection to various irrigant agitation techniques, there is a formation of the smear layer at the apical one-third [14]. Hence the apical one third is the most critical and difficult part of the root canal to shape and clean [13,15,16]. Only a small number of authors believe that clearly laid clinical research is required to completely comprehend the effects of eliminating the smear layer and treatment outcomes. According to the data from a systematic review, the results of root canal therapy seem to be improved with the elimination of the smear layer, [4,6]. The information that is now available therefore supports eliminating of the smear layer before proceeding with root canal obturation [17].

Previous studies have discussed the importance of chemo-mechanical debridement methods in removing the adherent inorganic and organic smear layer from the root canal system [18,19]. The use of sodium hypochlorite (NaOCl) followed by ethylenediaminetetraacetic acid (EDTA) for 1 min each is a standard smear layer removal protocol [20]. Various other factors such as building a pre-endodontic coronal wall before root canal debridement, [21] access cavity design, [22,23] choice of root canal irrigant [24,25], irrigant concentration, [26] usage of root canal agitation devices for final irrigant activation, [27,28] type of irrigant activation device, [29–31] activation protocols, [32] choice of instrument used for the root canal debridement, [33–35] canal curvature, and the apical root canal anatomy [36] determines the debridement efficacy and smear removal from the root canal system.

A recent report [37] has highlighted a novel automated root canal irrigation device which could be a potential alternative to current syringe needle irrigation. The claimed advantage of the automated irrigant delivery flow rates include the prevention of the operator's fatigue and inherent irrigant extrusions. Hence, our study aimed at assessing root canal cleanliness after automated root canal irrigation using scanning electron microscopy. The null hypothesis considered in the current study was that no statistically significant difference in the debris accumulation or smear layer formation would occur with automated root canal irrigation as compared to the conventional syringe needle irrigation.

2. Materials and Methods

Before commencing the study, ethical approval was obtained from the institutional human ethical committee of Saveetha Dental College (Institutional Human Ethical Committee/Saveetha Dental College/Faculty/21/Endodontics/135). The research was performed as a pilot study, and the sample size was calculated with an effect size of 0.62, maintaining an alpha error of 5% and a study power of 80%. Thirty freshly extracted single-rooted human mandibular premolar teeth were obtained. These teeth had closed apices and had undergone therapeutic orthodontic extractions. Teeth chosen for the study had curvatures less than 10°. Teeth having calcifications and open apices were excluded from the study. Following tooth extraction, a curette was used to remove debris and small pieces of soft tissue was stuck to the tooth surface. To rule out the potential of numerous canals, digital radiography was used to evaluate each sample.

Following collection, the teeth were kept at +4 °C in physiological saline until the experiment. The purpose of storing at a low temperature is that it preserves the properties of the tooth and also provides potential storage medium for a longer duration. Storing the teeth in physiological saline aid prevents the growth of bacteria and dehydration. The 30 mandibular premolars' root surfaces were dipped in a molten wax of approximately 0.2–0.3 mm thick to a depth of 1 mm apical to the cement–enamel junction (CEJ). The molten wax layer was created to mimic or replicate the alveolar bone and periodontal ligament. Once the resin was completely set, the wax was removed from the samples and embed 1 mm apical to the CEJ vertically in a self-cure acrylic. The mould cavity was filled with elastomeric impression material and the sample was then re-seated. With a no. 15 scalpel blade, the extruded material was cut to size.

With the aid of a high-speed handpiece, the access cavity was prepared using Endo Access Bur (Dentsply Maillefer, Ballaigues, Switzerland). With a fine-barbed broach, the pulp tissue was removed. A #10 stainless steel K-file (Dentsply Maillefer, Ballaigues, Switzerland), was used to negotiate the canal until the apex. The working length was determined, and the glide path was created. Based on the irrigation protocol of the study, the teeth were randomly allocated into the following into three study groups:

- Group 1: Manual syringe needle irrigation (*n* = 10);
- Group 2: Automated root canal irrigation (*n* = 10);
- Group 3: Un-instrumented group (Control) (*n* = 10).

2.1. Group 1: Manual Syringe Needle Irrigation

All the canals were enlarged to 30 0.06 using Protaper gold rotary files. A disposable syringe with a 30-gauge side-vented needle (NaviTip, Ultradent Products, South Jordan, UT, USA) was employed for irrigation during and at the end of the instrumentation procedure. Two milliliters of 5.25% sodium hypochlorite solution (Parcan, Septodont, France) was used before starting the filing and at every change of instrument. Additionally, 2 mL of 17.5% EDTA solution (MD Cleanser, MetaBiomed, South Korea) and 2 mL of 5.25% NaOCl were alternately used. Each root canal received 2 mL of 5.25% NaOCl followed by 5 mL of a 5.25% NaOCl solution for the final irrigation. Distilled water was used as the final flush, and paper points were used to dry the canals.

2.2. Group 2: Automated Root Canal Irrigation

All the canals were enlarged to 30 0.06 using Protaper gold rotary files. An automated root canal irrigation device was coupled to a disposable plastic syringe with an attached 30-gauge side-vented needle (NaviTip, Ultradent Products, South Jordan, UT, USA) for irrigation in between and at the completion of the instrumentation process. The entire irrigation procedure was identical to group 1, but it was performed using an automated irrigation system [37]. Following the completion of the entire irrigation technique, the crown portion was decoronated at the cement–enamel junction (CEJ). Additionally, using a microtome LEICA SP 1600 (Wetzlar, Germany), the roots were separated bucco-lingually. The root was sputter-coated with gold and examined under scanning electron microscopy (SEM).

Using the scoring system developed by Hülsmann et al. [38], the debris and smear layers were examined independently and scores ranging from 1 to 5 were given [39] (Tables 1 and 2). The debris and smear layer were evaluated separately using reference images and a five score-index for each. All of the samples were scored by two unbiased evaluators (KJ and KVT) using calibration data for debris and smear layer scores. In 1000× magnification, the debris and smear layers were scored (Figure 1).

Table 1. Hülsmann criteria for debris scoring.

Score 1	Clean root canal wall, very slight debris.
Score 2	Slight debris.
Score 3	Moderate amount of debris,
Score 4	Substantial debris, >50% of the sample surface covered.
Score 5	Root canal sample was almost completely covered with debris.

Table 2. Hülsmann criteria for smear layer scoring.

Score 1	No smear layer, open dentinal tubuli
Score 2	Slight smear layer, most tubuli were open
Score 3	Homogeneous smear layer covering the major part of the surface, a few dentinal tubuli open
Score 4	Homogeneous smear layer covering the surface, no open dentinal tubuli.
Score 5	Thick nonhomogeneous smear layer covering the surface.

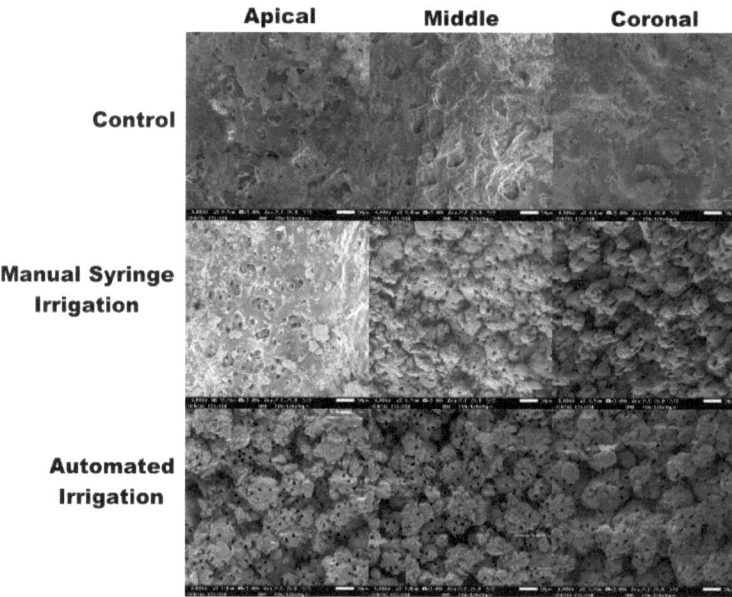

Figure 1. Scanning electron microscope images of the apical, middle and coronal third following irrigation of the control group, manual syringe irrigation group and automated irrigation group (1000× magnification).

2.3. Statistical Analysis

Using IBM SPSS Statistics for Windows, Version 23.0, the data was examined (Armonk, NY, IBM Corp, USA). The Kruskal–Wallis test was used to determine whether there was a significant difference between the independent groups. Dunn's pair-wise comparison test was used for an intra-group comparison.

3. Results

A significantly low mean debris and smear layer score ($p < 0.05$) was observed in both of study groups namely automated irrigation and control and manual syringe needle irrigation when they were individually compared with the control group. Additionally, no statistically significant difference was evident in the debris and smear layer scoring at the apical, middle or coronal region with regard to all three groups ($p > 0.05$). Nevertheless, no discernible difference between irrigation using a manual syringe needle and irrigation using an automated system was found (Tables 3 and 4).

Table 3. Mean distribution of debris and smear scores among different groups.

Group	Debris Score			p Value	Total	Smear Score			p Value	Total
	Apical	Middle	Coronal			Apical	Middle	Coronal		
Manual syringe needle irrigation	1.42 ± 0.50	1.43 ± 0.53	1.22 ± 0.41	0.11	4.01 ± 0.71	1.63 ± 0.82	1.42 ± 0.53	2.21 ± 0.86	0.23	5.22 ± 0.80
Automated root canal irrigation	1.31 ± 0.81	2.12 ± 1.02	2.24 ± 0.83	0.09	5.40 ± 2.13	1.13 ± 0.53	1.32 ± 0.84	2.02 ± 0.75	0.17	5.13 ± 1.60
Control	5.01 ± 0.72	5.41 ± 0.54	5.22 ± 0.85	0.26	13.61 ± 1.54	4.82 ± 0.82	5.21 ± 0.82	5.43 ± 1.13	0.50	13.44 ± 1.12
p value	0.00	0.01	0.01		0.04	0.02	0.00	0.01		0.01

Note: Results are expressed in Mean ± Standard Deviation; $p < 0.05$—Significant; $p > 0.05$—non-significant.

Table 4. Pair-wise Comparison of Mean debris and Smear layer scores.

Study Groups	Test Statistic	p Value
Automated irrigation vs. Manual syringe needle irrigation	0.60	0.10
Automated irrigation vs. Control	−10.50	0.01
Manual syringe needle irrigation vs. Control	−9.90	0.01

Note: $p < 0.05$—Significant; $p > 0.05$—non-significant.

4. Discussion

The current study results showed no statistically significant differences ($p > 0.05$) between the two different irrigation modes considered. Pair-wise comparison showed significant results ($p < 0.05$) with experimental irrigation modes as compared to control, with significant differences ($p > 0.05$) with syringe needle or automated irrigation. Despite irrigant activation developments, the usage of a syringe needle irrigation system has remained the main mode of supply during root canal disinfection [40]. Recent evidence states that there are various factors and parameters involved with the syringe needle irrigation which would alter the irrigant flow and apical pressures [41].

When preparing the root canal using manual or rotary instruments, the mineralized tissues are shredded, producing a large amount of debris. A significant portion of this, which is composed of extremely fine particles of mineralized collagen matrix, is applied to the surface to create the "smear layer".

Based on the previous periapical pressure assessment model, 1–4 mL/min is decided as an optimal irrigant flow rates to prevent the inherent apical pressures during irrigation [42,43]. However, it is impossible for an operator to maintain constant irrigant flow rates. Previous studies proved that syringe needle irrigation is difficult to standardize in the clinical scenario, as the irrigation efficiency varies based on the gender and clinical experience of the operator [44]. Hence, an automated root canal device could potentially benefit the operator by preventing the instant fatigue to operators and delivering the irrigant at constant flow rate.

To date, there is no data comparing the efficacy of the device for smear and debris removal. Hence, our study is the first one to assess smear removal and debris accumulation using automated root canal irrigation. Previous evidence clearly states the inefficiency of manual syringe needle irrigation in removal of debris and smear layer [27,28]. The current study aimed at assessing the manual syringe needle irrigation as compared to the automated root canal irrigation.

Histological evaluations of the amount of debris accumulation or residual smear layer in the root canal following instrumentation are used to measure the root canal cleanliness. The efficiency of rotary or reciprocating devices in canal cleanliness is still questionable [45,46]. Although some studies imply that reciprocating a approach leads to more debris accumulation [47], various other studies showed overall disinfection effectiveness almost comparable [45,46,48]. It has been proposed that it is the file design rather than a system's kinematics which is responsible for better disinfection [49]. We therefore attempted to standardize the rotary file system in the current study such that there might not be any differences in debris accumulation or smear formation.

In the present study, an un-instrumented group served as a control. As far as the irrigation protocol is concerned, the proposed irrigation regimen was standardized in all the groups with no activation protocol followed. A previous study stated that the smear layer and debris removal is partly attributed to the irrigation protocol followed too [50]. As the following protocol was similar in all the groups, the effect is negligible in the current study. The irrigation protocol for the current study was selected based on the previous research report which investigated various irrigants in smear removal [51], except for the concentration of sodium hypochlorite used during irrigation. As 5.25% sodium hypochlorite has been proved to be superior to any other concentrations in terms of both efficacy and effectiveness [52–58], and it is the most widely preferred by world-wide endodontists [59,60], we considered evaluating using 5.25% sodium hypochlorite.

To ensure complete removal of the smear layer, the smear layer must be correctly identified. The smear layer can be identified using an electron microprobe with a scanning electron microscope (SEM) and digital image analysis. In the present study, SEM was used for analysis of the smear layer. One of the limitations of this study is that extracted, single-rooted teeth with minimal curvature were used for evaluation. Another drawback was that the irrigant activation was not followed as it could be a confounding factor since our goal was to evaluate the accumulation of debris and smear when using various irrigation techniques. Although we adhered to a standardized root canal shaping methodology in the current investigation, we did not focus on analyzing the impact of access cavity sizes and types on the evaluated outcome. Therefore, future research should focus more on evaluating molars with complex anatomy and curvatures using a standardized approach that mimics a clinical setting.

5. Conclusions

Within the limitation of the study, it can be concluded that manual and automated irrigation devices showed similar results for the removal of the smear and debris layer with no difference elicited between both the groups. Future studies should be performed focusing the drawbacks addressed in the present study.

Author Contributions: Conceptualization, K.R., S.R., K.V.T., K.J., S.C. and J.J.; methodology, K.V.T., K.J., S.C. and J.J.; software, A.S.A., M.F.A., K.H.A., S.A.B. and S.P.; validation, A.S.A., M.F.A., K.H.A., S.A.B. and S.P.; formal analysis, K.R., K.V.T., K.J. and K.C.S.; investigation, K.R., S.R., K.V.T., K.J., S.C. and J.J.; data curation, A.S.A., M.F.A., K.H.A., S.A.B., K.C.S., D.S. and S.P.; writing—original draft preparation, K.R., S.R., K.V.T., K.J., K.C.S. and D.S.; writing—review and editing, K.R., S.R., K.V.T., A.S.A., M.F.A., K.H.A., S.A.B., K.J., S.C., J.J., K.C.S., D.S. and S.P.; visualization, M.F.A., K.H.A., S.A.B., D.S. and S.P.; supervision, S.R.; project administration, S.R. and K.C.S.; funding acquisition, K.C.S., A.S.A., M.F.A., K.H.A., S.A.B. and S.P. All authors have read and agreed to the published version of the manuscript.

Funding: This research received no external funding.

Institutional Review Board Statement: The study was conducted in accordance with the Declaration of Helsinki and approved by the Institutional Human Ethical Committee of Saveetha Dental College and Hospitals (IHEC/SDC/FACULTY/21/ENDO/135).

Informed Consent Statement: Informed consent was obtained from all subjects involved in the study.

Data Availability Statement: Data will be made available on reasonable request from the corresponding authors.

Conflicts of Interest: The authors declare no conflict of interest.

References

1. Hülsmann, M.; Peters, O.A.; Dummer, P.M.H. Mechanical preparation of root canals: Shaping goals, techniques and means. *Endod. Top.* **2005**, *10*, 30–76. [CrossRef]
2. Dhaimy, S.; Imdary, S.; Dhoum, S.; Benkiran, I.; El Ouazzani, A. Radiological Evaluation of Penetration of the Irrigant according to Three Endodontic Irrigation Techniques. *Int. J. Dent.* **2016**, *2016*, 3142742. [CrossRef] [PubMed]
3. Munoz, H.R.; Camacho-Cuadra, K. In vivo efficacy of three different endodontic irrigation systems for irrigant delivery to working length of mesial canals of mandibular molars. *J. Endod.* **2012**, *38*, 445–448. [CrossRef] [PubMed]
4. Torabinejad, M.; Handysides, R.; Khademi, A.A.; Bakland, L.K. Clinical implications of the smear layer in endodontics: A review. *Oral Surg. Oral Med. Oral Pathol. Oral Radiol. Endod.* **2002**, *94*, 658–666. [CrossRef]
5. Yang, G.; Wu, H.; Zheng, Y.; Zhang, H.; Li, H.; Zhou, X. Scanning electron microscopic evaluation of debris and smear layer remaining following use of ProTaper and Hero Shaper instruments in combination with NaOCl and EDTA irrigation. *Oral Surg. Oral Med. Oral Pathol. Oral Radiol. Endod.* **2008**, *106*, e63–e71. [CrossRef]
6. Violich, D.R.; Chandler, N.P. The smear layer in endodontics—a review. *Int. Endod. J.* **2010**, *43*, 2–15. [CrossRef]
7. Adorno, C.G.; Fretes, V.R.; Ortiz, C.P.; Mereles, R.; Sosa, V.; Yubero, M.F.; Escobar, P.M.; Heilborn, C. Comparison of two negative pressure systems and syringe irrigation for root canal irrigation: An ex vivo study. *Int. Endod. J.* **2016**, *49*, 174–183. [CrossRef]
8. Plotino, G.; Cortese, T.; Grande, N.M.; Leonardi, D.P.; Di Giorgio, G.; Testarelli, L.; Gambarini, G. New Technologies to Improve Root Canal Disinfection. *Braz. Dent. J.* **2016**, *27*, 3–8. [CrossRef]
9. Kokkas, A.B.; Boutsioukis, A.C.; Vassiliadis, L.P.; Stavrianos, C.K. The influence of the smear layer on dentinal tubule penetration depth by three different root canal sealers: An in vitro study. *J. Endod.* **2004**, *30*, 100–102. [CrossRef]
10. Çobankara, F.K.; Adanur, N.; Belli, S. Evaluation of the influence of smear layer on the apical and coronal sealing ability of two sealers. *J. Endod.* **2004**, *30*, 406–409. [CrossRef]
11. Shahravan, A.; Haghdoost, A.A.; Adl, A.; Rahimi, H.; Shadifar, F. Effect of smear layer on sealing ability of canal obturation: A systematic review and meta-analysis. *J. Endod.* **2007**, *33*, 96–105. [CrossRef]
12. Ruddle, C.J. Finishing the apical one third. Endodontic considerations. *Dent. Today* **2002**, *21*, 66–70, 72–73.
13. Park, E.; Shen, Y.A.; Haapasalo, M. Irrigation of the apical root canal. *Endod Top.* **2012**, *27*, 54–73. [CrossRef]
14. Kanaan, C.G.; Pelegrine, R.A.; da Silveira Bueno, C.E.; Shimabuko, D.M.; Pinto, N.M.V.; Kato, A.S. Can Irrigant Agitation Lead to the Formation of a Smear Layer? *J. Endod.* **2020**, *46*, 1120–1124. [CrossRef]
15. Yu, D.C.; Schilder, H. Cleaning and shaping the apical third of a root canal system. *Gen. Dent.* **2001**, *49*, 266–270.
16. Haapasalo, M.; Shen, Y.; Wang, Z.; Gao, Y. Irrigation in endodontics. *Br. Dent. J.* **2014**, *216*, 299–303. [CrossRef]
17. Pintor, A.V.; Dos Santos, M.R.; Ferreira, D.M.; Barcelos, R.; Primo, L.G.; Maia, L.C. Does Smear Layer Removal Influence Root Canal Therapy Outcome? A Systematic Review. *J. Clin. Pediatric Dent.* **2016**, *40*, 1–7. [CrossRef]
18. Alamoudi, R.A. The smear layer in endodontic: To keep or remove—an updated overview. *Saudi Endod. J.* **2019**, *9*, 71–81.
19. JOE Editorial Board. Root canal debridement: An online study guide. *J. Endod.* **2008**, *34*, e17–e31. [CrossRef]
20. Sen, B.H.; Wesselink, P.R.; Türkün, M. The smear layer: A phenomenon in root canal therapy. *Int. Endod. J.* **1995**, *28*, 141–148. [CrossRef]
21. Kharouf, N.; Pedullà, E.; La Rosa, G.R.M.; Bukiet, F.; Sauro, S.; Haikel, Y.; Mancino, D. In Vitro Evaluation of Different Irrigation Protocols on Intracanal Smear Layer Removal in Teeth with or without Pre-Endodontic Proximal Wall Restoration. *J. Clin. Med.* **2020**, *9*, 3325. [CrossRef] [PubMed]
22. Kulkarni, G.; Rajeev, K.G.; Ambalavanan, P.; Kidiyoor, K.H. Successful endodontic management of hypo, meso and hypertaurodontism: Two case reports. *Contemp. Clin. Dent.* **2012**, *3*, S253–S256. [PubMed]
23. Shabbir, J.; Zehra, T.; Najmi, N.; Hasan, A.; Naz, M.; Piasecki, L.; Azim, A.A. Access Cavity Preparations: Classification and Literature Review of Traditional and Minimally Invasive Endodontic Access Cavity Designs. *J. Endod.* **2021**, *47*, 1229–1244. [CrossRef] [PubMed]
24. Mohammadi, Z.; Shalavi, S.; Yaripour, S.; Kinoshita, J.I.; Manabe, A.; Kobayashi, M.; Giardino, L.; Palazzi, F.; Sharifi, F.; Jafarzadeh, H. Smear Layer Removing Ability of Root Canal Irrigation Solutions: A Review. *J. Contemp. Dent. Pract.* **2019**, *20*, 395–402. [CrossRef]
25. Gulati, S.; Mulay, S.; Shetty, R.; Bhosale, S. Comparative Evaluation of Chitosan and other Irrigating Solutions and Chelating Agents on their ability to Remove Smear Layer—A Systematic Review. *J. Crit. Rev.* **2020**, *7*, 4066–4072.
26. Orlowski, N.B.; Schimdt, T.F.; da Silveira Teixeira, C.; Garcia, L.D.F.R.; Savaris, J.M.; Tay, F.R.; Bortoluzzi, E.A. Smear Layer Removal Using Passive Ultrasonic Irrigation and Different Concentrations of Sodium Hypochlorite. *J. Endod.* **2020**, *46*, 1738–1744. [CrossRef]
27. Virdee, S.S.; Seymour, D.W.; Farnell, D.; Bhamra, G.; Bhakta, S. Efficacy of irrigant activation techniques in removing intracanal smear layer and debris from mature permanent teeth: A systematic review and meta-analysis. *Int. Endod. J.* **2018**, *51*, 605–621. [CrossRef]
28. Susila, A.; Minu, J. Activated Irrigation vs. Conventional non-activated Irrigation in Endodontics—A Systematic Review. *Eur. Endod. J.* **2019**, *4*, 96–110. [CrossRef]
29. Singh, A.K.; Khateeb, S.U.; Pathrose, S.P.; Kumar, A.S.; Haribaskar, S.; Thota, G. SEM Evaluation of Various Intracanal Irrigation Devices on Smear Layer Removal: A Comparative Study. *J. Contemp. Dent. Pract.* **2021**, *22*, 184–188.

30. Lauritano, D.; Moreo, G.; Carinci, F.; Della Vella, F.; Di Spirito, F.; Sbordone, L.; Petruzzi, M. Cleaning Efficacy of the XP-Endo®. Finisher Instrument Compared to Other Irrigation Activation Procedures: A Systematic Review. *Appl. Sci.* **2019**, *9*, 5001. [CrossRef]
31. Widbiller, M.; Keim, L.; Schlichting, R.; Striegl, B.; Hiller, K.A.; Jungbauer, R.; Buchalla, W.; Galler, K.M. Debris Removal by Activation of Endodontic Irrigants in Complex Root Canal Systems: A Standardized In-Vitro-Study. *Appl. Sci.* **2021**, *11*, 7331. [CrossRef]
32. Plotino, G.; Colangeli, M.; Özyürek, T.A.H.A.; DeDeus, G.; Panzetta, C.; Castagnola, R.; Grande, N.M.; Marigo, L. Evaluation of smear layer and debris removal by stepwise intraoperative activation (SIA) of sodium hypochlorite. *Clin. Oral Investig.* **2021**, *25*, 237–245. [CrossRef]
33. Campello, A.F.; Marceliano-Alves, M.F.; Siqueira, J.F.; Fonseca, S.C.; Lopes, R.T.; Alves, F.R. Unprepared surface areas, accumulated hard tissue debris, and dentinal crack formation after preparation using reciprocating or rotary instruments: A study in human cadavers. *Clin. Oral Investig.* **2021**, *25*, 6239–6248. [CrossRef]
34. Predin Djuric, N.; Van der Vyver, P.J.; Vorster, M.; Vally, Z.I. Factors influencing apical debris extrusion during endodontic treatment—A review of the literature. *S. Afr. Dent. J.* **2021**, *76*, 28–36. [CrossRef]
35. Dagna, A.; Gastaldo, G.; Beltrami, R.; Poggio, C. Debris evaluation after root canal shaping with rotating and reciprocating single-file systems. *J. Funct. Biomater.* **2016**, *7*, 28. [CrossRef]
36. Robberecht, L.; Dehurtevent, M.; Lemaitre, G.; Béhal, H.; Hornez, J.C.; Claisse-Crinquette, A. Influence of root canal curvature on wall cleanliness in the apical third during canal preparation. *Eur. Endod. J.* **2017**, *2*, 1–6. [CrossRef]
37. Teja, K.V.; Ramesh, S.; Vasundhara, K.A.; Janani, K.C.; Jose, J.; Battineni, G. A new innovative automated root canal device for syringe needle irrigation. *J. Taibah Univ. Med. Sci.* **2022**, *17*, 155–158. [CrossRef]
38. Metzger, Z.; Teperovich, E.; Cohen, R.; Zary, R.; Paqué, F.; Hülsmann, M. The self-adjusting file (SAF). Part 3: Removal of debris and smear layer—a scanning electron microscope study. *J. Endod.* **2010**, *36*, 697–702. [CrossRef]
39. Rödig, T.; Hülsmann, M.; Kahlmeier, C. Comparison of root canal preparation with two rotary NiTi instruments: ProFile. 04 and GT Rotary. *Int. Endod. J.* **2007**, *40*, 553–562. [CrossRef]
40. Sujith, I.L.; Teja, K.V.; Ramesh, S. Assessment of irrigant flow; apical pressure in simulated canals of single-rooted teeth with different root canal tapers and apical preparation sizes: An ex vivo study. *J. Conserv. Dent.* **2021**, *24*, 314–322.
41. Teja, K.V.; Ramesh, S.; Battineni, G.; Vasundhara, K.A.; Jose, J.; Janani, K. The effect of various in-vitro and ex-vivo parameters on irrigant flow and apical pressure using manual syringe needle irrigation: Systematic review. *Saudi Dent. J.* **2022**, *34*, 87–99. [CrossRef]
42. Park, E.; Shen, Y.; Khakpour, M.; Haapasalo, M. Apical pressure and extent of irrigant flow beyond the needle tip during positive-pressure irrigation in an in vitro root canal model. *J. Endod.* **2013**, *39*, 511–515. [CrossRef] [PubMed]
43. Khan, S.; Niu, L.N.; Eid, A.A.; Looney, S.W.; Didato, A.; Roberts, S.; Pashley, D.H.; Tay, F.R. Periapical pressures developed by nonbinding irrigation needles at various irrigation delivery rates. *J. Endod.* **2013**, *39*, 529–533. [CrossRef] [PubMed]
44. Boutsioukis, C.; Lambrianidis, T.; Kastrinakis, E.; Bekiaroglou, P. Measurement of pressure and flow rates during irrigation of a root canal ex vivo with three endodontic needles. *Int. Endod. J.* **2007**, *40*, 504–513. [CrossRef] [PubMed]
45. Amaral, P.; Forner, L.; Llena, C. Smear layer removal in canals shaped with reciprocating rotary systems. *J. Clin. Exp. Dent.* **2013**, *5*, e227. [CrossRef]
46. De-Deus, G.; Barino, B.; Zamolyi, R.Q.; Souza, E.; Júnior, A.F.; Fidel, S.; Fidel, R.A. Suboptimal debridement quality produced by the single-file F2 ProTaper technique in oval-shaped canals. *J. Endod.* **2010**, *36*, 1897–1900. [CrossRef] [PubMed]
47. Robinson, J.P.; Lumley, P.J.; Cooper, P.R.; Grover, L.M.; Walmsley, A.D. Reciprocating root canal technique induces greater debris accumulation than a continuous rotary technique as assessed by 3-dimensional micro–computed tomography. *J. Endod.* **2013**, *39*, 1067–1070. [CrossRef]
48. Dietrich, M.A.; Kirkpatrick, T.C.; Yaccino, J.M. In vitro canal and isthmus debris removal of the self-adjusting file, K3, and WaveOne files in the mesial root of human mandibular molars. *J. Endod.* **2012**, *38*, 1140–1144. [CrossRef]
49. Bürklein, S.; Hinschitza, K.; Dammaschke, T.; Schäfer, E. Shaping ability and cleaning effectiveness of two single-file systems in severely curved root canals of extracted teeth: Reciproc and WaveOne versus Mtwo and ProTaper. *Int. Endod. J.* **2012**, *45*, 449–461. [CrossRef]
50. Kim, J.-G.; Kum, K.-Y.; Kim, E.-S. Comparative study on morphology of cross-section and cyclic fatigue test with different rotary NiTi files and handling methods. *J. Korean Acad. Conserv. Dent.* **2006**, 96–102. [CrossRef]
51. Wadhwani, K.K.; Tikku, A.P.; Chandra, A.; Shakya, V.K. A comparative evaluation of smear layer removal using two rotary instrument systems with ethylenediaminetetraacetic acid in different states: A SEM study. *Indian J. Dent. Res.* **2011**, *22*, 10–15. [CrossRef]
52. Gomes, B.P.; Ferraz, C.C.; Vianna, M.E.; Berber, V.B.; Teixeira, F.B.; Souza-Filho, F.J. In vitro antimicrobial activity of several concentrations of sodium hypochlorite and chlorhexidine gluconate in the elimination of Enterococcus faecalis. *Int. Endod. J.* **2001**, *34*, 424–428. [CrossRef]
53. Vianna, M.E.; Gomes, B.P.; Berber, V.B.; Zaia, A.A.; Ferraz, C.C.; de Souza-Filho, F.J. In vitro evaluation of the antimicrobial activity of chlorhexidine and sodium hypochlorite. *Oral Surg. Oral Med. Oral Pathol. Oral Radiol. Endod.* **2004**, *97*, 79–84. [CrossRef]

54. Berber, V.B.; Gomes, B.P.; Sena, N.T.; Vianna, M.E.; Ferraz, C.C.; Zaia, A.A.; Souza-Filho, F.J. Efficacy of various concentrations of NaOCl and instrumentation techniques in reducing Enterococcus faecalis within root canals and dentinal tubules. *Int. Endod. J.* **2006**, *39*, 10–17. [CrossRef]
55. Oliveira, D.P.; Barbizam, J.V.; Trope, M.; Teixeira, F.B. In vitro antibacterial efficacy of endodontic irrigants against Enterococcus faecalis. *Oral Surg. Oral Med. Oral Pathol. Oral Radiol. Endod.* **2007**, *103*, 702–706. [CrossRef]
56. Mohammadi, Z. Sodium hypochlorite in endodontics: An update review. *Int. Dent. J.* **2008**, *58*, 329–341. [CrossRef]
57. Giardino, L.; Ambu, E.; Savoldi, E.; Rimondini, R.; Cassanelli, C.; Debbia, E.A. Comparative evaluation of antimicrobial efficacy of sodium hypochlorite, MTAD, and Tetraclean against Enterococcus faecalis biofilm. *J. Endod.* **2007**, *33*, 852–855. [CrossRef]
58. Jefferson, J.C.; Manhães, F.C.; Bajo, H.; Duque, T.M. Efficiency of different concentrations of sodium hypochlorite during endodontic treatment. *Dental Press Endod. J.* **2012**, *2*, 32–37.
59. Basudan, S.O. Sodium hypochlorite use, storage, and delivery methods: A Survey. *Saudi Endod. J.* **2019**, *9*, 27–33.
60. Cárdenas-Bahena, Á.; Sánchez-García, S.; Tinajero-Morales, C.; González-Rodríguez, V.M.; Baires-Várguez, L. Use of sodium hypochlorite in root canal irrigation. Opinion survey and concentration in commercial products. *Rev. Odontológica Mex.* **2012**, *16*, 252–258.

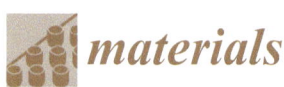 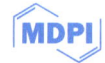

Article

The Impact of Citric Acid Solution on Hydraulic Calcium Silicate-Based Sealers and Root Dentin: A Preliminary Assessment

Saulius Drukteinis [1,*], Goda Bilvinaite [1,2] and Simas Sakirzanovas [2]

1. Institute of Dentistry, Faculty of Medicine, Vilnius University, Zalgirio 115, LT-08217 Vilnius, Lithuania; goda.bilvinaite@mf.stud.vu.lt
2. Department of Applied Chemistry, Institute of Chemistry, Vilnius University, Naugarduko 24, LT-03225 Vilnius, Lithuania; simas.sakirzanovas@chf.vu.lt
* Correspondence: saulius.drukteinis@mf.vu.lt; Tel.: +370-610-41808

Abstract: Hydraulic calcium silicate-based (HCS) sealers have recently gained tremendous popularity due to their unique properties. However, their removal during endodontic retreatment is challenging. The solvent, which could chemically deteriorate the material, would be highly desirable for endodontic retreatment procedures. This preliminary study assessed the interplay and dissolving capability of 10% and 20% citric acid, compared to 17% EDTA, on commonly used HCS sealers (AH Plus Bioceramic Sealer, Bio-C Sealer, BioRoot RCS, TotalFill BC Sealer), and evaluated the potential impact of these solutions on root dentin structure. The interaction between tested sealers and irrigating solutions was photographed, and solubility-related mass changes were determined. The surface morphology of treated filling materials and dentin was evaluated using a scanning electron microscope (SEM). One-way analysis of variance (ANOVA) along with Tukey's test were used to detect the statistically significant differences among groups at the confidence level of 0.95. Intense gas release was observed during the interaction of HCS materials and citric acid, with no evidently visible "bubbling" after the immersion in EDTA. The mass loss of HCS sealers equally confirmed the significantly higher dissolving characteristics of 10% and 20% citric acid solutions compared to EDTA. The surface structural changes, associated with pore and crack formation, were mainly seen for HCS sealers exposed to citric acid. Meanwhile, no severe erosion was detected for dentin after root canal preparation with 10% and 20% citric acid solutions. These findings demonstrate that citric acid has the potential to dissolve HCS sealers with minimal or no negative impact on root dentin, suggesting citric acid as a solvent for HCS sealers in endodontic retreatment procedures.

Keywords: calcium silicate; sealer; citric acid; EDTA; retreatment; root canal; SEM; solvent

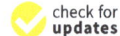

Citation: Drukteinis, S.; Bilvinaite, G.; Sakirzanovas, S. The Impact of Citric Acid Solution on Hydraulic Calcium Silicate-Based Sealers and Root Dentin: A Preliminary Assessment. *Materials* **2024**, *17*, 1351. https://doi.org/10.3390/ma17061351

Academic Editors: Lavinia Cosmina Ardelean and Laura-Cristina Rusu

Received: 14 February 2024
Revised: 9 March 2024
Accepted: 13 March 2024
Published: 15 March 2024

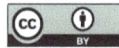

Copyright: © 2024 by the authors. Licensee MDPI, Basel, Switzerland. This article is an open access article distributed under the terms and conditions of the Creative Commons Attribution (CC BY) license (https:// creativecommons.org/licenses/by/ 4.0/).

1. Introduction

The success of endodontic treatments is significantly affected by the quality of root canal obturation and the materials used, including endodontic sealers [1]. These materials must ensure a three-dimensional seal within the root canal system, preventing re-infection and promoting the long-term success and survival of the endodontically treated tooth [2]. Despite meticulous efforts during the initial endodontic treatment procedures, the success rates of primary endodontics never reach 100% [3]. The need for endodontic retreatment usually arises if there is a persistent or recurrent infection and the tooth continues to exhibit symptoms, e.g., persistent pain, swelling, or inflammation [4]. Additionally, various problems and complications, such as missed root canals, incomplete removal of the pulp tissue, and non-hermetic root canal sealing, may warrant a second intervention [5].

The ability to completely remove the previous root canal filling material, typically the gutta-percha and the sealer, is crucial for precise root canal disinfection and subsequent re-obturation during endodontic retreatment. Factors such as the type of sealer, its chemical composition, and its interaction with root canal walls highly affect how easily the sealer can be dislodged and removed [6]. However, unlike the gutta-percha, most sealers do not have any specific solvent, facilitating their removal from the root canal system [6,7]. This problem equally applies to all types of hydraulic calcium silicate-based (HCS) materials, which are currently the most popular clinical choice and are highly recommended by various clinical guidelines and evidence-based data [8].

Over the years, various endodontic sealers have been developed, each possessing unique properties, advantages, and disadvantages [9]. The choice of sealer often depends on factors such as the specific clinical scenario, the clinician's experience and preference, and the desired properties of the material suitable to the particular biological conditions of every clinical case [10]. HCS sealers significantly changed the fundamental principles of root canal obturation, which focused on higher amounts of gutta-percha and less sealer [11]. Due to the lack of shrinkage and long-term dimensional stability, HCS materials overcame the need to increase the gutta-percha/sealer ratio and, thus, were advocated for the simplified obturation concept based on the single tapered gutta-percha point and HCS sealer [12]. This root canal filling technique highly simplified the daily clinical practice, even for operators with limited clinical experience, while equally providing high clinical success rates in primary endodontic treatment and retreatment [13].

However, the retreatment of root canals previously obturated with HCS sealers usually poses a significant challenge. Owing to the adhesion of HCS materials to the dentin via mineral infiltration zone formation and the deeper penetrability into dentinal tubules, these sealers are hardly removed from the root canal system, even mechanically [14]. The previously tested irrigating solutions, such as EDTA, NaOCl, carbonated water, and formic and acetic acids, could neither successfully dislodge nor dissolve the HCS sealers [15]. Therefore, the need for solvents for HCS materials still remains a clinically relevant topic.

Citric acid is a colorless organic acid commonly tested in endodontic research for different purposes [16]. However, little attention has been paid to citric acid as a potential solvent for HCS sealers. Based on the existing evidence-based literature on the chemistry of HCS cements, citric acid induces the gradual dissolution of calcium-based hydration products, eventually compromising the structural integrity of the material [17]. Therefore, it can be assumed that if the citric acid can dissolve the HCS materials, the solution could potentially be used as a solvent during endodontic retreatment when indicated.

The number of commercially available HCS materials, launched as powder/liquid formulations or premixed and ready-to-use pastes, has increased significantly within the last few years [12]. Five types of HCS materials are available. The first type of material is based on Portland cement, contains a radio-pacifier and no additives, and is mixed with water. The second type has various additives (e.g., calcium oxide, calcium carbonate), whereas, in the third type, the water is replaced by alternative vehicles [18]. The fourth and fifth types of HCS materials are the most widespread in modern endodontics. Although both types are tri-calcium silicate-based, type four has to be hand-mixed with water, while type five is already premixed and ready to use [18]. BioRoot RCS sealer (BR; Septodont, Saint-Maur-des-Fosses, France) is a widely investigated fourth-type material, which is provided in powder (tri-calcium silicate, zirconium oxide, povidone) and liquid (water, calcium chloride, polycarboxylate) formulations. It should be manually mixed before use [11]. TotalFill BC Sealer (TF; FKG, La Chaux-de-Fonds, Switzerland) is one of the first introduced premixed formulations (fifth generation) composed of tri-and dicalcium silicate, calcium phosphate monobasic, zirconium oxide, tantalum oxide, calcium hydroxide, filler, and thickening agents [11]. Bio-C Sealer (BIOC; Angelus, Londrina, Brazil) is another premixed fifth-generation HCS sealer containing tri-and dicalcium silicate, tri-calcium aluminate, calcium oxide, zirconium oxide, silicon oxide, polyethene glycol, and iron oxide [12]. AH, Plus Bioceramic Sealer (AHPB; Dentsply Sirona, Ballaiques, Switzerland) is a relatively new also premixed fifth-type HCS material composed of zirconium dioxide, tri-calcium silicate, dimethyl sulfoxide, lithium carbonate, and thickening agents [12]. However, it should be highlighted that all these materials have the same biological properties and differ slightly in their chemical compositions and physical properties [10].

The solvent must have a disintegrational and deterioration effect on the appropriate material and simultaneously avoid exerting detrimental effects on the dentin microstructure. It has been demonstrated that scanning electron microscopy (SEM) is a precise method widely used in endodontic research to observe the topographic profiles of the surfaces of instruments, materials, or root dentine [19–21]. Since little is known about the interaction of citric acid with commonly used HCS sealers and root canal dentine, the present study aimed to assess the potential impact of 10% and 20% citric acid solutions on HCS materials and root canal dentine using SEM. The tested hypothesis was that citric acid possesses dissolving capability on HCS sealers with no adverse effect on root canal dentine.

2. Materials and Methods

2.1. HCS Sealers Preparation

Four HCS materials to be tested (AH Plus Bioceramic Sealer, Bio-C Sealer, BioRoot RCS and TotalFill BC Sealer) were prepared according to the manufacturer's instructions. Plastic molds (5 mm diameter × 2 mm height) were used to standardize the samples. Molds filled with HCS sealers were incubated in culture tissue dishes sealed with polyethylene film at 37 °C. Samples were regularly sprayed with Hank's balanced salt solution (HBSS) for the first 12 h (2 sprays of 0.1 mL per application every hour at the 20 cm source-to-object distance), aiming to provide moisture for the initial setting of sealers. Full immersion into storage solution within the first hours was avoided due to a high risk of material washout. After the initial setting, samples were stored in gelatinized HBSS for 59 days at 37 °C. At the end of incubation, the surfaces of all samples were polished with fine polishing discs. Samples were then gently removed from molds, rinsed in distilled water, and incubated in gas-permeable culture tissue dishes for 24 h at 37 °C to allow for liquid evaporation. Samples with cracks and pores detected on the radiographs were discarded.

2.2. Visualization of HCS Exposure to EDTA and Citric Acid

Six samples of each completely set material were selected to visualize the interaction between HCS sealers and 17% EDTA (Cerkamed, Stalowa Wola, Poland), 10% citric acid, and 20% citric acid solutions. Both citric acid solutions were prepared by diluting 40% citric acid (Cerkamed, Stalowa Wola, Poland) with distilled water. Specimens were immersed in Eppendorf polypropylene tubes (Eppendorf, Hamburg, Germany) containing 2 mL of the tested irrigating solution. The experiment was repeated twice, and the visible outcome was recorded with a camera.

2.3. Solubility of HCS Sealers

The minimum sample size was calculated using G*Power v.3.1 software (Heinrich Heine, Dusseldorf, Germany) with α error probability of 0.05 and 1-β error probability of 0.90. A required size of 8 specimens per group was determined. A total of 24 samples completely set of each material were weighed to an accuracy of 0.0001 g, and the mass was recorded as M_1. Samples were then randomly allocated to three groups (n = 8): 17% EDTA (served as a control), 10% citric acid, and 20% citric acid.

HCS samples were fully immersed in 2 mL of test solution for 5 min. Afterwards, samples were rinsed in distilled water for 1 min and incubated in gas-permeable culture tissue dishes for 24 h at 37 °C. The mass determined after the incubation was marked as M_2. The percentage difference between the initial mass (M_1) and final mass (M_2) was calculated to express the material's solubility in the immersion solution.

2.4. Statistical Analysis

Statistical analysis was performed using RStudio software v.4.1.1 (RStudio Inc., Boston, MA, USA). The Shapiro–Wilk test, followed by the Levene's test, was applied to determine the assumption of normality and the homogeneity of variance, respectively. One-way analysis of variance (ANOVA) along with Tukey's test were selected to detect the statistically significant differences among groups at the confidence level of 0.95.

2.5. Root Canal Preparation

Nine intact and fully developed single-rooted lower premolars from patients aged 15–20 years were selected for this preliminary observation. Vital teeth were extracted for medical reasons and subsequently used in the study under the approval of the local ethics committee (protocol no. EK-2). Teeth were stored in 0.5% Chloramine-T trihydrate solution at 4 °C until the start of preparation.

Conventional endodontic access cavities were prepared using size No.2 EndoAccess burs (Dentsply Sirona, Ballaigues, Switzerland). The root canal length was determined by inserting a size 10 K-file into the canal until the tip was visible at the apical foramin, and the working length (WL) was established 1 mm short of the root canal length. Teeth were then randomly allocated to experimental groups (n = 3) depending on the irrigating solution applied during the preparation of root canals: 17% EDTA, 10% citric acid, or 20% citric acid.

The glide path was created using size 15 and 20 K-Flexofile (Dentsply Sirona, Ballaigues, Switzerland) instruments. Further root canal shaping was performed with Hylex EDM instruments (Coltene-Whaledent, Allstetten, Switzerland) to the full WL in the following sequence: 25/0.12 Orifice opener, 25/~HyFlex OneFile, 40/0.04 Finishing File, 50/0.03 Finishing File. EDM instruments, powered by CanalPro Cordless Handpiece (Coltene-Whaledent, Allstetten, Switzerland), were used at a rotation speed of 500 rpm and a torque control level of 2.5 N/cm according to the manufacturer's recommendations. During the shaping, root canals were repeatedly irrigated with 2 mL of appropriate irrigating solution for 2 min after each instrument change. As a final flush, 5 mL of sterile distilled water was used. The 5 mL syringes and 31-G NaviTip irrigation needles (Ultradent Products Inc., South Jordan, UT, USA) were used to deliver the irrigating solutions. All root canal shaping and cleaning procedures were performed by a single operator, an experienced endodontist.

After the preparation, root canals were dried with paper points. Teeth were carefully grooved longitudinally on the buccal and lingual surfaces without penetrating the root canal space. The specimens were then gently split into half and subjected to observation under a scanning electron microscope (SEM).

2.6. Scanning Electron Microscopy

The surface morphology of HCS sealers was evaluated using SEM Hitachi TM3000 (Hitachi, Tokyo, Japan), with an accelerating voltage of 15 kV. Three random specimens from each test group were attached to an aluminum stub and examined at ×1.0 k magnification.

Analysis of the dentin surface was performed using SEM Hitachi SU-70 (Hitachi, Tokyo, Japan). Specimens were dried in a vacuum desiccator, coated with silver, and examined at ×500, ×2.5 k, and ×5.0 k magnifications with an accelerating voltage of 2 kV.

3. Results

3.1. Visualization of HCS Exposure to EDTA and Citric Acid

Representative images visualizing the exposure of HCS sealers to 17% EDTA and 10% and 20% citric acid solution are shown in Figure 1. The more intense dissolution-related "bubbling" was visible in both citric acid solutions compared to EDTA. Meanwhile, the intensity of the gas release in 10% and 20% citric acid solutions was visually similar. The bubbling continued for all tested 5 min periods.

Considering the differences among the HCS sealers tested, all filling materials submerged in 17% EDTA revealed similar behavior, associated with the formation of only a few gas bubbles. On the contrary, the "bubbling" seen in citric acid solutions was apparently different, with the AHPB sealer demonstrating the most intense gas release.

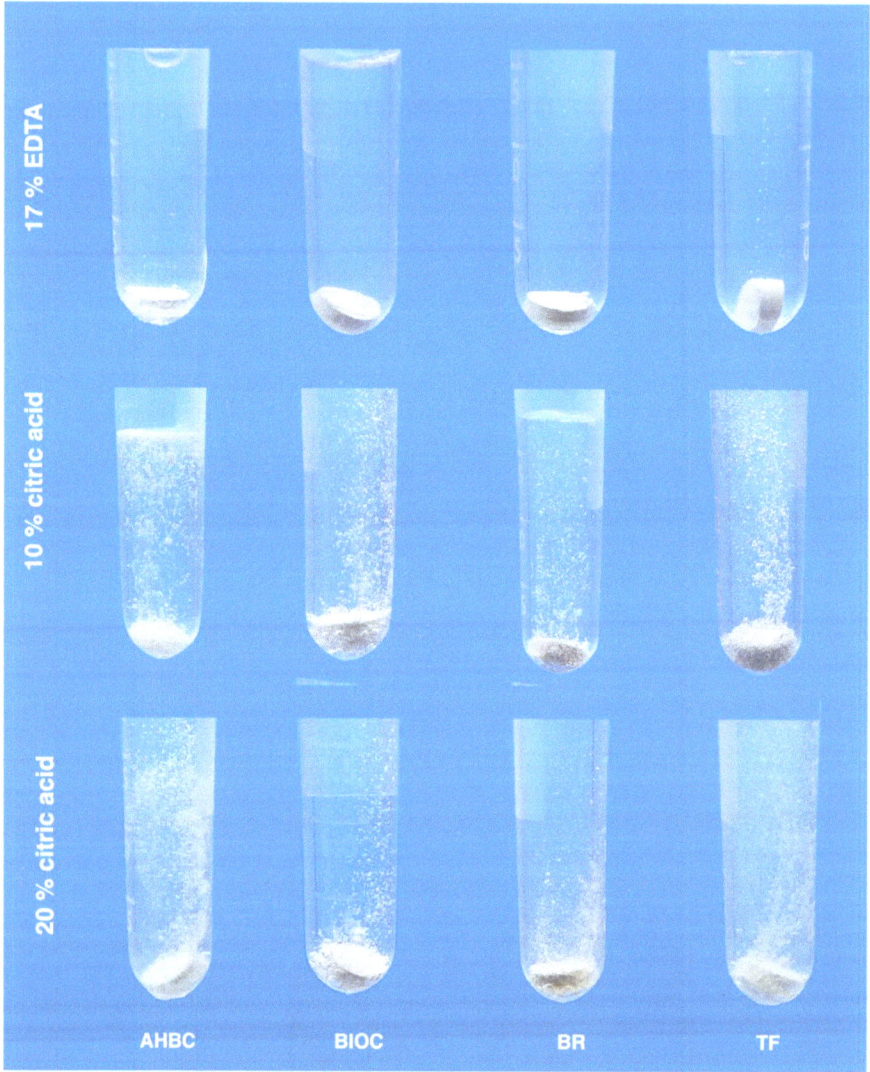

Figure 1. Representative images of HCS materials submerged into organic acids and demonstrating different intensities of "bubbling".

3.2. Solubility of HCS Sealers

The solubility of HCS sealers, to a certain degree, was determined for all tested solutions (Table 1). The highest solubility of all pre-mixed filling materials (AHPB, BIOC, and TF) was observed in 20% citric acid, followed by 10% citric acid. Meanwhile, BR demonstrated controversial results, being the most soluble in 10% citric acid. However, no tested HCS sealers showed statistically significant differences in mass loss between the 10% and 20% citric acid solutions. Further, both citric acid solutions were significantly more effective solvents for HCS materials compared to 17% EDTA.

Table 1. Mean and minimum–maximum percentages (%) of material mass loss in each immersion solution tested.

Sealer	17% EDTA	10% Citric Acid	20% Citric Acid
AHBC	14.19 (13.95–14.37) [A]	22.27 (21.45–23.75) [B]	23.42 (22.36–24.95) [B]
BIOC	7.11 (6.48–8.42) [C]	12.58 (11.08–15.01) [D]	13.62 (12.02–15.63) [D]
BR	3.05 (2.68–3.35) [E]	6.51 (5.98–7.17) [F]	6.29 (5.92–6.72) [F]
TF	4.32 (3.92–4.81) [G]	7.08 (6.61–7.42) [H]	7.72 (6.91–8.24) [H]

Values indexed with the same superscript letter in a row had no statistically significant differences ($p > 0.05$).

3.3. Surface Characterization of HCS Sealers

The superior dissolving properties of the 10% and 20% citric acid solutions were equally confirmed by SEM analysis of the treated HCS sealers (Figure 2). Morphological changes associated with pores and crack formation were clearly visible for all HCS materials exposed to citric acid solutions. Meanwhile, the damage to structural integrity provoked by EDTA was apparently less pronounced, and was mainly noticed for the AHPB sealer.

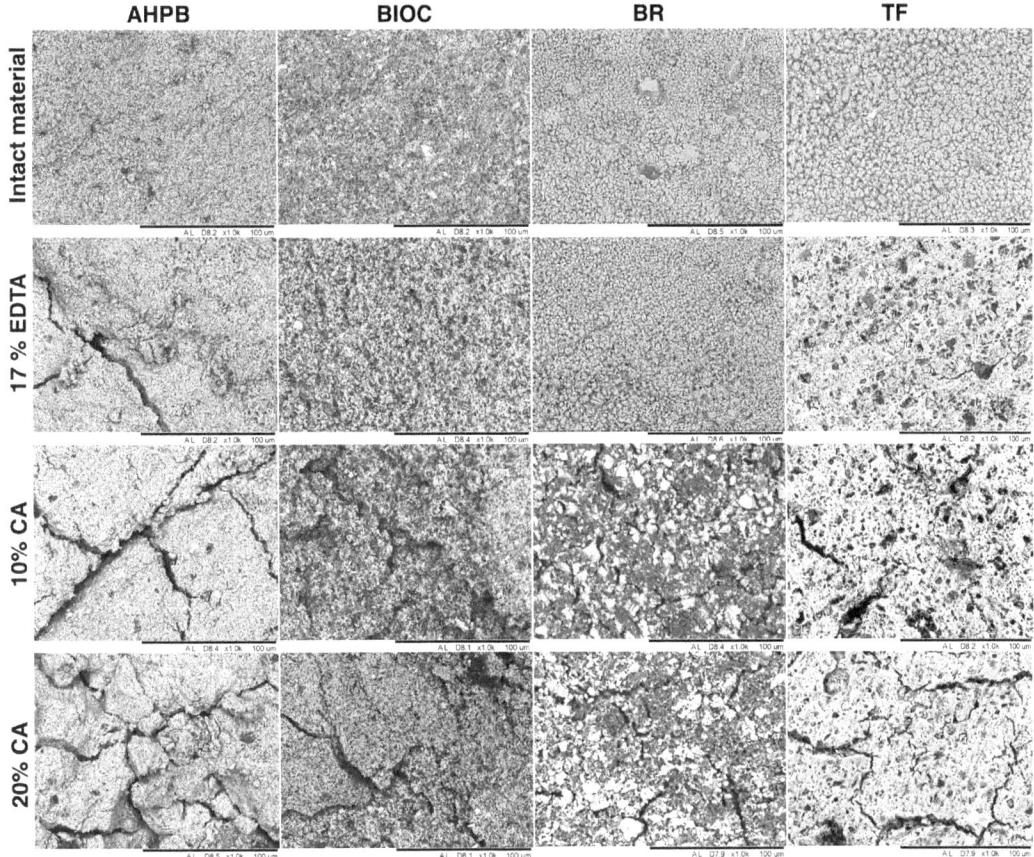

Figure 2. Representative SEM images of tested HCS materials before and after exposure to EDTA and citric acid (CA) solutions ($\times 1.0$ k magnification).

3.4. Surface Characterization of Root Dentin

Representative images of the root canal segments treated with 17% EDTA, 10% citric acid, and 20% citric acid solutions are shown in Figures 3–5, respectively. The EDTA mainly resulted in widening of the dentinal tubules, with some erosion and exposition of collagen fibrils. No evident structural changes were observed for 10% citric acid-treated dentine, demonstrating relatively regular and smooth outlines of most dentinal tubules. Meanwhile, the 20% citric acid resulted in relatively minimal peritubular and intertubular erosion, associated with rough and wider orifices of some dentin tubules. However, none of the tested groups demonstrated severe damage to dentine integrity nor to surface structure.

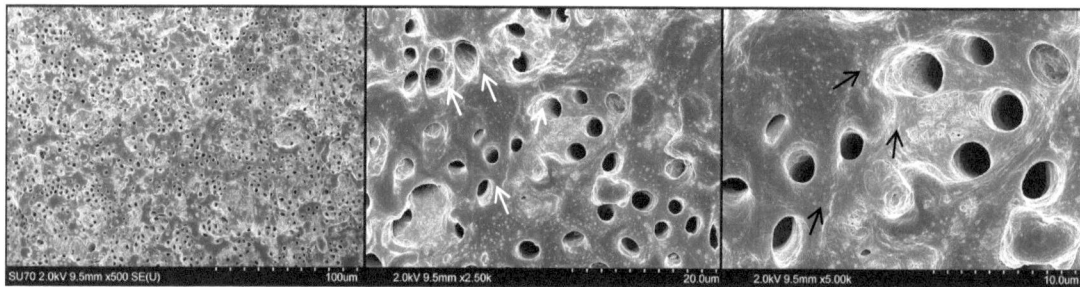

Figure 3. Representative SEM images of dentin surfaces conditioned with 17% EDTA. Magnifications at ×500, ×2.5 k, and ×5.0 k (**left** to **right**). White arrows indicate some widened and eroded dentinal tubules. Black arrows show areas of exposition of collagen fibrils.

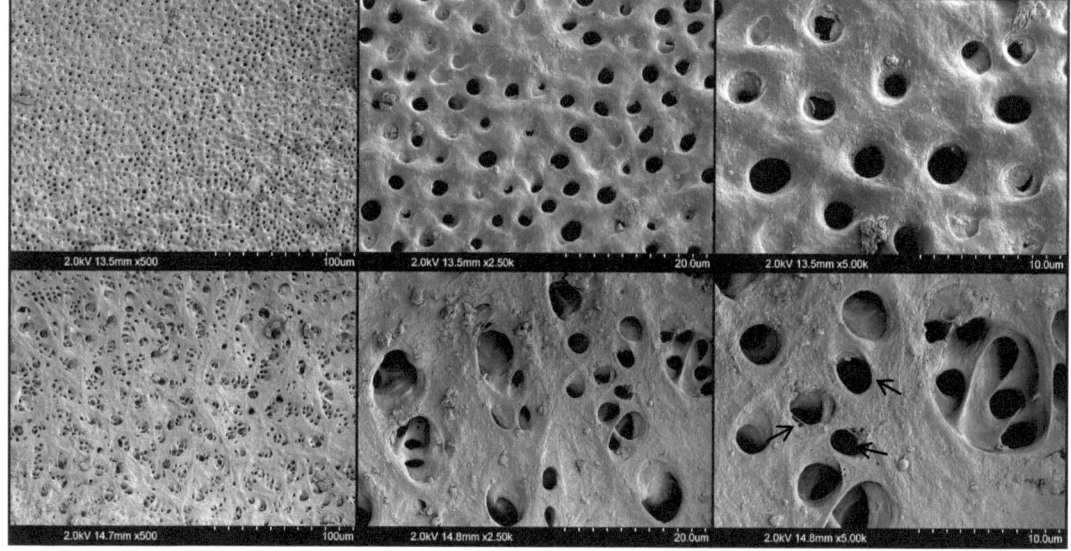

Figure 4. Representative SEM images of dentin surfaces conditioned with 10% citric acid. Magnifications set at ×500, ×2.5 k, and ×5.0 k (**left** to **right**). Arrows show areas of exposed collagen fibrils.

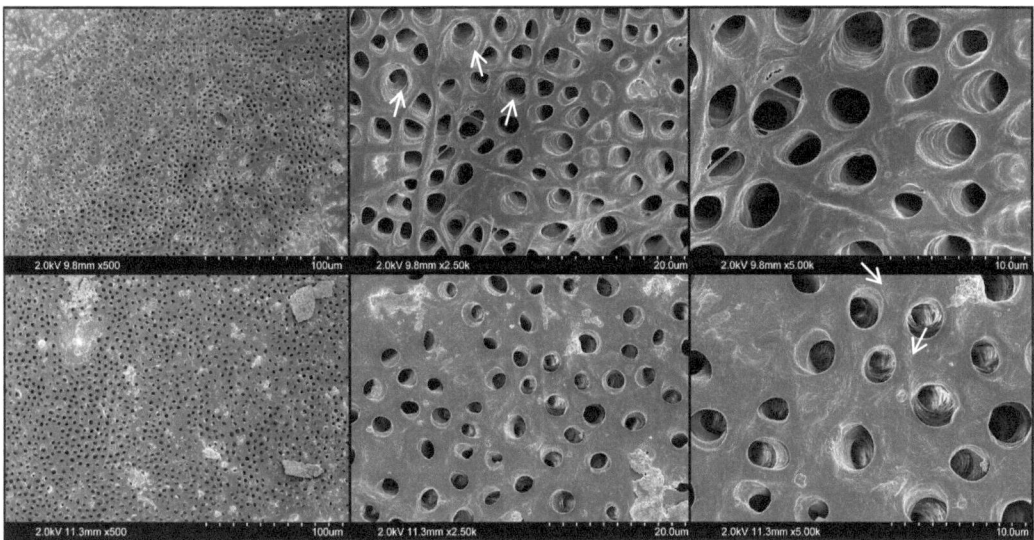

Figure 5. Representative SEM images of dentin surfaces conditioned with 20% citric acid. Magnifications at ×500, ×2.5 k, and ×5.0 k (**left** to **right**). Arrows indicate some widened and eroded dentinal tubules.

4. Discussion

This initial observation evaluated the dissolving potential of different concentrations of citric acid solutions on the fourth and fifth types of HCS sealers. Also, the potential detrimental impact of these irrigants on the microstructure of root dentine was examined. The findings indicated that citric acid at different concentrations could effectively dissolve all tested HCS materials without causing adverse effects on the root canal dentine. Therefore, the null hypothesis was accepted.

It has been shown that using different organic solvents or heat facilitates the removal of gutta-percha during endodontic retreatment [7]. However, the removal of root canal sealers, particularly based on HCS, is considerably more challenging owing to the higher physicochemical stability of these materials and, thus, the increased resistance to different solvents [6,15]. Currently, it is generally assumed that no specific and compelling solvent exists for HCS sealers [22]. Therefore, the mechanical removal of the previously placed HCS filling material remains the only clinically available option for endodontic retreatment procedures.

Published studies demonstrate that the retreatability of root canals filled with HCS sealers is possible, and that root canal patency can be regained in 91.67–100% of cases, depending on the tooth type [23,24]. However, the retreatment procedure is more challenging and time-consuming compared to some sealers with different chemical compositions [24]. It has been shown that removal of the HCS materials requires twice as much time as the resin-based or zinc oxide eugenol-based sealers [24]. Additionally, removing HCS sealers from larger root canals requires even more time, as the higher quantity of the sealer must be removed mechanically [23]. It should also be highlighted that internal root canal anatomy is usually very complex, and endodontic instruments cannot ensure complete root canal debridement and filling material removal [25,26]. Aiming to touch a higher surface area of the root canal walls, instruments bigger in size and taper might be used [25]. However, this generally results in excessive dentin removal, thereby weakening the root and increasing the risk of fracture. Therefore, a solvent capable of dissolving HCS materials would be a highly desirable clinical means to facilitate all these endodontic retreatment procedures [8,15].

Previously, M. Garrib and J. Camilleri (2020) [15] demonstrated that 10% formic acid and 17% EDTA might be efficient solvents, which, in conjunction with mechanical instrumentation, achieve over 95% removal of gutta-percha and HCS sealer [15]. However, other studies have not revealed any significant dissolving effect of irrigating solutions on HCS materials [8,27]. Surprisingly, citric acid as a potential solvent has not been tested until now, and there are no data available on the efficiency of citric acid for the dissolution of HCS sealers. Therefore, our preliminary findings, demonstrating the promising characteristics of 10% and 20% citric acid solutions, cannot be compared to previous investigations.

The hypothesis to test citric acid on HCS sealers mainly arose from the fact that the hydration products of di- and tri-calcium silicates become unstable and degradable at a pH below 8.8 [17]. Since the pH of citric acid solutions is typically below 2, it may explain the superior dissolving properties of citric acid compared to EDTA, which provides more alkaline conditions with a pH range from 7.5 to 9.5 [16]. Moreover, it should also be mentioned that in our study, the efficiency of citric acid solutions was clearly visible for both types of HCS sealers (mixed by hand or premixed), as dissolution and structural damage were objectively observed for all tested HCS materials, which were distinct in their chemical compositions and preparations.

The solvent's interaction with root canal dentin during endodontic retreatment procedures is also inevitable. Generally, the potential adverse effect of the irrigating solutions on the root dentin microstructure directly relates to the concentration and exposure time [16]. Regarding the longer time required for HCS sealers to be removed from root canals compared to other types of sealers, prolonged exposure of the solvent to root dentin should always be expected [23]. Therefore, aiming to mimic the clinical situation and simulate the possible time-dependent effect of citric acid on the root dentine, prolonged exposure time was applied in this preliminary observation by using repetitive citric acid irrigation after each instrument. During the root canal shaping procedures, no use of NaOCl was included, exceptionally evaluating only the citric acid's effect on the root dentin. The obtained results of SEM observations revealed that 10% and 20% citric acid solutions, even after a relatively long exposure, have no significant impact on the microstructure of root dentin. The exposed collagen fibers were observed only for EDTA-treated dentin in some areas. However, no significant erosive damage was noticed. These results agree with previous data demonstrating that EDTA alone does not adversely affect the dentin microstructure and that only additional subsequent application of NaOCl is related to erosion on the surface of the root dentine [16,28].

The interaction of HCS sealers and their behavior in citric acid solutions has not been investigated and visualized previously. Depending on HCS sealers' chemistry and the hypothetical assumption that these materials in contact with chelating solutions can start to degrade, the tested HCS sealers were submerged in 17% EDTA and 10% and 20% citric acid solutions. The intense gas release and material physical changes reflected the ongoing chemical reaction between the HCS material and citric acid solutions at both concentrations. On the contrary, no evident bubbling was seen in the EDTA solution, indicating the absence of an intense chemical reaction. These observations support the previous findings demonstrating that HCS materials have very minimal solubility in EDTA [15]. Therefore, this irrigating solution has no evident potential to be used as a solvent for HCS sealers during endodontic retreatment procedures.

Additionally, it should be highlighted that the intensity of gas release visually differed among the materials tested, and was apparently most intensive for AHPB. The different degree of solubility was equally confirmed by the assessment of mass changes and surface morphology, demonstrating the highest mass loss and structural damage for AHPB, followed by BIOC, TF, and BR, respectively. The different acid resistance might be related to differences in the chemical composition and preparation of these materials. However, all these differences did not change the fact that all tested HCS sealers were significantly more soluble in citric acid solutions than EDTA. Therefore, our primary results suggest 10% and 20% citric acid solutions as potential solvents for HCS sealers, which could facilitate endodontic retreatment procedures. Further comprehensive investigations must be conducted to confirm or deny these results and, potentially, to modify the current clinical retreatment approaches for teeth previously filled with HCS material.

Author Contributions: Conceptualization, S.D. and G.B.; methodology, S.D., G.B. and S.S.; software, G.B.; validation, S.D.; formal analysis, G.B.; investigation, G.B. and S.D.; resources, S.S.; data curation, S.D.; writing—original draft preparation, S.D. and G.B.; writing—review and editing, S.S.; visualization, S.D.; supervision, S.D. and S.S.; project administration, S.D. All authors have read and agreed to the published version of the manuscript.

Funding: This research received no external funding.

Institutional Review Board Statement: The study was conducted according to the guidelines of the Declaration of Helsinki and approved by the Ethics Committee of Vilnius University Hospital Zalgirio Clinics (protocol no. EK-2, 3 June 2016).

Informed Consent Statement: Informed consent was obtained from all subjects involved in the study.

Data Availability Statement: Data are contained within the article.

Conflicts of Interest: The authors declare no conflicts of interest.

References

1. Duncan, H.F.; Nagendrababu, V.; El-Karim, I.A.; Dummer, P.M.H. Outcome measures to assess the effectiveness of endodontic treatment for pulpitis and apical periodontitis for use in the development of European Society of Endodontology (ESE) S3 level clinical practice guidelines: A protocol. *Int. Endod. J.* **2021**, *54*, 646–654. [CrossRef] [PubMed]
2. Santos-Junior, A.; De Castro Pinto, L.; Mateo-Castillo, J.; Pinheiro, C. Success or failure of endodontic treatments: A retrospective study. *J. Conserv. Dent.* **2019**, *22*, 129. [CrossRef] [PubMed]
3. Azarpazhooh, A.; Sgro, A.; Cardoso, E.; Elbarbary, M.; Laghapour Lighvan, N.; Badewy, R.; Malkhassian, G.; Jafarzadeh, H.; Bakhtiar, H.; Khazaei, S.; et al. A Scoping Review of 4 Decades of Outcomes in Nonsurgical Root Canal Treatment, Nonsurgical Retreatment, and Apexification Studies—Part 2: Outcome Measures. *J. Endod.* **2022**, *48*, 29–39. [CrossRef] [PubMed]
4. Gulabivala, K.; Ng, Y.L. Factors that affect the outcomes of root canal treatment and retreatment—A reframing of the principles. *Int. Endod. J.* **2023**, *56*, 82–115. [CrossRef] [PubMed]
5. Zuolo, M.; Silva, E.J.N.L.; Souza, E.; De Deus, G.; Versiani, M.A. Shaping for cleaning in retreatment cases. In *Shaping for Cleaning the Root Canals: A Clinical-Based Strategy*; De Deus, G., Silva, E.J.N.L., Souza, E., Versiani, M.A., Zuolo, M., Eds.; Springer: Cham, Switzerland, 2021; pp. 249–293.
6. Martos, J.; Gastal, M.T.; Sommer, L.; Lund, R.G.; Del Pino, F.A.B.; Osinaga, P.W.R. Dissolving efficacy of organic solvents on root canal sealers. *Clin. Oral. Investig.* **2006**, *10*, 50–54. [CrossRef] [PubMed]
7. Dotto, L.; Sarkis-Onofre, R.; Bacchi, A.; Pereira, G.K.R. The use of solvents for gutta-percha dissolution/removal during endodontic retreatments: A scoping review. *J. Biomed. Mater. Res. B Appl. Biomater.* **2021**, *109*, 890–901. [CrossRef]
8. Arul, B.; Varghese, A.; Mishra, A.; Elango, S.; Padmanaban, S.; Natanasabapathy, V. Retrievability of bioceramic-based sealers in comparison with epoxy resin-based sealer assessed using microcomputed tomography: A systematic review of laboratory-based studies. *J. Conserv. Dent.* **2021**, *24*, 421–434. [CrossRef]
9. Pirani, C.; Camilleri, J. Effectiveness of root canal filling materials and techniques for treatment of apical periodontitis: A systematic review. *Int. Endod. J.* **2023**, *56*, 436–454. [CrossRef]
10. Fonseca, D.A.; Paula, A.B.; Marto, C.M.; Coelho, A.; Paulo, S.; Martinho, J.P.; Carrilho, E.; Ferreira, M.M. Biocompatibility of Root Canal Sealers: A Systematic Review of In Vitro and In Vivo Studies. *Materials* **2019**, *12*, 4113. [CrossRef]
11. Sfeir, G.; Zogheib, C.; Patel, S.; Giraud, T.; Nagendrababu, V.; Bukiet, F. Calcium Silicate-Based Root Canal Sealers: A Narrative Review and Clinical Perspectives. *Materials* **2021**, *14*, 3965. [CrossRef]
12. Camilleri, J.; Atmeh, A.; Li, X.; Meschi, N. Present status and future directions: Hydraulic materials for endodontic use. *Int. Endod. J.* **2022**, *55*, 710–777. [CrossRef]
13. Drukteinis, S.; Bilvinaite, G.; Tusas, P.; Shemesh, H.; Peciuliene, V. Porosity Distribution in Single Cone Root Canal Fillings Performed by Operators with Different Clinical Experience: A microCT Assessment. *J. Clin. Med.* **2021**, *10*, 2569. [CrossRef] [PubMed]
14. Carrillo, C.A.; Kirkpatrick, T.; Freeman, K.; Makins, S.R.; Aldabbagh, M.; Jeong, J.W. Retrievability of Calcium Silicate–based Root Canal Sealers During Retreatment: An Ex Vivo Study. *J. Endod.* **2022**, *48*, 781–786. [CrossRef] [PubMed]
15. Garrib, M.; Camilleri, J. Retreatment efficacy of hydraulic calcium silicate sealers used in single cone obturation. *J. Dent.* **2020**, *98*, 103370. [CrossRef] [PubMed]
16. Gómez-Delgado, M.; Camps-Font, O.; Luz, L.; Sanz, D.; Mercade, M. Update on citric acid use in endodontic treatment: A systematic review. *Odontology* **2023**, *111*, 1–19. [CrossRef] [PubMed]

17. Yang, H.; Che, Y.; Leng, F. Calcium leaching behavior of cementitious materials in hydrochloric acid solution. *Sci. Rep.* **2018**, *8*, 8806. [CrossRef] [PubMed]
18. Camilleri, J. Current Classification of Bioceramic Materials in Endodontics. In *Bioceramic Materials in Clinical Endodontics*, 1st ed.; Drukteinis, S., Camilleri, J., Eds.; Spinger: Cham, Germany, 2021; pp. 1–6.
19. Asawaworarit, W.; Pinyosopon, T.; Kijsamanmith, K. Comparison of apical sealing ability of bioceramic sealer and epoxy resin-based sealer using the fluid filtration technique and scanning electron microscopy. *J. Dent. Sci.* **2020**, *15*, 186–192. [CrossRef] [PubMed]
20. Wang, Y.; Liu, S.; Dong, Y. In vitro study of dentinal tubule penetration and filling quality of bioceramic sealer. *PLoS ONE* **2018**, *13*, e0192248. [CrossRef]
21. Wang, Z.; Shen, Y.; Haapasalo, M. Root Canal Wall Dentin Structure in Uninstrumented but Cleaned Human Premolars: A Scanning Electron Microscopic Study. *J. Endod.* **2018**, *44*, 842–848. [CrossRef]
22. Ballal, N.V.; Roy, A.; Zehnder, M. Effect of Sodium Hypochlorite Concentration in Continuous Chelation on Dislodgement Resistance of an Epoxy Resin and Hydraulic Calcium Silicate Sealer. *Polymers* **2021**, *13*, 3482. [CrossRef]
23. Marchi, V.; Scheire, J.; Simon, S. Retreatment of Root Canals Filled with BioRoot RCS: An In Vitro Experimental Study. *J. Endod.* **2020**, *46*, 858–862. [CrossRef]
24. Agrafioti, A.; Koursoumis, A.D.; Kontakiotis, E.G. Re-establishing apical patency after obturation with Gutta-percha and two novel calcium silicate-based sealers. *Eur. J. Dent.* **2015**, *9*, 457–461. [CrossRef]
25. Maria, B.; Silva-Sousa, Y.T.C.; de Macedo, L.M.D.; Oliveira, O.P.; Alfredo, E.; Leoni, G.B.; Rached-Junior, F.J.A. Removal of filling material using rotating or reciprocating systems with or without solvent: Microct analysis. *Braz. Oral. Res.* **2021**, *35*, e117. [CrossRef]
26. Karobari, M.I.; Arshad, S.; Noorani, T.Y.; Ahmed, N.; Basheer, S.N.; Peeran, S.W.; Marya, A.; Marya, C.M.; Messina, P.; Scardina, G.A. Root and Root Canal Configuration Characterization Using Microcomputed Tomography: A Systematic Review. *J. Clin. Med.* **2022**, *11*, 2287. [CrossRef] [PubMed]
27. Pedullà, E.; Abiad, R.S.; Conte, G.; Khan, K.; Lazaridis, K.; Rapisarda, E.; Neelakantan, P. Retreatability of two hydraulic calcium silicate-based root canal sealers using rotary instrumentation with supplementary irrigant agitation protocols: A laboratory-based micro-computed tomographic analysis. *Int. Endod. J.* **2019**, *52*, 1377–1387. [CrossRef]
28. Bosaid, F.; Aksel, H.; Makowka, S.; Azim, A.A. Surface and structural changes in root dentine by various chelating solutions used in regenerative endodontics. *Int. Endod. J.* **2020**, *53*, 1438–1445. [CrossRef] [PubMed]

Disclaimer/Publisher's Note: The statements, opinions and data contained in all publications are solely those of the individual author(s) and contributor(s) and not of MDPI and/or the editor(s). MDPI and/or the editor(s) disclaim responsibility for any injury to people or property resulting from any ideas, methods, instructions or products referred to in the content.

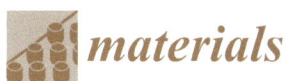

Article

Do the Mechanical Properties of Calcium-Silicate-Based Cements Influence the Stress Distribution of Different Retrograde Cavity Preparations?

Tarek Ashi [1,†], Raphaël Richert [2,3,†], Davide Mancino [1,4,5], Hamdi Jmal [6], Sleman Alkhouri [7], Frédéric Addiego [8], Naji Kharouf [1,4,*,‡] and Youssef Haïkel [1,4,5,*,‡]

1. Department of Biomaterials and Bioengineering, INSERM UMR_S, Strasbourg University, 67000 Strasbourg, France; tarekachi@live.com (T.A.); mancino@unistra.fr (D.M.)
2. Hospices Civils de Lyon, PAM Odontologie, 69100 Lyon, France; richertg@gmail.com
3. Laboratoire de Mécanique des Contacts et Structures, UMR 5259 CNRS/INSA Lyon, 69100 Lyon, France
4. Department of Endodontics, Faculty of Dental Medicine, Strasbourg University, 67000 Strasbourg, France
5. Pôle de Médecine et Chirurgie Bucco-Dentaire, Hôpital Civil, Hôpitaux Universitaire de Strasbourg, 67000 Strasbourg, France
6. ICube Laboratory, Mechanics Department, UMR 7357 CNRS, University of Strasbourg, 67000 Strasbourg, France; jmal@unistra.fr
7. Private Practice, 20097 Hamburg, Germany; slemanko@gmx.de
8. Department Materials Research and Technology (MRT), Luxembourg Institute of Science and Technology (LIST), ZAE Robert Steichen, 5 Rue Bommel, L-4940 Hautcharage, Luxembourg; frederic.addiego@list.lu

* Correspondence: dentistenajikharouf@gmail.com (N.K.); youssef.haikel@unistra.fr (Y.H.); Tel.: +33-(0)6-6752-2841 (N.K.)

† These authors contributed equally to this work as co-first authors.
‡ These authors contributed equally to this work as co-first authors.

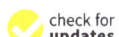

Citation: Ashi, T.; Richert, R.; Mancino, D.; Jmal, H.; Alkhouri, S.; Addiego, F.; Kharouf, N.; Haïkel, Y. Do the Mechanical Properties of Calcium-Silicate-Based Cements Influence the Stress Distribution of Different Retrograde Cavity Preparations? *Materials* 2023, *16*, 3111. https://doi.org/10.3390/ma16083111

Academic Editors: Lavinia Cosmina Ardelean and Laura-Cristina Rusu

Received: 16 March 2023
Revised: 6 April 2023
Accepted: 13 April 2023
Published: 14 April 2023

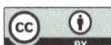

Copyright: © 2023 by the authors. Licensee MDPI, Basel, Switzerland. This article is an open access article distributed under the terms and conditions of the Creative Commons Attribution (CC BY) license (https://creativecommons.org/licenses/by/4.0/).

Abstract: The aim of the present study was to investigate the influence of the mechanical properties of three different calcium-silicate-based cements on the stress distribution of three different retrograde cavity preparations. Biodentine™ "BD", MTA Biorep "BR", and Well-Root™ PT "WR" were used. The compression strengths of ten cylindrical samples of each material were tested. The porosity of each cement was investigated by using micro-computed X-ray tomography. Finite element analysis (FEA) was used to simulate three retrograde conical cavity preparations with an apical diameter of 1 mm (Tip I), 1.4 mm (Tip II), and 1.8 mm (Tip III) after an apical 3 mm resection. BR demonstrated the lowest compression strength values (17.6 ± 5.5 MPa) and porosity percentages (0.57 ± 0.14%) compared to BD (80 ± 17 MPa–1.22 ± 0.31%) and WR (90 ± 22 MPa–1.93 ± 0.12%) ($p < 0.05$). FEA demonstrated that the larger cavity preparation demonstrated higher stress distribution in the root whereas stiffer cement demonstrated lower stress in the root but higher stress in the material. We can conclude that a respected root end preparation associated with cement with good stiffness could offer optimal endodontic microsurgery. Further studies are needed to define the adapted cavity diameter and cement stiffness in order to have optimal mechanical resistance with less stress distribution in the root.

Keywords: retrograde cavity; calcium silicate cement; stress distribution; compression strength

1. Introduction

Thanks to the use of magnification devices, micro-instruments, and biocompatible materials, endodontic microsurgery is an optimal option with a success rate of 89–94% when the nonsurgical treatment or retreatment fails to solve the problem [1–4]. Despite improvements in surgical techniques and materials, the retrograde cavity preparation design and the optimal root-end filling material which insure appropriate mechanical, biological, and physicochemical properties of steel need further investigations.

Different materials were used as root-end filling products such as glass ionomer, plaster of Paris, zinc oxide eugenol, and resin cements which were unable to confront the ideal characteristics of root-end filling materials [5–7]. Calcium-silicate-based materials were introduced in the dental market and could be considered the optimal materials for different endodontic treatments [8]. The putty form of these materials is used in several endodontic clinical situations such as pulp cupping, perforations, open apex, apicoectomy, and pulpotomy [4,9,10]. These materials are used in a wide range of endodontic treatments due to their good biological, mechanical, and physicochemical properties [8–11]. These materials compounds undergo hydrolysis in water to generate greatly soluble calcium hydroxide at the origin of Ca^{2+} ions and alkaline pH [9] which play an important role in the biological reactions and mineralization procedure [12]. Moreover, the mechanical properties of these cements are related to different factors such as the chemical compositions and the hydration process [3,9]. Hou et al. [13] reported that the silica chain and calcium interactions are the main factors of the mechanical strength of these materials.

It was reported that the retrograde cavity design could influence the stress distribution [14]. Until now, there is no study in the literature that has investigated the influence of using calcium silicate materials with different mechanical properties on the distribution of stress concentration. In the present in vitro experiment and finite element analysis (FEA), three calcium-silicate-based cements were mechanically compared. FEA was used previously in dental studies in several dental fields such as coronal restoration [15], root-end surgery [14,16], and implantology [17]. Mineral trioxide aggregate (MTA) and Biodentine™ are the most used calcium-silicate-based materials in putty form. MTA Biorep (Itena Clinical, Paris, France) and Biodentine™ (Septodont, Saint-Maur-des-fossés, France) are powder–liquid calcium-silicate-based cements and in our previous study [3], their biological and physicochemical properties were studied as well as the physicochemical and biological properties of the novel premixed calcium-silicate-based cement (Well-Root™ PT, Vericom, Chuncheon-si, Republic of Korea)). The mechanical properties of the novel premixed product were not found in the literature and the influence of their mechanical properties on the distribution of stress concentration should be investigated. Moreover, the relation between the different calcium-silicate-based cement stiffnesses and the retrograde cavity design should be investigated.

Therefore, the aim of the present study was to investigate the influence of the mechanical properties of three different calcium-silicate-based cements on the stress distribution of three different retrograde cavity preparations. The first null hypothesis was that there is no difference between the compression strength of the different cements and the second one was that the different retrograde cavity preparations could not affect the stress distribution.

2. Materials and Methods

2.1. Materials and Sample Preparations

Three different calcium-silicate-based cements were used in the study. Biodentine™ "BD" (Powder-liquid cement, Septodont, Saint-Maur-des-fossés, France), MTA Biorep "BR" (Powder-liquid cement, Itena Clinical, Paris, France), and Well-Root™ PT "WR" (Premixed cement, Vericom, Chuncheon-si, Republic of Korea) were prepared following the manufacturer's instructions [3].

Cylindrical samples (n = 10) were prepared using Teflon molds (height: 3.8 mm; diameter: 3 mm) [18]. After filling the molds with the different cements, the samples were put in the dark at 37 °C and 95% humidity for 48 h in a container. After the storage period, the specimens were immersed in distilled water before the mechanical test and porosity investigation at 37 °C for 24 h.

2.2. Porosity

After the storage in distilled water for 24 h at 37 °C, the interior texture of BD, BR, and WR were investigated in 3D by using micro-computed X-ray tomography (μCT) (EasyTom 160 from RX Solutions, Chavanod, France). A current of 125 μ and a voltage of 45 kV were used in the execution of imaging procedures using a micro-focused tube supplied with a lanthanum hexaboride (LaB$_6$) filament. The source-to-object distance (SOD) and the source-to-detector distance (SDD) were regulated to have a voxel size of around 2.3 µm. The software Xact64 (Version: 22.01.1 2022-03-14, RX Solutions, Chavanod, France) was used to perform the volume reconstruction after the application of ring artifact attenuation and the geometrical corrections. The Avizo software (Version: 3D 2022-2) was used in the image process to remove insignificant small objects, de-noise the images with a median filter, determine the 3D geometrical aspects of the objects of interest, and segment the image intensity in order to reveal the objects of interest [19].

2.3. Compression Strength and Modulus

After the storage in distilled water for 24 h at 37 °C, ten specimens from each group were tested through the uni-axial compression test. A universal compression/tensile testing machine (Instron 3345, Norwood, MA, USA) associated with a 1 kN cell force (Class 0.5 following ISO 7500-1) was used at a constant crosshead speed of 0.5 mm/min.

The crosshead displacement in mm and the force in n were registered during the test. The stress was calculated in MPa as force dived by the primary section. The strain was acquired by dividing the crosshead displacement by the sample's primary length. The stress–strain curve was then plotted. The linear section of the stress–strain curve represents the elastic behavior. The compression modulus (Young's modulus), for each sample is the slope of this linear section that is defined by a linear regression fitting.

The compression strength was calculated in megapascals (MPa) according to the following formula:

$$\sigma c = 4P/\pi D^2$$

where P is the maximum recorded force during the test and D is the initial sample diameter.

The results of mechanical tests were statistically analyzed using the Kruskal–Wallis test associated with the Tukey test. SigmaPlot release 11.2 (Systat Software, Inc., San Jose, CA, USA) was performed with a statistical significance set at $\alpha = 0.05$.

2.4. Finite Element Analysis (FEA)

An intact human maxillary central incisive, extracted for periodontics problems, was used in the present study. The tooth was scanned by the use of a cone beam computed tomography (CBCT; Vatech, Hwaseong, Republic of Korea) operating with a field of view = 80×80 mm^2 and voxel size = $200 \times 200 \times 200$ mm^3. The segmentation of the different anatomical structures was based on a previously validated protocol [20]. The segmented 3D image was adjusted to simulate three retrograde conical cavity preparations with an apical diameter of 1 mm (Tip I), 1.4 mm (Tip II), and 1.8 mm (Tip III) after an apical 3 mm resection with 0° bevel angle. The alveolar bone and a periodontal ligament of 0.2 mm around the root were simulated [15]. The segmented 3D image was then meshed using quadratic tetrahedral elements after a convergence test. All dental materials were supposed homogeneous and linearly elastic except the periodontal ligament, which was supposed hyper-elastic. The three root-end filling cements were considered: BD, BR, and WR, and the attributed material properties were referenced from the literature [15] (Table 1). There was a perfect bonding between each component and a vertical load of 150 n was applied on the top of the root following published protocols [14,16]. The nodes of the lateral faces of the cortical bone were constrained to prevent displacement. The FEA was conducted on the software Abaqus (Version: Abaqus 6.7 2021, Dassault Systèmes, Vélizy-Villacoublay, France) to calculate the von Mises stresses of the root-end filling.

Table 1. Material properties used for FEA analysis [15].

Material	Model
Dentine	Linear elastic isotropic E = 14,600 MPa, ν = 0.31
Gutta-Percha	Linear elastic isotropic E = 69 MPa, ν = 0.45
Ligament	Hyper-elastic Ogden order 1; μ = 0.12 MPa, α = 20.9 MPa, D = 10
Trabecular bone	Linear elastic isotropic E = 1300 MPa, ν = 0.3
Cortical bone	Linear elastic isotropic E = 13,000 MPa, ν = 0.3
Biodentine™	Linear elastic isotropic E = 5490 MPa, ν = 0.3
MTA Biorep	Linear elastic isotropic E = 3870 MPa, ν = 0.3
Well-Root PT	Linear elastic isotropic E = 6400 MPa, ν = 0.3

3. Results

3.1. Internal Structure (Porosity)

All three cements presented pores in their internal structures (Figure 1). BD (1.22 ± 0.31%) and WR (1.93 ± 0.12%) demonstrated slightly higher porosity volume percentages than BR (0.57 ± 0.14%). Therefore, both calcium-silicate-based cements (BD and WR) were characterized by a higher porosity compared to BR (Table 2).

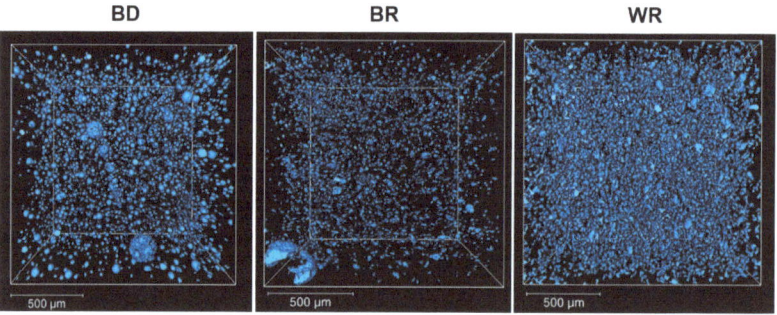

Figure 1. Volume rendering of the segmented pores (blue color) in Biodentine™ (BD), MTA Biorep (BR), and Well-Root PT (WR) obtained by X-ray tomography analysis. The scale bar corresponds to 500 μm in all the images.

Table 2. Pore volume fraction and average pore equivalent diameter obtained by X-ray tomography analysis in the case of Biodentine™ (BD), MTA Biorep (BR), and Well-Root PT (WR).

	BD	BR	WR
Pore volume fraction (%)	1.22 ± 0.31	0.57 ± 0.14	1.93 ± 0.12
Average pore equivalent diameter (μm)	16.80 ± 0.59	13.20 ± 0.09	18.51 ± 0.08

The distribution of equivalent diameters and the average equivalent diameter of the pores were calculated for the three types of samples. The most numerous size range is 14–16 μm in the case of BD, 12–14 μm in the case of BR, and 16–18 μm in the case of WR. For both BD and WR, pores with an equivalent diameter above 30 μm were observed, whereas BR did not exhibit significant pores larger than an equivalent diameter of 30 μm. On average, larger porosity was noted for BD (average equivalent diameter of 16.80 μm) and WR (average equivalent diameter of 18.51 μm) compared to BR (average equivalent diameter of 13.20 μm) (Figure 2).

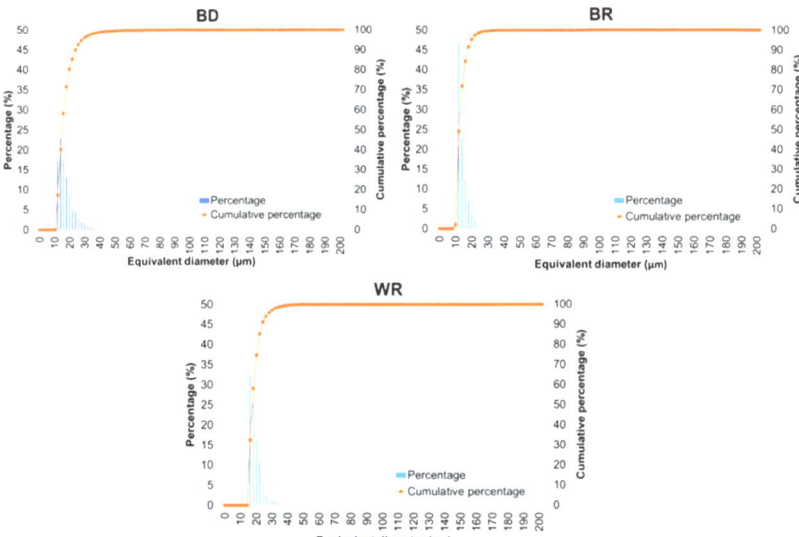

Figure 2. Histograms of the distribution of pore equivalent diameter obtained by X-ray tomography analysis in the case of Biodentine™ (BD), MTA Biorep (BR), and Well-Root PT (WR).

3.2. Compression Strength and Modulus

The compression strength values for BD (80 ± 17 MPa) and WR (90 ± 22 MPa) were significantly higher than for BR (17.6 ± 5.5 MPa) ($p < 0.05$) after the immersion in water at 37 °C for 24 h (Figure 3a). MTA Biorep presented the lowest compression strength whereas no significant difference was found between WR and BD ($p > 0.05$). For compression modulus, BR cement showed a significantly lower modulus (387 ± 80 MPa) compared to WR (640 ± 46 MPa) and BD (549 ± 117 MPa) after 24 h of immersion in water at 37 °C ($p < 0.05$). No significant difference was found between BD and WR ($p > 0.05$) (Figure 3b).

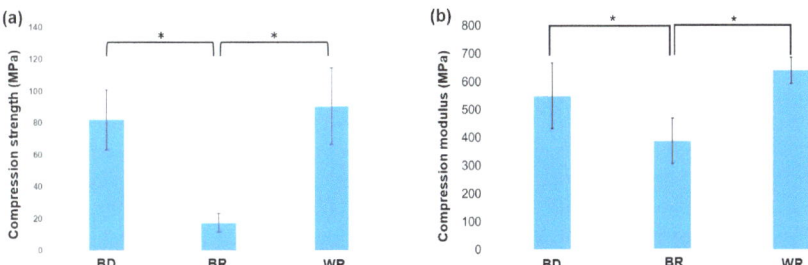

Figure 3. (**a**) Compression strength values (means and standard deviations "MPa") and (**b**) compression modulus values (means and standard deviations "MPa") for Biodentine™ (BD), MTA Biorep (BR), and Well-Root PT (WR). (* $p < 0.05$).

3.3. Finite Element Analysis (FEA)

Considering all FE models, the highest stress values were located on the apical part of the root and on the root-end filling. For large retrograde cavity preparations, the stress values significantly increase in the root, but significantly decrease in the root-end filling materials. For the same retrograde cavity preparation, the use of a stiffer root-end filling reduces the stress values in the root but increases the stress values in the root-end filling materials. For the smallest retrograde cavity preparation, the stress value varies from 8.56 ± 4.33 MPa to 7.20 ± 4.46 MPa in the root-end filling material. For the largest retrograde cavity preparation, the stress value varies from 5.92 ± 1.93 MPa to 4.87 ± 1.92 MPa in the root-end filling (Figure 4).

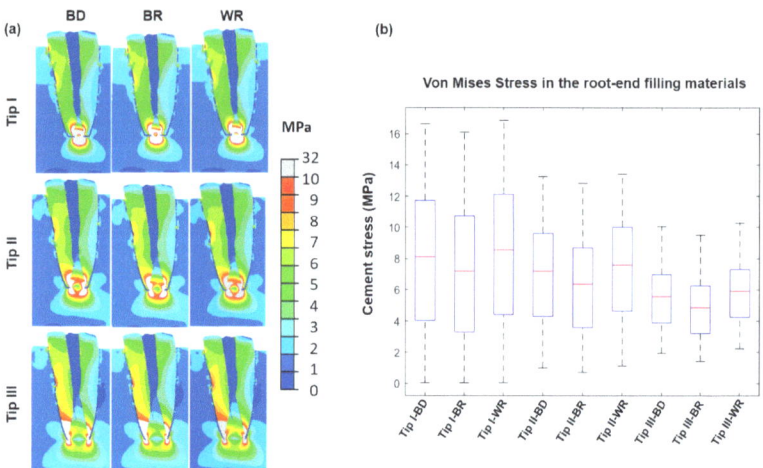

Figure 4. Biomechanical behavior of the resected root with (**a**) stress distribution and (**b**) boxplots presenting the cement stresses for different clinical situations with Biodentine™ (BD), MTA Biorep (BR), and Well-Root PT (WR) and apical diameter of 1 mm (Tip I), 1.4 mm (Tip II), and 1.8 mm (Tip III). On each box, the red central mark indicates the median, and the bottom and top edges of the box indicate the 25th and 75th percentiles, respectively.

4. Discussion

As previously described in the literature, bioceramic materials are bioactive products that could offer good biological reactions such as remineralization, antibacterial activity, and antioxidant properties [8,21]. The mechanical properties of endodontic materials could have [11] or no [22] importance due to the location of these materials through the tooth. In addition, the mechanical properties of an endodontic material were considered an unimportant factor in the root canal and as such, they are materials that do not receive high compressive stress [22]. Other studies reported that the mechanical properties of these materials have an important impact on reinforcing the prepared root as well as the resistance against the coronal forces [11,23]. Moreover, the most important factors that could influence the mechanical properties of bioceramic materials are their chemical composition such as the quantity of calcium silicate and the conditions in which these materials should be set up such as the temperature and the humidity [8,9,13,24]. These factors could explain the difference in the mechanical properties of bioceramic materials.

In the present study, BR demonstrated significantly lower compression and modulus strength compared to BD and WR ($p < 0.05$). Therefore, the first null hypothesis must be rejected. These differences could be due to the difference in the chemical composition and the different percentages of calcium silicate in each material [8,9,13]. Moreover, BR demonstrated lower pore percentages compared to BD and WR which could be related to the ability and the speed of hydration of these materials (setting time). Guo et al. [25] reported different setting times of the bioceramic materials and noted that most of the hydration phase occurs during the first several days, despite complete hydration may even take two years. In addition, we can assume that higher porosity percentages and the difference in sizes and pores distributions could affect the compression and modulus strength of calcium silicate materials [8,9]. Moreover, the porosity percentages and pores distribution values were closed in WR and BD which had no significant difference in their compression and modulus strength ($p > 0.05$).

The FEA method was used in the present study to investigate the influence of the mechanical properties of endodontic cements on the stress distribution in endodontic microsurgery. This method presents the advantage of controlling all the conditions and considers various factors that could influence the analysis by using computer software that is inaccessible to test in clinical research [26–28]. The applied force (150 n) was thought to be sufficient to stimulate the maximum bite force in clinical conditions [14]. All the anatomical considerations that the surgeon could find in a tooth could not be modifiable clinically [14]; therefore, the surgeon could play on the retrograde cavity design and the used bioactive material which could be chosen to ameliorate the quality of the microsurgery treatment and decrease the stress distribution in dentin. In the present study, the material stiffness and retrograde cavity designs affected the stress distribution; thus, the second null hypothesis must be rejected. The larger cavity preparation increased the stress distribution in the root and decreased the stress in the cement material. Therefore, Tip I demonstrated lesser stress in the root and higher stress in the cement material compared to Tip III. In contrast, Kim et al. [14,16] reported that larger retrograde cavity preparations decrease the stress in the root. The difference between these results is that Kim et al. used a higher stiffness for MTA (22 GPa) compared to lower stiffness for the dentin (14 GPa), whereas in our study the cement had lower stiffness values than that used in Kim's studies [14,16]. Considering that the cement is stiffer than the dentin in their study [14], the FEA will always advantage models presenting larger preparations and thinner dentin walls, which appears to be in contradiction with clinical considerations of preserving more tissue. In parallel, in our study, as the cements had less stiffness than the dentin, the results of FEA concluded that more preparation in dentin generates more stress values in the root. This implies more dentin preservation and again emphasizes the need for adequate retrograde preparation and the influence of this factor compared to other ones such as resection length [29,30]. Moreover, BD and WR generated less stress in the root than BR which had lower stiffness than the other cements ($p < 0.05$), but also a lower compressive strength evaluated experimentally. Therefore, the best choice to decrease the stress distribution in the root is to have a conservative retrograde cavity filled with a cement which presents a higher Young modulus.

Further studies should be performed using more stiffer materials and other retrograde cavity designs applied to different maxillary and mandibular teeth. As a perspective, subsequent research is needed to evaluate the impact of these bioceramic materials in the case of microcracks, a common event in endodontic microsurgery [31]. Moreover, it is important to note that the current study had some limitations that should be taken into account. One of these limitations is that only a single root was simulated, in accordance with previous protocols [14]. However, future studies should also investigate the biomechanical impact of the material on patient-specific models, taking into account the specific anatomy of the root and the dental occlusion, which are known to greatly affect stress distribution [32]. Additionally, the numerical method developed in this study should not lead clinicians to focus solely on the biomechanical aspects of the treatment outcome, as other important factors, such as the use of an operating microscope and ultrasonic instruments, are also crucial for improving the cleaning of the root canal space. Moreover, different immersion periods of calcium silicate materials should be performed to investigate the change of compression and modulus strength in time and their effects on the stress distribution in retrograde treatment. For further clinical applications, future studies should investigate the adapted cavity diameter and cement stiffness in order to have optimal mechanical resistance with less stress distribution in the root.

5. Conclusions

Calcium silicate cements have different chemical compositions that play an important role in their biological and mechanical properties. The stiffness of these materials influences the stress distribution in the root and material structure. Moreover, apical preparation design influences stress distribution and the quality of treatment. We can conclude that a respected root-end preparation associated with stiffer cement offer an optimal retrograde treatment with less stress in the root. Therefore, the decrease in stress distribution through the root generates less microfractures; thus, it ameliorates the clinical rate success of the retrograde procedure.

Author Contributions: Conceptualization, N.K. and Y.H; methodology, T.A., H.J., R.R. and F.A.; software, H.J. and R.R.; validation, S.A. and N.K.; writing—original draft preparation, N.K., H.J., T.A. and R.R.; writing—review and editing, N.K. and D.M.; visualization, R.R.; supervision, N.K.; project administration, N.K. and Y.H.; funding acquisition, Y.H. All authors have read and agreed to the published version of the manuscript.

Funding: This research received no external funding.

Institutional Review Board Statement: Not applicable.

Informed Consent Statement: Not applicable.

Data Availability Statement: Not applicable.

Conflicts of Interest: The authors declare no conflict of interest.

References

1. Tsesis, I.; Rosen, E.; Schwartz-Arad, D.; Fuss, Z. Retrospective evaluation of surgical endodontic treatment: Traditional versus modern technique. *J. Endod.* 2006, *32*, 412–416. [CrossRef]
2. Tsesis, I.; Rosen, E.; Taschieri, S.; Telishevsky Strauss, Y.; Ceresoli, V.; Del Fabbro, M. Outcomes of surgical endodontic treatment performed by a modern technique: An updated meta-analysis of the literature. *J. Endod.* 2013, *39*, 332–339. [CrossRef]
3. Ashi, T.; Mancino, D.; Hardan, L.; Bourgi, R.; Zghal, J.; Macaluso, V.; Al-Ashkar, S.; Alkhouri, S.; Haikel, Y.; Kharouf, N. Physicochemical and Antibacterial Properties of Bioactive Retrograde Filling Materials. *Bioengineering* 2022, *9*, 624. [CrossRef] [PubMed]
4. Wang, Z.H.; Zhang, M.M.; Wang, J.; Jiang, L.; Liang, Y.H. Outcomes of Endodontic Microsurgery Using a Microscope and Mineral Trioxide Aggregate: A Prospective Cohort Study. *J. Endod.* 2017, *43*, 694–698. [CrossRef]
5. Viswanath, G.; Tilakchand, M.; Naik, B.D.; Kalabhavi, A.S.; Kulkarni, R.D. Comparative evaluation of antimicrobial and antifungal efficacy of bioactive root-end filling materials: An in vitro study. *J. Conserv. Dent.* 2021, *24*, 148–152. [CrossRef]
6. Suhag, A.; Chhikara, N.; Pillania, A.; Yadav, P. Root end filling materials: A review. *Indian J. Dent. Sci.* 2018, *4*, 320–323.
7. Kharouf, N.; Mancino, D.; Zghal, J.; Helle, S.; Jmal, H.; Lenertz, M.; Viart, N.; Bahlouli, N.; Meyer, F.; Haikel, Y.; et al. Dual role of Tannic acid and pyrogallol incorporated in plaster of Paris: Morphology modification and release for antimicrobial properties. *Mater. Sci. Eng. C Mater. Biol. Appl.* 2021, *127*, 112209. [CrossRef] [PubMed]
8. Kharouf, N.; Sauro, S.; Eid, A.; Zghal, J.; Jmal, H.; Seck, A.; Macaluso, V.; Addiego, F.; Inchingolo, F.; Affolter-Zbaraszczuk, C.; et al. Physicochemical and Mechanical Properties of Premixed Calcium Silicate and Resin Sealers. *J. Funct. Biomater.* 2023, *14*, 9. [CrossRef]
9. Kharouf, N.; Zghal, J.; Addiego, F.; Gabelout, M.; Jmal, H.; Haikel, Y.; Bahlouli, N.; Ball, V. Tannic acid speeds up the setting of mineral trioxide aggregate cements and improves its surface and bulk properties. *J. Colloid Interface Sci.* 2021, *589*, 318–326. [CrossRef] [PubMed]
10. Eid, A.; Mancino, D.; Rekab, M.S.; Haikel, Y.; Kharouf, N. Effectiveness of Three Agents in Pulpotomy Treatment of Permanent Molars with Incomplete Root Development: A Randomized Controlled Trial. *Healthcare* 2022, *10*, 431. [CrossRef]
11. Kharouf, N.; Arntz, Y.; Eid, A.; Zghal, J.; Sauro, S.; Haikel, Y.; Mancino, D. Physicochemical and Antibacterial Properties of Novel, Premixed Calcium Silicate-Based Sealer Compared to Powder–Liquid Bioceramic Sealer. *J. Clin. Med.* 2020, *9*, 3096. [CrossRef] [PubMed]
12. Farrayeh, A.; Akil, S.; Eid, A.; Macaluso, V.; Mancino, D.; Haïkel, Y.; Kharouf, N. Effectiveness of Two Endodontic Instruments in Calcium Silicate-Based Sealer Retreatment. *Bioengineering* 2023, *10*, 362. [CrossRef]
13. Hou, D.; Zhu, Y.; Li, Z. Mechanical properties of calcium silicate hydrate (C–S–H) at nano-scale: A molecular dynamics study. *Mater. Chem. Phys.* 2014, *146*, 503–551. [CrossRef]
14. Kim, S.; Park, S.Y.; Lee, Y.; Lee, C.J.; Karabucak, B.; Kim, H.C.; Kim, E. Stress Analyses of Retrograde Cavity Preparation Designs for Surgical Endodontics in the Mesial Root of the Mandibular Molar: A Finite Element Analysis-Part I. *J. Endod.* 2019, *45*, 442–446. [CrossRef]
15. Richert, R.; Farges, J.-C.; Tamimi, F.; Naouar, N.; Boisse, P.; Ducret, M. Validated Finite Element Models of Premolars: A Scoping Review. *Materials* 2020, *13*, 3280. [CrossRef]
16. Kim, S.; Chen, D.; Park, S.Y.; Lee, C.J.; Kim, H.C.; Kim, E. Stress Analyses of Retrograde Cavity Preparation Designs for Surgical Endodontics in the Mesial Root of the Mandibular Molar: A Finite Element Analysis-Part II. *J. Endod.* 2020, *46*, 539–544. [CrossRef] [PubMed]
17. Bandela, V.; Kanaparthi, S. Finite Element Analysis and Its Applications in Dentistry. In *Finite Element Methods and Their Applications*; IntechOpen: London, UK, 2020. [CrossRef]

18. Kharouf, N.; Sauro, S.; Hardan, L.; Fawzi, A.; Suhanda, I.E.; Zghal, J.; Addiego, F.; Affolter-Zbaraszczuk, C.; Arntz, Y.; Ball, V.; et al. Impacts of Resveratrol and Pyrogallol on Physicochemical, Mechanical and Biological Properties of Epoxy-Resin Sealers. *Bioengineering* **2022**, *9*, 85. [CrossRef]
19. Kharouf, N.; Sauro, S.; Hardan, L.; Jmal, H.; Bachagha, G.; Macaluso, V.; Addiego, F.; Inchingolo, F.; Haikel, Y.; Mancino, D. Compressive Strength and Porosity Evaluation of Innovative Bidirectional Spiral Winding Fiber Reinforced Composites. *J. Clin. Med.* **2022**, *11*, 6754. [CrossRef]
20. Jacinto, H.; Kéchichian, R.; Desvignes, M.; Prost, R.; Valette, S. A web interface for 3D visualization and interactive segmentation of medical images. In Proceedings of the 17th International Conference on 3D Web Technology, Web3D, Paris, France, 2–4 November 2012; pp. 51–58. [CrossRef]
21. Kharouf, N.; Sauro, S.; Hardan, L.; Haikel, Y.; Mancino, D. Special Issue "Recent Advances in Biomaterials and Dental Disease" Part I. *Bioengineering* **2023**, *10*, 55. [CrossRef] [PubMed]
22. Gjorgievska, E.S.; Nicholson, J.W.; Coleman, N.J.; Booth, S.; Dimkov, A.; Hurt, A. Component Release and Mechanical Properties of Endodontic Sealers following Incorporation of Antimicrobial Agents. *Biomed. Res. Int.* **2017**, *2017*, 2129807. [CrossRef]
23. Branstetter, J.; von Fraunhofer, J.A. The physical properties and sealing action of endodontic sealer cements: A review of the literature. *J. Endod.* **1982**, *8*, 312–316. [CrossRef]
24. Hachem, C.E.; Chedid, J.C.A.; Nehme, W.; Kaloustian, M.K.; Ghosn, N.; Sahnouni, H.; Mancino, D.; Haikel, Y.; Kharouf, N. Physicochemical and Antibacterial Properties of Conventional and Two Premixed Root Canal Filling Materials in Primary Teeth. *J. Funct. Biomater.* **2022**, *13*, 177. [CrossRef] [PubMed]
25. Guo, Y.J.; Du, T.F.; Li, H.B.; Shen, Y.; Mobuchon, C.; Hieawy, A.; Wang, Z.J.; Yang, Y.; Ma, J.; Haapasalo, M. Physical properties and hydration behavior of a fast-setting bioceramic endodontic material. *BMC Oral Health* **2016**, *16*, 23. [CrossRef]
26. Belli, S.; Eraslan, O.; Eskitascioglu, G.; Karbhari, V. Monoblocks in root canals: A finite elemental stress analysis study. *Int. Endod. J.* **2011**, *44*, 817–826. [CrossRef]
27. Toparli, M.; Gökay, N.; Aksoy, T. Analysis of a restored maxillary second premolar tooth by using three-dimensional finite element method. *J. Oral Rehabil.* **1999**, *26*, 157–164. [CrossRef]
28. Eraslan, Ö.; Eraslan, O.; Eskitaşcıoğlu, G.; Belli, S. Conservative restoration of severely damaged endodontically treated premolar teeth: A FEM study. *Clin. Oral Investig.* **2011**, *15*, 403–408. [CrossRef] [PubMed]
29. Azim, A.A.; Albanyan, H.; Azim, K.A.; Piasecki, L. The Buffalo study: Outcome and associated predictors in endodontic microsurgery- a cohort study. *Int. Endod. J.* **2021**, *54*, 301–318. [CrossRef]
30. Richert, R.; Farges, J.C.; Maurin, J.C.; Molimard, J.; Boisse, P.; Ducret, M. Multifactorial Analysis of Endodontic Microsurgery Using Finite Element Models. *J. Pers. Med.* **2022**, *12*, 1012. [CrossRef] [PubMed]
31. von Arx, T.; Maldonado, P.; Bornstein, M.M. Occurrence of Vertical Root Fractures after Apical Surgery: A Retrospective Analysis. *J. Endod.* **2021**, *47*, 239–246. [CrossRef]
32. Lahoud, P.; Jacobs, R.; Boisse, P.; EzEldeen, M.; Ducret, M.; Richert, R. Precision medicine using patient-specific modelling: State of the art and perspectives in dental practice. *Clin. Oral Investig.* **2022**, *26*, 5117–5128. [CrossRef]

Disclaimer/Publisher's Note: The statements, opinions and data contained in all publications are solely those of the individual author(s) and contributor(s) and not of MDPI and/or the editor(s). MDPI and/or the editor(s) disclaim responsibility for any injury to people or property resulting from any ideas, methods, instructions or products referred to in the content.

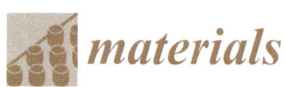 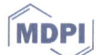

Article

Push-Out Bond Strength of Endodontic Posts Cemented to Extracted Teeth: An In-Vitro Evaluation

Syed Rashid Habib [1,*], Abdul Sadekh Ansari [2], Aleshba Saba Khan [3], Nawaf M. Alamro [4], Meshari A. Alzaaqi [4], Yazeed A. Alkhunefer [4], Abdulaziz A. AlHelal [1], Talal M. Alnassar [1] and Abdulaziz S. Alqahtani [1]

[1] Department of Prosthetic Dental Sciences, College of Dentistry, King Saud University, Riyadh 11545, Saudi Arabia
[2] Dentistry Hospital, King Saud University Medical City, Riyadh 11545, Saudi Arabia
[3] Department of Prosthodontics, Shahida Islam Dental College, Lodhran 59320, Pakistan
[4] College of Dentistry, King Saud University, Riyadh 11545, Saudi Arabia
* Correspondence: syhabib@ksu.edu.sa; Tel.: +966-534750834

Abstract: (1) Background: An ideal bond strength between endodontic posts and root canal dentin is essential for optimal retention and good prognosis. This study aimed to evaluate the push-out bond strength (PBS) of prefabricated fiber and metal posts, luted with resin cement to natural dentin. (2) Methods: Extracted premolars with similar root dimensions were assigned into two groups of 30 each for the metal and fiber posts. Teeth were mounted in acrylic blocks exposing 2 mm of the coronal root. Teeth were subjected to endodontic treatment and post-space preparations. Two groups were further subdivided into three sub-groups (n = 10) according to the size of the posts (# 4, 5 and 6). Posts were cemented with resin cement. Specimens were sectioned into 4 mm slices and subjected to the PBS test. (3) Results: The mean PBS was similar for the metal and fiber posts bonded with resin cement, showing a statistically significant result. An increase in post size increased the bond strength initially, but a further increase in size did not show any marked difference. A total of 71.66% of tested specimens failed with the adhesive failure mode. (4) Conclusions: Metal posts showed slightly higher retention compared to the fiber posts, although the *p*-value was similar for both types. An increase in the size of posts showed increased retention. The most common mode of failure was adhesive failure between cement and dentin.

Keywords: endodontic posts; dowel; fiber posts; prefabricated posts; titanium posts

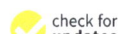

Citation: Habib, S.R.; Ansari, A.S.; Khan, A.S.; Alamro, N.M.; Alzaaqi, M.A.; Alkhunefer, Y.A.; AlHelal, A.A.; Alnassar, T.M.; Alqahtani, A.S. Push-Out Bond Strength of Endodontic Posts Cemented to Extracted Teeth: An In-Vitro Evaluation. *Materials* **2022**, *15*, 6792. https://doi.org/10.3390/ma15196792

Academic Editors: Lavinia Cosmina Ardelean and Laura-Cristina Rusu

Received: 25 August 2022
Accepted: 26 September 2022
Published: 30 September 2022

Publisher's Note: MDPI stays neutral with regard to jurisdictional claims in published maps and institutional affiliations.

Copyright: © 2022 by the authors. Licensee MDPI, Basel, Switzerland. This article is an open access article distributed under the terms and conditions of the Creative Commons Attribution (CC BY) license (https://creativecommons.org/licenses/by/4.0/).

1. Introduction

The preservation of sound tooth structure will ensure the strength of the teeth and is critical for the long-term success of endodontically treated teeth [1]. Root canal treatment, followed by the preparation of the post space, results in a reduction in the remaining tooth structure, which compromises the strength of the teeth [2]. Factors such as the amount and quality of tooth structure, tooth position in the arch, anatomy, function, absence of a periapical infection, a well-condensed root filling, the root filling extending to 2 mm within the radiographic apex and not beyond, a satisfactory coronal restoration and use of a rubber dam during treatment may also contribute to the success of endodontically treated teeth [3].

Root canal treatment, when carried out on badly damaged teeth, makes them feebler and less resistant to cracks or fractures under occlusal loads or stresses [4,5]. After endodontic treatment, already weak and broken-down teeth need a reconstruction of walls and tooth structure before the provision of fixed dental prosthesis. The greater the damage to the walls of teeth, the more the chances of incorporating endodontic posts are considered to retain the build-up of the tooth before crowning [4–7]. Different post systems, i.e., metal, zirconia, fiber and composite, are commercially available [8,9]. The difference in rigidity of different post materials and the structure of the tooth may compromise the endurance limit of the tooth treated with an endodontic post [4,10]. With advancements in mechanical properties, along with the benefit of esthetic properties, fiber posts are being increasingly considered, as their rigidity is comparable to the dentin [5,10]. In addition to good mechanical properties, the prefabricated metal and fiber posts also possess excellent biocompatibility properties [11].

The most common type of failures seen in the teeth restored with endodontic posts is the loss of bond between the post and the tooth structure, retention loss, post fracture or fracture of the tooth [12,13]. Fiber posts have the benefit of preventing the tooth from fracturing by taking the impact, and the post may get fractured by itself [12]. The most repeated issue seen when the root-canal-treated tooth receives a fiber post is debonding [5,8,10].

Resin-based adhesive cements are more extensively being adopted for the cementation of different fixed dental prosthesis and endodontic posts [5]. Multiple adhesive systems, such as self-cure or dual-cure treatments, are available [7]. Few studies have reported that a self-adhesive resin-based system provides a simple technique for adhesion, thus limiting the possible drawbacks. Meanwhile, some studies have reported that the conventional or dual-cure resin system shows less solubility and better bonding with dentin [12].

The choice of an appropriate cement for luting the posts to dentin in the root canal is a challenge [4,8]. The strength of bond formed is affected by several factors; nevertheless, higher success rates have been reported with resin-based cements and fiber posts [5]. Many factors affect the bond strength of the posts by influencing the bond formed between cement–tooth and cement–fiber posts, as well as factors that lead to difficulties in bonding [4–8]. The factors to keep in consideration are the anatomy and preparation of the canal, dentin dehydration, choice of cement for luting, type of sealer used during endodontic treatment, direction of tubules of dentin in the canal at various levels, controlling contamination with saliva, working in indirect vision inside the canals, stress caused by polymerization contraction of the cement, density of layer of the cement and cyclic loads during mastication [4,5,14].

Over the years, few tests such as the micro-tensile strength evaluation, as well as the pull-out and push-out tests have been devised to assess the bond strength among the posts and root canal dentin [5,13]. Some drawbacks associated with micro-tensile and pull-out test, as well as more reliable results with push-out tests, make this method more widely acceptable to evaluate adhesive strength [7,12].

The push-out strength test, or PBS, was first advocated by Roydhouse11 in 1970, and it is being frequently used to evaluate the shear bond strength of resin-based cements to root dentin in relatively thick cross-sectional specimens of root-canal-treated teeth. In this method, a compressive load is applied to the sliced-root specimen in an apico-coronal direction to push the post coronally. The stress applied in this analysis is more uniform, and it gives a better estimation of bond strength as it imitates the clinical conditions by debonding in small sections of the root [15,16].

This study aimed to assess the PBS of fiber and metal posts luted with dual-cure resin-based cement to the natural dentin. The study also evaluated the PBS for different sizes of fiber and metal posts. In addition, analysis for the methods of failure among the cemented posts, cement and dentin was performed. The null hypothesis tested stated that there is no variation between the PBS of fiber versus metal posts, and there is no effect of post size on the PBS.

2. Materials and Methods

Ethical Approval:

As this research study was performed on extracted human teeth, an ethical approval was obtained from the institutional review board at King Saud University, Riyadh (Registration # E-21-5804) before commencement of the study.

Specimen Preparation:

Sixty mandibular first premolar teeth with caries-free, single-straight roots, as well as almost-similar root dimensions extracted for orthodontic purposes, were collected for the present study. Obtained teeth were cleaned with water and disinfected with 5.25% NaOCl solution and stored in distilled water at 37 °C for 24 h. NaOCl, which is easily available in dental setups, was used for disinfection as it is considered one of the most potent agents against a wide range of pathogens such as Gram-positive and Gram-negative bacteria, fungi, viruses and spores, and it is even reported to be effective against HIV present in the oral micro-biofilm [17]. Then, each tooth was mounted in a clear acrylic resin cylinder (Orthoplast, Vertex dental, AV Soesterberg, The Netherlands) of 2 × 2 cm dimensions, exposing the anatomic crown and 2 mm of the coronal portion of the root. To obtain the study specimens, anatomic crowns of all the teeth were removed by transversely sectioning the cemento-enamel junction with a diamond disc (NTI Sintered, Kerr Corporation, Brea, CA, USA) in a high-speed air-turbine hand piece (NSK, Nakanishi Inc., Shinohinata, Kanuma Tochigi, Japan) under copious water irrigation (Figure 1a). All the obtained specimen roots were subjected to endodontic treatment using Protaper Ni-Ti rotary instruments (size S1, S2, F1, F2; Dentsply Maillefer, Tulsa, OK, USA) in a high-torque endodontic motor (X-Smart, Dentsply Maillefer, Tulsa, OK, USA) up to ISO size 35 and 0.06 taper, following the crown-down technique. A total of 17% EDTA (Pulpdent, Watertown, MA, USA) and 5.25% sodium hypochlorite (Ogna, Milan, Italy) were used for irrigation. All the root canals were obturated with gutta-percha (Kerr Corporation, Brea, CA, USA) and an endodontic sealer (AH plus, Dentsply Maillefer, Tulsa, OK, USA), using the warm vertical condensation technique (System B, SybronEndo, Orange, CA, USA), and backfilled with thermo-plasticized gutta-percha using Obtura II (Spartan, Fenton, MO, USA) (Figure 1b). Then, specimens were stored in 100% relative humidity at room temperature for 24 h. Specimens were randomly divided into two groups of thirty each (Group-A = Metal post and Group-B = Fiber post), according to the type of post. Further, each group was subdivided into three subgroups of ten specimens each (n = 10/post sizes #4, #5, #6) according to the size of post used, as shown in Table 1.

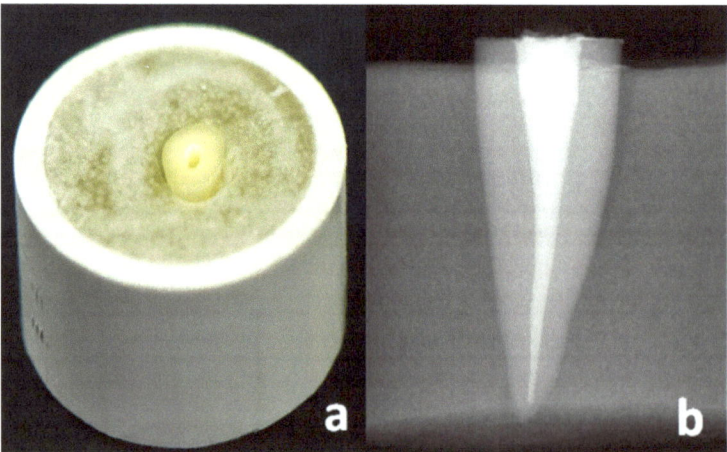

Figure 1. (**a**): Mounted tooth specimen sectioned at cemento-enamel junction; (**b**): Radiograph of specimen after endodontic treatment and before post space preparation.

After 24 h of storage, all the filled root canals were prepared for post spaces using Peeso reamers (Pulpdent Corp, Watertown, MA, USA) of sizes #2, #3 and #4, sequentially, for each specimen to remove gutta-percha, and then the specimens in each group were prepared for the final post spaces using Parapost drills (Coltene/Whaledent Inc. Feldwiesenstrasse, Altstätten, Switzerland) of sizes #4, #5 and #6, respectively, as recommended by the manufacturer for the similar size of posts used. All the post spaces were prepared uniformly at a standardized depth of 8 mm, leaving 5 mm of apical gutta-percha intact under copious water irrigation with a slow-speed dental handpiece (NSK, Nakanishi Inc., Shinohinata, Japan) attached to a customized dental surveyor (J. M. Ney Co., Hartford, Connecticut, CT, USA) to guide the post space preparation, parallel to the long axis of the teeth. Periapical radiographs were taken for all the specimens before and after post space preparations to confirm the optimal post space preparations and to ensure no traces of gutta-percha and sealant remained in the post spaces (Figure 2a,b).

Table 1. Details of the tested post materials for each group in the present study.

Groups	Subgroup N-10	Post Material	Trade Name	Manufacturer	Post Size	Drill Used	Lot Number
Group A (Metal)	A1	Titanium post parallel serrated	Parapost XP	Coltene/Whaledent Inc. Feldwiesenstrasse, Altstätten, Switzerland	Size 4 Ø 0.9 mm Yellow P-784-4	Parapost Drill size 4	H17858
	A2	Titanium post parallel serrated	Parapost XP	Coltene/Whaledent Inc. Feldwiesenstrasse, Altstätten, Switzerland	Size 5 Ø 1.15 mm Red P-784-5	Parapost Drill size 5	H17858
	A3	Titanium post parallel serrated	Parapost XP	Coltene/Whaledent Inc. Feldwiesenstrasse, Altstätten, Switzerland	Size 6 Ø 1.4 mm Black P-784-6	Parapost Drill size 6	H17858
Group B (Fiber)	B1	Fiber post parallel serrated	Parapost fiber Lux Plus	Coltene/Whaledent Inc. Feldwiesenstrasse, Altstätten, Switzerland	Size 4 Ø0.9 mm Yellow PF1714	Parapost Drill size 4	H65570
	B2	Fiber post parallel serrated	Parapost fiber Lux Plus	Coltene/Whaledent Inc. Feldwiesenstrasse, Altstätten, Switzerland	Size 5 Ø 1.15 mm Red PF1715	Parapost Drill size 5	H65570
	B3	Fiber post parallel serrated	Parapost fiber Lux Plus	Coltene/Whaledent Inc. Feldwiesenstrasse, Altstätten, Switzerland	Size 6 Ø 1.4 mm Black PF1716	Parapost Drill size 6	H65570

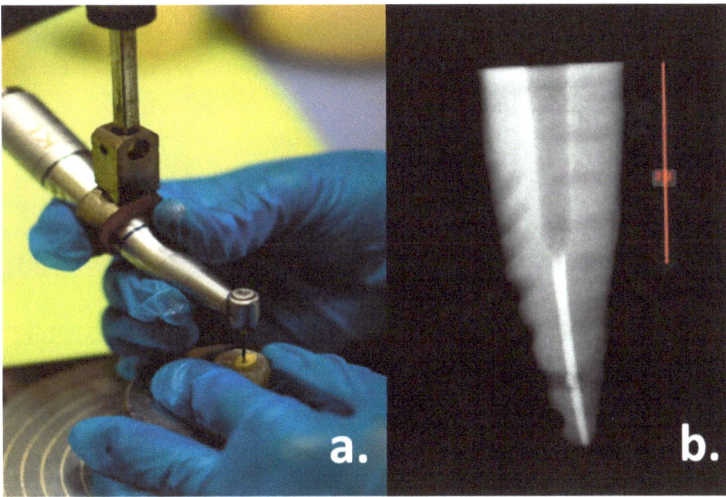

Figure 2. (**a**): Customized surveyor used during post space preparations; (**b**): Radiograph after post space preparation.

The cementation of endodontic posts was performed as per the recommendations of the manufacturer for each group. Root dentin in the prepared post spaces of all the specimens were etched with 37% orthophosphoric acid etching gel (DentoEtch, Itena-Clinical, Villepinte, France) for 5 s, cleaned with normal saline and dried using absorbent paper points. The posts were cleaned with 92.8% ethanol and silanized with Monobond N Primer (Ivoclar Vivadent AG, Schaan, Liechtenstein) before cementation. The prepared root canals were coated with Multilink primer (Ivoclar Vivadent AG, Schaan, Liechtenstein) using a microbrush, and any excess was blotted with absorbent paper points. Then, each post was cemented into the respective specimens using Multilink N (Ivoclar Vivadent AG, Schaan, Liechtenstein) dual-cure resin cement, as per the manufacturer's instructions. The required amount of resin cement was dispensed into a post space through the intracanal tip attached to an automix syringe. Then, each post was inserted into the prepared post space with light finger pressure and a dental surveyor (J. M. Ney Company, Hartford, Connecticut, CT, USA) was used to guide the cementation of posts parallel to the long axis of the root. Extruded excess cement was removed with a microbrush, leaving the cement flush with the coronal portion of the root, and it was then polymerized with a visible light curing unit (XL 2500; 3M ESPE, St. Paul, MN, USA) for 40 s at 300 mW/cm^2 intensity. Periapical radiographs were recorded to verify the post fit after cementation (Figure 3a,b). Then, all the specimens were stored in a distilled-water container at 37 °C for one week.

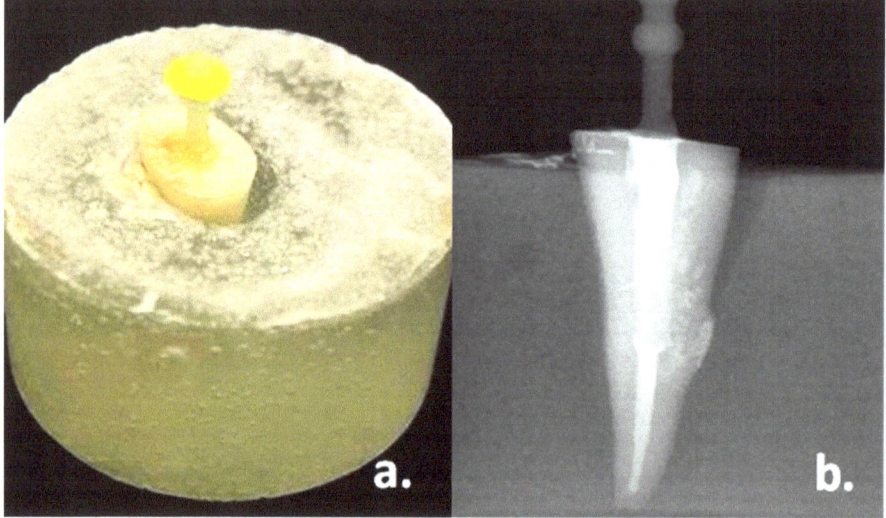

Figure 3. (**a**): Photograph of the specimen after cementation of post; (**b**): Radiograph of the specimen after cementation of post.

Slicing of specimens for Push-out test:

The specimens were transversely sectioned into 4 mm thick slices using a precision cutting saw (Isomet Low Speed Saw, Buehler Ltd., Lake Bluff, IL, USA) at a speed of 150 rpm with a diamond cutting blade under copious water cooling. A first transverse cut was made in the coronal part of the root, measuring 4 mm from the cemento-enamel junction, and the second transverse cut was carried out at 4 mm apical to the first cut, discarding 5 mm of the apical part of the root. Two slices of 4 ± 0.1 mm thickness were obtained from each specimen corresponding to the coronal and middle portion of each root. A slice thickness of 4 mm was chosen to keep sufficient dentin thickness that can withstand the push-out load without fracturing the specimen (Figure 4a,b).

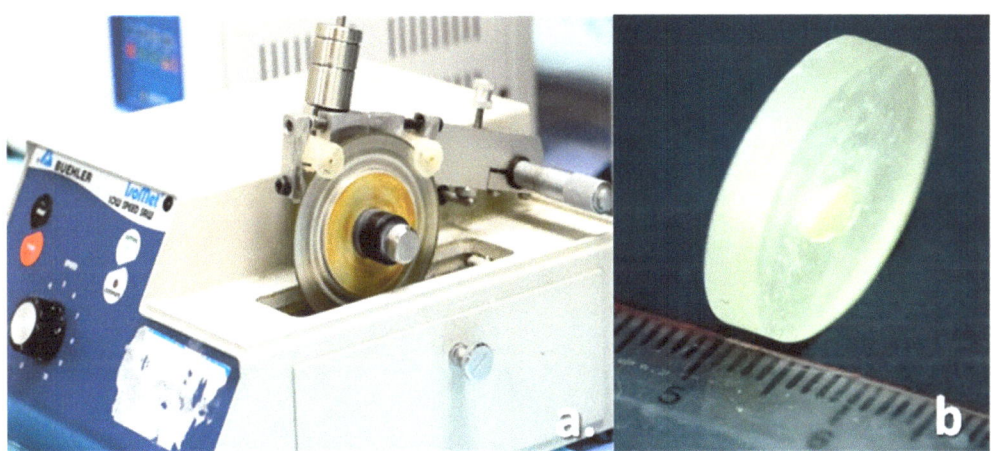

Figure 4. (**a**): Mounted specimen on Isomet precision machine for sectioning; (**b**): 4 mm slice of specimens obtained for push-out test.

Push-out test:

Each 4 mm thick slice was subjected to a push-out bond strength test using a universal testing machine (Instron, model 8500 Plus; Dynamic Testing System; Instron Corporation.; Norwood, MA, USA.) at a cell load of 50 kg and a crosshead speed of 0.5 mm/min until the post was debonded (Figure 5a). Each slice was secured on a push-out jig, and the load was applied from the apico-coronal direction so as to push the post towards the broader part of the root, thus avoiding any limitations to the post movement due to the root canal taper. The metallic end of the push-out plunger, measuring 0.8 mm in diameter, was positioned vertically on the slice so that it was centered on the post without creating any stress in the surrounding dentinal walls (Figure 5b). A constant vertical static load was applied until failure occurred. The maximum load recorded at the point of extrusion of the post from the slice was considered the point of bond failure. The push-out bond strength of each slice was recorded in megapascal (MPa). After the push-out test, specimens were individually stored in dry containers.

Failure mode analysis:

After the push-out test, all the slices were evaluated under a digital microscope ((HIROX, KH-7700, Digital microscope system, Tokyo, Japan) at 50× magnification to analyze the failure modes. Each tested slice was observed under a digital microscope and failure modes were determined to be an adhesive failure within the cement–dentin interface, adhesive failure within the cement–post interface and mixed failure (Figure 6a,b). Based on the failure mode, the percentage of the failed specimens were calculated and recorded.

Statistical analysis:

All the collected data were tabulated and analyzed using SPSS (Version 23.0, SPSS, Chicago, IL, USA) analysis software. ANOVA and post-hoc Tukey tests were used for the statistical analysis of the collected data.

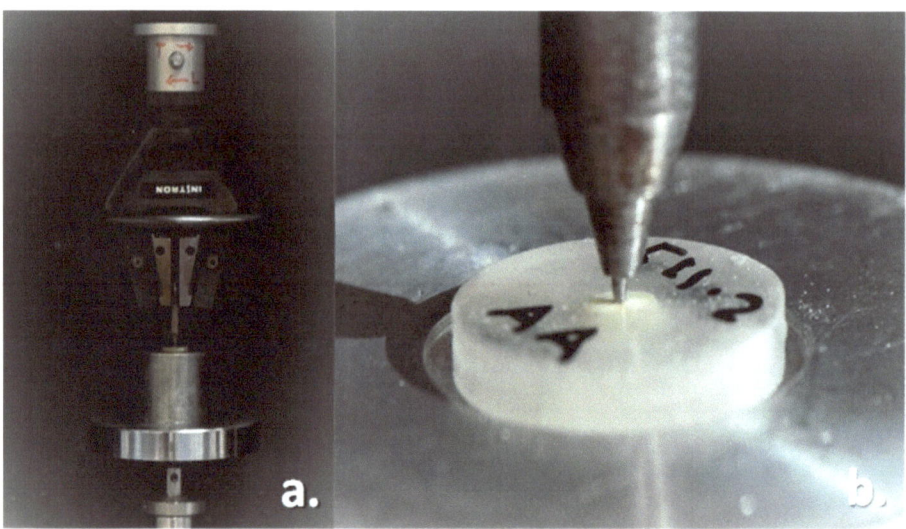

Figure 5. (**a**): Specimen attached to the universal testing machine for push-out test; (**b**): Close up view of the slice attached to push-out jig with plunger centered on the post.

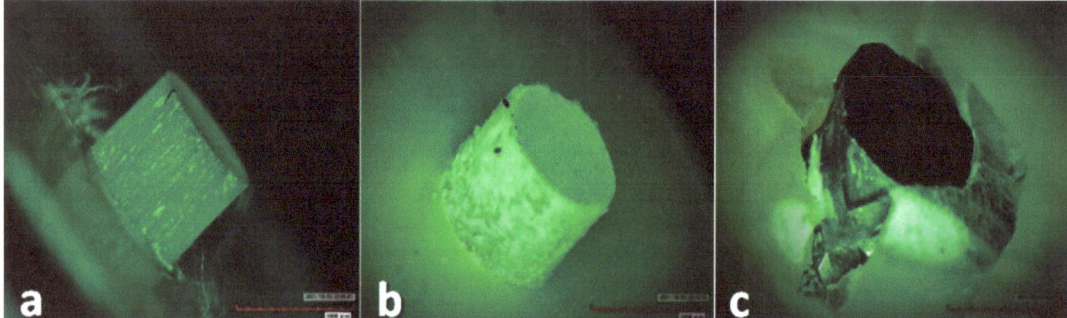

Figure 6. (**a**): Digital microscopic picture showing adhesive failure of cement–post interface; (**b**): Specimen showing adhesive failure of cement–dentin interfaces; (**c**): Specimen showing mixed failure.

3. Results

A total sample size of N = 60 teeth was included in the study. Metal and fiber posts of three different sizes were bonded with dual-cure resin-luting cement. A total of 30 (50%) teeth received fiber posts and 30 (50%) received metal posts. Three sizes (# 4, 5 and 6) were used for each endodontic post system (Table 2). Size 5 posts showed the highest push-out bond strength for both types, i.e., metal and fiber. The mean push-out bond strength for both types of post was almost similar: 225.45 ± 132.94 for the metal posts and 225.29 ± 109.67 for the fiber posts. Slightly higher values were observed for the metal posts, and the results were statistically significant, depicting an increased bond strength with an increased post size as shown in Table 2.

Table 2. Descriptive statistics for the *PBS of the tested groups.

Post Type	Groups	N	Mean POBS	Std. Deviation	95% Confidence Interval for Mean		Minimum	Maximum	** Anova Results
					Lower Bound	Upper Bound			
Metal	Size 4	10	142.08	73.80	89.27	194.87	63.61	286.38	0.039
	Size 5	10	283.24	119.65	197.64	368.83	143.90	561.10	
	Size 6	10	251.03	158.19	137.86	364.20	77.21	600.67	
	Total	30	225.45	132.94	175.80	275.09	63.61	600.67	
Fiber	Size 4	10	130.46	38.10	103.20	157.71	76.29	189.72	0.001
	Size 5	10	284.67	120.78	198.26	371.07	126.88	463.08	
	Size 6	10	260.73	86.11	199.12	322.33	193.81	473.12	
	Total	30	225.29	109.67	184.33	266.24	76.29	473.12	

*PBS = push-out bond strength; ** p value was considered significant ≤ 0.05.

The descriptive statistics show that, on comparison of push-out bond strength among different sizes of metal posts, a statistically significant increase in mean bond strength was observed when the size increased from 4 to 5. A slight rise in mean value was also seen in push-out bond strength when the size increased from size 4 to size 6. Mean push-out bond strength varied from 283.24 ± 119.65 for size 5 and 251.03 ± 158.19 for size 6, showing a slight further increase when considering the maximum values with standard deviation. Results were statistically significant (Table 2).

A comparison of push-out bond strength among variable sizes of posts in the fiber post system showed that significant results were observed when the size increased from size 4 to size 5, or from size 4 to size 6, depicting an increase in surface area for bonding, thus increasing the retention of the post with increasing sizes. An increase in the size of fiber posts from size 5 to 6 did not show a marked increase in push-out bond strength of the fiber posts. Results, as analyzed by the ANOVA test, were statistically significant (Tables 2 and 3).

Table 3. Multiple comparisons and mean differences of the *PBS by Tukey HSD post-hoc tests.

Dependent Variable	Groups	Compared to	Mean Difference	Sig.	95% Confidence Interval	
					Lower Bound	Upper Bound
Metal	Size 4	Size 5	−141.16 **	0.040	−276.65	−5.67
		Size 6	−108.95	0.133	−244.44	26.52
	Size 5	Size 4	141.16 **	0.040	5.67	276.65
		Size 6	32.20	0.827	−103.28	167.69
	Size 6	Size 4	108.95	0.133	−26.52	244.44
		Size 5	−32.20	0.827	−167.69	103.28
Fiber	Size 4	Size 5	−154.20 **	0.002	−252.25	−56.16
		Size 6	−130.27 **	0.008	−228.31	−32.22
	Size 5	Size 4	154.20 **	0.002	56.16	252.25
		Size 6	23.93	0.818	−74.11	121.98
	Size 6	Size 4	130.27 **	0.008	32.22	228.31
		Size 5	−23.93	0.818	−121.98	74.11

*PBS = push-out bond strength; ** The mean difference was significant at $p < 0.05$.

On comparison of metal with fiber posts, the mean difference in POBS (push-out bond strength) was 19.61 for size 4 posts, −1.43 for size 5 posts and −9.69. for size 6 posts A group comparison of both posts systems showed a marked increase in mean values as size increased but the results were insignificant (Table 4). Both the systems, i.e., metal and fiber, showed similar patterns. Thus, an insignificant difference was noticed in the push-out bond strength of the metal versus fiber post systems when bonded with dual-cure resin-based luting cement.

Table 4. Group statistics (independent sample's *t*-test) of the specimens based on the type of posts.

Post Size	Groups	N	Mean	Std. Deviation	Std. Error Mean	Mean Difference	Sig.	95% Confidence Interval of the Difference	
								Lower	Upper
Size 4	Metal	10	150.08	82.45	26.07	19.61	0.503	−40.73	79.95
	Fiber	10	130.46	38.10	12.04				
Size 5	Metal	10	283.24	119.65	37.83	−1.43	0.979	−114.32	111.52
	Fiber	10	284.67	120.78	38.19				
Size 6	Metal	10	251.03	158.19	50.02	−9.69	0.867	−129.36	109.96
	Fiber	10	260.73	86.11	27.23				

Analysis of Modes of Failure

The analysis of methods of failure (Figure 7) revealed that more than half of the total failures were observed within the cement and dentin interface, with the adhesive failures of cement–dentin accounting for 53.33%. Meanwhile, 18.33% of the specimens had failures within the cement–post interface (adhesive failures of cement–post), and mixed failures accounted for 28.33%.

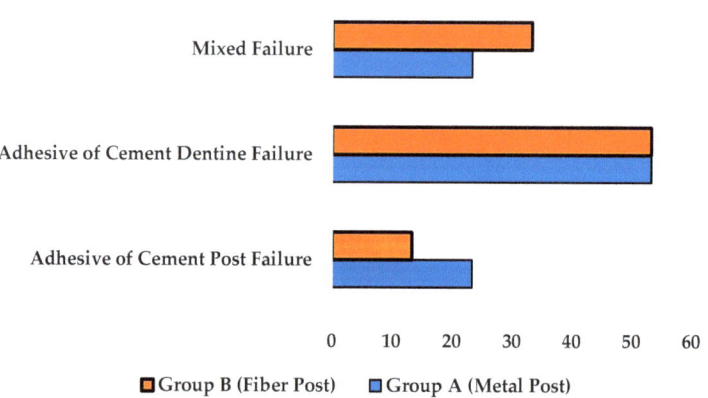

Figure 7. Graph showing analysis of failure modes for tested groups.

4. Discussion

In this research, the PBS of two different types of endodontic post systems and three variable sizes of each post system, bonded to natural teeth with resin-based cement, was evaluated and tested. In earlier published data, multiple methods, such as the pull-out and micro-tensile tests, have been performed to analyze the bond strength of endodontic posts cemented in the roots of natural teeth [5,18]. In the current study, the push-out test was applied to yield the gauging of the bond strength in two different parts of the root. This method put specimens under shear stresses between the dentin–cement and cement–post interfaces, which was comparable to clinical conditions [19,20]. In addition, a study by Goracci et al. [21] concluded that, when gauging the bond durability of fiber posts adhesively cemented to dentin of the root canal, the push-out test seemed to be more coherent and dependable than the micro-tensile technique [21]. Shear bond strength mainly depends on the degree and stability of the micromechanical intermesh and/or the chemical adherence between the dentin inside the root canal, the bonding cement and the post interface [21,22]. Therefore, for many reasons, the initial and long-term bond strengths achieved in clinical practice may be significantly less than optimal [21,22]. The adherence of an endodontic post cemented to the dentin in the root canal is largely dependent on various components, such as the type of luting cement used, the union among the cement–post and cement–dentin interface at different levels within the root canal, the physical or mechanical properties of the posts and the luting cements utilized and the impact of water-absorption on the cement, as well as the type, shape and surface characteristics of the post used [23,24]. Therefore, based on these observations, the investigation and correlation of the push-out bond durability of luted, prefabricated, parallel and serrated fiber or metal posts under homogenized conditions were performed in this research. A slight difference was seen in push-out bond strength where metal posts showed slightly better results, but the difference was statistically insignificant. This accepts the null hypothesis that there is no difference in the comparison between the bond strength of fiber posts versus the bond strength of metal posts.

In the current study, the variation in push-out bond strength amongst metal and fiber posts was insignificant, which is in accordance with other studies, such as those by Wang X and associates [22] and by R Sarkis et al. [25], which also reported similar results for metal and fiber posts [22]. R Sarkis et al. observed the performance of posts in clinical trials observed for five years [25,26]. Gbadebo and associates and Sterzenbach et al. also reported no variance in the performance of the two endodontic post systems, which is in accordance with the current study [27,28]. The basis for similarity may be that multiple other factors, i.e., frictional retention, shape of the post, micromechanical bond, etc. also play a role in the retention of posts, and not only the material for the post system is responsible for it [22].

The results of a study by Turker SA and associates reported that metal posts showed better bonding strength compared to fiber posts [22,29]. Other research by Singh A. et al. and Macros et al. reported that fiber endodontic posts had better bond durability in contrast to metal posts [22,30,31]. Schmitter et al. and King et al. reported a significant difference between the two post systems where fiber posts showed less bond strength and thus showed more debonding, and metal posts showed better bond strength and thus increases fractures in the metal post instead of debonding [22,32–34]. The findings of all these studies are in total contrast to the results of the current study. These differences in results might be due to the variation in the thickness of the cement layer as an intracanal site cannot be seen directly, thus resulting in a compromise in the adequate layer of thickness. This can lead to an increase in stress due to polymerization, as well as a reduced bond strength [35,36]. Although applying the cement in indirect vision with difficult access and a lack of adequate light to apply the cement makes the procedure technique sensitive, other factors such as the inherent nature of intra-canal dentin, the shape of the canal, the angulation and density of tubules in the dentin, smear layer, the remaining gutta-percha attached to walls of the canal and the role of the C-factor (proportion of bonded to un-bonded surface), result in variations in the results and standard deviation [19,29–31]. The choice of post diameter and taper according to shape of the canal also contributes to the variation in bond strength [17,21].

The current research showed that an increase in post size increased the push-out bond strength, as size was increased from 4 to 5 or 4 to 6 in both post systems. A study by Ulgey M et al. [37] showed that bond strength increased as the size of the post increased from 3 to 6, but the results were not statistically significant [36,37]. Another study by Amiri EM et al. [8] concluded the findings that the strength of the bond is higher in the cervical third in contrast to the apical region. This may be on the basis that, as surface area is increased for bonding, the bond strength is increased. Furthermore, a reduced number of tubules in the apical region compromised the bonding [8]. A thick layer of cement and an uncontrolled application of cement with different thicknesses in different canals also resulted in increased debonding [22,31]. A comparison of tapered posts versus cylindrical post- or pre-fabricated posts with custom posts also showed similar results in that that cylindrical posts and custom posts have a higher surface area available for bonding; thus, they yield better retention [26]. An increased surface roughness of posts or technique of application of cement in the canal might also affect the push-out bond durability of the posts by increasing the adherence [25,38].

Upon analysis of the mode of failure observed under a digital microscope, it was seen that 53.33% of failures were adhesive in nature and occurred between cement and dentin. Adhesive failure between cement and the post was 18.33% and 28.33%, respectively, which accounted for the mixed-type failure. Thus, adhesive failure was the most common failure seen in the present study. Similar results were reported by Aleisa K et al. [39] who reported adhesive failure to be 73.5% and thus predominant [39]. A study by Prisco et al. reported that debonding was mainly initiated by crack propagation at the junction of cement and post; thus, adhesive failure was considered to be the more common mode of failing [23]. The likely inference for this might be due to the remnants of gutta-percha, the smear layer or different thicknesses of cement in different areas [22]. The posts, i.e., fiber posts, have a modulus of elasticity near to dentin, which reduces the chances of tooth fracture; thus, failure is seen to be adhesive in nature.

Even though the adhesive failure is more likely to be observed under a digital microscope, other factors such as the type of cement, material of the post and its modulus, nature of prepared dentin in the canal and regions of stress concentration might lead to a variation in the mode of failure [39]. A study by Le Bell et al. observed that, as the bonding improved between posts and canals, the stress concentration shifted to the dentin instead of the junction, which might lead to a cohesive or mixed-failure types [40].

Despite an effort being made to standardize conditions to obtain accuracy in the results, a few factors cannot be controlled, such as the inherent nature of luting cement, polymerization stress, the role of the C-factor, the smear layer, technique sensitivity of cement application and the preparation of the post space, the remnants of sealer in the root canal and the nature of intra-canal dentin, which may have an impact on the outcome [22,39]. Another limitation was that this research was performed on extracted teeth, which might change characteristics of teeth due to ageing, thus affecting the bond strength [39]. Therefore, further research needs to be conducted in a clinical setting or by simulation of a clinical setting, i.e., by the artificial ageing of teeth, aside from using every possible mean to standardize the condition to obtain accurate responses from different post systems. Moreover, it was only performed on one type of tooth (premolars), so anterior as well as posterior teeth need to be incorporated in further research.

5. Conclusions

Fiber and metal endodontic posts bonded to extracted natural teeth with resin-based cement showed almost similar values of bond strength, with metal posts showing slightly higher values in contrast to that of fiber posts. An increase in the size of the post increased retention, which can be attributed to an increase in the bonding surface area. However, a further increase in post size limited the increase in strength of the bond at the expense of the root canal diameter or root dentin thickness. The most prevalent mode of failure observed was adhesive failure, i.e., failure among the dentin and cement, or between the post and cement.

Author Contributions: Conceptualization, S.R.H., A.S.A. (Abdul Sadekh Ansari) and A.S.K.; methodology, A.S.A. (Abdul Sadekh Ansari), N.M.A., M.A.A. and Y.A.A.; software, S.R.H.; validation, A.S.A. (Abdulaziz S. Alqahtani), A.A.A. and T.M.A.; formal analysis, S.R.H. and A.S.A. (Abdul Sadekh Ansari); investigation, N.M.A., M.A.A. and Y.A.A.; resources, A.A.A., T.M.A. and A.S.A.(Abdulaziz S. Alqahtani); writing—original draft preparation, S.R.H., A.S.A. (Abdul Sadekh Ansari) and A.S.K.;

writing—review and editing, A.A.A., T.M.A. and A.S.A. (Abdulaziz S. Alqahtani); supervision, S.R.H.; project administration, S.R.H.; funding acquisition, A.A.A., T.M.A. and A.S.A. (Abdulaziz S. Alqahtani). All authors have read and agreed to the published version of the manuscript.

Funding: The research project was approved and supported by the College of Dentistry Research Center (Registration number FR 0594) and Deanship of Scientific Research, King Saud University, Riyadh, KSA.

Institutional Review Board Statement: The study was conducted in accordance with the Declaration of Helsinki, and approved by the institutional review board, King Saud University, Riyadh (Registration # E-21-5804) before commencement of the study.

Informed Consent Statement: Not applicable.

Data Availability Statement: Data are available on request from corresponding author.

Acknowledgments: The authors are thankful to Bong, technician at CDRC for his help with specimen preparation and testing. The research project was approved and supported by the College of Dentistry Research Center (Registration number FR 0594) and Deanship of Scientific Research, King Saud University, Riyadh, KSA.

Conflicts of Interest: The authors declare no conflict of interest.

References

1. Baba, N.Z.; Goodacre, C.J.; Daher, T. Restoration of endodontically treated teeth: The seven keys to success. *Gen. Dent.* **2009**, *57*, 596–603. [PubMed]
2. Zarow, M.; Ramírez-Sebastià, A.; Paolone, G.; de Ribot Porta, J.; Mora, J.; Espona, J.; Durán-Sindreu, F.; Roig, M. A new classification system for the restoration of root filled teeth. *Int. Endod. J.* **2018**, *51*, 318–334. [CrossRef]
3. Chandra, A. Discuss the factors that affect the outcome of endodontic treatment. *Aust. Endod. J.* **2009**, *35*, 98–107. [CrossRef] [PubMed]
4. Allabban, M.N.; Youssef, S.A.; Nejri, A.A.; Qudaih, M.A. Evaluation of bond strength of aesthetic type of posts at different regions of root canal after application of adhesive resin cement. *Open Access Maced. J. Med. Sci.* **2019**, *7*, 2167. [CrossRef] [PubMed]
5. Pereira, J.R.; Pamato, S.; Santini, M.F.; Porto, V.C.; Ricci, W.A.; Só, M.V. Push-out bond strength of fiberglass posts cemented with adhesive and self-adhesive resin cements according to the root canal surface. *Saudi Dent. J.* **2019**, *33*, 22–26. [CrossRef]
6. Huber, L.; Cattani-Lorente, M.A.; Shaw, L.; Krejci, I.; Bouillaguet, S. Push-out bond strengths of endodontic posts bonded with different resin-based luting cements. *Am. J. Dent.* **2007**, *20*, 167–172. [PubMed]
7. Altmann, A.S.; Leitune, V.C.; Collares, F.M. Influence of eugenol-based sealers on push-out bond strength of fiber post luted with resin cement: Systematic review and meta-analysis. *J. Endod.* **2015**, *41*, 1418–1423. [CrossRef]
8. Amiri, E.M.; Balouch, F.; Atri, F. Effect of self-adhesive and separate etch adhesive dual cure resin cements on the bond strength of fiber post to dentin at different parts of the root. *J. Dent. (Tehran Iran)* **2017**, *14*, 153.
9. Purger, L.O.; Tavares, S.J.; Martinez, R.L.; Caldas, I.; Antunes, L.A.; Scelza, M.Z. Comparing Techniques for Removing Fiber Endodontic Posts: A Systematic Review. *J. Contemp. Dent. Pract.* **2021**, *22*, 587–595.
10. Alnaqbi, I.O.; Elbishari, H.; Elsubeihi, E.S. Effect of fiber post-resin matrix composition on bond strength of post-cement interface. *Int. J. Dent.* **2018**, *2018*, 4751627. [CrossRef]
11. Liu, P.; Deng, X.L.; Wang, X.Z. Use of a CAD/CAM-fabricated glass fiber post and core to restore fractured anterior teeth: A clinical report. *J. Prosthet. Dent.* **2010**, *103*, 330–333. [CrossRef]
12. Mastoras, K.; Vasiliadis, L.; Koulaouzidou, E.; Gogos, C. Evaluation of push-out bond strength of two endodontic post systems. *J. Endod.* **2012**, *38*, 510–514. [CrossRef] [PubMed]
13. Lee, Y.; Kim, J.; Shin, Y. Push-Out Bond Strength Evaluation of Fiber-Reinforced Composite Resin Post Cemented with Self-Adhesive Resin Cement Using Different Adhesive Bonding Systems. *Materials* **2021**, *14*, 3639. [CrossRef] [PubMed]
14. Vieira, L.C.; Araújo, É.; Baratieri, L.N.; Barrantes, J.C. Push-out bond Strength of quartz fiber posts luted with self-adhesive and conventional resin cements. *Odovtos-Int. J. Dent. Sci.* **2016**, *18*, 73–90.
15. Roydhouse, R.H. Punch-shear test for dental purposes. *J. Dent. Res.* **1970**, *49*, 131–136. [CrossRef]
16. Mitchell, C.A.; Orr, J.F.; Connor, K.N.; Magill, J.P.; Maguire, G.R. Comparative study of four glass ionomer luting cements during post pull-out tests. *Dent. Mater.* **1994**, *10*, 88–91. [CrossRef]
17. Dominici, J.T.; Eleazer, P.D.; Clark, S.J.; Staat, R.H.; Scheetz, J.P. Disinfection/sterilization of extracted teeth for dental student use. *J. Dent. Educ.* **2001**, *65*, 1278–1280. [CrossRef]
18. Drummond, J.L. In vitro evaluation of endodontic posts. *Am. J. Dent.* **2000**, *13*, 5–8B.
19. Schmage, P.; Pfeiffer, P.; Pinto, E.; Platzer, U.; Nergiz, I. Influence of oversized dowel space preparation on the bond strengths of FRC posts. *Oper. Dent.* **2009**, *34*, 93–101. [CrossRef]
20. Bitter, K.; Meyer-Lueckel, H.; Priehn, K.; Kanjuparambil, J.P.; Neumann, K.; Kielbassa, A.M. Effects of luting agent and thermocycling on bond strengths to root canal dentine. *Int. Endod. J.* **2006**, *39*, 809–818. [CrossRef]

21. Goracci, C.; Tavares, A.U.; Fabianelli, A.; Monticelli, F.; Raffaelli, O.; Cardoso, P.C.; Tay, F.; Ferrari, M. The adhesion between fiber posts and root canal walls: Comparison between microtensile and push-out bond strength measurements. *Eur. J. Oral. Sci.* **2004**, *112*, 353–361. [CrossRef] [PubMed]
22. Wang, X.; Shu, X.; Zhang, Y.; Yang, B.; Jian, Y.; Zhao, K. Evaluation of fiber posts vs metal posts for restoring severely damaged endodontically treated teeth: A systematic review and meta-analysis. *Quintessence Int.* **2019**, *50*, 8–20. [PubMed]
23. Prisco, D.; De Santis, R.; Mollica, F.; Ambrosio, L.; Rengo, S.; Nicolais, L. Fiber post adhesion to resin luting cements in the restoration of endodontically treated teeth. *Oper. Dent.* **2003**, *28*, 515–521. [PubMed]
24. Sokolowski, G.; Szczesio, A.; Bociong, K.; Kaluzinska, K.; Lapinska, B.; Sokolowski, J.; Domarecka, M.; Lukomska-Szymanska, M. Dental Resin Cements—The Influence of Water Sorption on Contraction Stress Changes and Hydroscopic Expansion. *Materials* **2018**, *11*, 973. [CrossRef]
25. Sarkis-Onofre, R.; Pinheiro, H.A.; Poletto-Neto, V.; Bergoli, C.D.; Cenci, M.S.; Pereira-Cenci, T. Randomized controlled trial comparing glass fiber posts and cast metal posts. *J. Dent.* **2020**, *96*, 103334. [CrossRef]
26. Marchionatti, A.M.; Wandscher, V.F.; Rippe, M.P.; Kaizer, O.B.; Valandro, L.F. Clinical performance and failure modes of pulpless teeth restored with posts: A systematic review. *Braz. Oral Res.* **2017**, *31*, e64. [CrossRef]
27. Gbadebo, O.S.; Ajayi, D.M.; Oyekunle, O.O.; Shaba, P.O. Randomized clinical study comparing metallic and glass fiber post in restoration of endodontically treated teeth. *Indian J. Dent. Res.* **2014**, *25*, 58. [CrossRef]
28. Sterzenbach, G.; Franke, A.; Naumann, M. Rigid versus flexible dentine-like endodontic posts—Clinical testing of a biomechanical concept: Seven-year results of a randomized controlled clinical pilot trial on endodontically treated abutment teeth with severe hard tissue loss. *J. Endod.* **2012**, *38*, 1557–1563. [CrossRef]
29. Türker, S.A.; Özçelik, B.; Yilmaz, Z. Evaluation of the Bond Strength and Fracture Resistance of Different Post Systems. *J Contemp Dent Pract.* **2015**, *16*, 788–793. [CrossRef]
30. Singh, A.; Logani, A.; Shah, N. An ex vivo comparative study on the retention of custom and prefabricated posts. *J. Conserv. Dent. JCD* **2012**, *15*, 183.
31. Marcos, R.M.; Kinder, G.R.; Alfredo, E.; Quaranta, T.; Correr, G.M.; Cunha, L.F.; Gonzaga, C.C. Influence of the resin cement thickness on the push-out bond strength of glass fiber posts. *Braz. Dent. J.* **2016**, *27*, 592–598. [CrossRef] [PubMed]
32. Schmitter, M.; Hamadi, K.; Rammelsberg, P. Survival of two post systems—Five-year results of a randomized clinical trial. *Quintessence Int.-J. Pract. Dent.-Engl. Ed.* **2011**, *42*, 843–850.
33. King, P.A.; Setchell, D.J.; Rees, J.S. Clinical evaluation of a carbon fibre reinforced carbon endodontic post. *J. Oral Rehabil.* **2003**, *30*, 785–789. [CrossRef] [PubMed]
34. Goracci, C.; Ferrari, M. Current perspectives on post systems: A literature review. *Aust. Dent. J.* **2011**, *56* (Suppl. 1), 77–83. [CrossRef]
35. Mjor, I.A.; Smith, M.R.; Ferrari, M.; Mannocci, F. The structure of dentine in the apical region of human teeth. *Int. Endod. J.* **2001**, *34*, 346–353. [CrossRef]
36. Ulgey, M.; Zan, R.; Hubbezoglu, I.; Gorler, O.; Uysalcan, G.; Cotur, F. Effect of different laser types on bonding strength of CAD/CAM-customized zirconia post to root canal dentin: An experimental study. *Lasers Med. Sci.* **2020**, *35*, 1385–1392. [CrossRef]
37. Bouillaguet, S.; Troesch, S.; Wataha, J.C.; Krejci, I.; Meyer, J.-M.; Pashley, D.H. Microtensile bond strength between adhesive cements and root canal dentin. *Dent. Mater.* **2003**, *19*, 199–205. [CrossRef]
38. Tuncdemir, A.R.; Buyukerkmen, E.B.; Celebi, H.; Terlemez, A.; Sener, Y. Effects of postsurface treatments including femtosecond laser and aluminum-oxide airborne-particle abrasion on the bond strength of the fiber posts. *Niger. J. Clin. Pract.* **2018**, *21*, 350.
39. Aleisa, K.; Habib, S.R.; Ansari, A.S.; Altayyar, R.; Alharbi, S.; Alanazi, S.A.; Alduaiji, K.T. Effect of Luting Cement Film Thickness on the Pull-Out Bond Strength of Endodontic Post Systems. *Polymers* **2021**, *13*, 3082. [CrossRef]
40. Le Bell, A.M.; Lassila, L.V.; Kangasniemi, I.; Vallittu, P.K. Bonding of fibre-reinforced composite post to root canal dentin. *J. Dent.* **2005**, *33*, 533–539. [CrossRef] [PubMed]

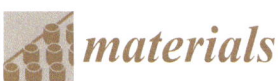

Article

Biomechanical Assessment of Endodontically Treated Molars Restored by Endocrowns Made from Different CAD/CAM Materials

Mhd Ayham Darwich [1,2], Abeer Aljareh [3], Nabil Alhouri [3], Szabolcs Szávai [4], Hasan Mhd Nazha [5,*], Fabian Duvigneau [5] and Daniel Juhre [5]

1. Faculty of Biomedical Engineering, Al-Andalus University for Medical Sciences, Tartous, Syria; a.darwich@au.edu.sy
2. Faculty of Technical Engineering, University of Tartous, Tartous, Syria
3. Faculty of Dentistry, Damascus University, Damascus, Syria; abeer1abeer92@gmail.com (A.A.); nalhouri@gmail.com (N.A.)
4. Faculty of Mechanical Engineering and Informatics, University of Miskolc, 3515 Miskolc, Hungary; szavai.szabolcs@uni-miskolc.hu
5. Faculty of Mechanical Engineering, Institute of Mechanics, Otto Von Guericke University Magdeburg, Universitätsplatz 2, 39106 Magdeburg, Germany; fabian.duvigneau@ovgu.de (F.D.); daniel.juhre@ovgu.de (D.J.)
* Correspondence: hasan.nazha@ovgu.de

Abstract: The aim of this study was to evaluate the deflection and stress distribution in endodontically treated molars restored by endocrowns from different materials available for the computer-aided design/computer-aided manufacturing (CAD/CAM) technique using three-dimensional finite element analysis. The models represented extensively damaged molars restored by endocrowns from the following materials: translucent zirconia; zirconia-reinforced glass ceramic; lithium disilicate glass ceramic; polymer-infiltrated ceramic network (PICN) and resin nanoceramic. Axial and oblique loadings were applied and the resulting stress distribution and deflection were analyzed. The Mohr–Coulomb (MC) ratio was also calculated in all models. The translucent zirconia endocrown showed the highest stress concentration within it and the least stress in dental structures. The resin nanoceramic model was associated with the greatest stress concentration in dental tissues, followed by the PICN model. Stress was also concentrated in the distal region of the cement layer. The MC ratio in the cement was higher than 1 in the resin nanoceramic model. Oblique loading caused higher stresses in all components and greater displacement than axial loading, whatever the material of the endocrown was. The translucent zirconia model recorded deflections of enamel and dentin (38.4 μm and 35.7 μm, respectively), while resin nanoceramic showed the highest stress concentration and displacement in the tooth–endocrown complex.

Keywords: dental crowns; finite element analysis; CAD-CAM; lithium disilicate; ceramics; zirconium oxide

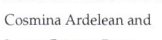

Citation: Darwich, M.A.; Aljareh, A.; Alhouri, N.; Szávai, S.; Nazha, H.M.; Duvigneau, F.; Juhre, D. Biomechanical Assessment of Endodontically Treated Molars Restored by Endocrowns Made from Different CAD/CAM Materials. *Materials* 2023, 16, 764. https://doi.org/10.3390/ma16020764

Academic Editors: Lavinia Cosmina Ardelean and Laura-Cristina Rusu

Received: 20 December 2022
Revised: 3 January 2023
Accepted: 11 January 2023
Published: 12 January 2023

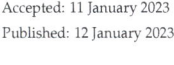

Copyright: © 2023 by the authors. Licensee MDPI, Basel, Switzerland. This article is an open access article distributed under the terms and conditions of the Creative Commons Attribution (CC BY) license (https://creativecommons.org/licenses/by/4.0/).

1. Introduction

The restoration of endodontically treated teeth is still a real challenge, particularly teeth with extensively damaged coronal tissues [1]. Although various types of intraarticular posts have been used widely to provide retention for the core material [1,2], they might weaken the restored teeth due to the additional removal of sound dental structures [3]. Moreover, the preparation of the post space may increase the risk of root perforation and root fracture [1].

Taking advantage of the increasing interest in minimally invasive treatment as well as the evolution of dental materials manufacturing, endocrowns had been introduced as a more conservative approach to rehabilitate endodontically treated teeth with large loss of coronal tissues [4,5]. It was first introduced by Pissis in 1995 as a monoblock ceramic restoration. This restoration is composed of a monoblock ceramic crown anchored on the cavity margins with an extension to the pulp chamber. Mechanical and micromechanical retention can be provided from the pulp chamber walls and the adhesive cement, respectively [6]. Endocrowns preserve dental tissues and reduce the risk of tooth fracture when compared to conventional treatment by post and core systems [7]. They also save costs and time, as they minimize the required clinical and technical procedures [8]. Furthermore, endocrowns are associated with less stress concentration and higher fracture strength than conventional crowns supported by different types of posts and cores [6,9,10].

The computer-aided design/computer-aided manufacturing (CAD/CAM) technique has been used widely in dentistry [11]. This manufacturing technology reduces needed time and procedures. Furthermore, its restorations are more accurate, with better marginal adaptation than restorations fabricated by conventional techniques [12]. Numerous CAD/CAM materials are utilized to fabricate various restorations, including endocrowns [5,11,12]. 3Y-TZP zirconia (yttrium-cation-doped tetragonal zirconia polycrystals: 2–3% mol Y2O3) [13] is known for its highest strength and toughness among dental ceramics [14]. However, the opacity of traditional zirconia has led to the generation of more translucent zirconia by reducing the alumina amount to 0.05% by weight and increasing the yttria content to 4% mol (4Y-PSZ: yttria partially stabilized zirconia), 5% mol (5Y-PSZ) and recently to 8% mol (e.g., DD Bio ZX2, Dental Direkt, Spenge, Germany) [13–15]. This new generation of zirconia has allowed for the production of full anatomical zirconia restorations with appropriate esthetic appearances, using CAD/CAM manufacturing technology [13]. On the other hand, lithium disilicate glass ceramic (LDS) is another example of ceramics that shows high mechanical and esthetic properties and could be fabricated by the CAD/CAM technique (e.g., IPS e.max CAD, Ivoclar Vivadent, Ellwangen, Germany) [16]. Thanks to the needle-shaped crystals that form within the glass ceramic during crystallization, the flexural strength and fracture toughness of the material are doubled [17].

Various types of CAD/CAM materials have been produced due to the combination of different components such as glass ceramic, zirconia crystals, and resin matrix. Polymer-infiltrated ceramic network (PICN) material has been introduced as a result of infiltrating a ceramic scaffold (86% by weight) with a resin network (14% by weight) (e.g., VITA ENAMIC, VITA Zahnfabrik, Bad Säckingen, Germany) [18]. This composition offers many benefits. For instance, PICN, which is described as a hybrid ceramic, is much easier to mill by the CAD/CAM technique compared to other ceramics. Moreover, its tendency to brittle fracture is lower than pure ceramics [18]. Zirconia-reinforced lithium silicate glass ceramic (ZLS) (e.g., VITA SUPRINITY, Vita Zahnfabrik, Germany) is another CAD/CAM material that is fabricated by adding zirconia crystals (10% by weight) to glass ceramic [19]. Not only does ZLS have high mechanical and esthetic properties due to its structure, but it also provides better milling and polishing procedures than LDS, according to the manufacturer [19]. Resin nanoceramic (RNC) (e.g., Lava Ultimate, 3M ESPE, St. Paul, MN, USA) was suggested to be classified as a type of resin-matrix ceramic as it contains 80% by weight silica and zirconia nanoparticles with a highly cured resin matrix [20,21]. This formulation allows for the fabrication of restorations with high strength and high polish retention. It also allows for faster manufacturing procedures [20].

The wide variation of available materials in the market, which are all alleged to be characterized by high esthetic and physical properties according to the manufacturers [16,18–20], makes it difficult to choose a suitable restorative material depending on its biomechanical behavior. Furthermore, there is no crucial conclusion about endocrown materials. An earlier study found that the facture load and the flexural strength of lithium disilicate ceramic (mean value 0.4 KN and 271.6 MPa, respectively) were the highest among studied materials (resin nanoceramic, feldspathic ceramic and PICN). It also found that the strength of feldspathic ceramic (137.8 MPa) was less than the strength of resin nanoceramic (164.3 MPa) [11]. However, another study concluded that resin nanoceramic endocrowns had significantly higher fracture resistance (1583.28 N) than LDS and feldspathic ceramic endocrowns (1340.92 N and 1368.76 N, respectively) [8]. Moreover, Aktas et al. [22] showed no differences in the mechanical failure of endocrowns from alumina-silicate, zirconia-reinforced lithium silicate ceramic and PICN. In addition to the conflicting results about endocrown materials, there is a lack of studies about the behavior of endocrowns from translucent zirconia. Sahebi et al. [23] concluded that translucent zirconia endocrowns showed higher fracture strength with lower retention than zirconium lithium silicate endocrowns. While a previous study found that resin composite endocrowns were a reliable approach to restoring endodontically treated teeth compared to lithium disilicate and translucent zirconia endocrowns or crowns with conventional posts [24], another study found that higher fracture strength was seen in lithium disilicate ceramic endocrowns, whereas translucent zirconia endocrowns showed more catastrophic failure types [25].

The biomechanical behavior of restorative materials could play an important role in choosing the suitable material for endocrowns to rehabilitate molars with excessively damaged coronal structures. The conflicting conclusions of previous studies about endocrown materials led us to carry out this study. To our knowledge, the present investigation is one of the first studies to assess stress distribution in molars restored by endocrowns from translucent zirconia. Thus, this study aimed to evaluate the biomechanical behavior of endocrowns from translucent zirconia and compare it with endocrowns from other CAD/CAM materials, using finite element analysis (FEA).

2. Materials and Methods
2.1. FEA Modeling

At first, mandibular molar was scanned using cone-beam computed tomography imaging technique (CBCT); (Pax-i3D Green; Vatech, Gyeonggi-do, Republic of Korea). Then, image slices were imported to Mimics 21.0 software (Materialise NV Technologielaan, Leuven, Belgium), and 186 slices were selected from a total of 416 slices. Separate masks were created to isolate dental tissues—enamel; dentin and pulp—in each slice of the image (Figure 1), depending on Hounsfield Units (HU) in the CBCT image (6830–7000 HU for enamel, 4179–6198 HU for dentin and 3499–4617 HU for pulp).

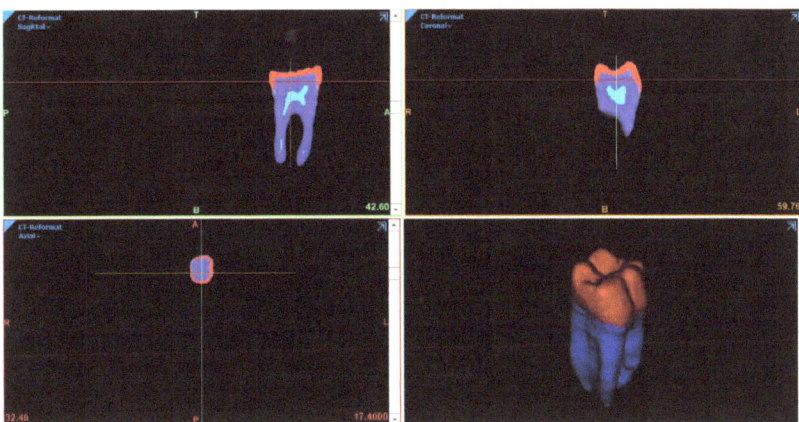

Figure 1. The isolated dental components.

Utilizing 3Matic software (Materialise NV Technologielaan, Leuven, Belgium), the periodontal ligament was created by the offset feature with a thickness of 0.25 mm. The 3D objects were exported as STL files to Geomagic Studio (Geomagic Inc., Morrisville, NC, USA) to refine them and generate NURBS (non-uniform rational B-spline) models in IGES format. Powershape Ultimate software (Autodesk Inc., San Rafael, CA, USA) was used then to convert the components to solids and export them in Parasolid (x.t) format. Afterwards, SolidWorks software (Dassault Systèmes SolidWorks Corporation,

Waltham, MA, USA) was used to create the preparation design and the surrounding bones. Cortical and trabecular bones were created according to the dimensions mentioned in the literature [26,27], as shown in Figure 2A.

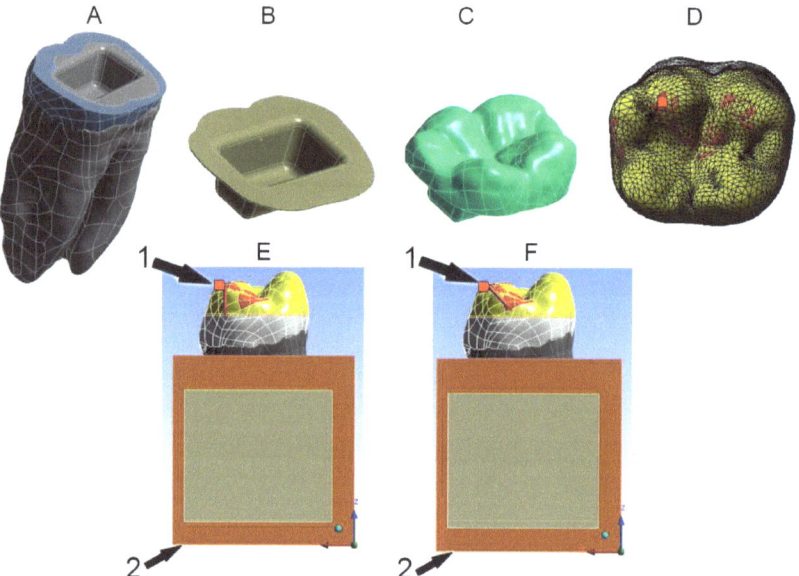

Figure 2. (**A**): dental tissues; (**B**): cement layer; (**C**): endocrown; (**D**): loading points on endocrown; (**E**): axial loading; (**F**): oblique loading. 1: applied force and 2: fixed support (inferior surface of cortical bone).

2.2. Preparation Design

Using SolidWorks, coronal tissues were cut 2 mm above the cementoenamel junction (CEJ) to simulate the extensive loss of coronal structures [5,28,29]. The occlusal margins were flat to represent butt joint preparation (Figure 2A) [5,29]. The pulp chamber was 3 mm in depth [30] with rounded angles and 10° internal wall divergence [4,28,29], (Figure 2B). A 0.1 mm thickness of the cement layer was also represented [10,31], as shown in Figure 2B.

Boolean operations were performed using Powershape Ultimate software to obtain the restorations and prepared dental structures separately. Five different CAD/CAM materials were used to represent the endocrown. Therefore, the models were: translucent zirconia endocrown (E-Z); zirconia-reinforced lithium silicate ceramic endocrown (E-S); lithium disilicate glass ceramic endocrown (E-E); polymer-infiltrated ceramic network endocrown (E-P) and resin nanoceramic endocrown (E-L). Table 1 shows the models and their materials.

Meshing was performed for each model by generating a mesh of tetrahedral quadratic elements. Based on mesh sensitivity analysis, the optimized number of elements is reported in Table 2, based on 1% convergence tolerance in model output for each component.

2.3. Material Properties

All materials and components were assumed to be linearly elastic, isotropic and homogenous. All components were also assumed to be bonded to each other in the model. Table 3 summarizes the mechanical properties of materials and structures taken from the literature [32–38].

Table 1. The models and their materials.

Model	Material	Abbreviation	Chemical Composition (%wt) *	Example	Manufacturer
E-E	Lithium disilicate glass ceramic	LDS	SiO_2 (80.0), Li_2O (19), K_2O (13), P_2O_5 (11), ZrO_2 (8), ZnO (8), Al_2O_3 (5), MgO (5) and coloring oxides	IPS e.max CAD	Ivoclar Vivadent GmbH, Germany
E-P	Polymer-infiltrated ceramic network	PICN	Ceramic part (86 wt%): SiO_2 (63), Al_2O_3 (23), Na_2O (6), B_2O_3 (2), ZrO_2 (<1), CaO (<1). Polymer part (14 wt%): UDMA and TEGDMA	VITA Enamic	VITA Zahnfabrik, Germany
E-S	Zirconia-reinforced lithium silicate glass ceramic	ZLS	SiO_2 (64), Li_2O (21), K_2O (4), P_2O_5 (8), Al_2O_3 (4), ZrO_2 (12), CeO_2 (4), La_2O_3 (0.1) and pigments (6)	VITA Suprinity	VITA Zahnfabrik, Germany
E-L	Resin nanoceramic	RNC	Nanomer and nanocluster fillers (nanoceramic material 80% wt). Nanoclusters (0.6–10 μm) of 20 nm silica and zirconia 4–11 nm.	Lava Ultimate	3M ESPE, USA
E-Z	Translucent zirconia	-	ZrO_2, HfO_2, Y_2O_3 (> 90), Al_2O_3 (<0.5) and other oxides ($\leq$1) **	DD Bio zx2	Dental Direkt GmbH, Germany

* Chemical compositions are according to the manufacturers. ** (Schatz et al. [13]).

Table 2. The number of nodes and elements in the models.

Model *	Elements	Nodes
E-E	56,274	110,644
E-L	64,796	126,213
E-S	64,796	126,213
E-P	64,796	126,213
E-Z	50,626	100,495

* E-E: lithium disilicate glass ceramic; E-L: resin nanoceramic; E-S: zirconia-reinforced lithium silicate glass ceramic; E-P: polymer-infiltrated ceramic network; E-Z: translucent zirconia.

Table 3. The mechanical properties of the materials.

Material	Young's Modulus (GPa)	Poisson Ratio	UTS * (MPa)	UCS ** (MPa)
Enamel	84	0.33	-	-
Dentin	18.6	0.30	-	-
Periodontal ligament	0.069	0.45	-	-
Resin cement	8.3	0.35	45	178
Cortical bone	13.7	0.30	-	-
Trabecular bone	1.37	0.30	-	-
Gutta percha	0.69	0.45	-	-
Translucent zirconia	210	0.307	745	904
Zirconia-reinforced lithium silicate ceramic	102.9	0.208	459 ‡	676 ‡
Lithium disilicate glass ceramic	83	0.21	173	448
Polymer-infiltrated network ceramic	30	0.23	100	370
Resin nanoceramic	12.7	0.47	100	516

* UTS: ultimate tensile strength. ** UCS: ultimate compressive stress. ‡ UTS and UCS are estimated.

2.4. Boundary Conditions

The inferior surface of the cortical bone was fixed in all directions. Axial and oblique loadings of 600 N were separately applied on the occlusal contact points—the buccal cusps tips, the central fossa and the distal marginal ridge [35]—as shown in Figure 2E. The axial loading was applied parallelly to the longitudinal axis of the tooth as a normal force on the molars, whereas the other loading was applied 45 degrees to the longitudinal axis of the tooth. The oblique loading simulated the force on molars during the closing phase of the mastication cycle [35]. Used in many studies to evaluate stresses in diverse restorative materials [39,40], the equivalent von Mises stresses are evaluated in molars restored by endocrowns from different CAD/CAM materials. Von Mises stress theory, based on the distortion energy theory in engineering, is a combination of the three principal stresses (σ_1, σ_2 and σ_3) in the studied field. If any of these stresses reach a critical value related to the property of the material, the material begins to fail [41]. Total deformation was analyzed to determine the total displacement in the endocrown as well as the dental structures. Maximum principal (tensile) stress, which is used as an index of failure in brittle materials, and minimum principal (compressive) stress were also calculated in the restorations and the tooth [31,35,39,40,42]. Depending on the peak values of maximum and minimum principal stresses [43], the Mohr–Coulomb ratio was calculated in each model. Maximum principal stress theory is used to predict failure in brittle materials; when this stress exceeds the ultimate strength, failure would occur in the material [44]. When the maximum principal stress exceeds the ultimate tensile strength of the material, or when the minimum principal stress exceeds the compressive strength of the material, the material is predicted to fail [43]. Failure is also predicted when the combination of the maximum principal stress and the minimum principal stress equals or exceeds the ultimate strengths [43]. The Mohr–Coulomb theory can predict failure in brittle materials, and its formula is given as follows:

$$\sigma_{MC} = \frac{\sigma_{MAX}}{UTS} + \frac{\sigma_{MIN}}{UCS} \qquad (1)$$

where UTS is the ultimate tensile strength and UCS is the ultimate compressive strength of the material, while σ_{MAX} and σ_{MIN} are the maximum and minimum principal stresses, respectively [43].

3. Results

The results obtained from the FEA are shown in Figures 3–12. The color scale in color maps ranges from purple and red (the highest stresses or deflection) to blue (the lowest stresses or deflection) in each model.

3.1. Endocrowns

Color maps of stress distribution in endocrowns are shown in Figures 3 and 4. The von Mises stresses in endocrowns when axial and oblique loadings were applied are cited in Figure 5. Von Mises stresses are mostly concentrated in the distal marginal ridge of endocrowns in all models. Furthermore, oblique loading causes much higher stress concentrations in endocrowns than axial loading (Figures 3 and 4). Under both loadings, stress concentration in endocrowns is the highest in the E-Z model, followed by the E-S and E-E models, whereas the lowest stresses in endocrowns are in the E-L model.

Maximum principal (tensile) stress is concentrated in the distal marginal ridge of endocrowns under axial loading (Figures 3 and 4). The E-L endocrown shows the least stress concentration and the lowest value of tensile stress (46.3 MPa). The greatest tensile stress concentration is in the E-Z endocrown under both loadings. The E-Z endocrown also shows the highest tensile stress (69.7 MPa) when oblique loading is applied. However, the values of tensile stress in endocrowns from all materials are similar under oblique loading (Figure 6).

The minimum principal (compressive) stress concentration is similar in all endocrowns regardless of the loading direction. The highest value of compressive stress is seen in the E-L and E-Z endocrowns under axial loading, while the lowest values are seen in the E-E endocrown under axial and oblique loadings (1.4 MPa and 1.3 MPa), respectively, as shown in Figure 7.

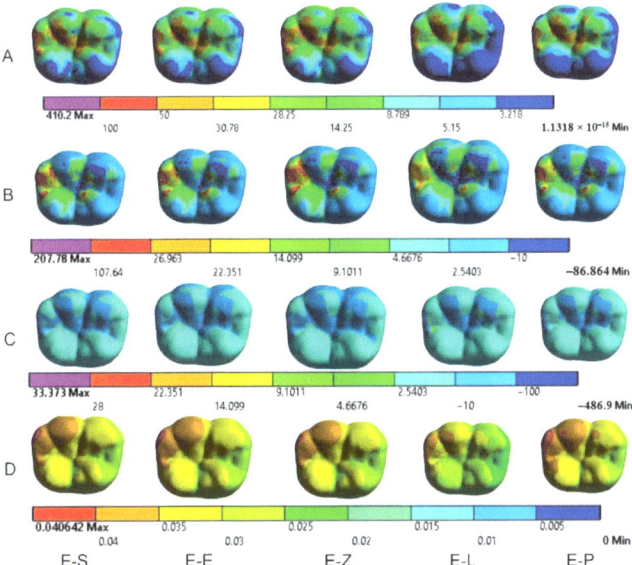

Figure 3. Stress distribution and displacement of endocrowns in all models under axial loading. (**A**) von Mises stress, (**B**) maximum principal stress, (**C**) minimum principal stress and (**D**) displacement. E-S: zirconia-reinforced lithium silicate ceramic model, E-E: lithium disilicate glass ceramic model, E-Z: translucent zirconia model, E-L: resin nanoceramic model and E-P: polymer-infiltrated ceramic network model.

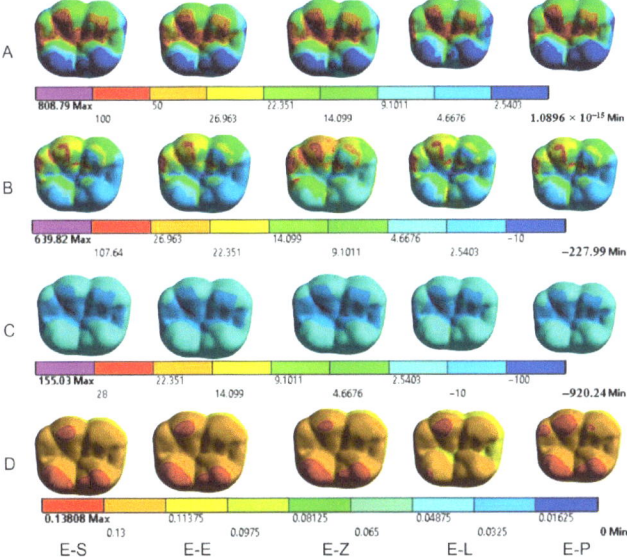

Figure 4. Stress distribution and displacement of endocrowns in all models under oblique loading. (**A**) von Mises stress, (**B**) maximum principal stress, (**C**) minimum principal stress and (**D**) displacement. E-S: zirconia-reinforced lithium silicate ceramic model, E-E: lithium disilicate glass ceramic model, E-Z: translucent zirconia model, E-L: resin nanoceramic model and E-P: polymer-infiltrated ceramic network model.

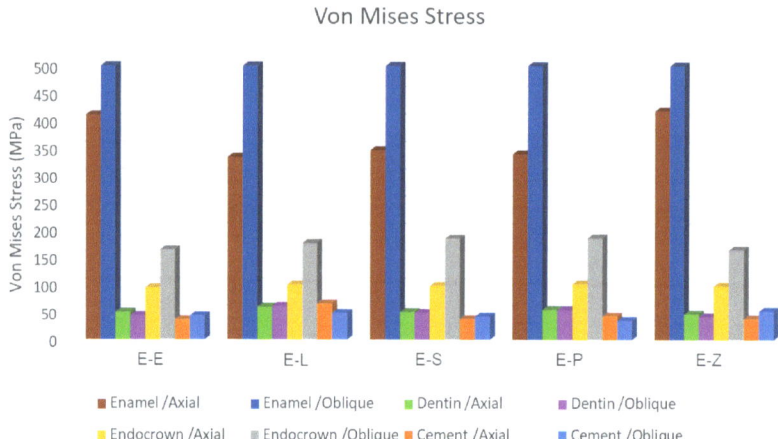

Figure 5. The maximum values of von Mises stress (MPa). E-Z: translucent zirconia model, E-P: polymer-infiltrated ceramic network model, E-S: zirconia-reinforced lithium silicate ceramic model, E-L: resin nanoceramic model and E-E: lithium disilicate glass ceramic model.

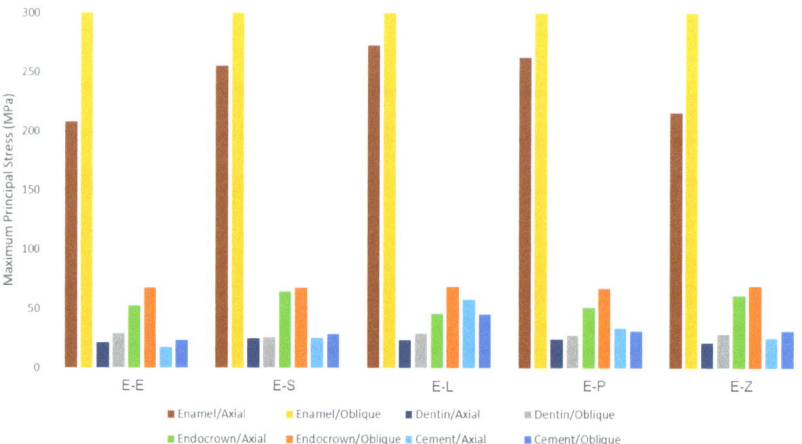

Figure 6. The maximum values of maximum principal stresses (MPa). E-E: lithium disilicate glass ceramic model, E-S: zirconia-reinforced lithium silicate ceramic model, E-L: resin nanoceramic model, E-P: polymer-infiltrated ceramic network model and E-Z: translucent zirconia model.

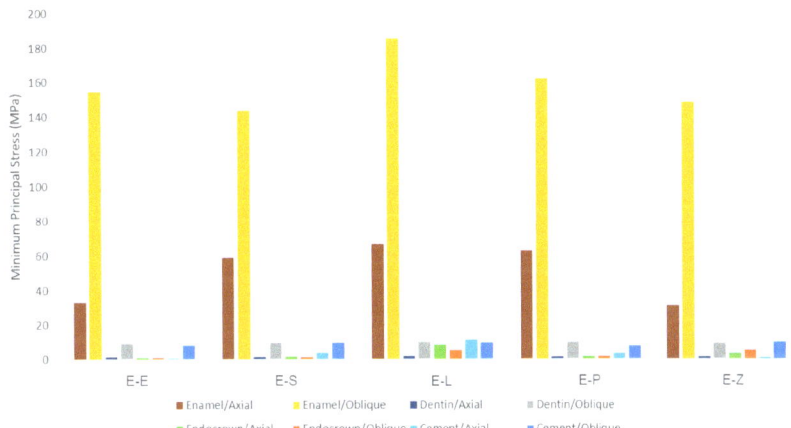

Figure 7. The maximum values of minimum principal stresses (MPa). E-E: lithium disilicate glass ceramic model, E-S: zirconia-reinforced lithium silicate ceramic model, E-L: resin nanoceramic model, E-P: polymer-infiltrated ceramic network model and E-Z: translucent zirconia model.

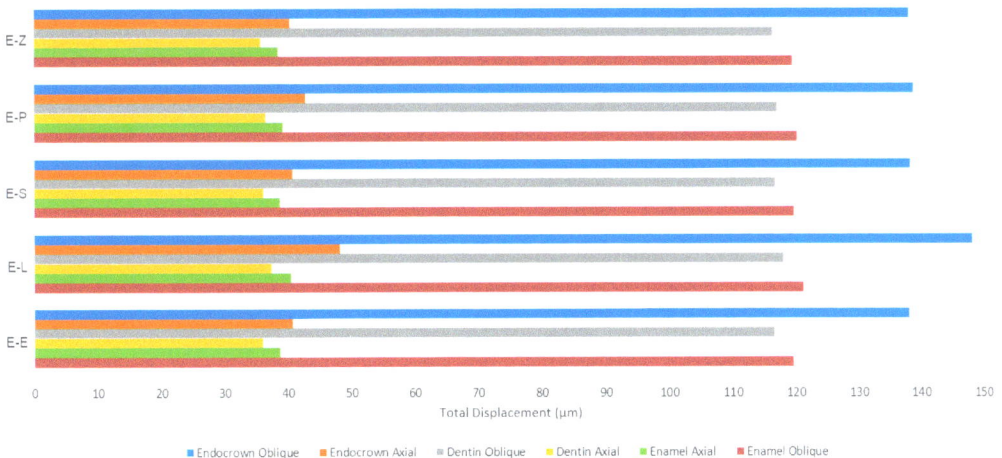

Figure 8. Maximum values of deflection (μm) of endocrowns, dental tissues and cement layer. E-Z: translucent zirconia model, E-P: polymer-infiltrated ceramic network model, E-S: zirconia-reinforced lithium silicate ceramic model, E-L: resin nanoceramic model and E-E: lithium disilicate glass ceramic model.

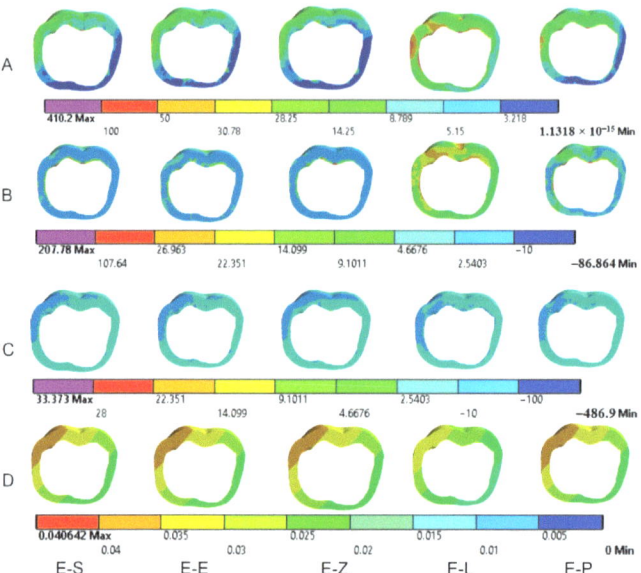

Figure 9. Stress distribution and displacement of enamel in all models under axial loading. (**A**) von Mises stress, (**B**) maximum principal stress, (**C**) minimum principal stress and (**D**) displacement. E-S: zirconia-reinforced lithium silicate ceramic model, E-E: lithium disilicate glass ceramic model, E-Z: translucent zirconia model, E-L: resin nanoceramic model and E-P: polymer-infiltrated ceramic network model.

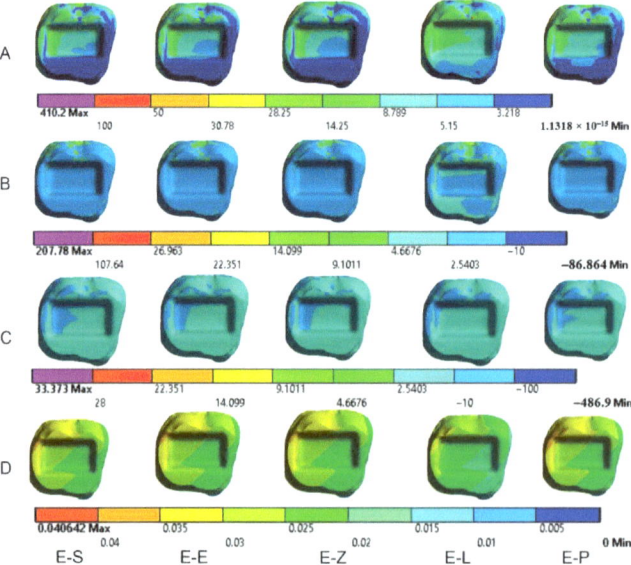

Figure 10. Stress distribution and displacement of dentin in all models under axial loading. (**A**) von Mises stress, (**B**) maximum principal stress, (**C**) minimum principal stress and (**D**) displacement. E-S: zirconia-reinforced lithium silicate ceramic model, E-E: lithium disilicate glass ceramic model, E-Z: translucent zirconia model, E-L: resin nanoceramic model and E-P: polymer-infiltrated ceramic network model.

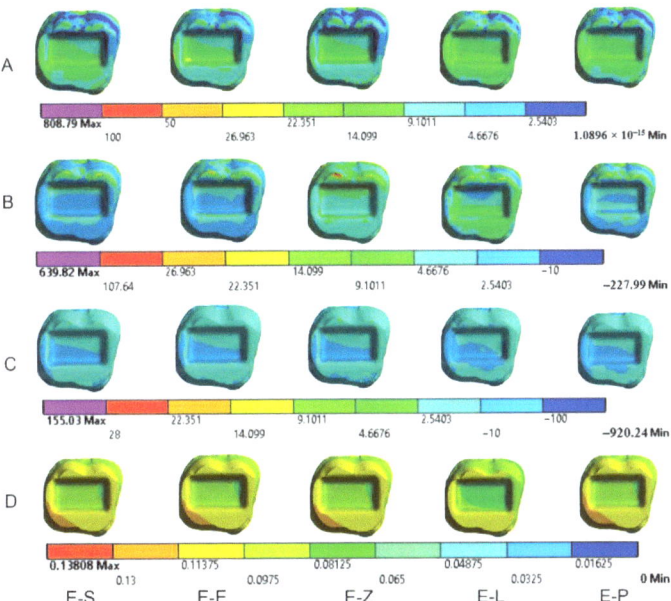

Figure 11. Stress distribution and displacement of dentin in all models under oblique loading. (**A**) von Mises stress, (**B**) maximum principal stress, (**C**) minimum principal stress and (**D**) displacement. E-S: zirconia-reinforced lithium silicate ceramic model, E-E: lithium disilicate glass ceramic model, E-Z: translucent zirconia model, E-L: resin nanoceramic model and E-P: polymer-infiltrated ceramic network model.

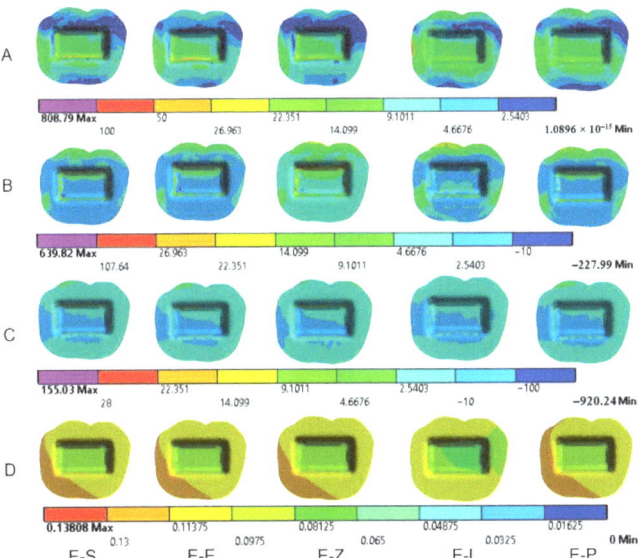

Figure 12. Stress distribution and displacement of cement in all models under oblique loading. (**A**) von Mises stress, (**B**) maximum principal stress, (**C**) minimum principal stress and (**D**) displacement. E-S: zirconia-reinforced lithium silicate ceramic model, E-E: lithium disilicate glass ceramic model, E-Z: translucent zirconia model, E-L: resin nanoceramic model and E-P: polymer-infiltrated ceramic network model.

The values of the Mohr–Coulomb (MC) ratio in endocrowns from all materials under axial and oblique loadings are shown in Table 4. The values under oblique loading are higher than axial loading. All values are lower than 1 in all models. However, the E-Z endocrown shows the lowest MC ratio, while the EL and E-P endocrowns show the highest MC ratios. The total displacement of endocrowns for most of the models is in the same range, except for the E-L endocrown, which shows the highest displacement (48.1 μm under axial loading and 148.0 μm under oblique loading). The E-Z endocrown records the lowest values of displacement (40.2 μm under axial loading and 138.0 μm under oblique loading), as shown in Figure 8. The maximum displacement occurs in the occlusal surface of the endocrown whatever the material and the direction of the loading were (Figures 3 and 4).

Table 4. The Mohr–Coulomb ratio in endocrowns from all materials when axial and oblique loadings were applied *.

Model	Axial Loading	Oblique Loading
E-E	0.30	0.39
E-S **	0.14	0.15
E-L	0.48	0.70
E-P	0.52	0.68
E-Z	0.08	0.09

* Mohr–Coulomb ratio was calculated based on the peak of maximum and minimum principal stresses in the restorations. ** The ultimate tensile and ultimate compressive strengths of zirconia lithium silicate ceramic were estimated to be in a range between the strength of LDS and zirconia ceramic.

Von Mises stress is concentrated in the distal surface of enamel in all models when axial loading is applied (Figure 9). Oblique loading is associated with greater stress concentration in the buccal part of the occlusal surface of enamel compared to axial loading. It also causes more stress concentration in the lingual wall of the pulp chamber (Figures 10 and 11). Moreover, oblique loading causes higher stress values in enamel and dentin than in axial loading (Figure 5). Not only does the E-L model record the highest values of von Mises stresses in dentin (60.1–61.8 MPa) under axial and oblique loadings (Figure 5), but it also shows the greatest stress concentration in dental tissues, followed by the E-P model. The lowest stress concentration in enamel and dentin is found in the E-Z model (Figures 9–11).

3.2. Dental Structures

Maximum principal (tensile) stress is concentrated in the distal region of enamel under axial loading (Figure 9). Oblique loading causes higher tensile stresses in dental structures than axial loading in all models (Figures 6 and 11). In addition, greater stress is concentrated in the occlusal surface under oblique loading. The highest maximum principal stress concentration in dental tissues is in the E-L model whatever the direction of the loading was.

Oblique loading increases the concentration of minimum principal stress in the lingual part of the occlusal surface in all models. The highest values of compressive stress in dental tissues are in the E-L model under both loadings (Figure 7).

The maximum deflection of dental tissues is in the distal buccal area of the preparation in all models under axial loading (Figure 9). It is greater in the lingual part of the coronal tissues when oblique loading was applied (Figure 11). The E-L model shows the highest displacement of dental structures under both loadings, followed by the E-P model, the E-S model, the E-E model and finally the E-Z model. The last model recorded the lowest deflection of enamel and dentin (38.4 μm and 35.7 μm, respectively, under axial loading), as shown in Figure 8.

3.3. Cement

The values and the distribution of von Mises stress in the cement layer are shown in Figures 5 and 12A. Stress is concentrated in the distal region of the cement layer. Oblique loading is associated with higher stresses in the cement than axial loading (Figures 6 and 12). The E-Z model shows the lowest stress concentration in the cement layer. In contrast, the greatest stress concentration in the cement layer is seen in the E-L model, followed by the E-P model.

The highest values of tensile stress in the cement layer are in the E-L model (58.0 MPa, 45.5 MPa), whereas the lowest values are in the E-E model (18.0 MPa, 23.6 MPa) under axial and oblique loadings, respectively (Figure 6). Oblique loading causes higher stress concentration, particularly in the buccal area of the cement in E-L and E-P models (Figure 12).

More minimum principal stress is concentrated in the buccal area of the cement under oblique loading (Figure 12). Although the values of compressive stresses are similar under oblique loading in all models, the highest values under axial loading are seen in the E-E model (1.0 MPa) as shown in Figure 7. The Mohr–Coulomb ratio in cement is higher than 1 in the E-L (resin nanoceramic) model (Table 5). The values of the MC ratio are lower than 1 in the cement layer in the other models.

Table 5. The Mohr–Coulomb ratio in cement layer in the models when axial and oblique loadings were applied.

Model	Axial Loading	Oblique Loading
E-E	0.40	0.57
E-S	0.59	0.69
E-L	1.35	1.06
E-P	0.78	0.73
E-Z	0.57	0.75

The values of deflection range from 38.647 μm to 41.019 μm under axial loading. However, these values increase to approximately 120.6 μm when oblique loading is applied (Figure 8). The displacement is the highest in the lingual area of the cement under oblique loading (Figure 12).

4. Discussion

Dentists still face difficulty when restoring endodontically treated posterior teeth with extensively damaged coronal tissues [45]. Endocrowns offer a good choice to rehabilitate such teeth [45], as they minimize contact interfaces between different materials within the restoration system and reduce the need for additional macroretentive features in comparison with the conventional post and core approach [29]. It could also be the best restoration when the interocclusal space is limited or the clinical crown length is inadequate [8]. Taking advantage of the development of CAD/CAM technology and the expansion of its materials, endocrowns from various CAD/CAM materials have been manufactured recently with more accurate marginal adaptation and high fracture strength [5,12].

Finite element analysis (FEA) is an effective tool that has been used widely to evaluate stress distribution in complex systems, such as tooth–restoration, and to expect their behavior under various conditions [40]. Using the Mohr–Coulomb ratio, which is based on maximum and minimum principal stresses, failure is expected if this ratio exceeds 1 [43]. The von Mises stress was evaluated in all models in this study. Minimum and maximum principal stresses were utilized to calculate stresses in endocrowns and restored teeth, too. The Mohr–Coulomb ratio and total displacement were also assessed in each model to evaluate the biomechanical behavior of endocrowns from different CAD/CAM materials that restore mandibular molars. Posterior teeth are subjected to various functional and parafunctional forces in different directions [46]. Normal bite forces on molars range from 520 N to 800 N [39]. Thus, 600 N was applied in two directions on the occlusal surface of the molar model in this FEA study.

Not surprisingly, oblique loading caused higher stress concentration and greater values of von Mises, tensile and compressive stresses in all structures than axial loading. It also increased the values of total displacement by approximately 32% in all components of the models. This finding, which is in line with other studies [31,39] confirms the harmful effects of nonaxial forces on the tooth–restoration complex [47]. Nonaxial loadings, including oblique loading, resolve to their axial and horizontal components. The axial component distributes stresses along the longitudinal axis of the structure subjected to the loading, while the horizontal component concentrates stresses in this structure.

While minimum principal (compressive) stress showed a similar pattern of distribution in all endocrowns, the concentration of von Mises stress and maximum principal stress in endocrowns was seen in the distal marginal ridge. The maximum deflection of the endocrown was in the occlusal surface; in the distal buccal cusp under axial loading and in the lingual cusps under oblique loading, respectively. This result partially corresponds with the findings of Hasan et al. [48], who found that the maximum deflection occurred at the occlusal third of the endocrown. The displacement and stress concentration could indicate that cracks would initiate in the loading points, particularly the distal marginal ridge during clinical function [4,39]. Furthermore, this pattern of stress concentration might clarify why cracks and fractures started at these points in previous mechanical studies [4,31,39]. Even though Pérez-González et al. [49] concluded that von Mises theory is not an appropriate criterion for brittle materials, as they found that von Mises theory had predicted failure in the compressive areas rather than in tensile areas, von Mises theory in this study predicted failure in the same areas as tensile stress theory did in endocrowns, and in most of the tensile stress areas in the dental tissues.

The greatest values of minimum principal (compressive) stress were seen in endocrowns in the E-L model under both loadings. The concentration of compressive stress in resin nanoceramic endocrowns caused by the occlusal compressive loading could be explained by the elastic behavior of this material, which allows the material to withstand high compressive stresses before distortion. Nevertheless, the level of tensile stresses is a critical concern for the potential failure of the material [50]. Although the highest values of maximum principal stress were seen in endocrowns from translucent zirconia, maximum principal stress in endocrowns in all models did not exceed the ultimate tensile strength of studied materials whatever the direction of the loading was. The greatest von Mises and tensile stresses in endocrowns were found in translucent zirconia endocrowns (E-Z), while they were the lowest in the dental tissues in the E-Z model. In contrast, the E-L model (resin nanoceramic) showed the greatest stress concentration in dental structures and the lowest stresses in endocrowns. This result may be attributed to the elastic moduli of the studied materials. Material with high elastic modulus is more probable to concentrate stress within it rather than transmit stresses to the surrounding structures [4,39]. Furthermore, the E-Z model showed the smallest values of total displacement in all components and the lowest value of the Mohr–Coulomb ratio in the endocrown, while the E-L and E-P models were associated with the highest values of deflection and the highest values of Mohr–Coulomb ratio. This displacement could be due to the stiffness of the restorative material and its elastic modulus. Stiff materials, whose elastic moduli are high [32], cause less displacement of dental structures. Thus, endocrowns from such materials could provide greater protection for the residual dental tissues than endocrowns from materials whose elastic moduli are low [41,51]. Furthermore, the results showed that the highest displacement occurred in the lingual part of the occlusal surface in the dental structures under oblique loading. This could be due to the direction of the loading, which was applied at 45 degrees to the longitudinal axis from the buccal area towards the lingual area of the tooth. This displacement of the dental structures might result in tooth fracture [41]. The high deflection and stress concentration in the dental structures in the E-L model, which are restored by elastic material (resin nanoceramic), might explain why teeth restored by resin nanoceramic endocrowns showed lower fracture strength than teeth restored by LDS endocrowns in a previous study [47]. This finding could also clarify the reason for cracks that occurred in the residual dental tissues restored by endocrowns in a previous study [39].

Regarding stresses in the cement layer, tensile stress concentrated in the buccal area of the cement near margins in the E-L and E-P models. The highest values of von Mises and tensile stresses in the cement were also in the E-L model. This could be attributed to the low elastic modulus of resin nanoceramic, which leads to the concentration of more stresses in the neighboring structures, including the cement. The values of the Mohr–Coulomb ratio in cement in the E-L model were greater than 1 under both loadings. Moreover, the maximum principal stresses in the cement in the E-L model were higher than the ultimate tensile strength of resin cement. Tensile stress values and their concentration in the marginal part of the cement layer might indicate that clinical failure of the resin nanoceramic endocrown would occur in the cement, resulting in debonding, marginal leakage or secondary caries [48]. On the other hand, the smallest von Mises stress and tensile stress in the cement layer were seen in the E-Z and E-E models, respectively. This could be attributed to the high elastic modulus of these materials. The higher the elastic modulus of the material is, the more protection is provided for the adjacent structures, including the cement layer [31].

Although the findings of this study are essential to evaluate the biomechanical behavior of endocrowns from CAD/CAM materials, the results of this FE analysis should be considered carefully, since all structures were assumed to be isotropic and linearly elastic, while their real properties might be different. Moreover, the properties of the bonding to the restorative material and dentin may influence the type of failure. Despite the complexity of the oral environment, only static loadings were applied in this study to simplify the conditions required to perform the analysis. Although mandibular molars were selected as they lose hard tissues repeatedly, the type of the tooth may influence the pattern of stress distribution, since teeth are subjected to different forces in various magnitudes and directions. Furthermore, more studies about translucent zirconia and zirconia-reinforced lithium silicate are highly suggested to be performed to assess their mechanical properties, which are crucial for implementing some failure criteria. Further numerical studies are also needed to stimulate the nonlinearly elastic and nonhomogeneous properties of some components. The influences of other patterns of occlusal contacts, such as cross-bite, and different groups of teeth are also suggested to be studied.

5. Conclusions

Resin nanoceramic caused high stress concentration and displacement in dental structures, which might not make it a suitable material for endocrowns. It also caused high tensile stress in the cement layer with a high Mohr–Coulomb ratio in it, and that may compromise the unity of the endocrown–tooth complex. Translucent zirconia might be the best material for endocrowns to preserve the tooth–restoration complex since it absorbed stresses and showed low displacement within it and in the dental tissues. Lithium disilicate ceramic and zirconia-reinforced lithium silicate could be used to manufacture endocrowns as they offer an acceptable range of stresses, Mohr–Coulomb ratio, and displacement in the endocrown and dental structures. According to stress distribution and levels of stresses and displacements, dental materials with high elastic modulus appear to protect dental structures and the endocrown–tooth complex under occlusal loadings more than materials whose elastic moduli are low.

Author Contributions: Conceptualization, data curation, software, formal analysis: M.A.D. and H.M.N.; data curation, visualization, validation, writing—original draft: A.A. and N.A.; supervision, writing—review and editing: S.S., D.J. and F.D. All authors have read and agreed to the published version of the manuscript.

Funding: This research received no external funding.

Institutional Review Board Statement: The study was conducted in accordance with the 1964 Helsinki declaration and its later amendments or comparable ethical standard.

Informed Consent Statement: Not applicable.

Data Availability Statement: Data are available on request from corresponding author.

Conflicts of Interest: The authors declare that they have no conflict of interest.

References

1. Schwartz, R.S.; Robbins, J.W. Post Placement and Restoration of Endodontically Treated Teeth: A Literature Review. *J. Endod.* **2004**, *30*, 289–301. [CrossRef] [PubMed]
2. Zhu, Z.; Dong, X.-Y.; He, S.; Pan, X.; Tang, L. Effect of Post Placement on the Restoration of Endodontically Treated Teeth: A Systematic Review. *Int. J. Prosthodont.* **2015**, *28*, 475–483. [CrossRef] [PubMed]
3. Sedrez-Porto, J.A.; da Rosa, W.L.D.O.; da Silva, A.F.; Münchow, E.A.; Pereira-Cenci, T. Endocrown Restorations: A Systematic Review and Meta-Analysis. *J. Dent.* **2016**, *52*, 8–14. [CrossRef]
4. Dartora, N.R.; Maurício Moris, I.C.; Poole, S.F.; Bacchi, A.; Sousa-Neto, M.D.; Silva-Sousa, Y.T.; Gomes, E.A. Mechanical Behavior of Endocrowns Fabricated with Different CAD-CAM Ceramic Systems. *J. Prosthet. Dent.* **2021**, *125*, 117–125. [CrossRef] [PubMed]
5. Taha, D.; Spintzyk, S.; Sabet, A.; Wahsh, M.; Salah, T. Assessment of Marginal Adaptation and Fracture Resistance of Endocrown Restorations Utilizing Different Machinable Blocks Subjected to Thermomechanical Aging. *J. Esthet. Restor. Dent.* **2018**, *30*, 319–328. [CrossRef]
6. Biacchi, G.R.; Basting, R.T. Comparison of Fracture Strength of Endocrowns and Glass Fiber Post-Retained Conventional Crowns. *Oper. Dent.* **2012**, *37*, 130–136. [CrossRef]
7. Belleflamme, M.M.; Geerts, S.O.; Louwette, M.M.; Grenade, C.F.; Vanheusden, A.J.; Mainjot, A.K. No Post-No Core Approach to Restore Severely Damaged Posterior Teeth: An up to 10-Year Retrospective Study of Documented Endocrown Cases. *J. Dent.* **2017**, *63*, 1–7. [CrossRef]
8. El-Damanhoury, H.M.; Haj-Ali, R.N.; Platt, J.A. Fracture Resistance and Microleakage of Endocrowns Utilizing Three CAD-CAM Blocks. *Oper. Dent.* **2015**, *40*, 201–210. [CrossRef]
9. Lin, J.; Lin, Z.; Zheng, Z. Effect of Different Restorative Crown Design and Materials on Stress Distribution in Endodontically Treated Molars: A Finite Element Analysis Study. *BMC Oral. Health* **2020**, *20*, 226. [CrossRef] [PubMed]
10. Helal, M.A.; Wang, Z. Biomechanical Assessment of Restored Mandibular Molar by Endocrown in Comparison to a Glass Fiber Post-Retained Conventional Crown: 3D Finite Element Analysis: Mandibular Molar Endocrown Biomechanical Behavior: 3D FEA. *J. Prosthodont.* **2019**, *28*, 988–996. [CrossRef] [PubMed]
11. Albero, A.; Pascual, A.; Camps, I.; Grau-Benitez, M. Comparative Characterization of a Novel Cad-Cam Polymer-Infiltrated-Ceramic-Network. *J. Clin. Exp. Dent.* **2015**, *7*, e495–e500. [CrossRef] [PubMed]
12. Kanat-Ertürk, B.; Saridağ, S.; Köseler, E.; Helvacioğlu-Yiğit, D.; Avcu, E.; Yildiran-Avcu, Y. Fracture Strengths of Endocrown Restorations Fabricated with Different Preparation Depths and CAD/CAM Materials. *Dent. Mater. J.* **2018**, *37*, 256–265. [CrossRef] [PubMed]
13. Schatz, C.; Strickstrock, M.; Roos, M.; Edelhoff, D.; Eichberger, M.; Zylla, I.-M.; Stawarczyk, B. Influence of Specimen Preparation and Test Methods on the Flexural Strength Results of Monolithic Zirconia Materials. *Materials* **2016**, *9*, 180. [CrossRef] [PubMed]
14. Yan, J.; Kaizer, M.R.; Zhang, Y. Load-Bearing Capacity of Lithium Disilicate and Ultra-Translucent Zirconias. *J. Mech. Behav. Biomed. Mater.* **2018**, *88*, 170–175. [CrossRef]
15. Ghodsi, S.; Jafarian, Z. A Review on Translucent Zirconia. *Eur. J. Prosthodont. Restor. Dent.* **2018**, *26*, 62–74. [CrossRef]
16. Ivoclar Vivadent, Liechtenstein, IPS e.max CAD. IPS e.max CAD, Scientific Documentation. Available online: http://www.ivoclarvivadent.com/en/dental-professional-/ips-emax-cad-for-programill (accessed on 14 December 2020).
17. Mclaren, E.A.; Cao, P.T. Ceramics in Dentistry-Part I: Classes of Materials. *Inside Dent.* **2009**, *5*, 94–103.
18. VITA ENAMIC, Vita Zahnfabrik, Germany, Technical and Scientific Documentation. Available online: https://www.vita-zahnfabrik.com/en/VITA-ENAMIC-24970.html (accessed on 21 March 2018).
19. VITA SUPRINITY® PC, Vita Zahnfabrik, Germany, Technical and scientific documentation. Available online: https://www.vita-zahnfabrik.com/en/VITA-SUPRINITY-PC-44049.html (accessed on 4 March 2022).
20. 3M, ESPE, Lava Ultimate, USA. Lava™ Ultimate CAD/CAM Restorative, Technical Product Profile. Available online: https://www.3m.com/3M/en_US/p/d/b00008161/ (accessed on 4 March 2022).
21. Gracis, S.; Thompson, V.P.; Ferencz, J.L.; Silva, N.R.; Bonfante, E.A. A new classification system for all-ceramic and ceramic-like restorative materials. *Int. J. Prosthodont.* **2015**, *28*, 227–235. [CrossRef]
22. Aktas, G.; Yerlikaya, H.; Akca, K. Mechanical Failure of Endocrowns Manufactured with Different Ceramic Materials: An in Vitro Biomechanical Study: Mechanical Failure of Endocrowns. *J. Prosthodont.* **2018**, *27*, 340–346. [CrossRef]
23. Sahebi, M.; Ghodsi, S.; Berahman, P.; Amini, A.; Zeighami, S. Comparison of Retention and Fracture Load of Endocrowns Made from Zirconia and Zirconium Lithium Silicate after Aging: An in Vitro Study. *BMC Oral. Health* **2022**, *22*, 41. [CrossRef]
24. Hassouneh, L.; Jum'ah, A.A.; Ferrari, M.; Wood, D.J. Post-Fatigue Fracture Resistance of Premolar Teeth Restored with Endocrowns: An in Vitro Investigation. *J. Dent.* **2020**, *100*, 103426. [CrossRef]
25. Haralur, S.B.; Alamrey, A.A.; Alshehri, S.A.; Alzahrani, D.S.; Alfarsi, M. Effect of Different Preparation Designs and All Ceramic Materials on Fracture Strength of Molar Endocrowns. *J. Appl. Biomater. Funct. Mater.* **2020**, *18*, 2280800020947329. [CrossRef] [PubMed]

26. Meijer, H.J.; Kuiper, J.H.; Starmans, F.J.; Bosman, F. Stress Distribution around Dental Implants: Influence of Superstructure, Length of Implants, and Height of Mandible. *J. Prosthet. Dent.* **1992**, *68*, 96–102. [CrossRef] [PubMed]
27. Menicucci, G.; Mossolov, A.; Mozzati, M.; Lorenzetti, M.; Preti, G. Tooth-Implant Connection: Some Biomechanical Aspects Based on Finite Element Analyses: Biomechanical Aspects of Tooth-Implant Connection. *Clin. Oral. Implant. Res.* **2002**, *13*, 334–341. [CrossRef] [PubMed]
28. Amini, A.; Zeighami, S.; Ghodsi, S. Comparison of Marginal and Internal Adaptation in Endocrowns Milled from Translucent Zirconia and Zirconium Lithium Silicate. *Int. J. Dent.* **2021**, *2021*, 1544067. [CrossRef] [PubMed]
29. Zou, Y.; Bai, J.; Xiang, J. Clinical Performance of CAD/CAM-Fabricated Monolithic Zirconia Endocrowns on Molars with Extensive Coronal Loss of Substance. *Int. J. Comput. Dent.* **2018**, *21*, 225–232.
30. Fages, M.; Bennasar, B. The Endocrown: A Different Type of All-Ceramic Reconstruction for Molars. *J. Can. Dent. Assoc.* **2013**, *79*, d140.
31. Tribst, J.P.M.; Dal Piva, A.M.D.O.; de Jager, N.; Bottino, M.A.; de Kok, P.; Kleverlaan, C.J. Full-Crown versus Endocrown Approach: A 3D-Analysis of Both Restorations and the Effect of Ferrule and Restoration Material. *J. Prosthodont.* **2021**, *30*, 335–344. [CrossRef]
32. Sakaguchi, R.L.; Powers, J.M. *Craig's Restorative Dental Materials*, 13th ed.; Elsevier: Mosby, MO, USA, 2012.
33. Dejak, B.; Mlotkowski, A. Three-Dimensional Finite Element Analysis of Strength and Adhesion of Composite Resin versus Ceramic Inlays in Molars. *J. Prosthet. Dent.* **2008**, *99*, 131–140. [CrossRef]
34. Weinstein, A.M.; Klawitter, J.J.; Cook, S.D. Implant-Bone Interface Characteristics of Bioglass Dental Implants. *J. Biomed. Mater. Res.* **1980**, *14*, 23–29. [CrossRef]
35. Köycü, B.Ç.; Imirzalioğlu, P.; Oezden, U.A. Three-Dimensional Finite Element Analysis of Stress Distribution in Inlay-Restored Mandibular First Molar under Simultaneous Thermomechanical Loads. *Dent. Mater. J.* **2016**, *35*, 180–186. [CrossRef]
36. Holmes, D.C.; Diaz-Arnold, A.M.; Leary, J.M. Influence of Post Dimension on Stress Distribution in Dentin. *J. Prosthet. Dent.* **1996**, *75*, 140–147. [CrossRef] [PubMed]
37. Cousland, G.P.; Cui, X.Y.; Smith, A.E.; Stampfl, A.P.J.; Stampfl, C.M. Mechanical Properties of Zirconia, Doped and Undoped Yttria-Stabilized Cubic Zirconia from First-Principles. *J. Phys. Chem. Solids* **2018**, *122*, 51–71. [CrossRef]
38. Belli, R.; Wendler, M.; de Ligny, D.; Cicconi, M.R.; Petschelt, A.; Peterlik, H.; Lohbauer, U. Chairside CAD/CAM Materials. Part 1: Measurement of Elastic Constants and Microstructural Characterization. *Dent. Mater.* **2017**, *33*, 84–98. [CrossRef]
39. Zheng, Z.; He, Y.; Ruan, W.; Ling, Z.; Zheng, C.; Gai, Y.; Yan, W. Biomechanical Behavior of Endocrown Restorations with Different CAD-CAM Materials: A 3D Finite Element and in Vitro Analysis. *J. Prosthet. Dent.* **2021**, *125*, 890–899. [CrossRef] [PubMed]
40. Gulec, L.; Ulusoy, N. Effect of Endocrown Restorations with Different CAD/CAM Materials: 3D Finite Element and Weibull Analyses. *Biomed. Res. Int.* **2017**, *2017*, 5638683. [CrossRef]
41. Mei, M.L.; Chen, Y.M.; Li, H.; Chu, C.H. Influence of the Indirect Restoration Design on the Fracture Resistance: A Finite Element Study. *Biomed. Eng. Online* **2016**, *15*, 3. [CrossRef]
42. Costa, A.; Xavier, T.; Noritomi, P.; Saavedra, G.; Borges, A. The Influence of Elastic Modulus of Inlay Materials on Stress Distribution and Fracture of Premolars. *Oper. Dent.* **2014**, *39*, E160–E170. [CrossRef] [PubMed]
43. Dartora, G.; Rocha Pereira, G.K.; Varella de Carvalho, R.; Zucuni, C.P.; Valandro, L.F.; Cesar, P.F.; Caldas, R.A.; Bacchi, A. Comparison of Endocrowns Made of Lithium Disilicate Glass-Ceramic or Polymer-Infiltrated Ceramic Networks and Direct Composite Resin Restorations: Fatigue Performance and Stress Distribution. *J. Mech. Behav. Biomed. Mater.* **2019**, *100*, 103401. [CrossRef]
44. Sarkar, R. Investigation of Structural Integrity of Normal& Extreme Loading Conditions. Master's Thesis, Homi Bhabha National Institute, Mumbai, India, 2012.
45. Govare, N.; Contrepois, M. Endocrowns: A Systematic Review. *J. Prosthet. Dent.* **2020**, *123*, 411–418.e9. [CrossRef]
46. Ausiello, P.; Rengo, S.; Davidson, C.L.; Watts, D.C. Stress Distributions in Adhesively Cemented Ceramic and Resin-Composite Class II Inlay Restorations: A 3D-FEA Study. *Dent. Mater.* **2004**, *20*, 862–872. [CrossRef]
47. Gresnigt, M.M.M.; Özcan, M.; van den Houten, M.L.A.; Schipper, L.; Cune, M.S. Fracture Strength, Failure Type and Weibull Characteristics of Lithium Disilicate and Multiphase Resin Composite Endocrowns under Axial and Lateral Forces. *Dent. Mater.* **2016**, *32*, 607–614. [CrossRef] [PubMed]
48. Hasan, I.; Frentzen, M.; Utz, K.-H.; Hoyer, D.; Langenbach, A.; Bourauel, C. Finite Element Analysis of Adhesive Endo-Crowns of Molars at Different Height Levels of Buccally Applied Load. *J. Dent. Biomech.* **2012**, *3*, 1758736012455421. [CrossRef] [PubMed]
49. Pérez-González, A.; Iserte-Vilar, J.L.; González-Lluch, C. Interpreting Finite Element Results for Brittle Materials in Endodontic Restorations. *Biomed. Eng. Online* **2011**, *10*, 44. [CrossRef]
50. Holberg, C.; Winterhalder, P.; Wichelhaus, A.; Hickel, R.; Huth, K. Fracture Risk of Lithium-Disilicate Ceramic Inlays: A Finite Element Analysis. *Dent. Mater.* **2013**, *29*, 1244–1250. [CrossRef] [PubMed]
51. Souza, A.C.O.; Xavier, T.A.; Platt, J.A.; Borges, A.L.S. Effect of Base and Inlay Restorative Material on the Stress Distribution and Fracture Resistance of Weakened Premolars. *Oper. Dent.* **2015**, *40*, E158–E166. [CrossRef] [PubMed]

Disclaimer/Publisher's Note: The statements, opinions and data contained in all publications are solely those of the individual author(s) and contributor(s) and not of MDPI and/or the editor(s). MDPI and/or the editor(s) disclaim responsibility for any injury to people or property resulting from any ideas, methods, instructions or products referred to in the content.

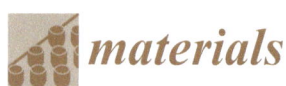 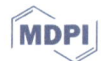

Article

Evaluation of Human Gingival Fibroblasts (HGFs) Behavior on Innovative Laser Colored Titanium Surfaces

Susi Zara [1,†], Giulia Fioravanti [2,†], Angelo Ciuffreda [3], Ciro Annicchiarico [4], Raimondo Quaresima [5] and Filiberto Mastrangelo [3,*]

1. Department of Pharmacy, University G. D'Annunzio of Chieti-Pescara, 66100 Chieti, Italy; susi.zara@unich.it
2. Department of Physical and Chemical Sciences, University of L'Aquila, 67100 L'Aquila, Italy; giulia.fioravanti@univaq.it
3. Clinical and Experimental Medicine Department, University of Foggia, 71122 Foggia, Italy; angelo_ciuffreda.555104@unifg.it
4. Independent Researcher, Bari 70124, Italy; annicchiarico.ciro63@gmail.com
5. Department of Civil, Construction-Architectural and Environmental Engineering, University of L'Aquila, 67100 L'Aquila, Italy; raimondo.quaresima@univaq.it
* Correspondence: filiberto.mastrangelo@unifg.it
† These authors contributed equally to this work.

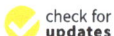

Citation: Zara, S.; Fioravanti, G.; Ciuffreda, A.; Annicchiarico, C.; Quaresima, R.; Mastrangelo, F. Evaluation of Human Gingival Fibroblasts (HGFs) Behavior on Innovative Laser Colored Titanium Surfaces. *Materials* 2023, 16, 4530. https://doi.org/10.3390/ma16134530

Academic Editors: Lavinia Cosmina Ardelean and Laura-Cristina Rusu

Received: 16 May 2023
Revised: 16 June 2023
Accepted: 18 June 2023
Published: 22 June 2023

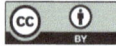

Copyright: © 2023 by the authors. Licensee MDPI, Basel, Switzerland. This article is an open access article distributed under the terms and conditions of the Creative Commons Attribution (CC BY) license (https://creativecommons.org/licenses/by/4.0/).

Abstract: The use of ytterbium laser to obtain colored titanium surfaces is a suitable strategy to improve the aesthetic soft tissue results and reduce implant failures in oral rehabilitation. To investigate the relationship between novel laser-colored surfaces and peri-implant soft tissues, Human Gingival Fibroblasts (HGFs) were cultured onto 12 colored titanium grade 1 light fuchsia, dark fuchsia, light gold, and dark gold disks and their viability (MTT Assay), cytotoxicity (lactate dehydrogenase release), and collagen I secretion were compared to the machined surface used as control. Optical and electronic microscopies showed a HGF growth directly correlated to the roughness and wettability of the colored surfaces. A higher viability percentage on dark fuchsia (125%) light gold (122%), and dark gold (119%) samples with respect to the machined surface (100%) was recorded. All specimens showed a statistically significant reduction of LDH release compared to the machined surface. Additionally, a higher collagen type I secretion, responsible for an improved adhesion process, in light fuchsia (3.95 μg/mL) and dark gold (3.61 μg/mL) compared to the machined surface (3.59 μg) was recorded. The in vitro results confirmed the innovative physical titanium improvements due to laser treatment and represent interesting perspectives of innovation in order to ameliorate aesthetic dental implant performance and to obtain more predictable osteo and perio-osteointegration long term implant prognosis.

Keywords: Human Gingival Fibroblasts; colored titanium surfaces; laser-induced coloration; biocompatibility; surface free energy; wettability

1. Introduction

According to the Oral Health Program of the WHO, oral diseases result in a major health burden for many countries and affect approximately 3.5 billion people worldwide throughout their lifetime [1].

It is estimated that oral health conditions treatment is expensive and usually not part of universal health coverage (UHC) [2].

Nowadays, in developing countries, tooth loss is considered a negative condition with social and psychological as well as functional implications associated with self-image loss and a reduction of the quality of life [3].

Among the most frequent conditions of oral disorders, it is possible to include edentulism. The results of the Global Burden of Disease Study 2010 showed a constant decrease in DALY rates for edentulism in the population standardized by age (Disability Adjusted

Life Year), from 144/100,000 in 1990 to 89/100,000 [4], which is related to the development of osseointegrated implantology in the last thirty years [5].

The rapid evolution of dental implantology has made maxillary edentulism solvable in a predictable way [6].

However, even after osseointegration of the implant, there are several clinical conditions, due to a thin gingival biotype of the patient, such as gingival retraction, mucositis, or peri-implantitis, especially in aesthetic areas of the maxilla, which are responsible for showing a portion of the implant screw or the titanium prosthetic neck of the abutment [7].

These conditions of aesthetic failure of implant rehabilitation are increasingly frequent, representing an important limitation in long-term rehabilitation success, and are related to the specific color characteristics of the titanium screw currently on the market [8].

Furthermore, the accepted criteria for implant success are defined by Branemark and Albrecktsson predicted a physiologic marginal bone loss (MBL) of 1–1.5 mm around dental implants during the first year after loading, and <0.2 mm annually thereafter [9–11].

Recently, several technologies and treatments have been developed for the production of coloured titanium surfaces, such as electrodeposition [12] and the zirconia ceramic implants, which seem to demonstrate the best results in terms of the color panel.

However, the color electrodeposition or the zirconia ceramic implants produced smooth surfaces, which seem to demonstrate inadequate results in terms of soft and hard tissue cell adhesion and titanium osseo- and perio-integration [8,13].

In 2009, Pae et al. [14] showed comparable biological responses of Human Gingival fibroblasts (HGFs) on titanium and zirconia surfaces, and Matthes et al. [15] concluded that plasma treatment supported cell covering on titanium and zirconia disks and both abutment surfaces. Currently, few scientific studies have been promoted to evaluate the color of implant surfaces and abutments. In 2022, Bass [12] and Seyidaliyeva [16] showed interesting results on the titanium color palette, comparing different surfaces after anodizing treatment with zirconia surfaces.

However, recently, Mastrangelo F. et al. showed how the laser use applied to modify titanium surfaces have obtained a wide panel of colors and creates specific micro-roughness surfaces able to promote osseo- and perio-integration [8].

Currently, the scientific literature recommends rough implant surfaces because they are able to promote osseointegration with a high percentage of success [17–19].

However, to favor an adequate aesthetic response in implantology it would be interesting to produce colored titanium surfaces, and, currently, the laser treatment with ytterbium seems to be the only alternative treatment to the anodization process, which, however, produces smooth surfaces, or to the use of abutments or zirconia implants.

The role of surface, physical, and chemical properties has been thoroughly evaluated in soft and hard tissue integration. Wettability, roughness, and biological response in dental implant clinical evaluation is receiving increased interest and is still under investigation [20]. Surface wettability, hydrophilicity, and roughness can affect adsorption of proteins onto the surface, cell adhesions, bacterial adhesion and subsequent biofilm formation, and the rate of osseointegration in vivo [21]. Different chemical, thermal, and electrochemical methods have been used to produce different titanium surfaces' properties and colors by means of the formation of a Ti oxide film in order to achieve osseointegration properties [22]. Within the different coloring methods used for aesthetic colored coatings or layers, the use of chemicals could produce allergic reactions, while the use of heat treatments could generate a uniform and non-reproducible color with low resistance to corrosion [23,24]. Furthermore, some studies have shown that the use of anodic oxidation could favor the color formation of the abutments, giving a better gingival aesthetic response [25], as well as increase the thickness of the oxide layer [26], thus obtaining a better resistance to surface corrosion.

However, anodic coloring has several disadvantages in terms of environmental and working risk, also producing smooth surfaces [27], which are not very suitable for some bioprocesses such as, for example, osseointegration [13,28]. It has been demonstrated that innovative and alternative titanium laser treatments having various colors are possible and able to produce a complete palette of colors [8] with different optical and physical features [13,23,24,29,30]. The coloring procedure itself is simple and based on the adopted laser power. No contaminants are induced on the native cp Ti surface as demonstrated by the EDX measures and there are no porous or marked grooves and pits. The novel laser coloring technique is ecofriendly, highly replicable, cheap, and cell compatible. Surface laser irradiation is able to modify all those chemical (oxide layer and periodic), physical (wettability), and mechanical (topography and roughness) features capable of positively improving cell adhesion, proliferation, and viability [31–37]. Even technologically simple [33], laser surface modification is a very complex process depending on many correlated parameters (speed and number of scans, energy density, spot size and variation of focal plane, pulse mode and repetition rate, power, fluency) [20,38]. Finished machined titanium surfaces have a roughness of micrometers, while in this case, the turning manufacturing produces a macro roughness of hundreds of nanometers. On the colored surface, compared with the machined one, the parameters, under patent and with a low power with high repetition rate, did not increase the roughness [34,39] and they did not produce any significant variation of the topography (pits, craters, or grooves) [40,41]. At high magnification, the electron microscopy shows that all the colored titanium surfaces produced appeared melted and cooled [42].

At atmospheric pressure, the different oxygen diffusions on the laser irradiated melted surface produce oxidized nanometer layers [33,35] able to interfere with the light and produce the colored aspect [8]. To titanium oxides and their thickness, authors attribute the absorption of albumin and fibrinogen blood proteins, which influences cell osseointegration or growth [33,43,44]. In order to better understand the behaviour of HGFs cultured on textured titanium surfaces, we deepened the analysis on the aforementioned materials by firstly performing a wettability test through the contact angle measurements. The liquid wets the surface of a solid by maximizing its area in contact.

The aim of the present in vitro study is to evaluate the behavior of primary HGFs cultured on different ytterbium laser-stained surfaces compared to smooth titanium surfaces.

2. Materials and Methods

A total of 15 commercial pure titanium (CpTi) Grade 1 disks (10 mm in diameter 0.5 thick) (Titanium Alloy-EuropaAcciai, Chieti, Italy) mechanically obtained by turning were ultrasonically cleaned (Elma Elmasonic S 60/H Gottlieb-Daimler-Straße 17 78224 Singen) in acetone (Carlo Erba, Milan, Italy) followed by Millipore water for 10 min for each step) and dried in a thermostatic oven (20 °C for 2 h). In a cleaning chamber, using an ytterbium laser with different selected sequences of nano-second pulses, the titanium surfaces were treated. Among all the colored titanium specimens obtained only light fuchsia, dark fuchsia, light gold, and dark gold colors were selected for the study. The laser-colored surfaces were compared to the titanium machined surface turning obtained.

2.1. Surface Analysis

The surface topographic features were analyzed by stereo (AXIO ZOOM, V16 Zeiss, Jena, Germany) and optical microscopy (Nikon Optiphot2, Tokyo, Japan). The surface color analysis was performed by spectrophotometry (X-Rite SP64, X-Rite Inc., Grand Rapids, MI, USA) with a diffuse illumination integrating sphere system (illuminant and reference angle for the output values of D50 2°). Colorimetric coordinates were expressed in the CIELAB standard colorimetric space defined by the International Commission on Illumination as lightness (L*) ranging from black (0) to white (100), as green (−) to red (+) (a*) and as blue (−) to yellow (+) (b*). The CIELAB system is able to define the numerical change in the Lab values and allows having a color measure that approximates human subjective vision (L* = 0 yields black and L* = 100 indicates diffuse white; specular white may be higher); values between red and green defined by a* (negative values indicate green, while positive values indicate red), between yellow and blue by b* (negative values indicate blue and positive values yellow).

The color variations between colored surfaces were detected by the CIELAB recommendations as (Equation (1)):

$$\Delta E_{ab}^* = \sqrt{(L_2^* - L_1^*)^2 + (a_2^* - a_1^*)^2 + (b_2^* - b_1^*)^2} \quad (1)$$

2.2. Contact Angle Measurements

For wetting analysis, the static contact angle (CA) of liquids on surfaces was measured using a contact angle analyzer (Kruss, DSA100, Kehl, Germany). Contact angles (CA) of distilled water (polar) and diiodomethane (Prod. 158429, Sigma Aldrich, Merck, St. Louis, MO, USA, 99%) (apolar) liquids were measured both on Ti surfaces, to examine the wettability of surfaces by liquids with different surface energy components. For CA measurement, 2.0 µL of liquid drops was placed on a surface, and CA was measured within 1 s after the droplet settlement. After each measurement, the surfaces were cleaned with isopropyl alcohol (Prod. W292907, Sigma Aldrich, Merck, 99.7%) and dried with compressed air. At least three measurements were obtained from different spots of the surfaces, and the mean value was used for analysis.

When a liquid is placed on a solid surface there can be two cases: the liquid can spread to form a continuous film or form discrete droplets or, in the second case, the drop on the three-phase contact line, where the solid (S), the liquid (L), and the vapor (V) meet, can generate an angle called contact angle (θ). A range of different contact angle values can be observed, from 0° (called perfect wetting and, hence, spontaneous spreading) up to 180° (perfectly non-wetted surface). Water contact angles lower than 90° indicate hydrophilic surfaces, where wetting is favourable and the fluid spreads over a large surface area. Wetting phenomena on a macroscopic scale can be illustrated using Young's Equation (Equation (2)).

$$\gamma_{SV} = \gamma_{SL} + \gamma_{LV} \cos\theta \quad (2)$$

where θ is the contact angle, γSV is the solid surface free energy, γSL is the solid/liquid interfacial free energy, and γ_{LV} is the liquid/vapor interfacial tension (liquid surface tension). Contact angle measurements of a surface using a probe liquid provides information about its wettability and Surface Free Energy (SFE). The SFE of a solid surface can provide information about how different liquids will interact with said surface and can be calculated using several models including the Owens–Wendt–Rabel–Kaelble (OWRK) model [45]. In the OWRK model, the solid SFE, γ_{SV}, and the liquid surface tension, γ_{LV}, are a sum of dispersive (e.g., London dispersion forces) and polar (e.g., hydrogen bonding) components, such that $\gamma = \gamma^d + \gamma^p$. Then, the relationship between liquid surface tension, solid SFE, and the contact angle between the liquid and the solid is described by the OWRK Equation (Equation (3)):

$$\gamma_{LV}(1 + \cos\theta) = 2\left[\left(\gamma_{SV}^d \gamma_{LV}^d\right)^{1/2} + \left(\gamma_{SV}^p \gamma_{LV}^p\right)^{1/2}\right] \quad (3)$$

where θ is the contact angle between the liquid and the solid. At least two liquids with well-defined characteristics are required in the OWRK method, as there are two unknowns (solid/liquid interfacial free energy and solid surface free energy) that need to be solved to determine the solid surface free energy. At least one of the two liquids must have a polar part in addition to the disperse one. Water and diiodomethane are most often utilized. Distilled water is a highly polar liquid as its polar component is 51.0 mN/m with total liquid surface tension of 72.8 mN/m [46]. Diiodomethane has only dispersive contribution (apolar solvent), with a value of total liquid surface tension of 50.8 mN/m [46].

2.3. Profilometer Analysis

Ti surfaces were analysed using a Dektak 6M Surface Profiler (Veeco Instruments, Inc., Plainview, NY, USA). The stylus radius was 12.5 µm, force of 3.0 mg. Measurements of

2 mm length along the North-South and West-East directions were performed back and forward in triplicate.

2.4. Scanning Electron Microscopy (SEM) and Energy-Dispersive X-ray Spectroscopy (EDX) Analysis

Scanning electron microscopy analysis (Gemini 5000, Zeiss, Germany) of the light fuchsia surface after HGF culture was performed. Chemical surface composition of Ti machined surface and light fuchsia was assessed by Energy-dispersive X-ray spectroscopy (EDX) (Atzec Live, High Wycombe, Oxford, UK) and Ultim Max 100 detector (Oxford Instruments, High Wycombe Buckinghamshire, UK) at a voltage of 20 kV. Cells were fixed in glutaraldehyde 2.5% in 0.1 M Cacodylate Buffer, pH 7.2, for 20 min at 4 °C. Then, samples were subjected to 3 washes in the cacodylate buffer and subsequently dehydrated with increasing alcohol solutions (25–50–70–90–100% EtOH). Final drying was performed by two passages of 15 min each in hexamethyldisilazane (HSMDA), and then left overnight in a fume hood to allow complete reagent evaporation.

2.5. Cell Culture

The project has obtained the approval of the Local Ethics Committee of the University of Chieti (approval number 1173, approval date 31 March 2016), in accordance with the Declaration of Helsinki. HGFs were isolated from gingival tissue fragments, as already reported elsewhere [47]. Titanium disks were sterilized with an UV lamp (1 h for each side) and placed in a sterile 48-well plate not treated for cell culture. Then, 20,000 cells were seeded on each titanium disc and cultured for 48 h. After 48 h, the culture supernatants were collected and frozen at -80 °C for subsequent analyses.

2.6. MTT Assay

The cell viability was evaluated after 48 h of culture by MTT (3-[4,5-dimethyl- thiazol-2-yl-]-2,5-diphenyl tetrazolium bromide) assay (Merck, Darmstadt, Germany), based on the ability of the mitochondrial dehydrogenase of viable cells to transform MTT into colored formazan salts. At established time points, the medium was replaced with a fresh one containing 0.4 mg/mL MTT, and the cells were incubated for 5 h at 37 °C. After a further incubation of the samples in DMSO for 20 min at 37 °C, 200 µL of each medium were transferred into a 96-well plate, and the absorbance was measured at 570 nm wavelength using a Multiscan GO microplate spectrophotometer (Thermo Fisher Scientific, Waltham, MA, USA). The values obtained without cells were subtracted from the values obtained from the samples. Three independent experiments were performed under the same experimental conditions.

2.7. Lactate Dehydrogenase (LDH) Cytotoxicity Assay

For the purpose of quantifying the cytotoxic effect exerted on HGFs by titanium discs, the CytoTox 96 Non-Radioactive Assay (Promega Corporation, Fitchburg, WI, USA) was performed. The assay quantitatively measures LDH release within the culture medium. Supernatants (50 µL) were pipetted in a 96 well plate with a flat bottom (Falcon, Corning Incorporated, New York, NY, USA) and the volume was doubled adding the LDH reaction mixture. After 30 min of incubation at room temperature in the dark, 50 µL of stop solution were added and the absorbance was measured at 490 and 690 nm wavelength; the values obtained were normalized on MTT values.

2.8. Collagen Type I (Col I) ELISA

Collagen type I released by HGFs, cultured on the aforementioned titanium surfaces, in the culture medium was evaluated using a Human Collagen Type 1 ELISA kit (Cosmo Bio Co., Ltd., Tokyo, Japan) following the manufacturer instructions. The absorbance was spectrophotometrically measured at 450 nm wavelength by Multiskan GO (Thermo Scientific, Waltham, MA, USA). The concentration of Col I (µg/mL) was calculated using a standard curve generated with specific standards provided by the manufacturer and normalized with the MTT values.

2.9. Statistical Analysis

Statistical analysis was carried out by one-way ANOVA, through Prism 5.0 software (GraphPad) followed by Tukey's post-hoc test. Statistically significant values were established for $p < 0.05$.

3. Results

3.1. Optical Microscopy

The titanium surfaces were observed by stereomicroscope, as reported in Figure 1. All the surfaces are characterized by typical circular tracks produced by the turning working. Colors are produced by powered micro pulses applied through laser scanning. This operation produces thin layers of titanium oxide able to interfere with the light and generating the visible color [8].

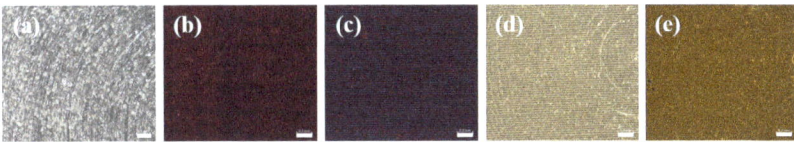

Figure 1. Aspect at the stereomicroscope of the Ti surfaces: (**a**) Machined, (**b**) light fuchsia, (**c**) dark fuchsia, (**d**) light gold, and (**e**) dark gold. Scale bar for all the surfaces is 0.2 mm.

The titanium machined surface, shown in Figure 1a, is characterized by typical circular tracks produced by the turning working. By increasing the applied power laser it is possible to produce higher titanium oxidation with a shifting from, respectively, Fuchsia to Gold and from light to dark hue (Figure 1b–e). The direction of the laser scanning is clearly visible on the surface (Figure 1c,d) while in the case of the gold color, the turning finishing is still observable (Figure 1d) or not (Figure 1e). Colorimetric coordinates were expressed in the CIELAB standard colorimetric space defined by the International Commission on Illumination. In Table 1, the three values of the CIELAB color space for Ti surfaces are reported. L* represents lightness from black to white on a scale of zero to 100, while a* and b* represent chromaticity with no specific numeric limits.

Table 1. Chromatic coordinates, expressed in the L*a*b* system, of Ti surfaces machined, light fuchsia, dark fuchsia, light gold, dark gold, and color variation (ΔE) compared with the machined titanium surface.

Sample	L*	a*	b*	ΔE
Machined	68.49	−0.40	−0.91	-
Light Fuchsia	27.49	+41.04	+55.21	48.91
Dark Fuchsia	17.42	+40.34	+50.31	38.84
Light Gold	88.12	−07.32	+34.05	25.33
Dark Gold	50.02	+09.32	+52.63	28.58

3.2. Contact Angle

Figure 2 shows the water and diiodomethane CA for all the Ti surfaces. The contact angle increases from a value of about 66.21° for the machined Ti surface up to 81.45° for the dark gold surface.

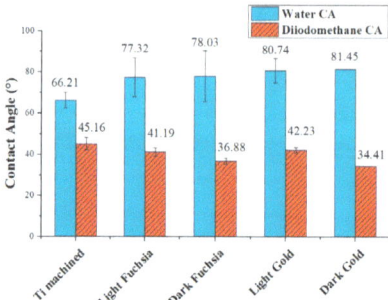

Figure 2. Water and diiodomethane Contact Angle measurement on Ti surfaces.

Figure 3 shows the polar and dispersive components of the surface free energy, calculated using the Owens Wendt approach, and the total SFE for all Ti surfaces. To better highlight the different components, a histogram graph was chosen, where the dispersive contributions are shown in blue, the polar contributions in red, and the total SFE in violet.

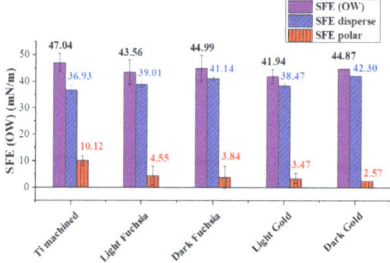

Figure 3. Surface Free Energy analysis for Ti surfaces (violet). Disperse (blue) and polar (red) components are also reported.

As observed in Figure 3, the overall SFE of laser-treated Ti surfaces is lower than the machined one, and the polar component has decreased, a trend most evident in the dark gold surface. The total SFE appears to have the same order of magnitude for all treated samples, considering the experimental errors.

Table 2 reports the values of the contact angles with the two selected solvents (water and diiodomethane), the dispersed and polar components of the surface energies, and the total SFE. The polar ratio is also shown for all samples, i.e., the ratio of the polar component to the total SFE.

Table 2. Water and diiodomethane Contact Angle data for coloured Ti discs. Surface free energy is also reported, together with dispersive and polar contributes, and polar ratio.

Sample	Water CA (°)	Diiodo Methane CA (°)	SFE (mN/m)	SFE Disperse (mN/m)	SFE Polar (mN/m)	Polar Ratio (%)
Ti machined	66.21 (±3.68)	45.16 (± 2.92)	47.04 (±3.55)	36.93 (±1.56)	10.12 (±1.98)	21.5
Light Fuchsia	77.32 (±9.44)	41.19 (±2.07)	43.56 (±4.56)	39.01 (±1.06)	4.55 (±3.5)	10.4
Dark Fuchsia	78.03 (±12.26)	36.88 (±1.48)	44.99 (± 4.9)	41.14 (±0.71)	3.84 (±4.19)	8.5
Light Gold	80.74 (±5.91)	42.23 (±1.36)	41.94 (±2.65)	38.47 (±0.71)	3.47 (±1.94)	8.3
Dark Gold	81.45 (±0.02)	34.41 (±0.02)	44.87 (±0.02)	42.30 (±0.01)	2.57 (±0.01)	5.7

The small differences between the SFEs are explained by the presence of a different polar component from surface to surface, the dispersive component being almost the same for all laser colored samples. All colored surfaces show higher SFE values than the machined surface. The ratio of polarity to the overall surface energy of solids was calculated, and reported in this table. The polar ratio decreased from 21.5% for the machined Ti surface to 5.7% of the dark gold surface.

3.3. Wetting Envelope

Liquid surface tension, solid SFE, and the contact angle a liquid droplet makes on the surface are all related, and their relationship can be visualized by the Wetting Envelope plot.

The polar and dispersive components are calculated using the Owens–Wendt equation and to highlight the differences between the various surfaces in terms of wettability, the polar contribution is plotted against the total surface tension in Figure 4. The envelope created for the case of a contact angle of $0°$ (complete wetting) is shown. All liquids whose surface tension falls below the wetting envelope have a high tendency to wet the solid surface.

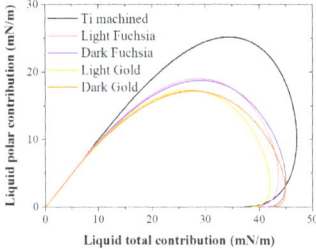

Figure 4. Wetting Envelope for Ti surfaces for complete wetting ($\theta = 0$). In the horizontal axis is the total surface tension of liquids γ_L and in the vertical axis is the polar surface tension component γ_{Lp}.

3.4. Profilometer

Ti surfaces were analyzed using a Dektak 6M Surface Profiler to profile surface topography and waviness, as well as measuring surface roughness in the sub-micrometer range. The arithmetic mean roughness (Ra) and the root-mean-square roughness (Rq) over the evaluation length (Table 3). Roughness profiles were reported in Figure 5 (panel a–e). Two different profiles were reported in black and red lines for any surfaces, obtained along the North-South and West-East scanning directions. A tiny contaminant causes a sharp peak in the profile line. The mean roughness values were calculated on at least four profile lines for each surface, and the standard deviation value is equal to ±50 nm for all surfaces.

Table 3. Roughness measurements on Ti discs. The arithmetic mean roughness (Ra) and the root-mean-square roughness (Rq) of the Ti surfaces were reported. The standard deviation value is equal to ± 50 nm for all surfaces.

Sample	Ra (nm)	Rq (nm)
Ti machined	191 (±50)	247 (±50)
Light Fuchsia	254 (±50)	311 (±50)
Dark Fuchsia	259 (±50)	324 (±50)
Light Gold	254 (±50)	315 (±50)
Dark Gold	215 (±50)	278 (±50)

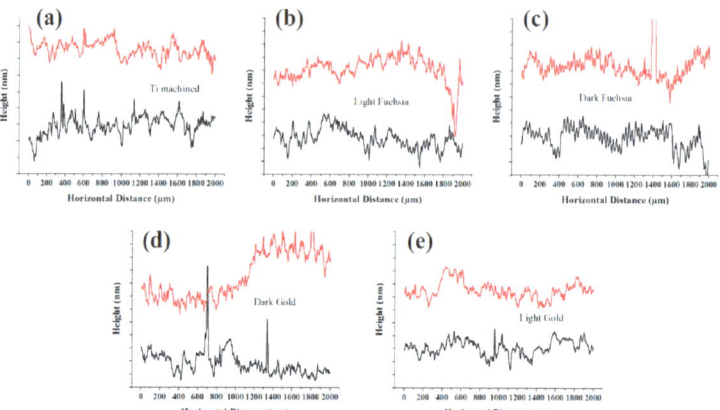

Figure 5. Surface profiles of (**a**) Ti machined, (**b**) light fuchsia, (**c**) dark fuchsia, (**d**) light gold, and (**e**) dark gold discs. Two profiles were reported for any surfaces (red and black lines), where each major vertical tick corresponds to 200 nm.

3.5. Scanning Electron Microscopy (SEM)—Energy-Dispersive X-ray Spectroscopy (EDX)

The electron scanning microscopy better shows the turning finishing of the surface with rip stack defects, as evidenced in Figure 6, where the machined Ti surface (Figure 6a) and the light fuchsia surface (Figure 6b) are reported. The laser treatment is able to produce a "craquelle-like" surface (Figure 6b) due to the fast cooling of the titanium. Since we are interested in highlighting the colored surfaces of relevant interest for clinical practice and not the influence of all colors, we show only the light fuchsia surface, which is the most promising, and the machined one, taken as a control.

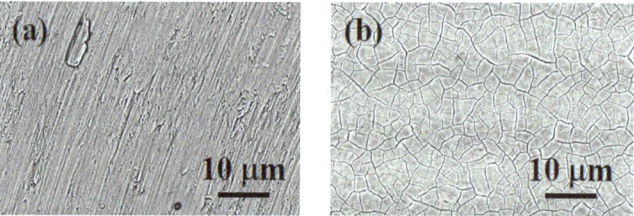

Figure 6. SEM of Ti surfaces: (**a**) machined and (**b**) light fuchsia. Magnification 2000×. Scale bar 10 µm.

Energy-dispersive X-ray spectroscopy (EDX) is an analytical technique used for the elemental analysis or chemical characterization of a sample. Figure 7 shows the EDX spectra of the machined Ti surface and the light fuchsia surface. The laser treatment did not produce impurities as confirmed by the EDX measures reported in Figure 7a (only Ti peaks are evidenced for Ti machined surface), but favors the formation of a surface layer of oxide, as shown in Figure 7b. The titanium surface is oxidized through the diffusion of oxygen into the molten metal and the presence of oxygen was verified by SEM/EDX analysis. Analyzing in detail the peaks of the colored sample in Figure 7b, it is possible to notice the presence of oxygen in the spectrum, represented by a resolved peak at about 0.52 keV. The same peak is absent in the worked Ti sample, as shown in Figure 7a.

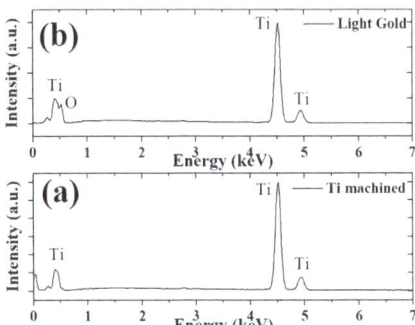

Figure 7. Energy-dispersive X-ray spectroscopy on the surface of (**a**) titanium machined and (**b**) light gold samples.

3.6. Viability Evaluation

HGF viability was measured after 48 h of culture on selected titanium discs by MTT test. A cell viability increase is recorded in Dark Fuchsia, Light Gold, and Dark Gold surfaces compared to the machined sample (control), even if not statistically significant (Figure 8).

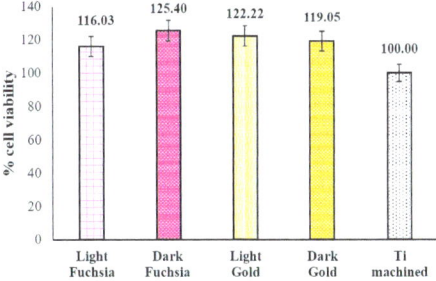

Figure 8. MTT test performed on HGFs cultured for 48 h on titanium surfaces. The most representative of three different experiments is shown. Data are presented as the mean ± standard deviation.

3.7. Cytotoxicity Evaluation

Cytotoxicity evaluation was carried out by means of LDH assay after 48 h of culture on previously selected titanium discs. The light fuchsia, dark fuchsia, light gold, and dark gold samples all show a statistically significant reduction in LDH release compared to the machined sample (Figure 9).

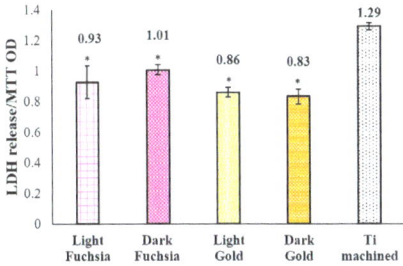

Figure 9. LDH assay of HGFs cultured for 48 h on titanium surfaces. LDH released is reported as OD LDH/OD MTT ratio. Data are presented as the mean ± standard deviation. * vs. CTRL $p < 0.05$.

3.8. Collagen I Release

The release of collagen I within the culture medium was evaluated by means of an ELISA assay after 48 h of culture on previously selected titanium discs. HGFs grown on light fuchsia and dark gold samples show a higher, even if not statistically significant, collagen I release, compared to machined secretion level (Figure 10).

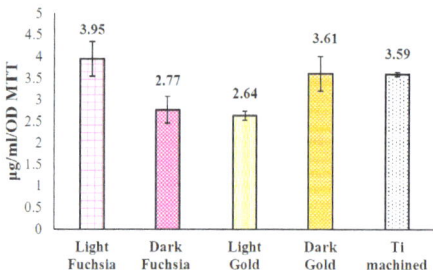

Figure 10. ELISA assay for collagen I secretion in HGFs cultured for 48 h on titanium surfaces. Secretion levels are reported as µg/mL/OD MTT. The bar graph displays densitometric values expressed as mean ± standard deviation.

3.9. Optical (OM) and Electron Microscopy (SEM) of Laser Colored Surfaces Seeded with HGF

Fibroblast adhesion and growth was observed by stereomicroscope and SEM, on the machined (a) and light fuchsia (b) surfaces. Once again, we show only the light fuchsia surface, which is the most promising, and the machined one, taken as a control.

The stereo microscopy shows that fibroblasts colonization starts from the edges of the specimens (Figure 11). This feature is probably due to the thickness of the specimens. The directions and the orienteering of fibroblasts appear more interesting: in all samples, the circular grooves produced by the lathe rough machining at the edge of the diskettes cause cells to move in circular orientations. At the interface with the colored surface, cells start to tilt their aligning incoming to a direction parallelly aligned with the laser scanning process. After 48 h HGFs of culture, the Optical and SEM analyses at lower magnification showed a small number of cells on the titanium machined surface (Figure 12a). At higher magnification, a small number of "stellate" cells showed thin cell-to-cell connections such as several lamellopodia and filopodia that tightly adhere to the machined surface (Figure 12b). At the same time, it was possible to observe the light fuchsia specimens completely colonized by HGFs (Figure 12c). At higher magnification, a higher number of cells adhered to the surface was observed. Furthermore, a tight network of interconnected cells along with only small areas free from HGFs were also detected (Figure 12d).

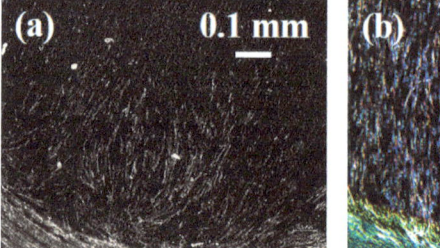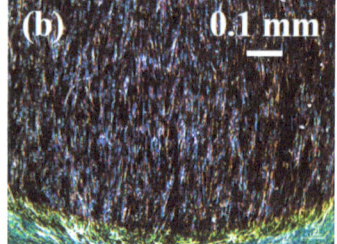

Figure 11. HGF optical images cultured for 48 h on (**a**) Ti machined and (**b**) light fuchsia surfaces by stereomicroscope. Scale bar 0.1 mm.

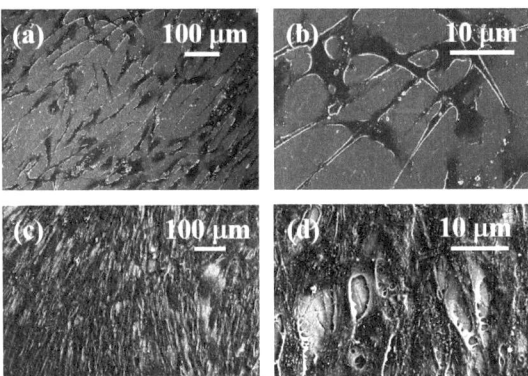

Figure 12. SEM images of HGFs cultured for 48 h on Ti machined surface at 150× (**a**) and 1000× (**b**) magnification, and on light fuchsia surface at 150× (**c**) and 1000× (**d**) magnification.

4. Discussion

Wettability was evaluated by measuring the contact angles of the surfaces with water, and the coloured surfaces showed an increase of contact angle, after laser treatment, with respect to the machined one. All the observed surfaces show a hydrophilic behavior (water contact angle less than 90°), even if it seems that the laser processing decreases the hydrophilic character of the surface itself. It can be noticed that all surfaces have a modest wettability, and wetting is not complete as the measured contact angles are far greater than 0°. Although an increase in the angle was verified, the values obtained are still compatible with those of a modest hydrophilic surface. The order of hydrophilicity of the surfaces is: machined Ti > light fuchsia > dark fuchsia > light gold > dark gold.

By carefully observing the contact angle data, it is possible to divide the series of treated surfaces into two subgroups, which appear to have similar wettability characteristics. The fuchsia surface series is more hydrophilic than the gold ones, but less than the solely machined Ti surface. Since the wetting is the result of surface interactions between a liquid and a solid in contact, it is necessary to measure the surface energies of both liquids and solids to predict wettability. The SFE of a solid surface and its components can provide useful information on how different liquids will interact with the solid surface and is probably the prevailing surface factor influencing cell adhesion strength and proliferation. SFEs with its dispersive and polar components for the Ti surfaces were estimated using the Owens–Wendt–Rabel–Kaelble (OWRK) model [45], by measuring the CA of water (w) and diiodomethane (dim). As observed in Figure 3 and Table 2, the overall SFE of laser-treated Ti surfaces is of the same order of magnitude for all the colored samples, considering the experimental errors, but lower than the machined one.

The small differences between the SFEs are explained by the presence of a different polar component from surface to surface, the dispersive component being almost the same for all laser colored samples. As observed in Figure 3 and Table 2, the overall SFE of laser-treated Ti surfaces is of the same order of magnitude for all the colored samples, considering the experimental errors, but lower than machined one. The polar ratio decreased from 21.5% for the machined Ti surface to 5.7% for the dark gold surface.

The polar component decreased, a trend most evident in the dark gold surface. The laser treatment led to a decrease in the wettability of these surfaces, as the SFE is lowered, and in particular the light gold surface is the one that has less cell adhesion, as demonstrated by collagen I secretion level. Furthermore, in the case of the light fuchsia surface it is possible to observe a much more significant polar contribution compared to the other treated surfaces. It has been previously already reported that cell attachment and spreading are better promoted on surfaces with higher hydrophilic characteristics [48].

Our biological results are in accordance with this assumption and with wettability analyses as they show that HGF adhesion and spreading processes on fuchsia series surfaces appear ameliorated compared to standard machined control. In fact, collagen I secretion and viability percentages, explanatory of adhesion and spreading events, respectively, seem to be enhanced on the aforementioned colored surfaces, which possess, at the same time, the more emphasized hydrophilic/wettable characteristics. Therefore, a positive connection between hydrophilicity of the surface, as well as cell spreading and adhesion, can be established, even if, considering the lack of statistically significant differences among the tested surfaces, further and deepened investigations, including the analysis of a broad panel of adhesion proteins, will be required to confirm this hypothesis. The interfacial energy of a liquid in contact with a solid depends on the dispersive and polar components of the surface energy of the liquid and the solid. From this relationship between the different components, it can be predicted that wettability is generally reduced when the overall surface energy of the solid surface is reduced. For a given liquid with a total surface tension γ_{LV}, the contact angle will be minimized if the polar and dispersive ratios of the liquid surface tension match those of the solid SFE. Plotting the polar component, plotted along the y-axis against the total surface tension along the x-axis (Wetting Envelope, WE), for all the Ti surface can provide a visual investigation of the factors affecting their wettability (Figure 4).

Wetting Envelope plots are particularly useful when studying the effect that the polar and dispersive components of liquid surface tension have on contact angle and wettability. The surface area under the wetting envelope of the machined Ti surface is the largest one. Once again, it is possible to observe a very similar behavior between the two series of colored surfaces, fuchsia and gold, supporting the hypothesis that the wettability is very similar for these two pairs of samples. However, fuchsia surfaces have a larger envelope area than gold surfaces, so they are more wettable. This indicates that the wettability of the latter surfaces is minimal; therefore, the liquid that wets the titanium surface will have a smaller solid–liquid contact area, i.e., less spreading. The polar ratio decreased from 21.5% for the machined Ti surface to 5.7% of the dark gold surface, as reported previously (Table 2). In conclusion, from the contact angle data, the light gold colored surface would appear to be the one in which there is the least spreading of a liquid (such as, for example, a body fluid), therefore the least area of adhesion of the liquid. The light and dark fuchsia surfaces would instead appear to be the ones showing greater wettability. A minor polar component would seem not to assist the adhesion of a liquid to the surface, and this could minimize cell adhesion and proliferation.

However, we must also consider another factor that can influence these phenomena, namely the roughness of the studied surfaces. To highlight the effect of the roughness of these surfaces, measurements were made with a profilometer. In Figure 5, roughness measurements on Ti surfaces are reported. Figure 5a shows the arithmetic mean roughness (Ra) and root mean square roughness (Rq) of the Ti surfaces. The arithmetic mean roughness (Ra) is calculated from the average of the individual heights and depths from the mean elevation of the profile. The root mean square roughness (Rq) is instead calculated from the square root of the sum of the squares of the individual heights and depths. The arithmetic mean roughness values for all surfaces are between 0.15 and 0.3 micron, while the root mean square roughness is between 0.2 and 0.4 micron. The standard deviation values are equal to ± 50 nm for all surfaces. A preliminary analysis of the profiles shows that laser treatment of the titanium surfaces increases the roughness of all observed samples (by about 20–25%), but in the case of the dark gold colored surface, the roughness increase is less pronounced (11%). Several studies have shown that fibroblasts do not attach easily to smooth titanium surfaces and that faster osseointegration has been observed on machined rather than smooth surfaces [21,49,50]. Surface roughness is a factor that can influence not only cell adhesion but also the bacteria adhesion to the titanium surface. Some studies have demonstrated a correlation between the increase in bacterial adhesion, and the consequent formation of biofilm, with surface roughness, and in some cases an arithmetic mean roughness threshold (Ra) of 0.2 μm has been proposed [51,52]. By their nature, bacteria with hydrophobic cell surfaces prefer surfaces of hydrophobic material while those with hydrophilic cell surfaces prefer surfaces of hydrophilic material. Bacterial adhesion increased with higher surface free energies and hydrophobicity of the material. Our laser treated Ti surfaces showed that modest hydrophilicity and biofilm formation should be minimized. Starting from the experimental data, we verified if there could be a correlation between surface parameters and cell viability, cytotoxicity and adhesion. R^2 values of < 0.3 mean a weak effect on the dependent variable, a value between 0.3 and 0.5 means moderate, and a value > 0.7 means strong effect, i.e., correlation. By analysing in detail the roughness data of the different surfaces in relation to the cellular response, it can be seen that there is not a good correlation between the roughness of the samples and the cellular assays with respective R^2 below 0.6.

From what was observed with the profilometer, there are no such substantial variations in the roughness of the samples, and this data is confirmed by the biological response.

A strong correlation between water contact angle and MTT/LDH assay was observed ($R^2 = 0.8433$ for MTT and $R^2 = 0.9585$ for LDH), as reported in Figure 13a. We can assume that a decrease in cell viability/cytotoxicity is observed as the water contact angle of the samples increases, i.e., surfaces become less hydrophilic. No correlation was observed with total SFE or disperse contribution. Only the polar contribution of SFE correlates with MTT/LDH assays ($R^2 = 0.830$ for MTT and $R^2 = 0.897$ for LDH), as reported in Figure 13b. Cell viability and cytotoxicity decrease with decreasing polar contribution, i.e., a decrease in hydrophilicity and adhesion. As revealed by ELISA essay, the surface that shows the best adhesion is the light fuchsia surface. Light fuchsia is also the most hydrophilic (lower water contact angle), the one with higher polar contribute to SFE (polar ratio 10.4%), and the one with higher wettability (higher area under WE). These results confirm the fact that cell adhesion and proliferation cannot be accurately predicted by a single factor, such as roughness, water Contact Angle values (hydrophilicity), Surface Free Energy (spreading), and Wetting Envelope (wettability). Laser irradiation varies the morphology of the titanium surfaces, increasing their roughness and promoting adhesion, cell proliferation, and viability, as it increases the contact area between implant and bone. The effect of the laser is also to allow the formation of a superficial layer of oxide, which favors the wettability of body fluids and consequently the compatibility with blood, which leads to better osseointegration. The laser treatment, therefore, has the multiple function of improving the interaction between bone and implant, but also the possibility of obtaining a colored implant, which blends better with the color of the regrowth dental gum, compared to the gray machined Ti.

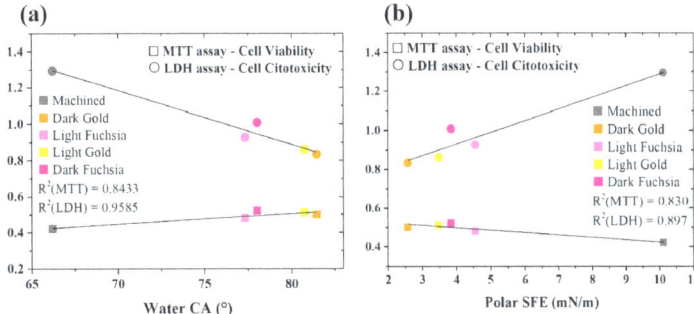

Figure 13. Correlation between (**a**) water CA and (**b**) polar component of SFE of Ti surfaces and cell viability, cytotoxicity, and adhesion.

5. Conclusions

The present study demonstrated that the technique used to obtain the titanium surfaces colored with laser ytterbium has the advantage of having produced, in an ecological way, surfaces that are all biocompatible with HGFs. This was especially confirmed by LDH assay, highlighting that the recorded cytotoxicity on all tested surfaces is reduced compared to the uncolored one (machined). Furthermore, cell viability is very high on all studied surfaces, as confirmed by both MTT test and by SEM analysis, which clearly evidences a dense cell network, despite these surfaces showing a modest hydrophilic behavior, and do therefore not become too wet in contact with an aqueous fluid such as those of the body. The laser treatment has led to a decrease in the wettability of the surfaces, as the SFE is lowered for all the colored surfaces compared to the machined one, but the decrease in wettability did not affect HGF growth. Thanks to the lathe rough machining, fibroblasts start to proliferate in oriented directions at the edge of the disks, aligned parallelly to the laser grooves. Laser treatment of the titanium surfaces increases the roughness of all observed samples, compared to the machined one, amplifying this beneficial effect towards cell growth.

Although all the colored surfaces show excellent biocompatibility and a very high rate of cell viability, light fuchsia appears to be the more promising as it further guarantees, on one hand, a higher collagen I secretion, which could be predictive of an ameliorated cell adhesion, and, on the other hand, a higher hydrophilicity (lower water contact angle), polar contribute to SFE (higher polar ratio), and wettability (higher area under WE).

In addition, from a purely aesthetic point of view, the choice of a fuchsia-colored surface in a dental implant is the most suitable to obtain color integration with the gums.

All in all, the obtained results underline that the best performance was evidenced for the light fuchsia colored Ti surface in terms of biocompatibility, cell viability, and adhesion, but also from an aesthetic point of view.

Therefore, the laser coloring methods adopted can be properly used for aesthetic, colored dental implants with gingival aesthetic features that are highly replicable, contaminant free, eco-friendly, and cheap. Further and extensive in vivo studies will be required to increase the statistical significance of all the data, and to clarify the molecular mechanisms underlying the biological processes, such as cell adhesion, proliferation, and cytotoxicity, on which the authors focused in this paper. However, the present study can help dental clinicians and oral implantologists to evaluate the impact of titanium surface modifications on the color of titanium implants and abutments. The ytterbium laser treatment of the titanium surfaces is biocompatible and allows for the creation of a complete color palette while maintaining the roughness of the titanium surface and it is able to promote the growth of soft tissues in all the evaluated samples with some interesting aesthetic differences without significance statistics.

Author Contributions: Conceptualization, F.M., S.Z.; Methodology, G.F., S.Z., R.Q.; Software, S.Z., C.A., A.C.; Validation, C.A., A.C., R.Q.; Formal Analysis, S.Z., G.F., R.Q.; Investigation, F.M., S.Z., G.F., C.A.; Resources, F.M., S.Z., G.F., R.Q.; Data Curation, C.A., A.C.; Writing—Original Draft Preparation, S.Z., G.F., C.A., R.Q., A.C., F.M.; Writing—Review & Editing, C.A., Visualization, R.Q., C.A.; Supervision, G.F., S.Z., F.M., R.Q.; Project Administration, F.M.; Funding Acquisition, S.Z. All authors have read and agreed to the published version of the manuscript.

Funding: This research was funded by FAR 2020, 2021 Zara. This research was partially founded by the European Union—NextGenerationEU under the Italian Ministry of University and Research (MUR) National Innovation Ecosystem grant ECS00000041—VITALITY (CUP E13C22001060006). This research was partially funded by Abruzzo—European Regional Development Fund Regional Programme (ERDF RP) 2014–2020; POR FESR Abruzzo 2018–2020 "Studio di soluzioni innovative di prodotto e di processo basate sull'utilizzo industriale dei materiali avanzati" (CUP: C17H18000100007).

Institutional Review Board Statement: The study was conducted in accordance with the Declaration of Helsinki, and approved by the Ethics Committee of Local Ethical Committee of the University of Chieti, Italy (protocol number 1173, approved on 31 March 2016).

Informed Consent Statement: Informed consent was obtained from all subjects involved in the study.

Data Availability Statement: No new data were created or analyzed in this study. Data sharing is not applicable to this article.

Conflicts of Interest: The authors declare no conflict of interest.

Sample Availability: Samples of the Titanium discs are available from the authors.

References

1. Salari, N.; Darvishi, N.; Heydari, M.; Bokaee, S.; Darvishi, F.; Mohammadi, M. Global prevalence of cleft palate, cleft lip and cleft palate and lip: A comprehensive systematic review and meta-analysis. *J. Stomatol. Oral. Maxillofac. Surg.* **2022**, *123*, 110–120. [CrossRef] [PubMed]
2. Wu, C.Z.; Yuan, Y.H.; Liu, H.H.; Li, S.S.; Zhang, B.W.; Chen, W.; An, Z.J.; Chen, S.Y.; Wu, Y.Z.; Han, B.; et al. Epidemiologic relationship between periodontitis and type 2 diabetes mellitus. *Bmc Oral. Health* **2020**, *20*, 204. [CrossRef] [PubMed]
3. Matsuyama, Y.; Jurges, H.; Dewey, M.; Listl, S. Causal effect of tooth loss on depression: Evidence from a population-wide natural experiment in the USA. *Epidemiol. Psych. Sci.* **2021**, *30*, e38. [CrossRef] [PubMed]
4. Mojon, P.; Thomason, J.M.; Walls, A.W.G. The impact of falling rates of edentulism. *Int. J. Prosthodont.* **2004**, *17*, 434–440.
5. Peltzer, K.; Hewlett, S.; Yawson, A.E.; Moynihan, P.; Preet, R.; Wu, F.; Guo, G.; Arokiasamy, P.; Snodgrass, J.J.; Chatterji, S.; et al. Prevalence of Loss of All Teeth (Edentulism) and Associated Factors in Older Adults in China, Ghana, India, Mexico, Russia and South Africa. *Int. J. Env. Res. Pub He* **2014**, *11*, 11308–11324. [CrossRef]
6. Duong, H.Y.; Roccuzzo, A.; Stahli, A.; Salvi, G.E.; Lang, N.P.; Sculean, A. Oral health-related quality of life of patients rehabilitated with fixed and removable implant-supported dental prostheses. *Periodontology 2000* **2022**, *88*, 201–237. [CrossRef]
7. Fuentealba, R.; Jofre, J. Esthetic failure in implant dentistry. *Dent. Clin. N. Am.* **2015**, *59*, 227–246. [CrossRef]
8. Mastrangelo, F.; Quaresima, R.; Abundo, R.; Spagnuolo, G.; Marenzi, G. Esthetic and Physical Changes of Innovative Titanium Surface Properties Obtained with Laser Technology. *Materials* **2020**, *13*, 1066. [CrossRef]
9. Albrektsson, T.; Zarb, G.; Worthington, P.; Eriksson, A.R. The long-term efficacy of currently used dental implants: A review and proposed criteria of success. *Int. J. Oral. Maxillofac. Implants* **1986**, *1*, 11–25.
10. Smith, D.E.; Zarb, G.A. Criteria for success of osseointegrated endosseous implants. *J. Prosthet. Dent.* **1989**, *62*, 567–572. [CrossRef]
11. Misch, C.E.; Perel, M.L.; Wang, H.L.; Sammartino, G.; Galindo-Moreno, P.; Trisi, P.; Steigmann, M.; Rebaudi, A.; Palti, A.; Pikos, M.A.; et al. Implant success, survival, and failure: The International Congress of Oral Implantologists (ICOI) Pisa Consensus Conference. *Implant. Dent.* **2008**, *17*, 5–15. [CrossRef]
12. Bas, B.B.; Cakan, U. Evaluation of the effect of anodization-colored titanium abutments and zirconia substructure thickness on zirconia substructure color: An In vitro study. *Niger. J. Clin. Pract.* **2022**, *25*, 2024–2029. [CrossRef]
13. Tete, S.; Mastrangelo, F.; Quaresima, R.; Vinci, R.; Sammartino, G.; Stuppia, L.; Gherlone, E. Influence of novel nano-titanium implant surface on human osteoblast behavior and growth. *Implant. Dent.* **2010**, *19*, 520–531. [CrossRef]
14. Pae, A.; Lee, H.; Kim, H.S.; Kwon, Y.D.; Woo, Y.H. Attachment and growth behaviour of human gingival fibroblasts on titanium and zirconia ceramic surfaces. *Biomed. Mater.* **2009**, *4*, 025005. [CrossRef]
15. Matthes, R.; Jablonowski, L.; Holtfreter, B.; Gerling, T.; von Woedtke, T.; Kocher, T. Fibroblast Growth on Zirconia Ceramic and Titanium Disks After Application with Cold Atmospheric Pressure Plasma Devices or with Antiseptics. *Int. J. Oral. Maxillofac. Implants* **2019**, *34*, 809–818. [CrossRef]
16. Seyidaliyeva, A.; Rues, S.; Evagorou, Z.; Hassel, A.J.; Busch, C.; Rammelsberg, P.; Zenthofer, A. Predictability and outcome of titanium color after different surface modifications and anodic oxidation. *Dent. Mater. J.* **2022**, *41*, 930–936. [CrossRef]
17. Matos, G.R.M. Surface Roughness of Dental Implant and Osseointegration. *J. Maxillofac. Oral. Surg.* **2020**, *20*, 1–4. [CrossRef]
18. Dank, A.; Aartman, I.H.A.; Wismeijer, D.; Tahmaseb, A. Effect of dental implant surface roughness in patients with a history of periodontal disease: A systematic review and meta-analysis. *Int. J. Implant. Dent.* **2019**, *5*, 12. [CrossRef]
19. Mastrangelo, F.; Parma-Benfenati, S.; Quaresima, R. Biologic Bone Behavior During the Osseointegration Process: Histologic, Histomorphometric, and SEM-EDX Evaluations. *Int. J. Periodontics Restorative Dent.* **2023**, *43*, 65–72. [CrossRef]
20. Simoes, I.G.; Reis, A.C.D.; da Costa Valente, M.L. Analysis of the influence of surface treatment by high-power laser irradiation on the surface properties of titanium dental implants: A systematic review. *J. Prosthet. Dent.* **2021**, *129*, 863–870. [CrossRef]
21. Ponsonnet, L.; Reybier, K.; Jaffrezic, N.; Comte, V.; Lagneau, C.; Lissac, M.; Martelet, C. Relationship between surface properties (roughness, wettability) of titanium and titanium alloys and cell behaviour. *Mater. Sci. Eng. C* **2003**, *23*, 551–560. [CrossRef]
22. Chen, J.; Mwenifumbo, S.; Langhammer, C.; McGovern, J.P.; Li, M.; Beye, A.; Soboyejo, W.O. Cell/surface interactions and adhesion on Ti-6Al-4V: Effects of surface texture. *J. Biomed. Mater. Res. B. Appl. Biomater.* **2007**, *82B*, 360–373. [CrossRef] [PubMed]
23. Liu, J.; Alfantazi, A.; Asselin, E. A new method to improve the corrosion resistance of titanium for hydrometallurgical applications. *Appl. Surf. Sci.* **2015**, *332*, 480–487. [CrossRef]
24. Minetti, E.; Giacometti, E.; Gambardella, U.; Contessi, M.; Ballini, A.; Marenzi, G.; Celko, M.; Mastrangelo, F. Alveolar Socket Preservation with Different Autologous Graft Materials: Preliminary Results of a Multicenter Pilot Study in Human. *Materials* **2020**, *13*, 1153. [CrossRef]
25. Diamanti, M.V.; Del Curto, B.; Masconale, V.; Passaro, C.; Pedeferri, M.P. Anodic coloring of titanium and its alloy for jewels production. *Color. Res. Appl.* **2012**, *37*, 384–390. [CrossRef]
26. Wadhwani, C.; Brindis, M.; Kattadiyil, M.T.; O'Brien, R.; Chung, K.-H. Colorizing titanium-6aluminum-4vanadium alloy using electrochemical anodization: Developing a color chart. *J. Prosthet. Dent.* **2018**, *119*, 26–28. [CrossRef]
27. Karambakhsh, A.; Afshar, A.; Ghahramani, S.; Malekinejad, P. Pure Commercial Titanium Color Anodizing and Corrosion Resistance. *J. Mater. Eng. Perform.* **2011**, *20*, 1690–1696. [CrossRef]

28. Al-Nawas, B.; Hangen, U.; Duschner, H.; Krummenauer, F.; Wagner, W. Turned, machined versus double-etched dental implants in vivo. *Clin. Implant. Dent. Relat. Res.* **2007**, *9*, 71–78. [CrossRef]
29. Belser, U.C.; Schmid, B.; Higginbottom, F.; Buser, H. Outcome analysis of implant restorations located in the anterior maxilla: A review of the recent literature. *Int. J. Oral. Max Impl* **2004**, *19*, 30–42.
30. Marenzi, G.; Impero, F.; Scherillo, F.; Sammartino, J.C.; Squillace, A.; Spagnuolo, G. Effect of Different Surface Treatments on Titanium Dental Implant Micro-Morphology. *Materials* **2019**, *12*, 733. [CrossRef]
31. Yu, Z.; Yang, G.; Zhang, W.; Hu, J. Investigating the effect of picosecond laser texturing on microstructure and biofunctionalization of titanium alloy. *J. Mater. Process. Technol.* **2018**, *255*, 129–136. [CrossRef]
32. Rafiee, K.; Naffakh-Moosavy, H.; Tamjid, E. The effect of laser frequency on roughness, microstructure, cell viability and attachment of Ti6Al4V alloy. *Mater. Sci. Eng. C* **2020**, *109*, 110637. [CrossRef]
33. Tsai, M.-H.; Haung, C.-F.; Shyu, S.-S.; Chou, Y.-R.; Lin, M.-H.; Peng, P.-W.; Ou, K.-L.; Yu, C.-H. Surface modification induced phase transformation and structure variation on the rapidly solidified recast layer of titanium. *Mater. Charact.* **2015**, *106*, 463–469. [CrossRef]
34. Lee, B.E.J.; Exir, H.; Weck, A.; Grandfield, K. Characterization and evaluation of femtosecond laser-induced sub-micron periodic structures generated on titanium to improve osseointegration of implants. *Appl. Surf. Sci.* **2018**, *441*, 1034–1042. [CrossRef]
35. Stango, S.A.X.; Karthick, D.; Swaroop, S.; Mudali, U.K.; Vijayalakshmi, U. Development of hydroxyapatite coatings on laser textured 316 LSS and Ti-6Al-4V and its electrochemical behavior in SBF solution for orthopedic applications. *Ceram. Int.* **2018**, *44*, 3149–3160. [CrossRef]
36. Santos, L.C.P.D.; Malheiros, F.C.; Guarato, A.Z. Surface parameters of as-built additive manufactured metal for intraosseous dental implants. *J. Prosthet. Dent.* **2020**, *124*, 217–222. [CrossRef]
37. Rupp, F.; Liang, L.; Geis-Gerstorfer, J.; Scheideler, L.; Hüttig, F. Surface characteristics of dental implants: A review. *Dent. Mater.* **2018**, *34*, 40–57. [CrossRef]
38. Menci, G.; Demir, A.G.; Waugh, D.G.; Lawrence, J.; Previtali, B. Laser surface texturing of β-Ti alloy for orthopaedics: Effect of different wavelengths and pulse durations. *Appl. Surf. Sci.* **2019**, *489*, 175–186. [CrossRef]
39. Jaritngam, P.; Tangwarodomnukun, V.; Qi, H.; Dumkum, C. Surface and subsurface characteristics of laser polished Ti6Al4V titanium alloy. *Opt. Laser Technol.* **2020**, *126*, 106102. [CrossRef]
40. Mastrangelo, F.; Quaresima, R.; Canullo, L.; Scarano, A.; Muzio, L.L.; Piattelli, A. Effects of Novel Laser Dental Implant Microtopography on Human Osteoblast Proliferation and Bone Deposition. *Int. J. Oral. Maxillofac. Implant.* **2020**, *35*, 320–329. [CrossRef]
41. Cunha, A.; Serro, A.P.; Oliveira, V.; Almeida, A.; Vilar, R.; Durrieu, M.-C. Wetting behaviour of femtosecond laser textured Ti–6Al–4V surfaces. *Appl. Surf. Sci.* **2013**, *265*, 688–696. [CrossRef]
42. Ciganovic, J.; Stasic, J.; Gakovic, B.; Momcilovic, M.; Milovanovic, D.; Bokorov, M.; Trtica, M. Surface modification of the titanium implant using TEA CO2 laser pulses in controllable gas atmospheres—Comparative study. *Appl. Surf. Sci.* **2012**, *258*, 2741–2748. [CrossRef]
43. Yoruç, A.B.H.; Keleşoğlu, E.; Yıldız, H.E. In vitro bioactivity of laser surface-treated Ti6Al4V alloy. *Lasers Med. Sci.* **2019**, *34*, 1567–1573. [CrossRef] [PubMed]
44. Allegrini, S.; Yoshimoto, M.; Salles, M.B.; Allegrini, M.R.F.; Pistarini, L.C.Y.; Braga, F.J.C.; Bressiani, A.H.D.A. Evaluation of bone tissue reaction in laser beamed implants. *Appl. Surf. Sci.* **2014**, *307*, 503–512. [CrossRef]
45. Owens, D.K.; Wendt, R.C. Estimation of the surface free energy of polymers. *J. Appl. Polym. Sci.* **1969**, *13*, 1741–1747. [CrossRef]
46. González-Martín, M.L.; Jańczuk, B.; Labajos-Broncano, L.; Bruque, J.M. Determination of the Carbon Black Surface Free Energy Components from the Heat of Immersion Measurements. *Langmuir* **1997**, *13*, 5991–5994. [CrossRef]
47. Ricci, A.; Gallorini, M.; Feghali, N.; Sampo, S.; Cataldi, A.; Zara, S. Snail Slime Extracted by a Cruelty Free Method Preserves Viability and Controls Inflammation Occurrence: A Focus on Fibroblasts. *Molecules* **2023**, *28*, 1222. [CrossRef]
48. Webb, K.; Hlady, V.; Tresco, P.A. Relative importance of surface wettability and charged functional groups on NIH 3T3 fibroblast attachment, spreading, and cytoskeletal organization. *J. Biomed. Mater. Res.* **1998**, *41*, 422–430. [CrossRef]
49. Martinez, M.A.F.; Balderrama, I.F.; Karam, P.; de Oliveira, R.C.; de Oliveira, F.A.; Grandini, C.R.; Vicente, F.B.; Stavropoulos, A.; Zangrando, M.S.R.; Sant'Ana, A.C.P. Surface roughness of titanium disks influences the adhesion, proliferation and differentiation of osteogenic properties derived from human. *Int. J. Implant. Dent.* **2020**, *46*, 6. [CrossRef]
50. Stoilov, M.; Stoilov, L.; Enkling, N.; Stark, H.; Winter, J.; Marder, M.; Kraus, D. Effects of Different Titanium Surface Treatments on Adhesion, Proliferation and Differentiation of Bone Cells: An In Vitro Study. *J. Funct. Biomater.* **2022**, *13*, 143. [CrossRef]
51. Xing, R.; Lyngstadaas, S.P.; Ellingsen, J.E.; Taxt-Lamolle, S.; Haugen, H.J. The influence of surface nanoroughness, texture and chemistry of TiZr implant abutment on oral biofilm accumulation. *Clin. Oral. Implant. Res.* **2015**, *26*, 649–656. [CrossRef]
52. Zheng, S.; Bawazir, M.; Dhall, A.; Kim, H.E.; He, L.; Heo, J.; Hwang, G. Implication of Surface Properties, Bacterial Motility, and Hydrodynamic Conditions on Bacterial Surface Sensing and Their Initial Adhesion. *Front. Bioeng. Biotechnol.* **2021**, *9*, 643722. [CrossRef]

Disclaimer/Publisher's Note: The statements, opinions and data contained in all publications are solely those of the individual author(s) and contributor(s) and not of MDPI and/or the editor(s). MDPI and/or the editor(s) disclaim responsibility for any injury to people or property resulting from any ideas, methods, instructions or products referred to in the content.

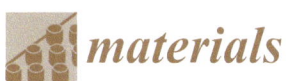

Article

A Comparison of Conical and Cylindrical Implants Inserted in an In Vitro Post-Extraction Model Using Low-Density Polyurethane Foam Blocks

Luca Comuzzi [1,†], Margherita Tumedei [2,3,†], Natalia Di Pietro [4,5,*], Tea Romasco [4,5], Hamid Heydari Sheikh Hossein [4,5,6], Lorenzo Montesani [7], Francesco Inchingolo [8], Adriano Piattelli [9,10] and Ugo Covani [11]

1. Independent Researcher, San Vendemiano-Conegliano, 31020 Treviso, Italy; luca.comuzzi@gmail.com
2. Department of Medical, Surgical, and Dental Sciences, University of Milan, 20122 Milan, Italy; margherita.tumedei@unimi.it
3. Maxillo-Facial Surgery and Dental Unit, Fondazione IRCCS Ca' Granda Ospedale Maggiore Policlinico, 20122 Milan, Italy
4. Department of Medical, Oral and Biotechnological Sciences, "G. D'Annunzio" University of Chieti-Pescara, 66013 Chieti, Italy; tea.romasco@unich.it (T.R.); hamidheydari93@gmail.com (H.H.S.H.)
5. Center for Advanced Studies and Technology-CAST, "G. D'Annunzio" University of Chieti-Pescara, 66013 Chieti, Italy
6. Villa Serena Foundation for Research, Via Leonardo Petruzzi 42, 65013 Città Sant'Angelo, Italy
7. Independent Researcher, 00187 Rome, Italy; lomonte@bu.edu
8. Interdisciplinary Department of Medicine, University of Bari "Aldo Moro", 70121 Bari, Italy; francesco.inchingolo@uniba.it
9. School of Dentistry, Saint Camillus International University of Health and Medical Sciences, 00131 Rome, Italy; apiattelli51@gmail.com
10. Facultad de Medicina, UCAM Universidad Católica San Antonio de Murcia, 30107 Murcia, Spain
11. Department of Stomatology, Tuscan Stomatologic Institute, Foundation for Dental Clinic, Research and Continuing Education, 55041 Camaiore, Italy; covani@covani.it
* Correspondence: natalia.dipietro@unich.it
† These authors contributed equally to this work.

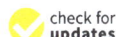

Citation: Comuzzi, L.; Tumedei, M.; Di Pietro, N.; Romasco, T.; Heydari Sheikh Hossein, H.; Montesani, L.; Inchingolo, F.; Piattelli, A.; Covani, U. A Comparison of Conical and Cylindrical Implants Inserted in an In Vitro Post-Extraction Model Using Low-Density Polyurethane Foam Blocks. *Materials* 2023, 16, 5064. https://doi.org/10.3390/ma16145064

Academic Editors: Lavinia Cosmina Ardelean and Laura-Cristina Rusu

Received: 8 June 2023
Revised: 11 July 2023
Accepted: 15 July 2023
Published: 18 July 2023

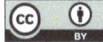

Copyright: © 2023 by the authors. Licensee MDPI, Basel, Switzerland. This article is an open access article distributed under the terms and conditions of the Creative Commons Attribution (CC BY) license (https://creativecommons.org/licenses/by/4.0/).

Abstract: Combining tooth extraction and implant placement reduces the number of surgical procedures that a patient must undergo. Thus, the present study aimed to compare the stability of two types of conical implants (TAC and INTRALOCK) and another cylindrical one (CYROTH), inserted with a range of angulation of 15–20 degrees in low-density polyurethane blocks (10 and 20 pounds per cubic foot, PCF) with or without a cortical lamina (30 PCF), which potentially mimicked the post-extraction in vivo condition. For this purpose, a total of 120 polyurethane sites were prepared (10 for each implant and condition) and the Insertion Torque (IT), Removal Torque (RT), and Resonance Frequency Analysis (RFA) were measured, following a Three-Way analysis of variance followed by Tukey's post hoc test for the statistical analysis of data. The IT and RT values registered for all implant types were directly proportional to the polyurethane density. The highest IT was registered by INTRALOCK implants in the highest-density block (32.44 ± 3.28 Ncm). In contrast, the highest RFA, a well-known index of Implant Stability Quotient (ISQ), was shown by TAC implants in all clinical situations (up to 63 ISQ in the 20 PCF block without the cortical sheet), especially in lower-density blocks. Although more pre-clinical and clinical studies are required, these results show a better primary stability of TAC conical implants in all tested densities of this post-extraction model, with a higher ISQ, despite their IT.

Keywords: artificial bone; conical implants; cylindrical implants; dental implants; implant stability quotient; insertion torque; polyurethane; post-extraction sites; removal torque

1. Introduction

Nowadays, advances in clinical techniques and biomaterials have facilitated the broadening of indications for immediate implant treatment [1,2]. Over the years, different types of implants and their positioning and loading protocols have evolved from the first protocols with the aim to obtain faster and easier surgical treatment times [3]. The immediate placement of dental implants in extraction sockets was described for the first time by Schulte and Heimke more than 40 years ago [4]. Since then, and as recently reported, preclinical, clinical, and radiological studies have allowed significant advances in understanding hard and soft tissue alterations in post-extraction sites [5]. Furthermore, it has been reported that the immediate dental implant loading procedure provides substantial advantages for the patient [6]. Thus, the immediate implant placement and provisionalization in post-extractive sockets have been proposed. As an example, Mura and collaborators [6], in a retrospective 5—year analysis of immediately loaded tapered implants placed in post-extraction sockets, have shown promising results concerning implant survival, soft tissue response, and peri-implant marginal bone conditions. Moreover, Han et al. [7] performed a comparison between survival, stability, and possible complications of immediately loaded tapered implants placed either in post-extraction or in healed sockets, and complications and failures were not reported to be significantly different between these two groups.

On the other hand, Mello et al. [8] conducted a systematic review with meta-analysis on the implant survival and possible peri-implant tissue modifications. Comparing immediate implant insertion in fresh extraction sockets and implant positioning in healed sites, they found that delayed implants reported a significantly higher survival in respect to immediate implants. In contrast, no differences were reported between the two groups as regards the marginal bone loss, the Implant Stability Quotient (ISQ) values, and the pocket probing depth. Similar results were reported in a recent systematic review [9] that compared post-extraction alveolar ridge preservation and the immediate implant insertion. Other authors, instead, asserted that an immediate implant insertion placement could be considered in post-extraction sites, since a limited amount of bone resorption was described [10]. However, other techniques, such as socket preservation using biomaterials and/or membranes, may be preferred when these conditions are not present [11].

Nowadays, polyurethane foam sheets have been used as a valuable substitute material for human bone in order to perform mechanical testing on instruments and orthopedic devices, as reported by the American Society for Testing and Materials [12], which recognized this material as a standard for in vitro tests. Recently, several authors started to use this artificial bone for mechanical testing on oral instruments and dental implants, especially for assessing implant primary stability [13,14]. Indeed, given the difficulties of working with human cadaver bones and animal bones, synthetic polyurethane foam has been widely used as alternative material in several biomechanical tests, as this material exhibits a similar cellular structure and consistent biomechanical characteristics [12,15–18]. In particular, a summary of the mechanical properties concerning the polyurethane foams used in this study (density, compression, and shear) and the corresponding ASTM F-1839-08 specifications have been reported in a previous study of this group [19]. Low- to high-density polyurethane foams are representative of different natural bone densities, according to the D1—D4 bone tissue classification proposed by Misch [20], since the ease and non-invasive nature of this model make it particularly valuable for predicting and evaluating the primary stability and osseointegration of implants in respect to other models, such as ex vivo or in vivo ones [21–23].

Specifically, in 2015, Kashi et al. [24] led an in vitro study with the aim to evaluate the primary stability of titanium implants inserted with different angle degrees in polyurethane foam sheets. For this purpose, polyurethane foam sheets mimicking artificial bone types II and IV, as well as angulations of 0, 10, and 20 degrees were used in this study, finding that implants placed with 10 degrees of angulation in a type II artificial bone showed a better primary stability. It should also be considered that, when using an in vitro polyurethane model also mimicking an extraction site, the implant design could have a pivotal role in achieving an adequate primary stability in challenging situations [25]. Moreover, Yim et al. [26], in a bovine bone in vitro study, reported that in peri-implant bone defects varying from 2 to 8 mm, decreased ISQ values and increased Periotest values were observed with the increase in the defect width.

Thus, the aim of the present study was to compare the stability of two types of conical implants (TAC and INTRALOCK) and a cylindrical one (CYROTH) when inserted with an angulation of 15–20 degrees in 10 and 20 Pounds per Cubic Foot (PCF) low-density polyurethane blocks with or without the presence of a cortical lamina (30 PCF in density), potentially mimicking the in vivo post-extraction condition. From this, the null hypothesis of the study would be the absence of differences in terms of Insertion Torque (IT), Removal Torque (RT), and Reference Frequency Analysis (RFA) values among conical and cylindrical implant macro-morphologies in order to guarantee a better implant behavior and primary stability in simulated extraction sites on polyurethane bone blocks.

2. Materials and Methods

2.1. Implant Description

Three types of implants were used for testing each experimental condition:

- TAC conical implants (Aon Implants, Grisignano di Zocco, Italy);
- INTRALOCK conical implants (Intra-Lock System Europa Spa, Salerno, Italy);
- CYROTH cylindrical implants (Aon Implants, Grisignano di Zocco, Italy).

All implants had the same dimensions (4×15 mm).

TAC implant macromorphology showed a more tapered and less aggressive collar shape, whereas threads were sharper and more aggressive. They presented a single-threaded design and there was a flat implant apex.

INTRALOCK implants had a more pronounced conical shape and the enlargement of the profile was 2 mm wider on the most coronal portion. The threads presented a triple pitch of the coil and there was a round apex.

CYROTH cylindrical implants had a slightly tapered collar with less aggressive threads, which tended to compress and deform the material rather than cutting it. They also presented a conical apex (Figure 1).

2.2. Drilling Protocol and Implant Insertion

The drilling protocol was performed by using an initial lanceolate bur at 300 rpm for all implants, followed by a 2.2 mm bur (AUN22300DR000, Aon Implants, Grisignano di Zocco, Italy) for TAC and CYROTH implants and a 2.0 mm bur (D-2015, Intra-Lock System Europa Spa, Salerno, Italy) for INTRALOCK implants, both used at 300 rpm. In order to finalize protocols, TAC and CYROTH implants were drilled with a 3.2 mm bur (AUN32000DR000, Aon Implants, Grisignano di Zocco, Italy), whereas INTRALOCK implants were drilled with a 4 mm conical bur (D-CT4D, Intra-Lock System Europa Spa, Salerno, Italy), both at 300 rpm. For this purpose, a Bien Air Chiropro (Bien Air SA, Bienne, Switzerland) surgical implant motor was used. The final implant insertion was performed at 30 rpm with a calibrated torque with a maximum range value of 50 Ncm and an inclination of 15–20 degrees; then, the Insertion Torque (IT) and the Removal Torque (RT) were evaluated in the last 1 mm during the implant seating, considered at 2 mm below the polyurethane block superficial profile. The n° 78 Smart Peg (Osstell AB, Gothenburg, Sweden) was used to evaluate the Resonance Frequency Analysis (RFA) values in the Bucco–Lingual (RFA-BL) and Mesial–Distal (RFA-MD) orientations (Figures 2 and 3).

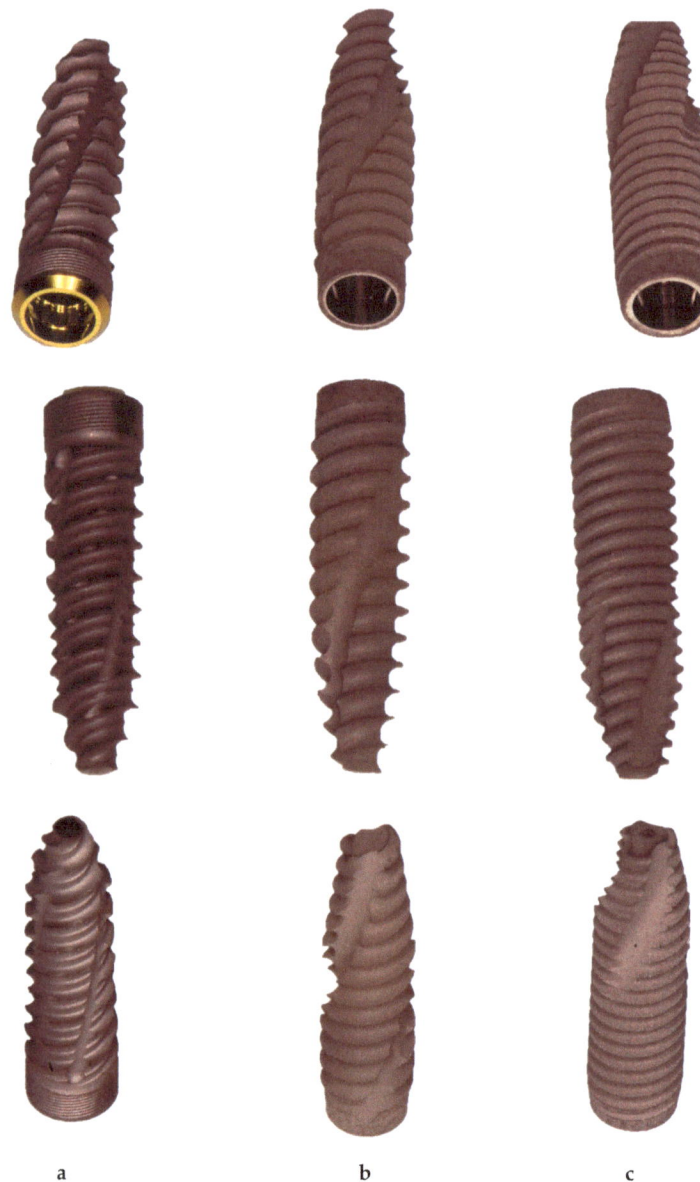

Figure 1. Representative images of the implants used in the present study: (**a**) INTRALOCK, (**b**) TAC, and (**c**) CYROTH implants from the bottom (first line), lateral (second line), and top (third line) views.

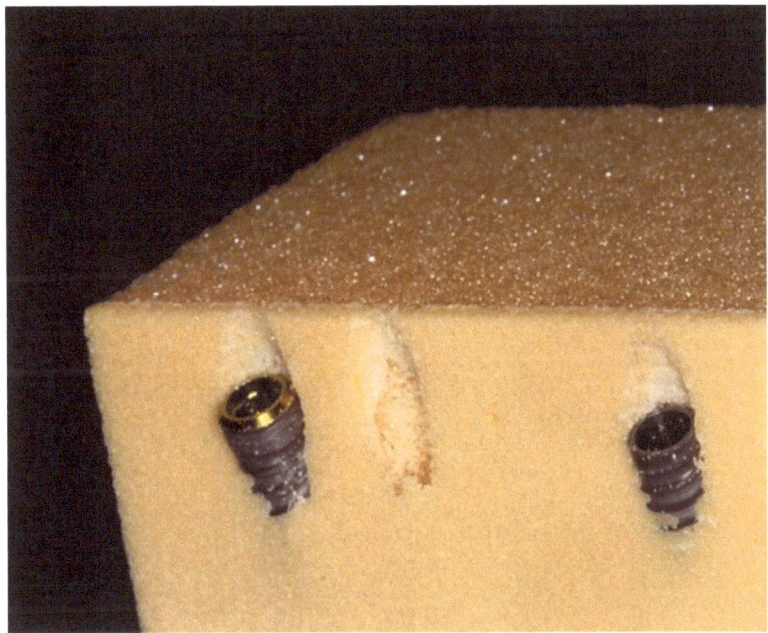

Figure 2. An example of the insertion of INTRALOCK (on the left) and TAC (on the right) implants up to 2 mm below the polyurethane profile and at 15–20 degrees of inclination.

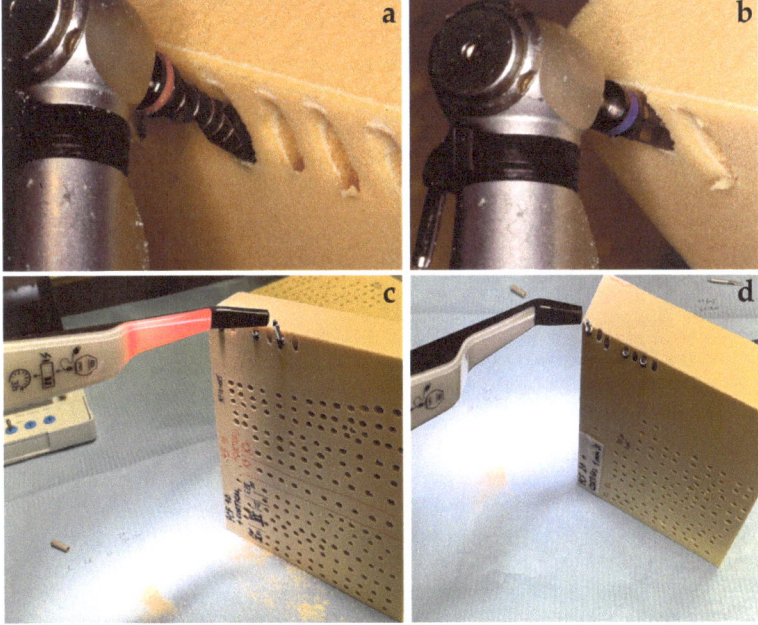

Figure 3. Representative images of the implant site preparation, implant insertion, and measurements: (**a**) Implant site preparation with 15–20 degrees of inclination; (**b**) Implant insertion; (**c**,**d**) Resonance Frequency Analysis (RFA) measurements.

The protocol described above was conducted in order to mimic an immediate post-tooth extraction condition with implant placement in an aesthetic zone. In particular, this aimed to represent the implant positioning in fresh sites, where the residual non-healed alveolar bone usually requires drilling through the palatal wall of the inclined socket.

As regards polyurethane foam blocks, they are constituted by a well-known material used to mimic the natural bone, since it has pronounced mechanical characteristics, avoiding human variables or particular handling and preservation treatments whilst preserving similar bone properties [12,13,27]. Nowadays, it is also preferred to cadaver or animal bones for ethical reasons, and it is used as an alternative material to perform biomechanical tests regarding orthopedic or dental medical devices [14,28].

In this study 4-mm thick blocks with densities of 10 and 20 PCF (Sawbones Europe AB, Malmö, Sweden) were used, corresponding to a density of 0.16 g/cm^3 and 0.32 g/cm^3, mimicking D3 and D2 natural bone types, respectively. In addition, a 1-mm thick sheet with a density of 30 PCF (corresponding to a density of 0.48 g/cm^3, similar to the D1 bone type) was added to the previous blocks when used to mimic the cortical bone [19] (Figure 4).

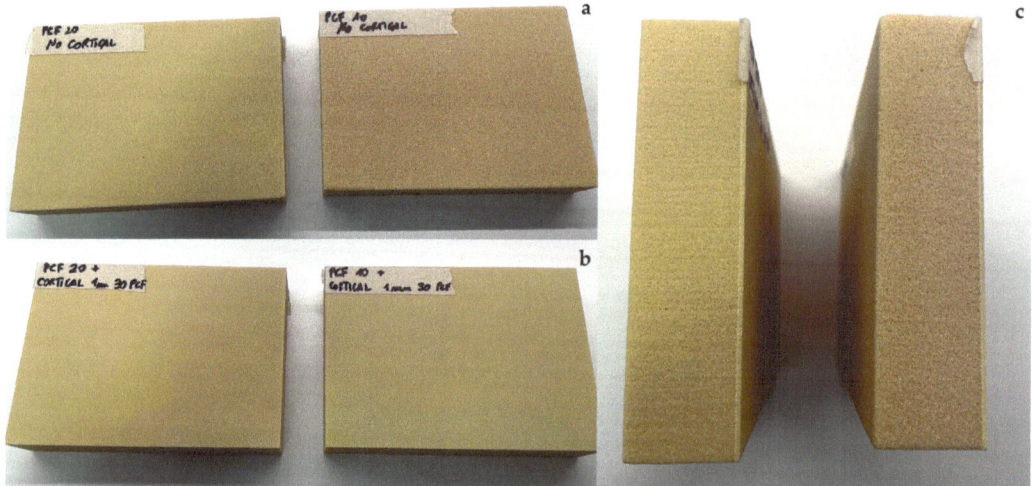

Figure 4. Representative images of the different blocks used: (**a**,**b**) polyurethane blocks of 20 and 10 Pounds per Cubic Foot (PCF) in density without and with the cortical sheets; (**c**) a detail of 20 and 10 PCF polyurethane blocks and the cortical sheets.

2.3. Study Design

To better clarify the dependent and independent variables analyzed in the present work, the different implant types, the different polyurethane densities, and the presence of a lamina could be identified as independent variables, whereas measurements of IT and RT have to be considered as dependent variables. In particular, the assessment of IT and RFA constitutes a non-destructive method to provide information on implant primary stability and survival [13,29], as the RT indirectly defines as well, representing a positive correlation with the degree of bone-to-impact contact (BIC) [23].

Thus, in Figure 5, the study design has been resumed: 10 implant sites were prepared for each implant type in all polyurethane densities, obtaining a total of 120 osteotomies.

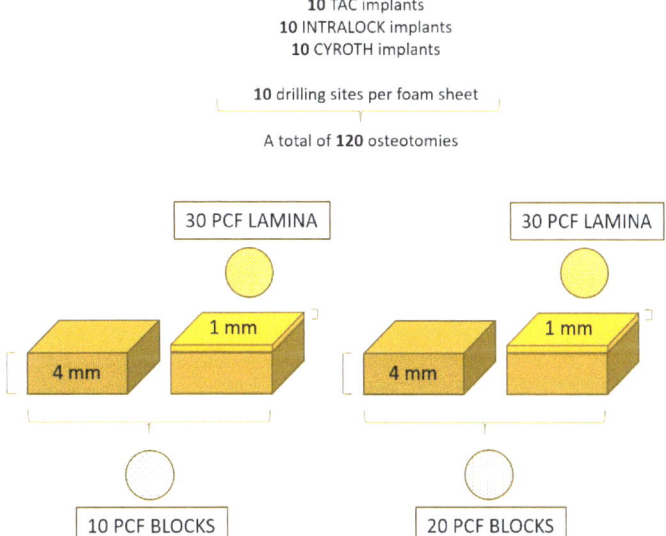

Figure 5. Schematic illustration of the osteotomies performed and the study design.

2.4. Statistical Analysis

Power analysis and sample size planning were calculated using the ANOVA: fixed effects, special, main effects, and interactions statistical test. If we consider 4 conditions and 3 testing groups, the following chart turns out: effect size: 0.4, α err: 0.05; power $(1-\beta)$: 0.9; numerator df: 6; number of groups: 12, using the G*Power 3.1.9.4 program to define it. The result of the minimum sample size necessary to achieve a statistically significant output was 116 implant sites and a total of 120 sites were performed in this study. The Shapiro–Wilk test was applied to evaluate the normal distribution of data. Subsequently, the differences among IT, RT, and RFA values expressed by the study groups were evaluated using a Three-Way analysis of variance (ANOVA) test, followed by Tukey's post hoc test. A p-value < 0.05 was considered statistically significant. The research data and the statistical analysis were elaborated using the statistical software package GraphPad 9.0 (Prism, San Diego, CA, USA). Data were expressed as the mean ± Standard Deviation (SD).

3. Results

The experimental results related to the IT, RT, RFA-BL, and RFA-MD values evaluation and comparison are reported in Table 1. These values were obtained from independent measurements related to different implants inserted in each artificial bone condition.

Table 1. Statistic values of the Insertion Torque (IT), Removal Torque (RT), and Resonance Frequency Analysis in the Bucco–Lingual (RFA-BL) and Mesial–Distal (RFA-MD) orientations related to the different experimental conditions tested for each type of implant (TAC, INTRALOCK, and CYROTH). SD: Standard Deviation.

IT		10 PCF						20 PCF					
		No Cortical			Cortical			No Cortical			Cortical		
	TAC	INTRALOCK	CYROTH	TAC	INTRALOCK	CYROTH	TAC	INTRALOCK	CYROTH	TAC	INTRALOCK	CYROTH
Min	5.90	6.90	6.50	14.70	15.70	16.60	24.50	22.50	24.50	23.50	28.40	25.50
Max	6.90	7.80	6.90	15.70	16.70	17.60	25.50	24.50	27.40	25.50	37.20	28.40
Mean	6.39	7.44	6.73	15.16	16.23	17.06	24.93	23.83	26.42	24.63	32.44	26.87
SD (±)	0.41	0.34	0.16	0.30	0.36	0.30	0.34	0.59	0.96	0.72	3.28	1.04

RT		10 PCF						20 PCF					
		No Cortical			Cortical			No Cortical			Cortical		
	TAC	INTRALOCK	CYROTH	TAC	INTRALOCK	CYROTH	TAC	INTRALOCK	CYROTH	TAC	INTRALOCK	CYROTH
Min	4.70	4.90	4.80	12.70	10.00	12.00	16.60	16.90	18.60	20.50	21.50	19.70
Max	4.90	4.90	5.10	13.70	11.00	13.00	18.60	18.60	21.50	22.50	23.50	22.50
Mean	4.81	4.90	4.95	13.20	10.72	12.40	17.70	17.94	20.33	21.60	22.41	21.15
SD (±)	0.10	0.00	0.08	0.31	0.36	0.34	0.63	0.57	0.98	0.75	0.72	1.14

RFA—BL		10 PCF						20 PCF					
		No Cortical			Cortical			No Cortical			Cortical		
	TAC	INTRALOCK	CYROTH	TAC	INTRALOCK	CYROTH	TAC	INTRALOCK	CYROTH	TAC	INTRALOCK	CYROTH
Min	50.00	35.00	44.00	60.00	55.00	56.00	62.00	53.00	61.00	61.00	52.00	62.00
Max	52.00	38.00	46.00	61.00	56.00	57.00	63.00	55.00	63.00	62.00	55.00	64.00
Mean	51.00	36.80	45.40	60.20	55.50	56.40	62.30	54.20	62.20	61.50	53.30	62.60
SD (±)	0.82	1.23	0.70	0.42	0.53	0.52	0.48	0.92	0.63	0.53	0.95	0.84

RFA—MD		10 PCF						20 PCF					
		No Cortical			Cortical			No Cortical			Cortical		
	TAC	INTRALOCK	CYROTH	TAC	INTRALOCK	CYROTH	TAC	INTRALOCK	CYROTH	TAC	INTRALOCK	CYROTH
Min	50.00	35.00	44.00	60.00	55.00	56.00	62.00	53.00	61.00	61.00	52.00	62.00
Max	52.00	38.00	46.00	61.00	57.00	57.00	63.00	55.00	63.00	62.00	58.00	64.00
Mean	51.20	37.00	45.30	60.40	56.00	56.50	62.20	54.40	62.10	61.50	54.30	62.90
SD (±)	0.92	1.25	0.82	0.52	0.82	0.53	0.42	0.70	0.74	0.53	2.21	0.74

3.1. Insertion Torque Evaluation

IT values appeared to be directly proportional to the polyurethane density, showing lower values in the lowest-density block, of 10 PCF in density, without the cortical sheet for all implant types, with a mean ± SD of 6.39 ± 0.41, 7.44 ± 0.34, and 6.73 ± 0.16 Ncm for TAC, INTRALOCK, and CYROTH implants, respectively. Specifically, TAC implants showed the lowest IT value (5.90 Ncm), but without statistically significant differences in respect to the other implants in the lowest-density condition. On the other hand, higher values were found in the block of 10 PCF density with the cortical sheet (with a mean ± SD of 15.16 ± 0.30 Ncm for TAC, 16.23 ± 0.36 Ncm for INTRALOCK, and 17.06 ± 0.30 Ncm for CYROTH implants) not reporting significant differences among groups, in the block of 20 PCF density without the cortical sheet (with a mean ± SD of 24.93 ± 0.34 Ncm for TAC, 23.83 ± 0.59 Ncm for INTRALOCK, and 26.42 ± 0.96 Ncm for CYROTH implants), reporting significant differences only between INTRALOCK and CYROTH ($p < 0.0001$), as well as in the block of 20 PCF density with the cortical sheet (with a mean ± SD of 24.63 ± 0.72 Ncm for TAC, 32.44 ± 3.28 Ncm for INTRALOCK, and 26.87 ± 1.04 Ncm for CYROTH implants). In particular, in this latter condition, INTRALOCK implants showed the highest IT value (37.20 Ncm), exhibiting significant differences in respect to the other implants ($p < 0.0001$).

Figure 6 reports all the statistically significant and non-significant differences concerning IT measurements expressed by the implant types in the different experimental artificial bone densities.

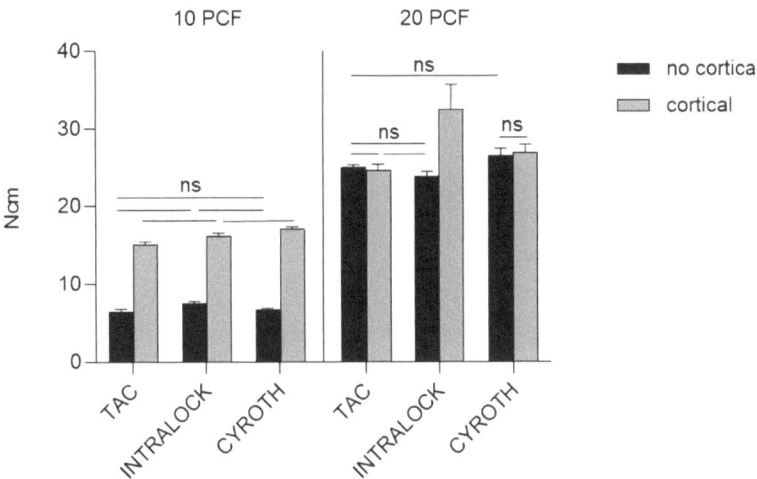

Figure 6. Bar graphs related to the distribution of Insertion Torque (IT) values expressed by each implant type in the different artificial bone conditions. Data were expressed as means ± Standard Deviation (SD). Non-significant differences were reported as "ns", whereas the other comparisons were considered significant with a $p < 0.05$.

Statistically significant higher values ($p < 0.01$) were found for CYROTH implants when inserted in the block of 10 PCF density with the cortical sheet and in the blocks of 20 PCF density without the cortical sheet ($p < 0.0001$) compared to TAC and INTRALOCK implants, respectively, as well as for those inserted in the block of 20 PCF density with the cortical sheet when compared to TAC implants ($p < 0.001$). As previously stated, INTRALOCK implants showed a statistical significance ($p < 0.0001$) only when inserted in the highest-density block, conversely reporting comparable results to the other implants in the blocks of 10 PCF density with and without the cortical sheet. Comparing blocks with the same density, added or not with the cortical sheet, statistical significances were found for all the implant types except for TAC and CYROTH in the block of 20 PCF in density. Similarly, each implant type inserted in the 20 PCF density blocks, with or without the cortical sheet, reported statistically significant higher values if compared with the corresponding one inserted in the 10 PCF blocks, added or not with the cortical sheet.

Overall, TAC implants resulted in slightly lower IT values in all the experimental conditions, except for the blocks of 10 and 20 PCF densities with the cortical sheet. However, they exhibited good IT values in all situations (14.7–25.5 Ncm) that were compatible with the mechanical implant stability, except for the block of 10 PCF density without the cortical sheet but showing no statistical differences with other implants' values.

3.2. Removal Torque Evaluation

RT values were proportional to the polyurethane density as well, showing the highest values in the block of 20 PCF with the cortical sheet (with a mean ± SD of 21.60 ± 0.75 Ncm for TAC, 22.41 ± 0.72 Ncm for INTRALOCK, and 21.15 ± 1.14 Ncm for CYROTH implants) and the lowest ones in the block of 10 PCF density without the cortical sheet (with a mean ± SD of 4.81 ± 0.10 Ncm for TAC, 4.90 ± 0.00 Ncm for INTRALOCK, and 4.95 ± 0.08 Ncm for CYROTH implants). TAC implants showed the lowest RT values in the latest mentioned block (4.70 Ncm), whereas the highest results were reported by INTRALOCK implants in the thickest block of 20 PCF density with the cortical sheet (23.50 Ncm).

Figure 7 shows that the RT values of all implant types inserted in the block of 10 PCF density without the cortical sheet were very low (about 5.00 Ncm), without reaching a statistical significance among groups.

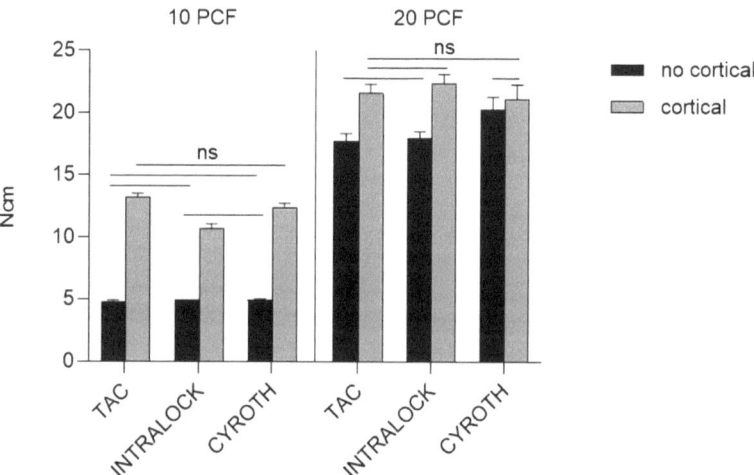

Figure 7. Bar graphs related to the distribution of Removal Torque (RT) values expressed by all the implant types in different artificial bone conditions. Data are expressed as means ± SD. Non-significant differences were reported as "ns", whereas the other comparisons were considered significant with a $p < 0.05$.

INTRALOCK and TAC implants reported comparable values in all experimental conditions, except for the 10 PCF density block with the cortical sheet, where both TAC and CYROTH implants showed significantly higher results ($p < 0.0001$). CYROTH implants also showed significantly higher RT values in respect to both other implants in the block of 20 PCF density without the cortical sheet ($p < 0.0001$). On the other hand, INTRALOCK implants reported the highest results in the block of 20 PCF density with the cortical sheet but showing a statistical significance only when compared to CYROTH implants ($p < 0.001$). In addition, for each implant type, the RT values registered in the 20 PCF blocks with and without the cortical sheet were significantly higher than those registered by the same implant in the 10 PCF blocks, and if considering each implant inserted in the same-density blocks but with or without the cortical sheet, the RT values showed by the block with the cortical always reported significantly higher results, except for CYROTH implants in the 20 PCF blocks.

For all implants, the RT was always lower than the corresponding IT. Higher differences between IT and RT values were found for INTRALOCK implants (more than 10 Ncm in the 20 PCF density block with the cortical sheet) compared with TAC and CYROTH implants (4–6 Ncm lower). In the lowest-density block there were lower differences between IT and RT values.

3.3. Resonance Frequency Analysis Evaluation

RFA values, instead, were consistently higher for conical TAC implants in all the experimental conditions, especially in the lowest-density blocks (for example, with a mean ± SD of 51.20 ± 0.92 ISQ in the 10 PCF density block without the cortical sheet and 60.40 ± 0.52 ISQ in the 10 PCF density block with the cortical sheet, compared to 37.00 ± 1.25 and 56.00 ± 0.82 ISQ of INTRALOCK, and 45.30 ± 0.82 and 56.50 ± 0.53 ISQ of CYROTH implants in the same conditions), always reaching statistical significance ($p < 0.0001$). Only the 20 PCF density blocks, with and without the cortical sheet ISQ values, were similar for conical TAC (61.50 ± 0.53 and 62.20 ± 0.42 ISQ, respectively) and cylindrical CYROTH implants (62.90 ± 0.74 and 62.10 ± 0.74 ISQ, respectively); both were significantly higher than those of INTRALOCK implants (Figure 8).

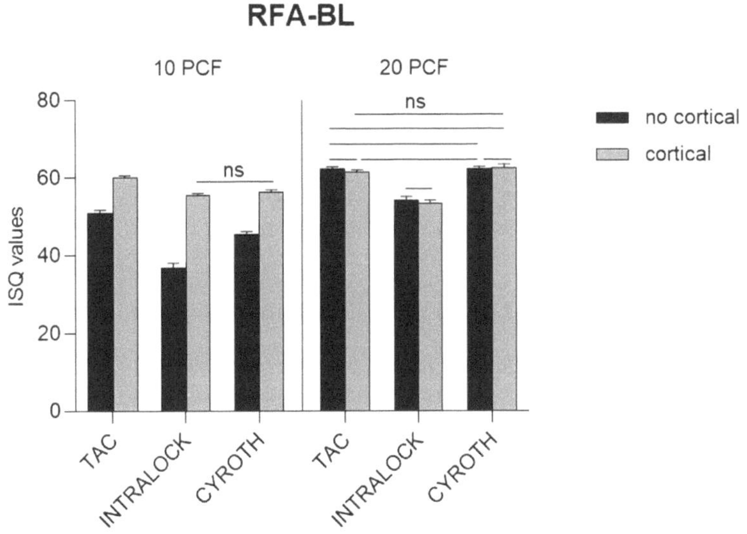

Figure 8. Cont.

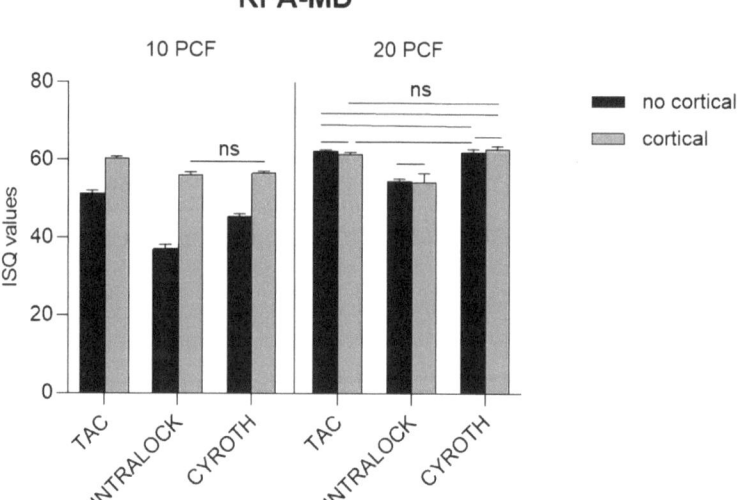

Figure 8. Bar graphs related to the distribution of RFA values in the Bucco–Lingual (BL, in the first line) and Mesial–Distal (MD, in the second line) orientations expressed by each implant type in the different artificial bone conditions. Data are expressed as means ± SD. Non-significant differences were reported as "ns", whereas the other comparisons were considered significant with a $p < 0.05$.

Related to the 10 PCF block without the cortical sheet, INTRALOCK implants exhibited significantly lower ISQ values compared to CYROTH implants ($p < 0.0001$); this was different from the same implants in the 20 PCF block with the cortical sheet. In addition, TAC implants also reported statistically significant higher values in the latest mentioned condition.

Overall, only between the lowest-density blocks (10 PCF with and without the cortical sheet) did all implants show a statistical significance ($p < 0.0001$).

4. Discussion

In light of what the above results, the null hypothesis of the study (which considered the absence of differences in terms of IT, RT, and RFA values expressed by these conical and cylindrical implants in order to guarantee a better primary stability in the simulated extraction sites of the tested polyurethane foams) could be considered rejected.

In detail, primary stability is considered as the crucial factor to reach implant success and it was demonstrated to be mostly affected by implant macro-geometry and IT [30,31]. In particular, reaching an ideal primary stability in the posterior maxilla, corresponding to a D3 bone, represents a key factor for an immediate implant loading protocol, due to the low density of the bone [32]. Thus, in this in vitro study, the effects of different dental implant macro-morphologies on the IT, RT, and RFA, that directly or indirectly represented the implant primary stability, has been evaluated after their insertion in polyurethane foam blocks with different densities and simulating poor natural bone and post-extraction sites.

In the past, other authors [33] proposed the use of a tapered implant shape in order to improve the primary stability in a low-quality bone, since this macro-geometry was able to increase the pressure on the cortical bone in poor-bone regions. This fact could be relevant when implants are immediately or early loaded in poor-quality bone districts.

In this study, TAC implants are characterized by a more tapered shape and a less aggressive coronal portion compared to the other implants used. As a result, the implant insertion proceeded easily and progressively increased the IT until the final position, without undergoing deviations and preserving the surface profile of the material. Compared to INTRALOCK and CYROTH implants, there was a reduction in IT values that, however, allowed a more precise implant positioning without affecting the prepared site or excessively stressing the internal portion of the Cone–Morse connection. Interestingly, the registered ISQ values were the highest in all situations, even in low-density blocks (51.20 ± 0.92, 60.40 ± 0.52, 62.30 ± 0.48, and 61.50 ± 0.53 ISQ for 10 and 20 PCF density blocks without and with the cortical sheet, respectively), more likely due to the precise fitting of the implant during the insertion process, without being subjected to deviations. Regarding the implant threads and their difference from the INTRALOCK profile and apex, these implants had a more cutting and aggressive thread profile. This enabled them to penetrate the polyurethane material even without the use of a drilling protocol. This behavior could be especially useful in post-extraction conditions since it could help to direct the implant insertion and its adjustment when necessary, without the affection of the coronal portion.

On the other hand, the INTRALOCK macro-geometry is more conical than that of TAC implants and it has a profile that is 2 mm wider in the most coronal portion. This latter characteristic could be probably responsible for the higher IT values in the 20 PCF density block with the cortical sheet. In fact, the torque value increases when this part of the implant engages the polyurethane, even if it may cause a slight deviation of the implant during the insertion towards the extraction defect. This phenomenon is frequently seen when, inserting a post-extraction implant in the maxilla of a patient, the implant used has a wider profile in its coronal portion and meets a higher density in the palatal bone [34]. This fact could also contribute to decreasing the ISQ values, because the implant does not exactly fit into the prepared site, but undergoes a slight deviation, in part losing contact with the polyurethane. This phenomenon becomes more evident in lower-density blocks (36.80 ± 1.23 ISQ in the 10 PCF block without the cortical sheet).

CYROTH cylindrical implants, instead, presented a tapered coronal portion and a slight conicity when moving towards the apex, as well as less aggressive threads that tended to compress and deform the material rather than cutting it. This morphology resulted in good IT values, except for the lowest-density block (6.73 ± 0.16 Ncm), but produced a slight deviation toward the defect, as for INTRALOCK implants. This fact, together with the macro-geometry, could determine a significant decrease in ISQ values in respect to TAC implants, especially in 10 PCF density blocks (45.30 ± 0.82 and 56.50 ± 0.53 ISQ in blocks without and with the addition of the cortical sheet), but never lower than INTRALOCK implants, and they did not report statistical significance when inserted into the 10 PCF block with the cortical sheet.

As described in the literature [35], a high IT does not always correspond to a high ISQ, but high RFA values may be more desirable than a high IT for an immediate loading protocol to guarantee a better bone-to-implant contact. In this context, analyzing data reported in this study for post-extraction conditions, it was possible to assess that all implants presented IT values > 15 Ncm in all polyurethane densities, except for the 10 PCF block without the cortical sheet, with the highest values for INTRALOCK implants (32.44 ± 3.28 Ncm in the 20 PCF block with the cortical sheet) but considering a possible loss of direction during implant insertion. Contrarily, they always showed the lowest ISQ values in all situations (from 36.80 ± 1.23 to a maximum of 56.00 ± 0.82 ISQ in 10 PCF blocks without and with the cortical sheet, respectively) when compared to CYROTH and TAC implants. Specifically, these latter also showed higher ISQ values than CYROTH, especially when reaching significance in the lowest-density bones (51.20 ± 0.92 in comparison with 45.30 ± 0.82 ISQ and 60.40 ± 0.52 compared to 56.50 ± 0.53 in 10 PCF blocks without and with the addition of the cortical sheet, respectively). Thanks to their thread profile and apex shape, besides the conical macro-morphology, TAC implants may be considered as the best-performing implants for immediate loading simulation in post-extraction sites in all the artificial bone densities tested, as also corroborated by previous studies [36]. Probably, when using TAC implants in low-density bones, a higher value of under-preparation (from 3.2 mm to 2.2 mm) may also help to reach a higher IT value, which in combination with their high ISQ values makes these implants also appropriate for immediate loading in low-density bones [19].

In summary, it becomes necessary to shed light on the due limitations of this in vitro study that, albeit presenting comfortable data and a standardized artificial bone model [12], could obviously never be comparable to an ex vivo or clinical study. Even if the use of a polyurethane material could offer preliminary information on the biomechanical behavior of dental implants in different bone consistencies [14], further experimental and clinical studies are needed to corroborate these results on implant stability. The analyzed parameters could be affected by a patient's physiological or pathological conditions and by other variables concerning bone density, such as the presence of natural bone or other grafting materials.

5. Conclusions

The present in vitro study performed in low-density polyurethane foam blocks demonstrated that the conical implant shape could be considered the best-performing in artificial post-extraction conditions, due to the higher primary stability values reported, despite the IT ones. In particular, the TAC implant's macro-morphology reported the best results in terms of ISQ in all the polyurethane conditions and especially in lower-density blocks, aside from adequate values of IT and RT. Although further experimental studies are needed, in future a more standardized site under-preparation could help in obtaining higher IT values to make these implants ideal for an immediate loading protocol in low-density bones.

Author Contributions: Conceptualization, L.C., U.C. and A.P.; methodology, L.C. and M.T.; software, T.R.; validation, T.R., N.D.P. and L.M.; formal analysis, T.R. and H.H.S.H.; investigation, L.C.; resources, L.C. and U.C.; data curation, T.R., H.H.S.H. and N.D.P.; writing—original draft preparation, L.C., M.T., A.P., T.R. and N.D.P.; writing—review and editing, A.P., U.C. and N.D.P.; visualization, F.I.; supervision, L.C. and A.P.; project administration, L.C. All authors have read and agreed to the published version of the manuscript.

Funding: This research received no external funding.

Institutional Review Board Statement: Not applicable.

Informed Consent Statement: Not applicable.

Data Availability Statement: Data are contained within the article and available on request from the corresponding author.

Acknowledgments: We thank AoN Implants S.r.l. Company (Grisignano di Zocco, Vicenza, Italy) and Intra-Lock System Europa SpA Company (Salerno, Italy) for providing implants.

Conflicts of Interest: The authors declare no conflict of interest.

References

1. Gautam, S.; Bhatnagar, D.; Bansal, D.; Batra, H.; Goyal, N. Recent Advancements in Nanomaterials for Biomedical Implants. *Biomed. Eng. Adv.* **2022**, *3*, 100029. [CrossRef]
2. Araújo, M.G.; Silva, C.O.; Souza, A.B.; Sukekava, F. Socket Healing with and without Immediate Implant Placement. *Periodontology 2000* **2019**, *79*, 168–177. [CrossRef]
3. Dhami, B.; Shrestha, P.; Gupta, S.; Pandey, N. Immediate Implant Placement: Current Concepts. *J. Nepal. Soc. Periodontol. Oral Implantol.* **2019**, *3*, 18–24. [CrossRef]
4. Schulte, W.; Heimke, G. The Tübinger Immediate Implant. *Quintessenz* **1976**, *27*, 17–23. [PubMed]
5. Buser, D.; Chappuis, V.; Belser, U.C.; Chen, S. Implant Placement Post Extraction in Esthetic Single Tooth Sites: When Immediate, When Early, When Late? *Periodontology 2000* **2017**, *73*, 84–102. [CrossRef]
6. Mura, P. Immediate Loading of Tapered Implants Placed in Postextraction Sockets: Retrospective Analysis of the 5-year Clinical Outcome. *Clin. Implant Dent. Relat. Res.* **2012**, *14*, 565–574. [CrossRef]
7. Han, C.-H.; Mangano, F.; Mortellaro, C.; Park, K.-B. Immediate Loading of Tapered Implants Placed in Postextraction Sockets and Healed Sites. *J. Craniofac. Surg.* **2016**, *27*, 1220–1227. [CrossRef]
8. Mello, C.C.; Lemos, C.A.A.; Verri, F.R.; Dos Santos, D.M.; Goiato, M.C.; Pellizzer, E.P. Immediate Implant Placement into Fresh Extraction Sockets versus Delayed Implants into Healed Sockets: A Systematic Review and Meta-Analysis. *Int. J. Oral Maxillofac. Surg.* **2017**, *46*, 1162–1177. [CrossRef]

9. Yu, X.; Teng, F.; Zhao, A.; Wu, Y.; Yu, D. Effects of Post-Extraction Alveolar Ridge Preservation versus Immediate Implant Placement: A Systematic Review and Meta-Analysis. *J. Evid. Based. Dent. Pract.* **2022**, *22*, 101734. [CrossRef]
10. Chappuis, V.; Araújo, M.G.; Buser, D. Clinical Relevance of Dimensional Bone and Soft Tissue Alterations Post-extraction in Esthetic Sites. *Periodontology 2000* **2017**, *73*, 73–83. [CrossRef]
11. Romasco, T.; Tumedei, M.; Inchingolo, F.; Pignatelli, P.; Montesani, L.; Iezzi, G.; Petrini, M.; Piattelli, A.; Di Pietro, N. A Narrative Review on the Effectiveness of Bone Regen-eration Procedures with OsteoBiol® Collagenated Porcine Grafts: The Translational Research Experience over 20 Years. *J. Funct. Biomater.* **2022**, *13*, 121. [CrossRef]
12. *ASTM F-1839-08*; Standard Specification for Rigid Polyurethane Foam for Use as a Standard Material for Testing Orthopedic Devices and Instruments. ASTM International: West Conshohocken, PA, USA, 2021.
13. Arosio, P.; Arosio, F.; Di Stefano, D.A. Implant Diameter, Length, and the Insertion Torque/Depth Integral: A Study Using Polyurethane Foam Blocks. *Dent. J.* **2020**, *8*, 56. [CrossRef] [PubMed]
14. Tsolaki, I.N.; Tonsekar, P.P.; Najafi, B.; Drew, H.J.; Sullivan, A.J.; Petrov, S.D. Comparison of Osteotome and Conventional Drilling Techniques for Primary Implant Stability: An In Vitro Study. *J. Oral Implant.* **2016**, *42*, 321–325. [CrossRef] [PubMed]
15. Calvert, K.L.; Trumble, K.P.; Webster, T.J.; Kirkpatrick, L.A. Characterization of Commercial Rigid Polyurethane Foams Used as Bone Analogs for Implant Testing. *J. Mater. Sci. Mater. Med.* **2010**, *21*, 1453–1461. [CrossRef]
16. Nagaraja, S.; Palepu, V. Comparisons of Anterior Plate Screw Pullout Strength Between Polyurethane Foams and Thora-columbar Cadaveric Vertebrae. *J. Biomech. Eng.* **2016**, *138*, 104505. [CrossRef] [PubMed]
17. Gehrke, S.A.; Guirado, J.L.C.; Bettach, R.; Fabbro, M.D.; Martínez, C.P.-A.; Shibli, J.A. Evaluation of the insertion torque, implant stability quotient and drilled hole quality for different drill design: An in vitro Investigation. *Clin. Oral Implants Res.* **2018**, *29*, 656–662. [CrossRef] [PubMed]
18. Romanos, G.E.; Delgado-Ruiz, R.A.; Sacks, D.; Calvo-Guirado, J.L. Influence of the implant diameter and bone quality on the primary stability of porous tantalum trabecular metal dental implants: An in vitro biomechanical study. *Clin. Oral Implants Res.* **2018**, *29*, 649–655. [CrossRef]
19. Comuzzi, L.; Tumedei, M.; Covani, U.; Romasco, T.; Petrini, M.; Montesani, L.; Piattelli, A.; Di Pietro, N. Primary Stability Assessment of Conical Implants in Under-Prepared Sites: An In Vitro Study in Low-Density Polyurethane Foams. *Appl. Sci.* **2023**, *13*, 6041. [CrossRef]
20. Misch, C.E. Bone density: A key determinant for clinical success. *Contemp. Implant. Dent.* **1999**, *8*, 109–111.
21. Romanos, G.; Damouras, M.; Veis, A.A.; Hess, P.; Schwarz, F.; Brandt, S. Comparison of histomorphometry and microradiography of different implant designs to assess primary implant stability. *Clin. Implant Dent. Relat. Res.* **2020**, *22*, 373–379. [CrossRef]
22. Mirzaie, T.; Rouhi, G.; Mehdi Dehghan, M.; Farzad-Mohajeri, S.; Barikani, H. Dental implants' stability dependence on rotational speed and feed-rate of drilling: In-vivo and ex-vivo investigations. *J. Biomech.* **2021**, *127*, 110696. [CrossRef] [PubMed]
23. Gehrke, S.A.; Treichel, T.L.E.; Pérez-Díaz, L.; Calvo-Guirado, J.L.; Aramburú Júnior, J.; Mazón, P.; de Aza, P.N. Impact of Different Titanium Implant Thread Designs on Bone Healing: A Biomechanical and Histometric Study with an Animal Model. *J. Clin. Med.* **2019**, *8*, 777. [CrossRef] [PubMed]
24. Kashi, A.; Gupta, B.; Malmstrom, H.; Romanos, G.E. Primary Stability of Implants Placed at Different Angulations in Artificial Bone. *Implant Dent.* **2015**, *24*, 92–95. [CrossRef] [PubMed]
25. Karl, M.; Irastorza-Landa, A. Does Implant Design Affect Primary Stability in Extraction Sites. *Quintessence Int.* **2017**, *48*, 219–224. [CrossRef]
26. Yim, H.; Lim, H.-C.; Hong, J.-Y.; Shin, S.-I.; Chung, J.-H.; Herr, Y.; Shin, S.-Y. Primary Stability of Implants with Peri-Implant Bone Defects of Various Widths: An in Vitro Investigation. *J. Periodontal Implant Sci.* **2019**, *49*, 39–46. [CrossRef]
27. Hollensteiner, M.; Fürst, D.; Esterer, B.; Augat, P.; Schrödl, F.; Hunger, S.; Malek, M.; Stephan, D.; Schrempf, A. Novel Bone Surrogates for Cranial Surgery Training. *J. Mech. Behav. Biomed. Mater.* **2017**, *72*, 49–51. [CrossRef]
28. Patel, P.S.; Shepherd, D.E.; Hukins, D.W. Compressive properties of commercially available polyurethane foams as mechanical models for osteoporotic human cancellous bone. *BMC Musculoskelet. Disord.* **2008**, *9*, 137. [CrossRef]
29. Meredith, N.; Alleyne, D.; Cawley, P. Quantitative Determination of the Stability of the Implant-Tissue Interface Using Resonance Frequency Analysis. *Clin. Oral Implants Res.* **1996**, *7*, 261–267. [CrossRef]
30. Staedt, H.; Palarie, V.; Staedt, A.; Wolf, J.M.; Lehmann, K.M.; Ottl, P.; Kämmerer, P.W. Primary Stability of Cylindrical and Conical Dental Implants in Relation to Insertion Torque—A Comparative Ex Vivo Evaluation. *Implant Dent.* **2017**, *26*, 250–255. [CrossRef]
31. Dos Santos, M.V.; Elias, C.N.; Cavalcanti Lima, J.H. The Effects of Superficial Roughness and Design on the Primary Stability of Dental Implants. *Clin. Implant Dent. Relat. Res.* **2011**, *13*, 215–223. [CrossRef]
32. Pommer, B.; Hof, M.; Fädler, A.; Gahleitner, A.; Watzek, G.; Watzak, G. Primary implant stability in the atrophic sinus floor of human cadaver maxillae: Impact of residual ridge height, bone density, and implant diameter. *Clin. Oral Implants Res.* **2014**, *25*, 109–113. [CrossRef] [PubMed]
33. Wilson Jr, T.G.; Miller, R.J.; Trushkowsky, R.; Dard, M. Tapered Implants in Dentistry: Revitalizing Concepts with Technology: A Review. *Adv. Dent. Res.* **2016**, *28*, 4–9. [CrossRef] [PubMed]
34. Chu, S.J.; Levin, B.P.; Egbert, N.; Saito, H.; Nevins, M. Use of a Novel Implant with an Inverted Body-Shift and Prosthetic Angle Correction Design for Immediate Tooth Replacement in the Esthetic Zone: A Clinical Case Series. *Int. J. Periodontics Restor. Dent.* **2021**, *41*, 195–204. [CrossRef] [PubMed]

35. Lages, F.S.; Douglas-de Oliveira, D.W.; Costa, F.O. Relationship between implant stability measurements obtained by insertion torque and resonance frequency analysis: A systematic review. *Clin. Implant Dent. Relat. Res.* **2018**, *20*, 26–33. [CrossRef]
36. Comuzzi, L.; Tumedei, M.; Di Pietro, N.; Romasco, T.; Montesani, L.; Piattelli, A.; Covani, U. Are Implant Threads Important for Implant Stability? An In Vitro Study Using Low-Density Polyurethane Sheets. *Eng* **2023**, *4*, 1167–1178. [CrossRef]

Disclaimer/Publisher's Note: The statements, opinions and data contained in all publications are solely those of the individual author(s) and contributor(s) and not of MDPI and/or the editor(s). MDPI and/or the editor(s) disclaim responsibility for any injury to people or property resulting from any ideas, methods, instructions or products referred to in the content.

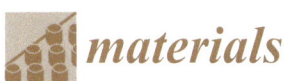

Article

Biological Performance of Titanium Surfaces with Different Hydrophilic and Nanotopographical Features

Barbara Illing [†], Leila Mohammadnejad [†], Antonia Theurer, Jacob Schultheiss, Evi Kimmerle-Mueller, Frank Rupp and Stefanie Krajewski *

Department Medical Materials Science & Technology, University Hospital Tübingen, Osianderstr. 2-8, 72076 Tübingen, Germany; barbara.illing@med.uni-tuebingen.de (B.I.); jacob.schultheiss@med.uni-tuebingen.de (J.S.); evi.kimmerle-mueller@med.uni-tuebingen.de (E.K.-M.)
* Correspondence: stefanie.krajewski@med.uni-tuebingen.de
[†] These authors contributed equally to this work.

Abstract: The micro- and nanostructures, chemical composition, and wettability of titanium surfaces are essential for dental implants' osseointegration. Combining hydrophilicity and nanostructure has been shown to improve the cell response and to shorten the healing time. This study aimed to investigate the biological response to different wettability levels and nanotopographical modifications in aged and non-aged titanium surfaces. By plasma etching titanium surfaces with the fluorine gas 2,3,3,3-tetrafluoropropene (R1234yF), additional nanostructures were created on the sample surfaces. Furthermore, this treatment resulted in sustained superhydrophilicity and fluoride accumulation. We examined the effect of various nanostructuring processes and aging using scanning electron microscopy, roughness analyses, and wettability measurement. In addition, all the surface modifications were tested for their effects on fibroblast adhesion, proliferation, and viability as well as osteoblast differentiation. Our study indicates that the plasma etching, with 2,3,3,3-tetrafluoropropene, of the machined and SLA surface neither favored nor had an adverse effect on the biological response of the SAOS-2 osteoblast cell line. Although the fluorine-plasma-etched surfaces demonstrated improved fibroblast cell viability, they did not lead to improved early osseointegration. It is still unclear which surface properties mainly influence fibroblast and osteoblast adhesion. Further physiochemical aspects, such as electrostatic interaction and surface tension, are crucial to be analyzed along with wettability and roughness.

Keywords: dental-implant interface; titanium; hydrophile; nanostructure; osseointegration; human gingival fibroblasts; plasma etching; R1234yF

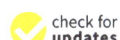

Citation: Illing, B.; Mohammadnejad, L.; Theurer, A.; Schultheiss, J.; Kimmerle-Mueller, E.; Rupp, F.; Krajewski, S. Biological Performance of Titanium Surfaces with Different Hydrophilic and Nanotopographical Features. *Materials* 2023, *16*, 7307. https://doi.org/10.3390/ma16237307

Academic Editors: Lavinia Cosmina Ardelean and Laura-Cristina Rusu

Received: 3 November 2023
Revised: 19 November 2023
Accepted: 21 November 2023
Published: 24 November 2023

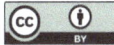

Copyright: © 2023 by the authors. Licensee MDPI, Basel, Switzerland. This article is an open access article distributed under the terms and conditions of the Creative Commons Attribution (CC BY) license (https:// creativecommons.org/licenses/by/ 4.0/).

1. Introduction

The insertion of bone-anchored titanium implants is, nowadays, the treatment of choice for patients suffering from tooth loss [1,2]. To guarantee long-term survival and functionality, two biological responses to the implant are essential. The first is proper osseointegration to provide a structural and functional connection between the bone tissue and the implant surface without the interference of soft-tissue cells [3,4]. The second process is the formation of a tight soft-tissue seal created by gingival cells, such as fibroblasts and oral keratinocytes, around the implants' neck to provide protection against invading pathogens and bacteria [5–7]. Among others, hydrophilicity is described to influence the biological response to the implant and, hence, may play a crucial role in the performance and success of dental implants [8]. Hydrophilicity can improve osseointegration; the process of implant integration into the surrounding bone tissue; as well as the adhesion and proliferation of gingival cells, such as fibroblasts and oral keratinocytes [9]. Hydrophilic surfaces promote better wetting and fluid transport at the implant–tissue interface, thereby enhancing protein adsorption from surrounding saliva and blood and resulting in improved clot formation on the implant surface. In addition, surface wettability affects the quantity and binding strength of bound proteins, their conformation and orientation, as well as the composition of the macromolecular films formed on them. Adsorbed proteins interact with cell-membrane receptors and activate biological pathways. The expression of the receptors on cells' surfaces varies depending on their type and differentiation stage. Additionally, these receptors control short- and long-term processes, such as proliferation and differentiation as well as initial cellular attachment [10]. Furthermore, hydrophilic implant surfaces with high wettability form a stable and uniform liquid film when in contact with biological fluids, which can improve cell proliferation and differentiation [11,12]. Hence, the hydrophilic surface properties of dental-implant materials can significantly impact their long-term performance and success rate.

The second implant surface characteristic that plays a crucial role in long-term success is the micro- and nanostructures. Nano- and microstructured implant surfaces have a larger surface area compared to smooth ones, which can increase the availability of protein-based recognition sequences for cell integrin binding, thereby promoting cell adhesion [13–15]. The size, shape, and distribution of these structures can also provide a topographical cue for cells to align and differentiate along the direction of the surface structures, further promoting cell adhesion, proliferation, and differentiation [16,17]. For example, studies have shown that micro- and nanoscaled topographical cues on the implant surface can enhance osteoblast adhesion and proliferation by providing them with a favorable microenvironment for cell attachment, growth, and function [18]. Similarly, nanostructured surfaces have been shown to promote the better adhesion and proliferation of fibroblasts, the key cells involved in the survival and function of the gingival tissue surrounding and sealing dental implants [19].

Various techniques have been developed to modify the surface properties of implant materials, like titanium, and to introduce micro- and nanostructures to them. The most common method is blasting, which refers to a procedure in which abrasive materials, like sand, glass, or aluminum oxide, are used to achieve a rough surface texture on an implant [20,21]. Blasting can be combined with acid etching, which involves immersing the implant in an acidic solution to dissolve the surface material and to create further pores and grooves [22,23]. These procedures increase the surface area and create surface features that improve cell adhesion and promote tissue integration. Moreover, plasma etching can efficiently generate nanostructured surfaces [24]. Using fluorinated gases, such as carbon tetrafluoride (CF_4), the surfaces of polymers, like polystyrene, or metals, like aluminum, can be modified to improve cellular responses [25,26]. A study targeting plasma-etched titanium revealed the formation of a two-tier hierarchical topography, which supports cell growth and osteogenic differentiation [27]. Overall, providing cells with favorable micro- and nanostructures on the surface of dental-implant materials can play a decisive role in regulating cell behavior, promoting osseointegration and gingival health, and ultimately enhancing the stability and longevity of dental implants.

These findings so far suggest that combined hydrophilic surfaces and nanostructures in dental implants exert synergistic effects on cell performance. This may result in the better cell adhesion and proliferation of soft-tissue cells and osteoblasts than that with either feature alone. Therefore, the present study aimed to assess the effect of different nanotopographical features and varied wettability in non-aged and aged titanium surfaces on their biological performance in vitro. In detail, machined titanium discs were used as an original substrate, and the effects of different nanostructuring processes and aging were investigated using scanning electron microscopy as well as roughness and wettability measurements. All the surfaces were further evaluated in terms of the adhesion, proliferation, and viability of fibroblasts as well as osteoblast differentiation.

2. Materials and Methods

2.1. Surface Modifications

Machined grade 2 titanium (Ti) discs (15 mm in diameter and 1 mm in thickness; Institute Straumann AG, Basel, Switzerland) was used as the basic material. In addition to the machined reference samples (M), four different groups, which were divided due to their processing, were included in this study (Table 1). The SLA titanium discs, with their coarsely grit-blasted and acid-etched surfaces, as well as an M_{nano} titanium surface, which was generated by plasma cleaning machined titanium, treating it with sodium chloride (saline) in a hydrothermal process, and storing it in saline for several weeks, were also supplied by Institute Straumann AG. The treatment process of the M_{nano} discs resulted in the development of small nanodots on the smooth machined surface. Moreover, the M and SLA discs underwent plasma etching with 2,3,3,3-tetrafluoropropene (Diener electronic GmbH + Co. KG, Ebhausen, Germany). For plasma etching of the R1234yF-modified surfaces, 20% R1234yF and 80% O_2 gas were used (generator frequency, MHz; RF power, 100 W; gas pressure, 0.4 mbar) for 15 min.

Table 1. Overview of specimen groups evaluated in the present study.

Group	Surface Modification
M	Machined surface without further surface treatment
M_{nano}	Plasma cleaning followed by hydrothermal treatment with sodium chloride
M_{RyF}	Plasma etching of machined surface with 2,3,3,3-tetrafluoropropene
SLA	Blasted with large grits of 0.25–0.50 mm corundum and acid-etched in a mixture of HCl and H_2SO_4.
SLA_{RyF}	Plasma etching of SLA surface with 2,3,3,3-tetrafluoropropene

2.2. Pre-Treatment of Samples

To exclude contaminations caused by different manufacturing processes and ambient conditions during manufacturing and storage of the samples, all samples were cleaned for 20 min in oxygen plasma (100% O_2; generator frequency, 40 kHz; RF power, 80 W; gas pressure of approximately 0.3 mbar) in a plasma chamber (DENTAPLAS PC, Diener electronic GmbH, Ebhausen, Germany) before the respective biological experiments. To further simulate aging and, thus, recontamination and re-hydrophobization, the samples were stored directly after cleaning in glass petri dishes under ambient conditions for 14 days before experiments started (referred to as "aged"). Sample discs, which were used directly after cleaning, are called "new".

2.3. Surface Characterization

2.3.1. Scanning Electron Microscopy (SEM) of the Different Surfaces

Nanotopographical surface features of each sample were characterized via field emission scanning electron microscopy (JSM-6500F, Jeol, Tokyo, Japan).

To assess the morphology and location of the cells on the test surfaces, the samples were fixed in 2% (v/v) glutaraldehyde overnight followed by ascending ethanol dehydration. Subsequently, the samples were critically point-dried. Samples were sputtered with Au-Pd and were characterized via scanning electron microscopy (LEO 1430, Zeiss, Oberkochen, Germany).

The chemical composition of the researched surfaces was detected via energy-dispersive X-ray spectroscopy (EDX) (EDX-ZKK-31 Detector, Röntec/Bruker, Berlin, Germany).

2.3.2. Roughness

The topography of the different surface modifications was determined via confocal microscopy (MarSurf CM Explorer, Mahr GmbH, Göttingen, Germany). For this purpose, five discs for each surface modification were evaluated. On each disc, six different areas of 800×800 µm were measured with a 20× objective (0.6 numeric aperture). Roughness was analyzed using MountainsMap Imaging Topography Software (Version 9.1.9957, Digital Surf, Besançon, France). First, the surface was leveled using the least square plane leveling method and then an S-Filter (λs): Gauss of 300:1 (800 µm) was applied to remove noise. Additionally, an L-Filter (λc): Gauss of 0.05 mm was used to remove possible waviness.

Arithmetic mean roughness heights (Sa) were calculated for each surface modification and were statistically analyzed.

2.3.3. Surface Wettability

Hydrophilicity was quantified by measuring static water contact angle with a high-resolution drop shape analysis system (OCA 200, DataPhysics Instruments GmbH, Filderstadt, Germany). A 1 µL drop of ultrapure water (Milli-Q; Merck Millipore, Darmstadt, Germany) was automatically placed on the sample disc surface and was video-recorded at 25 frames/s during an evaluation period of 30 s. The apparent contact angle at the equilibrated state (at 10 s) was chosen to characterize the hydrophilicity of the surface. Contact angles were measured immediately after oxygen plasma cleaning (0 h) and 1 h, 2 h, 3 h, 1 d, 2 d, 3 d, 7 d, and 14 d after cleaning. In total, 5 samples per surface modification and timepoint were measured. In this study, we define contact angles between 0° and 10° as superhydrophilic, contact angles of 10° to 30° as strong hydrophilic, contact angles of 30° to 60° as moderately hydrophilic, and contact angles of 60° to 90° as low hydrophilic. Contact angles between 90° and 180° indicate increasingly worse wetting conditions.

2.3.4. Biological Tests

In order to screen for biofunctionality and to test the suitability of the modified surfaces for the specific requirements of the different implantation sites, interactions with primary human gingival fibroblasts (HFG) and a human osteoblast-like cell line (SAOS-2) were investigated.

2.3.5. Cultivation of Cells

Human gingival fibroblasts (HGF) (HFIB-G, Cat.-No. 121 0412, Provitro AG, Berlin, Germany) cultured at 37 °C and 5% CO_2 in fibroblast growth medium (Provitro), containing 14% fetal calf serum and 1% antibiotics as supplements, were used between passages three and eight. Human primary osteogenic sarcoma (SAOS-2) cell lines (DSMZ GmbH, Braunschweig, Germany) were cultured at 37 °C and 5% CO_2 in McCoy's 5A medium (Sigma-Aldrich Chemie GmbH, Steinheim, Germany), containing 15% fetal bovine serum (Thermo Fisher Scientific, Darmstadt, Germany), 1% L-glutamine (Thermo Fisher Scientific, Darmstadt, Germany), and 1% penicillin and streptomycin (Thermo Fisher Scientific, Darmstadt, Germany).

2.3.6. Adhesion, Viability, and Proliferation Assay

Initial cell adhesion of HGF cells was determined 1 h after seeding using Alamar blue dye (Fisher Scientific, Schwerte, Germany) and was measured via UV photometry (Berthold Technologies, Bad Wildbad, Germany) (according to the manufacturer's instructions). Before staining, non-adhering cells were removed via rinsing. The proliferation of HGF cells on the different surface modifications was determined using the cell counting kit-8 (CCK-8) assay (Dojindo Laboratories, Kumamoto, Japan). After 10,000 cells/cm^2 were pre-incubated for 24 h on the different specimens, the CCK-8 solution was added according to the manufacturer's instructions, and the spectral absorbance was measured at 450 nm. This process was repeated 48 h and 72 h after the cells were seeded on the sample surfaces. Afterwards, crystal violet (Sigma-Aldrich, Taufkirchen, Germany) staining was performed and was macroscopically analyzed. To quantify the cell coverage rate, the dye eluate was measured photometrically at 550 nm (Tecan, Crailsheim, Germany). For each experiment, three independent experiments with four samples per surface modification, respectively, were carried out.

2.3.7. Differentiation of SAOS-2

To simulate bone healing, osteoblasts at a density of 10,000 SAOS-2 cells/cm^2 were seeded onto the different test surfaces and were incubated for 24 h to allow adhesion. The differentiation process was initiated by adding vitamin C, b-glycerophosphate, and dexamethasone (10 µL each per ml of medium) (Sigma-Aldrich, Taufkirchen Germany) After 7 d, 14 d, and 21 d, osteogenesis (mineralized deposits) of the osteoblasts was determined using alizarin red (Sigma-Aldrich, Taufkirchen, Germany) staining as described before [28]. The eluate was quantified via photometric measurement at 405 nm. (Tecan, Crailsheim, Germany) Each experiment was performed independently three times with three samples per surface modification.

2.3.8. Statistical Analysis

Unless otherwise specified, data are represented as mean ± standard deviation (SD). Student's t test was used to compare the means between two groups. Statistically significant differences between the means of three or more groups were determined using one-way analysis of variance (ANOVA). Afterwards, comparison of machined control groups with all other groups, corrected via post hoc Tukey's test, was performed. All statistical analyses were performed with the statistical software package GraphPad Prism (version 9.4.1, GraphPad Software, San Diego, CA, USA). Statistical significance was defined as $p < 0.05$.

3. Results

3.1. Surface Characteristics

For this study, five different modified titanium surfaces were selected (M, M_{nano}, SLA, M_{RyF}, and SLA_{RyF}). On all three machined-based surfaces, parallel grinding marks are visible in the SEM micrographs, indicating typical anisotropy. The M surface (Figure 1A(a)) showed no additional nanostructures, while on the M_{nano} surface (Figure 1A(b)), clear nanostructures and fine spherical particles were visible. In the case of the M_{RyF} (Figure 1A(c)), a cauliflower-like secondary structure developed on the machined surface. The grinding grooves of the M surface were still clearly visible. The typical three-dimensional structure with different-sized pits, sharp ridges, and crevices formed by etching and sand blasting was seen on the SLA (Figure 1A(d)) surface. On the SLA_{RyF} (Figure 1A(e)) samples, the cauliflower-like structure already seen on the M_{RyF} was superimposed onto the original pits and crevices from the SLA base. The recorded EDX spectra show an additional fluorine peak in the spectrum for the R1234yF-fluorine-plasma-etched samples. While all the surfaces based on machined titanium were relatively smooth (Sa values shown in Figure 1B: M, 0.145 ± 0.015 µm; M_{nano}, 0.131 ± 0.004 µm; M_{RyF}, 0.116 ± 0.007 µm), those based on SLA appeared significantly rougher (SLA, 1.651 ± 0.245 µm; SLA_{RyF}, 3.494 ± 0.321 µm) ($p < 0.0001$).

In order to investigate the wettability of the different surfaces, contact angle measurement was performed up to 14 days after cleaning with O_2 plasma (Figure 2). Immediately after plasma treatment, all the surfaces tested had a contact angle of $0°$, indicating initial superhydrophilic behavior. The machined surface displayed contact angles over $50°$ and already moderate hydrophilicity after only three days of storage. The contact angle reached $60.8° \pm 1.8°$ (M) after 14 days, which is comparable with the wettability of the SLA surface ($63.9° \pm 0.9°$ after 14 days). According to our suggested wetting classification of the measured contact angles, both M and SLA were categorized as low wettable after 14 days. In contrast, the R1234yF plasma etching of both the M and SLA surfaces resulted in water contact angles below $20°$ for at least 14 days. M_{RyF}, with contact angles of $15.4 \pm 0.9°$, was classified as strong hydrophilic and SLA_{RyF}, with contact angles of even $0°$, was classified as superhydrophilic (Figure 2B). The M_{nano} surface showed moderate hydrophilicity after 14 days, with contact angles of $33.8 \pm 1.7°$. Thus, a 14-day aging time led to a range of different hydrophilic titanium surfaces, from superhydrophilic to low-hydrophilic surfaces. None of the surfaces under investigation showed any hydrophobic wetting state after plasma cleaning or aging.

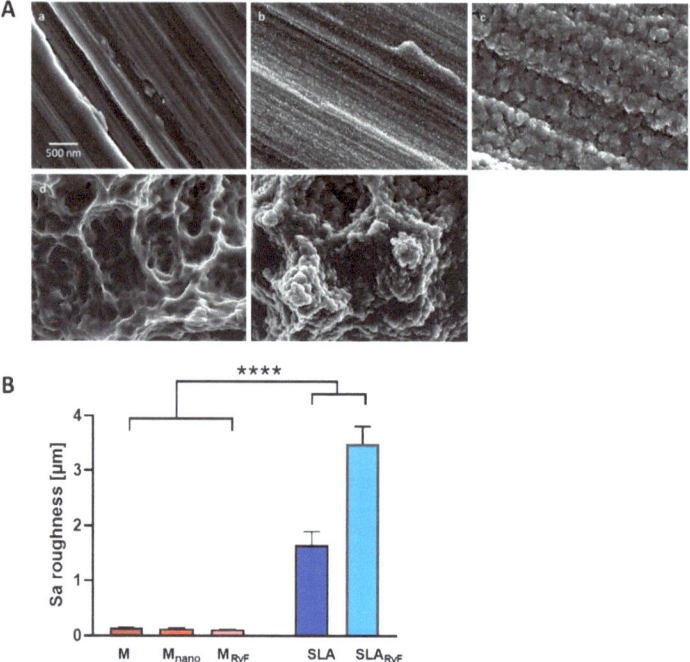

Figure 1. Scanning electron microscopy and roughness characterization of different surfaces. (**A**) Representative SEM images of the experimental titanium surfaces: (a) machined (M), (b) M_{nano}, (c) M_{RyF}, (d) SLA, and (e) SLA_{RyF}. (**B**) Quantitation of the average surface roughness of the different surfaces (n = 5 independent samples per group analyzed via one-way ANOVA with Tukey's post hoc test for multiple comparisons). Data are reported as mean ± SD (**** $p < 0.0001$).

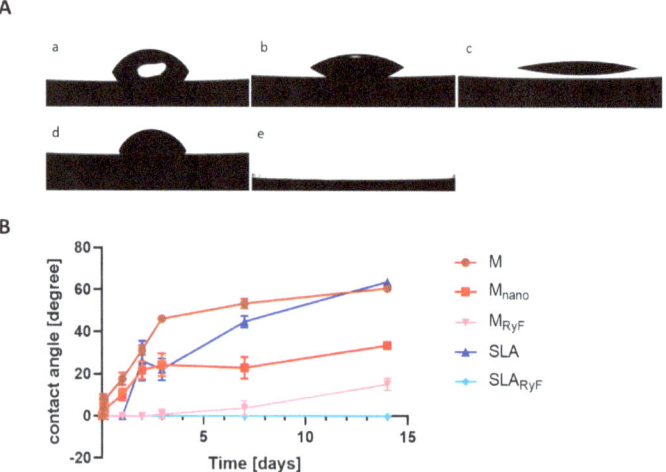

Figure 2. Contact angle measurement of the test samples at different time points: (**A**) Representative contact angle photos taken 14 days after O_2 plasma cleaning: M (a), M_{nano} (b), M_{RyF} (c), SLA (d), and SLA_{RyF} (e). The SLA_{RyF} surface (e) was so hydrophilic that the water drop immediately spread over the surface and the initial contact with the surface could not be captured photographically. (**B**) Quantitative analysis of surface angles. Data are reported as mean ± SD; n = 3.

3.2. Fibroblast Attachment and Proliferation

Since soft-tissue attachment to the implants' neck is as important as osseointegration for implantation success, the surfaces were also analyzed for the cellular response of human gingival fibroblasts (HGF).

To quantify the initial attachment of fibroblasts to different surfaces, Alamar blue staining was used to measure cell adhesion 1 h after seeding. It was observed that cells attached equally well to smooth and nanostructured surfaces. In addition, no significant differences were detected between the freshly O_2-plasma-cleaned (new) and the 14-day-aged (aged) surfaces (Figure 3). As can be seen in Figure 4A, the fibroblasts tended to grow in a structured linear way following the parallel grinding marks of the surface when seeded on M, M_{nano}, or M_{RyF}, whereas they showed a more widespread morphology when cultivated for 24 h on the pits, sharp ridges, and crevices of the SLA and SLA_{RyF} surfaces.

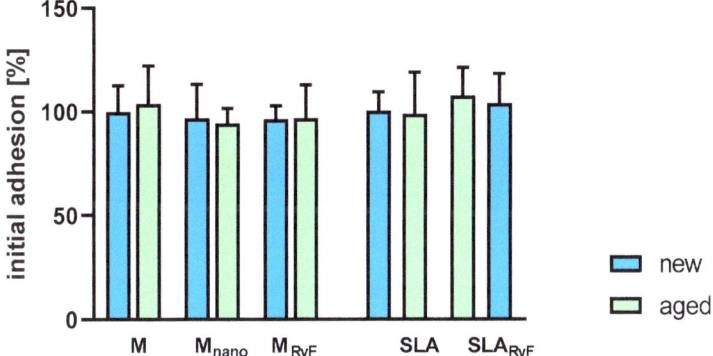

Figure 3. Initial adhesion of HGF cells was quantitatively determined with Alamar blue staining 1 h after seeding of the cells on the different titanium surfaces. The machined group (M new), after 24 h of cell incubation, was used as a control, set to 100%, and all other groups are referred to this. Three independent tests were performed with 4 discs per surface modification to be tested. The bar graph shows the mean ± SD.

The viability of the cells was monitored for a period of 72 h (Figure 4B). Even though the cells similarly attached to the different surfaces after 1 h of incubation, the cells growing on the SLA surfaces (SLA and SLA_{RyF}) displayed lower metabolic activity compared to the M, M_{nano}, or M_{RyF} surfaces after 24 h, 48 h, and 72 h of incubation. While viability remained low for the cells growing on SLA for 72 h, it increased over time for the cells growing on SLA_{RyF}, reaching 70% (new) or 67% (aged) of the reference viability on the M surface after 72 h; meanwhile, SLA reached only 28% (new) and 24% (aged). A comparison of the viability of the cells on the SLA surface with the SLA_{RyF} showed significantly higher viability for the fluorine-plasma-etched surfaces on both the "new" and the "aged" surfaces (SLA "new" vs. SLA_{RyF} "new": after 24 h, $p = 0.0132$; after 48 h, $p = 0.0002$; after 72 h, $p = 0.0049$) (SLA "aged" vs. SLA_{RyF} "aged": after 24 h, $p = 0.0118$; after 48 h, $p = 0.0006$; after 72 h, $p = 0.0016$). However, no differences in cell viability were found between "new" and "aged" surfaces of the same surface modification in all the specimen groups.

The results of the metabolic activity measurement could also be visualized via crystal violet staining (Figure 4C), which showed that the lower metabolic activity of the cells on the rougher SLA surfaces was caused by the degree of occupancy, that is, the number of cells on the surface.

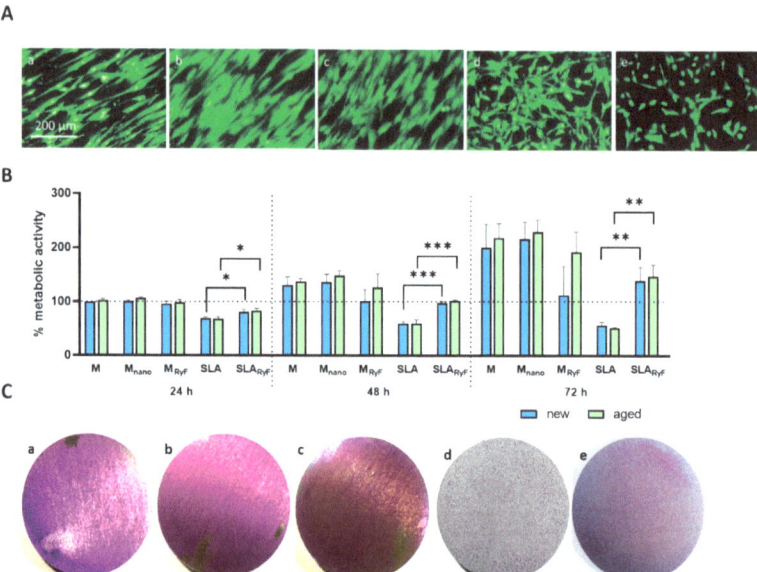

Figure 4. Evaluation of the cytocompatibility of different surfaces. (**A**) Representative fluorescent images of live/dead stained HGF cells seeded for 24 h on the different non-aged (new) sample discs (green = living; red = dead cells (not observed)). (**B**) Quantitative comparison of the metabolic activity of fibroblasts after 24 h, 48 h, and 72 h measured using CCK-8 assay. The machined group (M new), after 24 h of cell incubation, was used as a control and was set to 100%, and all other groups are displayed in relation to it. Three independent tests were performed, with 4 discs per surface modification to be tested. The bar graph shows the mean ± SD (* $p < 0.05$; ** $p < 0.01$; *** $p < 0.001$). (**C**) Representative images of crystal-violet-stained HGF fibroblasts growing on the non-aged sample discs for 72 h: (a) machined; (b) machined nano (M_{nano}); (c) machined R1234yF (M_{RyF}); (d) SLA; and (e) SLA R1234yF (SLA_{RyF}).

3.3. Osteoblast Differentiation

To investigate the osteogenic properties of the surface variants, the human-derived SAOS-2 osteoblast cell line was used. To test potential bone formation on the surfaces in vitro, SAOS-2 cells were stimulated to produce extracellular calcium phosphate deposits over 21 days. On the macroscopic imaging of the Alizarin-red-stained samples after 7, 14, or 21 days, there was no clear difference between the "new" surface (Figure 5A) and the "aged" surface (Figure S1), nor did the smooth surface and the nanostructured surface result in any substantial differences in calcium phosphate formation.

According to calcium quantification, mineralization occurred continuously on all the surfaces. After 14 days of differentiation, the cells on the M-based surfaces had deposited at least six times the amount of calcium phosphate than the cells on the SLA-based surfaces. This difference disappeared after 21 days since, at this time point, the quantity of mineral nodules was comparable between the SLA-based and the M-based surfaces, indicating similar calcium phosphate deposition in all the groups. Again, no differences between the "new" and the "aged" surfaces with the same modification could be detected (Figure 5B). The SEM images taken at the same timepoints as the calcium measurements show very clear morphological changes in the cells during the increasing calcium phosphate deposition (Figure 6). As with fibroblasts, SAOS-2 cells spread according to the surface structure.

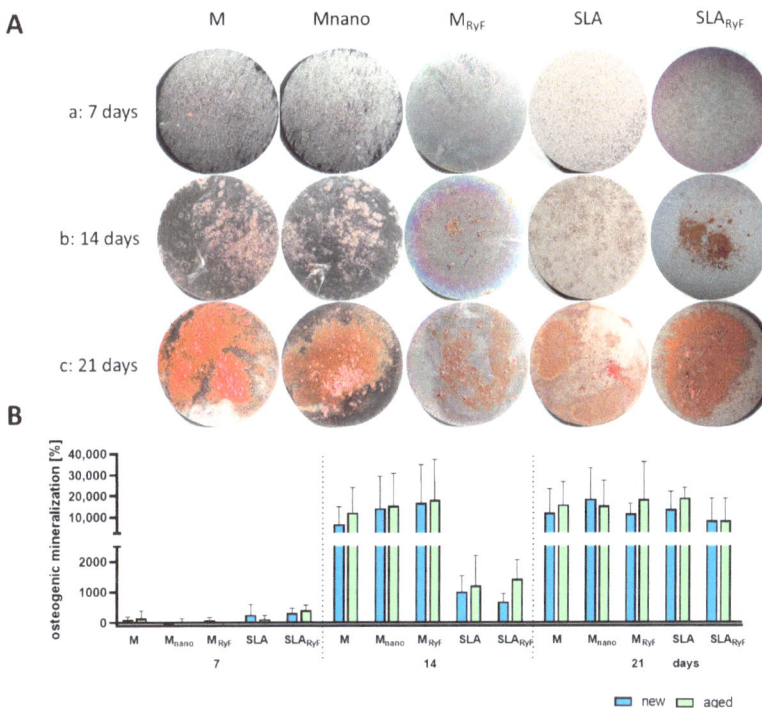

Figure 5. Osteogenic differentiation of osteoblasts on different "new" and "aged" titanium surfaces. (**A**) Representative images of the different "new" titanium discs with seeded SAOS-2 cells at different time points since the onset of differentiation. With prolonged differentiation, after (a) 7 days, (b) 14 days, and (c) 21 days, a visible increase in calcium phosphate formation stained with alizarin red was seen (disc diameter: 1.5 cm). (**B**) After photo documentation, the dye was dissolved from the cells and was quantified in a spectrophotometer. The machined "new" group, after 7 days, was used as a control and was set to 100%. The bar graph shows the mean ± SD ($n = 3$).

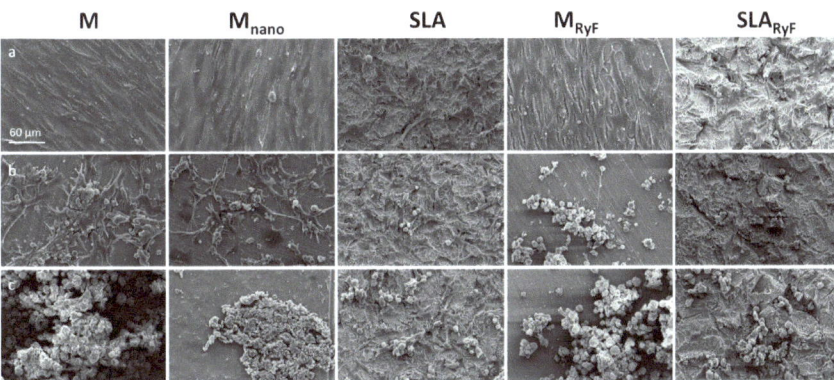

Figure 6. Representative scanning electron microscopy images showing the adhesion of SAOS-2 cells on the experimental non-aged titanium surfaces 7 days (**a**), 14 days (**b**), and 21 days (**c**) after the onset of osteogenic differentiation. With prolonged differentiation, morphological changes occurred, and calcium phosphate formation increased.

4. Discussion

The physicochemical surface properties of an implant material are proven to influence the cellular response, thus influencing the long-term success of implantation [29–32]. Various surface modification techniques, like blasting, acid etching, or coating, have been developed in the last decades to modulate the physicochemical and biological properties of titanium implants [33,34]. Titanium implants' topographical micro-/nanofeatures, in combination with their wettability, have been shown to modulate biological responses in in vitro and animal studies [16,35–37]. Highly structured implant surfaces are assumed to increase the implant–bone surface contact area, thus promoting the biological fixation [38]. Hence, the micro- and nanoscaled structuring of implant surfaces aims to enhance cell attachment and tissue healing, which are critical steps in osseointegration [35]. However, while the role of surface topography in bioresponses has received extensive attention, only a few studies have explored the relationship between implant wettability and cellular response [10,35,38].

This study focused on investigating two physical and chemical modification strategies that may impact implant healing. Firstly, the commercially available surfaces (machined and SLA) were additionally plasma-etched with fluorine gas (R1234yF) to create an additional and novel nanoroughness on the surfaces, as can be seen on the SEM images. Besides topography and roughness, the surface wettability or hydrophilicity of implants can also play a role in osseointegration. All the surfaces tested in our study were freshly O_2-plasma-cleaned (new) and were compared to the "aged" surfaces (14 days after plasma cleaning) to further investigate how hydrophilicity affects cell attachment, viability, and osteoblast differentiation.

It was shown that the O_2-plasma-cleaned surfaces had a water contact angle of $0°$ and were thus superhydrophilic. During storage in the ambient atmosphere (aging), the initial hydrophilicity of the material decreased over time. The superhydrophilicity of the fluorine-gas-etched surfaces, however, was maintained over a longer period of time. Several in vitro and in vivo studies showed that increased hydrophilicity is a crucial factor for fast implant healing since initial protein adhesion is promoted. It is well known that hydrophilicity is the main driving force in protein folding [39,40].

Hydrophilic surfaces maintain protein conformation and function, while hydrophobic surfaces seem to induce denaturation [41]. As a critical factor determining cell attachment and proliferation, rapid protein attachment should provide an advantage and can influence tissue–implant integration. In this study, we did not find significant differences between the hydrophilic and "aged" surfaces. Neither the initial attachment nor the viability of the HGF cells over 72 h showed a significant difference. There was also no difference in SAOS-2 osteoblast differentiation over 21 days between the "new" and "aged" surfaces. Despite higher mineralization on the M-based surfaces after 14 days (increased by a factor of 12,360 for M "new" within 7 days) compared to the SLA-based surfaces (SLA "new" increased by a factor of 394, where SLA_{RyF} "new" increased by 216), the values were comparable after 21 days in all the groups, indicating no profound impact neither of the different surface topographies nor of different wettability on osteoblast differentiation. Some published long-term in vivo studies on animals also showed no significant positive effect of hydrophilized implant surfaces [42]. On the other hand, a number of in vivo studies have demonstrated that hydrophilicity enhances early osseointegration [9,42,43].

It has to be considered that, even though aging lowered the superhydrophilic state of all the surfaces except plasma-etched SLA, none of the investigated surfaces were hydrophobic after aging and at the time point of biological testing. In this respect, our study did not compare real hydrophobic surfaces with superhydrophilic ones but different surface types, each with individual lowered hydrophilicity after aging.

Taken together, our results as well as findings from other groups suggest that hydrophilicity may not be the only determining factor regarding cell attachment and osseointegration. Other factors may play a decisive role in biological responses. These include surface charge, chemical composition, oxidation state, carbonate levels, and hydrocarbon contaminants.

Nanostructures, along with microstructures, accelerate osseointegration and reduce the healing time by improving adhesion and the proliferation time. In search of new, improved surfaces, this study investigated the plasma etching of titanium surfaces with the fluorine gas 2,3,3,3-tetrafluoropropene (R1234yF), which resulted in an additional nanostructure on the sample surfaces. Subsequently, it led to sustained superhydrophilicity and to fluorine accumulation on the surface.

Our study indicates that the plasma etching, with 2,3,3,3-tetrafluoropropene, of the machined and SLA surfaces did not have an adverse effect on the biological performance of the osteoblast cell line SAOS-2. In the osteoblasts, neither the additional nanostructure on the surfaces nor the fluorine content affected the differentiation or performance of the cells. These results agree with Pham et al.'s study [44], who examined the influence of fluoride on the proliferation and differentiation of primary human osteoblasts on HF-etched, untreated TiO_2 and Ti surfaces.

Moreover, there were no differences in cell differentiation over 21 days in this study as well. This contrasts with the results of Lamolle et al. [45]. When comparing titanium discs etched with increasing HF etching times with those not etched, it was shown that surfaces with a higher fluoride content had a less cytotoxic effect and that more cells were present on the surfaces. However, they used the mouse osteoblast cell line MC3T3-E1 for this study rather than human cells, which could explain the different findings. It is also difficult to conclude whether the observed differences are due to the fluoride content of the surfaces, the increased hydrophilicity, or the enlarged roughness caused by etching. However, these contradictory results could also be due to the fact that fluorine plasma etching, rather than wet chemical HF etching, was carried out in this study.

Other studies hypothesize that fluorine-containing surfaces propagate the host-to-implant reaction in early osseointegration [43,46,47], which we could not confirm for the SAOS-2 cell line. In the fibroblast cell line HGF, however, higher viability was detected on the fluorine-plasma-etched samples after 24, 48, and 72 h (SLA_{RyF} "new": after 24 h, 1.18 × increase; after 48 h, 1.64 × increase; after 72 h, 2.85 × increase) (SLA_{RyF} "aged": after 24 h, 1.22 × increase; after 48 h, 1.71 × increase; after 72 h, 2.85 × increase). This contradictory result could be due to the additional nanostructure or to the fluorine content on the fluorine-plasma-etched sample surfaces to which osteoblasts react differently than fibroblasts.

Overall, which surface characteristics are the key players influencing the cascade of biological reactions towards osseointegration and soft-tissue sealing is still controversially discussed. Next to wettability and roughness, it is pivotal to analyze the influence of further physiochemical aspects, like surface tension or surface energy [48].

5. Conclusions

In this study, the biological responses to different wettability levels and nanoscaled structures, which were superimposed, e.g., via plasma fluorine etching, on experimental machined (M) and combined blasted and acid-etched (SLA) titanium implant surfaces were examined. These surface-modifying processes resulted in different surface roughness values. All the surfaces were superhydrophilic directly after a plasma-cleaning process, whereas the hydrophilicity moderately decreased again with aging on the M, M_{nano}, and SLA surfaces. In contrast, the surfaces etched with fluorine gas (M_{RyF} and SLA_{RyF}) showed a long-term, strong hydrophilicity that lasted for at least 14 days.

Although different in surface roughness and hydrophilicity, the initial adhesion of fibroblasts was comparable on all the surfaces. However, after 72 h, the cell coverage rate of fibroblasts and their viability were clearly reduced on the SLA surface. Interestingly, this decrease was not observed on fluorine-gas-etched SLA, indicating that the SLA_{RyF} surface shows better biocompatibility for fibroblasts.

Calcium phosphate deposition by osteoblasts on all the surfaces did not show any significant differences after 21 days. We therefore conclude that other factors are likely to be decisive for cell attachment, cell viability, and osseointegration in addition to surface roughness and wettability. Surface energy and fluorine compounds are two factors that might play a role. Considering the lack of further characterization in terms of surface energy, charge, and contamination or the fact that every surface modification changes several parameters, it seems very difficult to systematically modify a single parameter as a whole. In order to determine the main factors influencing the observed cell reaction or bacterial adhesion and colonization, future analysis will need to be performed.

Supplementary Materials: The following supporting information can be downloaded at: https://www.mdpi.com/article/10.3390/ma16237307/s1, Figure S1: Osteogenic differentiation of osteoblasts on different hydrophobic titanium surfaces. Representative images of the different hydrophobic titanium disks with seeded SAOS-2 at different time points since onset of differentiation. With prolonged differentiation after (a) 7 days, (b) 14 days and (c) 21 days a visible increase in calcium phosphate formation stained with alizarin red is seen (disks diameter: 1.5 cm).

Author Contributions: Conceptualization, B.I. and F.R.; methodology, B.I., J.S. and E.K.-M.; validation, B.I., L.M., A.T., J.S. and S.K.; formal analysis, B.I., J.S. and E.K.-M.; investigation, B.I., J.S. and E.K.-M.; resources, F.R.; data curation, B.I. and S.K.; writing—original draft preparation, B.I., L.M., A.T. and S.K.; writing—review and editing, B.I., L.M., F.R. and S.K.; visualization, B.I. and S.K.; supervision, B.I., F.R. and S.K.; project administration, B.I., S.K. and F.R.; funding acquisition, F.R. All authors have read and agreed to the published version of the manuscript.

Funding: This research was funded by the International Team of Implantology (ITI, Basel, Switzerland), grant number ITI 1232_2017, and by the Federal Ministry for Economic Affairs and Climate Action, Germany, via the Central Innovation Program for small- and medium-sized enterprises (SMEs), grant number ZF4325308.

Institutional Review Board Statement: Not applicable.

Informed Consent Statement: Not applicable.

Data Availability Statement: Data are contained within the article.

Acknowledgments: The authors would like to thank Institute Straumann AG, Basel, Switzerland, for supplying materials and Diener electronic GmbH + Co. KG, Ebhausen, Germany, for the technical implementation of plasma etching with 2,3,3,3-tetrafluoropropene.

Conflicts of Interest: The authors declare no conflict of interest.

References

1. Amoroso, P.F.; Adams, R.J.; Waters, M.G.J.; Williams, D.W. Titanium surface modification and its effect on the adherence of *Porphyromonas gingivalis*: An in vitro study. *Clin. Oral Implant. Res.* **2006**, *17*, 633–637.
2. Palmquist, A.; Johansson, A.; Suska, F.; Brånemark, R.; Thomsen, P. Acute inflammatory response to laser-induced micro- and nano-sized titanium surface features. *Clin. Implant. Dent. Relat. Res.* **2013**, *15*, 96–104. [CrossRef] [PubMed]
3. Wennerberg, A.; Albrektsson, T.; Chrcanovic, B. Long-term clinical outcome of implants with different surface modifications. *Eur. J. Oral Implantol.* **2018**, *11*, S123–S136. [PubMed]
4. Brånemark, P.-I.; Breine, U.; Adell, R.; Hansson, B.O.; Lindström, J.; Ohlsson, Å. Intra-Osseous Anchorage of Dental Prostheses: I. Experimental Studies. *Scand. J. Plast. Reconstr. Surg.* **1969**, *3*, 81–100. [CrossRef] [PubMed]
5. Albrektsson, T.; Zarb, G.; Worthington, P.; Eriksson, A.R. The long-term efficacy of currently used dental implants: A review and proposed criteria of success. *Int. J. Oral Maxillofac. Implant.* **1986**, *1*, 11–25.
6. Kim, J.-J.; Lee, J.-H.; Kim, J.C.; Lee, J.-B.; Yeo, I.-S.L. Biological Responses to the Transitional Area of Dental Implants: Material- and Structure-Dependent Responses of Peri-Implant Tissue to Abutments. *Materials* **2019**, *13*, 72. [CrossRef] [PubMed]
7. Zhang, Z.; Ji, C.; Wang, D.; Wang, M.; Song, D.; Xu, X.; Zhang, D. The burden of diabetes on the soft tissue seal surrounding the dental implants. *Front. Physiol.* **2023**, *14*, 1136973. [CrossRef] [PubMed]
8. Smeets, R.; Stadlinger, B.; Schwarz, F.; Beck-Broichsitter, B.; Jung, O.; Precht, C.; Kloss, F.; Gröbe, A.; Heiland, M.; Ebker, T. Impact of Dental Implant Surface Modifications on Osseointegration. *BioMed Res. Int.* **2016**, *2016*, 6285620. [CrossRef]
9. Schwarz, F.; Wieland, M.; Schwartz, Z.; Zhao, G.; Rupp, F.; Geis-Gerstorfer, J.; Schedle, A.; Broggini, N.; Bornstein, M.M.; Buser, D.; et al. Potential of chemically modified hydrophilic surface characteristics to support tissue integration of titanium dental implants. *J. Biomed. Mater. Res. Part B Appl. Biomater.* **2009**, *88*, 544–557. [CrossRef]

10. Gittens, R.A.; Scheideler, L.; Rupp, F.; Hyzy, S.L.; Geis-Gerstorfer, J.; Schwartz, Z.; Boyan, B.D. A review on the wettability of dental implant surfaces II: Biological and clinical aspects. *Acta Biomater.* **2014**, *10*, 2907–2918. [CrossRef]
11. Toffoli, A.; Parisi, L.; Tatti, R.; Lorenzi, A.; Verucchi, R.; Manfredi, E.; Lumetti, S.; Macaluso, G.M. Thermal-induced hydrophilicity enhancement of titanium dental implant surfaces. *J. Oral Sci.* **2020**, *62*, 217–221. [CrossRef] [PubMed]
12. Zhao, G.; Schwartz, Z.; Wieland, M.; Rupp, F.; Geis-Gerstorfer, J.; Cochran, D.L.; Boyan, B.D. High surface energy enhances cell response to titanium substrate microstructure. *J. Biomed. Mater. Res. Part A* **2005**, *74A*, 49–58. [CrossRef] [PubMed]
13. Feller, L.; Jadwat, Y.; Khammissa, R.A.G.; Meyerov, R.; Schechter, I.; Lemmer, J. Cellular Responses Evoked by Different Surface Characteristics of Intraosseous Titanium Implants. *BioMed Res. Int.* **2015**, *2015*, 171945. [CrossRef] [PubMed]
14. Choi, J.Y.; Jung, U.W.; Lee, I.S.; Kim, C.S.; Lee, Y.K.; Choi, S.H. Resolution of surgically created three-wall intrabony defects in implants using three different biomaterials: An in vivo study. *Clin. Oral Implant. Res.* **2011**, *22*, 343–348. [CrossRef] [PubMed]
15. Zhao, L.; Mei, S.; Chu, P.K.; Zhang, Y.; Wu, Z. The influence of hierarchical hybrid micro/nano-textured titanium surface with titania nanotubes on osteoblast functions. *Biomaterials* **2010**, *31*, 5072–5082. [CrossRef]
16. Liang, J.; Xu, S.; Shen, M.; Cheng, B.; Li, Y.; Liu, X.; Qin, D.; Bellare, A.; Kong, L. Osteogenic activity of titanium surfaces with hierarchical micro-/nano-structures obtained by hydrofluoric acid treatment. *Int. J. Nanomed.* **2017**, *2017*, 1317–1328. [CrossRef] [PubMed]
17. Zhu, M.; Zhang, R.; Mao, Z.; Fang, J.; Ren, F. Topographical biointerface regulating cellular functions for bone tissue engineering. *Biosurface Biotribology* **2022**, *8*, 165–187. [CrossRef]
18. Zhang, J.; Xie, Y.; Zuo, J.; Li, J.; Wei, Q.; Yu, Z.; Tang, Z. Cell responses to titanium treated by a sandblast-free method for implant applications. *Mater. Sci. Eng. C* **2017**, *78*, 1187–1194. [CrossRef]
19. Guida, L.; Oliva, A.; Basile, M.A.; Giordano, M.; Nastri, L.; Annunziata, M. Human gingival fibroblast functions are stimulated by oxidized nano-structured titanium surfaces. *J. Dent.* **2013**, *41*, 900–907. [CrossRef]
20. Schünemann, F.H.; Galárraga-Vinueza, M.E.; Magini, R.; Fredel, M.; Silva, F.; Souza, J.C.M.; Zhang, Y.; Henriques, B. Zirconia surface modifications for implant dentistry. *Mater. Sci. Eng. C Mater. Biol. Appl.* **2019**, *98*, 1294–1305. [CrossRef]
21. Ivanoff, C.J.; Hallgren, C.; Widmark, G.; Sennerby, L.; Wennerberg, A. Histologic evaluation of the bone integration of TiO_2 blasted and turned titanium microimplants in humans. *Clin. Oral Implant. Res.* **2001**, *12*, 128–134. [CrossRef] [PubMed]
22. Wang, Q.; Zhou, P.; Liu, S.; Attarilar, S.; Ma, R.L.W.; Zhong, Y.; Wang, L. Multi-scale surface treatments of titanium implants for rapid osseointegration: A review. *Nanomaterials* **2020**, *10*, 1244. [CrossRef] [PubMed]
23. Abraham, C.M. A Brief Historical Perspective on Dental Implants, Their Surface Coatings and Treatments. *Open Dent. J.* **2014**, *8*, TODENTJ-8-50. [CrossRef] [PubMed]
24. Ostrikov, K.; Neyts, E.C.; Meyyappan, M. Plasma Nanoscience: From Nano-Solids in Plasmas to Nano-Plasmas in Solids. *Adv. Phys.* **2013**, *62*, 113–224. [CrossRef]
25. Dowling, D.P.; Miller, I.S.; Ardhaoui, M.; Gallagher, W.M. Effect of Surface Wettability and Topography on the Adhesion of Osteosarcoma Cells on Plasma-modified Polystyrene. *J. Biomater. Appl.* **2011**, *26*, 327–347. [CrossRef] [PubMed]
26. Asaduzzaman, A. Atomic-Scale Etching Mechanism of Aluminum with Fluorine-Based Plasma. *J. Phys. Chem. C* **2022**, *126*, 14180–14186. [CrossRef]
27. Clainche, T.L.; Linklater, D.; Wong, S.; Le, P.; Juodkazis, S.; Guével, X.L.; Coll, J.-L.; Ivanova, E.P.; Martel-Frachet, V. Mechano-Bactericidal Titanium Surfaces for Bone Tissue Engineering. *ACS Appl. Mater. Interfaces* **2020**, *12*, 48272–48283. [CrossRef]
28. Liang, L.C.; Krieg, P.; Rupp, F.; Kimmerle-Muller, E.; Spintzyk, S.; Richter, M.; Richter, G.; Killinger, A.; Geis-Gerstorfer, J.; Scheideler, L. Osteoblast Response to Different UVA-Activated Anatase Implant Coatings. *Adv. Mater. Interfaces* **2019**, *6*, 1801720. [CrossRef]
29. Engstrand, T.; Kihlström, L.; Lundgren, K.; Trobos, M.; Engqvist, H.; Thomsen, P. Bioceramic implant induces bone healing of cranial defects. *Plast. Reconstr. Surg.—Glob. Open* **2015**, *3*, e491. [CrossRef]
30. Omar, O.; Lennerås, M.; Svensson, S.; Suska, F.; Emanuelsson, L.; Hall, J.; Nannmark, U.; Thomsen, P. Integrin and chemokine receptor gene expression in implant-adherent cells during early osseointegration. *J. Mater. Sci. Mater. Med.* **2010**, *21*, 969–980. [CrossRef]
31. Taylor, S.R.; Gibbons, D.F. Effect of surface texture on the soft tissue response to polymer implants. *J. Biomed. Mater. Res.* **1983**, *17*, 205–227. [CrossRef] [PubMed]
32. Stanford, C.M. Surface modification of biomedical and dental implants and the processes of inflammation, wound healing and bone formation. *Int. J. Mol. Sci.* **2010**, *11*, 354–369. [CrossRef] [PubMed]
33. Yeo, I.S. Reality of dental implant surface modification: A short literature review. *Open Biomed. Eng. J.* **2014**, *8*, 114–119. [CrossRef] [PubMed]
34. Rupp, F.; Liang, L.; Geis-Gerstorfer, J.; Scheideler, L.; Hüttig, F. Surface characteristics of dental implants: A review. *Dent. Mater.* **2018**, *34*, 40–57. [CrossRef] [PubMed]
35. Dalby, M.J.; Gadegaard, N.; Oreffo, R.O. Harnessing nanotopography and integrin–matrix interactions to influence stem cell fate. *Nat. Mater.* **2014**, *13*, 558–569. [CrossRef] [PubMed]
36. Jia, F.; Zhou, L.; Li, S.; Lin, X.; Wen, B.; Lai, C.; Ding, X. Phosphoric acid and sodium fluoride: A novel etching combination on titanium. *Biomed. Mater.* **2014**, *9*, 035004. [CrossRef] [PubMed]
37. Im, J.S.; Choi, H.; An, H.W.; Kwon, T.Y.; Hong, M.H. Effects of Surface Treatment Method Forming New Nano/Micro Hierarchical Structures on Attachment and Proliferation of Osteoblast-like Cells. *Materials* **2023**, *16*, 5717. [CrossRef]

38. Cruz, M.B.; Silva, N.; Marques, J.F.; Mata, A.; Silva, F.S.; Caramês, J. Biomimetic implant surfaces and their role in biological integration—A concise review. *Biomimetics* **2022**, *7*, 74. [CrossRef]
39. Kauzmann, W. Some factors in the interpretation of protein denaturation. In *Advances in Protein Chemistry*; Academic Press: Cambridge, MA, USA, 1959; Volume 14, pp. 1–63.
40. Tengvall, P. Protein Interactions with Biomaterials. *Compr. Biomater.* **2017**, *4*, 63–73.
41. Terheyden, H.; Lang, N.P.; Bierbaum, S.; Stadlinger, B. Osseointegration—Communication of cells. *Clin. Oral Implant. Res.* **2012**, *23*, 1127–1135. [CrossRef]
42. Eriksson, C.; Nygren, H.; Ohlson, K. Implantation of hydrophilic and hydrophobic titanium discs in rat tibia: Cellular reactions on the surfaces during the first 3 weeks in bone. *Biomaterials* **2004**, *25*, 4759–4766. [CrossRef] [PubMed]
43. Coelho, P.G.; Granjeiro, J.M.; Romanos, G.E.; Suzuki, M.; Silva, N.R.; Cardaropoli, G.; Thompson, V.P.; Lemons, J.E. Basic research methods and current trends of dental implant surfaces. *J. Biomed. Mater. Res. B Appl. Biomater.* **2009**, *88*, 579–596. [CrossRef] [PubMed]
44. Pham, M.H.; Landin, M.A.; Tiainen, H.; Reseland, J.E.; Ellingsen, J.E.; Haugen, H.J. The effect of hydrofluoric acid treatment of titanium and titanium dioxide surface on primary human osteoblasts. *Clin. Oral Implant. Res.* **2014**, *25*, 385–394. [CrossRef] [PubMed]
45. Lamolle, S.F.; Monjo, M.; Rubert, M.; Haugen, H.J.; Lyngstadaas, S.P.; Ellingsen, J.E. The effect of hydrofluoric acid treatment of titanium surface on nanostructural and chemical changes and the growth of MC3T3-E1 cells. *Biomaterials* **2009**, *30*, 736–742. [CrossRef]
46. Ellingsen, J.E.; Johansson, C.B.; Wennerberg, A.; Holmen, A. Improved retention and bone-tolmplant contact with fluoride-modified titanium implants. *Int. J. Oral Maxillofac. Implant.* **2004**, *19*, 659–666.
47. Collaert, B.; Wijnen, L.; De Bruyn, H. A 2-year prospective study on immediate loading with fluoride-modified implants in the edentulous mandible. *Clin. Oral. Implants Res.* **2011**, *22*, 1111–1116. [CrossRef] [PubMed]
48. Elias, C.N.; Oshida, Y.; Lima, J.H.C.; Muller, C.A. Relationship between surface properties (roughness, wettability and morphology) of titanium and dental implant removal torque. *J. Mech. Behav. Biomed.* **2008**, *1*, 234–242. [CrossRef]

Disclaimer/Publisher's Note: The statements, opinions and data contained in all publications are solely those of the individual author(s) and contributor(s) and not of MDPI and/or the editor(s). MDPI and/or the editor(s) disclaim responsibility for any injury to people or property resulting from any ideas, methods, instructions or products referred to in the content.

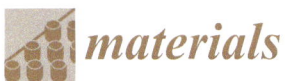

Review

Current Advances of Three-Dimensional Bioprinting Application in Dentistry: A Scoping Review

Nurulhuda Mohd [1], Masfueh Razali [1,*], Mariyam Jameelah Ghazali [2] and Noor Hayaty Abu Kasim [3]

1. Department of Restorative Dentistry, Faculty of Dentistry, Universiti Kebangsaan Malaysia, Jalan Raja Muda Abdul Aziz, Kuala Lumpur 50300, Malaysia
2. Department of Mechanical & Manufacturing Engineering, Faculty of Engineering & Built Environment, Universiti Kebangsaan Malaysia, Bangi 43600, Selangor, Malaysia
3. DLima Dental Clinic, 44-A, Jalan Plumbum N7/N, Seksyen 7, Shah Alam 40000, Selangor, Malaysia
* Correspondence: masfuah@ukm.edu.my

Abstract: Three-dimensional (3D) bioprinting technology has emerged as an ideal approach to address the challenges in regenerative dentistry by fabricating 3D tissue constructs with customized complex architecture. The dilemma with current dental treatments has led to the exploration of this technology in restoring and maintaining the function of teeth. This scoping review aims to explore 3D bioprinting technology together with the type of biomaterials and cells used for dental applications. Based on PRISMA-ScR guidelines, this systematic search was conducted by using the following databases: Ovid, PubMed, EBSCOhost and Web of Science. The inclusion criteria were (i) cell-laden 3D-bioprinted construct; (ii) intervention to regenerate dental tissue using bioink, which incorporates living cells or in combination with biomaterial; and (iii) 3D bioprinting for dental applications. A total of 31 studies were included in this review. The main 3D bioprinting technique was extrusion-based approach. Novel bioinks in use consist of different types of natural and synthetic polymers, decellularized extracellular matrix and spheroids with encapsulated mesenchymal stem cells, and have shown promising results for periodontal ligament, dentin, dental pulp and bone regeneration application. However, 3D bioprinting in dental applications, regrettably, is not yet close to being a clinical reality. Therefore, further research in fabricating ideal bioinks with implantation into larger animal models in the oral environment is very much needed for clinical translation.

Keywords: 3D bioprinting; tissue engineering; cell-laden; bioink; dental tissue regeneration

1. Introduction

Defects in the craniofacial region including the alveolar bone can occur because of periodontitis, motor vehicle accidents, tumor and genetic factors. Periodontitis is the sixth most prevalent disease worldwide and the leading cause of missing teeth, followed by caries and trauma [1,2]. The dilemma of current clinical treatments in treating periodontitis cases is that therapies cannot repair the alveolar bone destruction and restore the functionality of the periodontally involved teeth [3]. In addition, the selection case of the suitable treatment such as guided tissue generation and bone graft strongly depend on the shape and size of the osseous defects. Moreover, rehabilitating the function of the oral cavity by means of dental implant in a severely resorbed alveolar bone may pose a challenge. Several approaches have been utilized for bone regeneration, such as employing the autogenous bone block, allograft and xenograft, however, these conventional treatments come with limitations. The drawbacks of these approaches include (i) donor site morbidity, lack of tissue availability, difficulty to shape and conform to the defect, and graft resorption of the autogenous bone [4–6]; and (ii) high rates of infection and increase risk of host immune response caused by allograft and xenograft [7]. These clinical challenges faced by clinicians and surgeons have led to the exploration of new technology in oral tissue engineering to fabricate functional dental tissue constructs, such as periodontal ligament, dentin–pulp complex and alveolar and craniomaxillofacial bone with patient-specific shape and size [8].

Three-dimensional (3D) bioprinting is an emerging combination technology of 3D printing and tissue engineering [9]. It is an ideal approach to fabricating customized complex 3D tissue constructs with defect-specific architectures through computer-aided design modeling to mimic native tissues [10]. It involves layer-by-layer precise deposition of cell-laden constructs from various biomaterials, cells and bioactive molecules with spatial control of the placement of functional components onto predefined locations (extracellular matrix, cells and pre-organized microvessels) [11–13]. The main advantage of 3D bioprinting is its ability to control the delivery of cells and materials in complex fabricated tissue-like structures. Hence, 3D bioprinted structures can provide cell-to-cell growth interconnectivity for better tissue regeneration [14].

The application of 3D bioprinting techniques that are widely used includes extrusion-based [15,16], inkjet-based [17], laser-assisted [18] and stereolithography [14], as shown in Figure 1. Extrusion-based bioprinting deposits the bioink either using a pneumatic, piston or screw-based system. It is the frequently preferred strategy for the development of multilayer scaffolds in tissue engineering because of the wide range of biomaterials selected for printing, such as natural and synthetic polymers, cell-laden hydrogel and cell aggregates [19,20]. In addition, it can manage high cell density, different material viscosities and crosslinking mechanisms [21]. Meanwhile, in inkjet bioprinting or drop-on-demand technique, it utilizes heating reservoirs, piezoelectric actuators, and electrostatic or electrohydrodynamic methods in order to deposit cells and/or biomaterials in the form of droplets onto the substrates. The advantages of this technique are fast printing speed and low cost. However, nozzle clogging caused by high cell density is one of the disadvantages of this method [11]. Laser-assisted bioprinting (LAB) utilizes a laser as the energy source and consists of an energy-absorbing layer, a donor ribbon and a receiving substrate [22]. This technology employs a noncontact bioprinting method and is nozzle-free, which can be used to deposit high viscosity bioink with a high resolution without nozzle clogging issues [11]. Although this approach results in high cell viability during printing, the effect of laser exposure onto the cells is still not known [23]. Stereolithography (SLA) uses ultraviolet light or an electron beam to initiate a polymerization reaction to place biomaterials onto a substrate. SLA is able to print complex architectures at extremely high resolutions. However, the drawbacks of SLA are its slow printing speed, high cost and limited selection of materials with suitable processing properties [24].

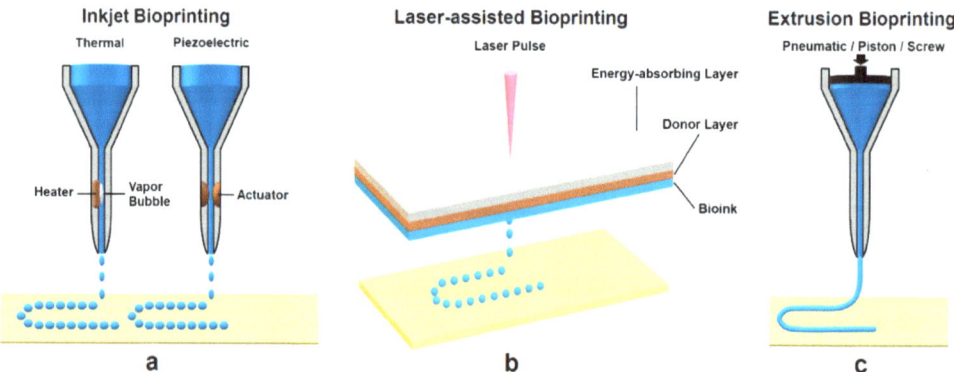

Figure 1. Common 3D bioprinting techniques: (**a**) inkjet bioprinting, (**b**) laser-assisted bioprinting (LAB) and (**c**) extrusion bioprinting [24].

One of the important components of 3D bioprinting is the bioink because of the effect it has on the outcome of the tissue engineering technology. Bioink refers to a formulation of cells that may contain biomaterials and biologically active components suitable for processing by an automated biofabrication technology [25] (see Figure 2). The use of bioinks enables the study of the effects of geometry and spatial organization on cell behavior and function in vitro, which can later be developed into in vivo models for applications in regenerative dentistry. At present, cell printing technology has become the preferred choice for a new biofabrication approach as compared to the conventional method of seeding cells on scaffolds. Three-dimensional bioprinting techniques are now able to incorporate living cells in bioprinted scaffolds, which enhance the position of cells. However, the disadvantage of the approach using scaffolds seeded with cells is that it could cause cell loss, which leads to poor cellular performance [26].

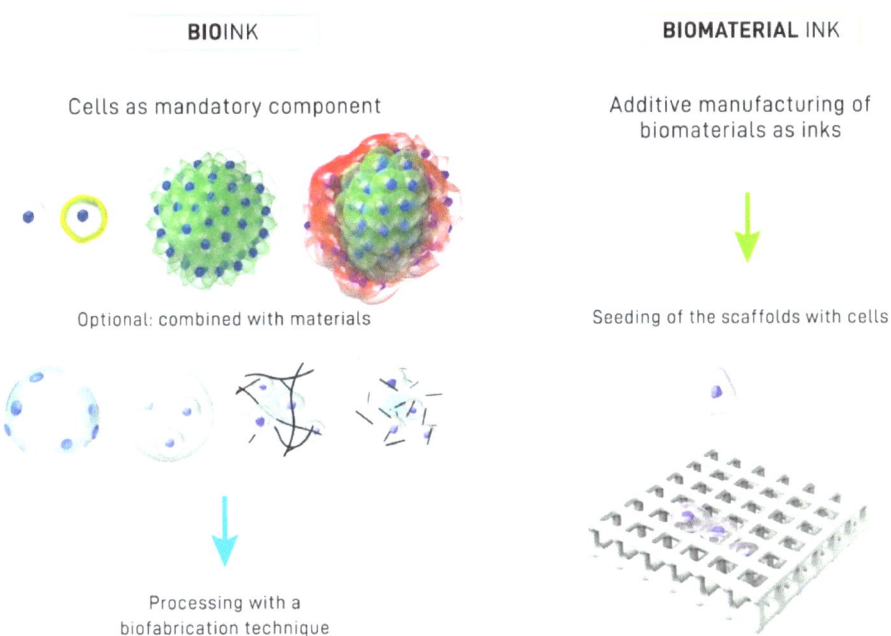

Figure 2. The characteristics distinction between bioink and biomaterial ink. In a bioink, cells are the mandatory component of the printing formulation, which can be in the form of single cells, coated cells and cell aggregates (one or several type of cells). The bioink may contain biomaterials and biologically active components. Meanwhile, the biomaterial ink is where the seeding cells are introduced within biomaterial scaffolds after printing. Reproduced with permission [25]. Copyright 2018 IOP publishing under a Creative Commons Attribution 3.0 Unported (CC BY 3.0). https://creativecommons.org/licenses/by/3.0/ (accessed on 21 August 2022).

Mesenchymal stem cells (MSCs), also known as "universal cells" are the most preferable cell source for tissue regeneration because they have self-renewal capability and can differentiate into various functional cell types under certain conditions [27,28]. MSCs can be isolated from embryonic stem cells or adult stem cells [29]. In addition, they are also easily extracted from almost all tissues (e.g., bone marrow, adipose tissue, umbilical cord and placenta), including dental tissues. Dental stem cells can be obtained from different parts of tissues such as periodontal ligaments (PDLSCs), dental pulp (DPSCs), from apical papilla (SCAPs) or exfoliated deciduous teeth (SHED) [28]. Rich sources of stem cells from the oral cavity have led to the great application and potential use in oral tissue engineering [28] (see Figure 3). Moreover, MSCs are also the most suitable cell source because of their immunomodulatory properties and ability to secrete protective biological factors [30,31].

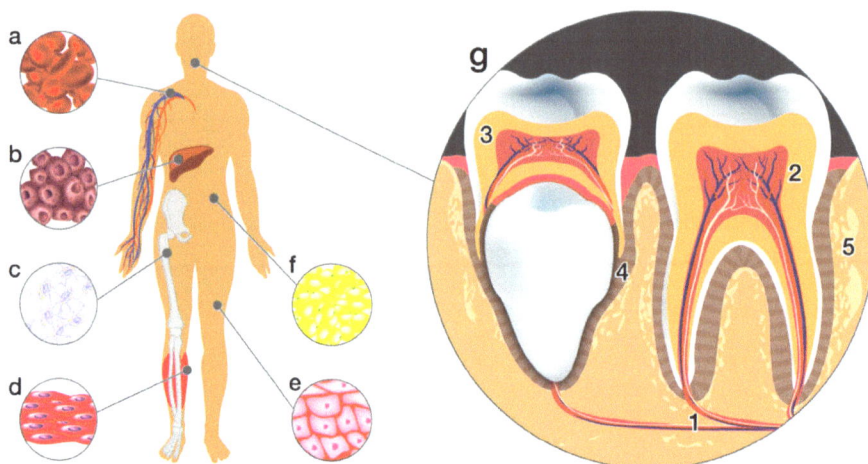

Figure 3. Sources of mesenchymal stem cells. This illustration shows human tissue sources: (**a**) peripheral blood, (**b**) liver, (**c**) bone marrow, (**d**) muscles, (**e**) skin, (**f**) adipose tissue and (**g**) dental tissues: (1. apical dental papilla, 2. dental pulp, 3. pulp from the exfoliated deciduous tooth, 4. periodontal ligament, 5. alveolar bone) [29].

The most common bioink materials are hydrogel-based bioprinted constructs. They have gained popularity in recent years because of similar characteristics to natural extracellular matrix (ECM), homogenous distribution of cells in the scaffolds, their ability to hold live cells, and enhancement of the cell viability in a hydrated 3D environment [32–34]. They can be derived from natural polymers (alginate, agarose, collagen, chitosan, gelatin, hyaluronic acid) or synthetic polymers including poly(ethylene glycol) (PEG), polyglycolic acid (PGA), poly(lactic-co-glycolic acid) (PDGA) and polycaprolactone (PCL). The advantages of natural polymers are the ability to biomimick ECM structure composition, the ability to self-assemble and also their biocompatibility [35], whereas, for synthetic polymers, they have proper degrading rate and photocrosslinking ability, which is not present in the natural polymer [36].

Three-dimensional bioprinting has emerged as a promising treatment strategy for fabricating complex biological constructs in oral tissue engineering, thus solving the issues associated with current therapies and overcoming the limitations of conventional techniques [37]. However, there is limited literature that has reported on the 3D bioprinting applications in dentistry. Therefore, this scoping review aimed to identify the gaps based on the available literature to answer the following questions: (i) How has 3D bioprinting technology been applied in dentistry? (ii) What are the types of biomaterials and cells used in 3D bioprinting?

2. Materials and Methods

2.1. Search Strategy

This review implemented the methodological framework from the Joanna Briggs Institute guidelines for scoping reviews and was carried out based on the Preferred Reporting Items for Systematic Reviews and Meta-Analyses extension for Scoping Review (PRISMA-ScR) [38,39]. The research questions for this review follow: (i) How has 3D bioprinting technology been applied in dentistry? (ii) What are the types of biomaterials and cells used in 3D bioprinting?

A search of the literature published through May 2022 was performed using four databases: Ovid, PubMed, EBSCOhost and Web of Science. The following search terms were used: ("3D bioprinting" OR "3D-bioprint*" OR "3D print*" OR "3D-print*" OR

"Bioprinting" OR "Three-dimensional bioprint*") AND ("Tissue engineering" OR "Tissue regeneration" OR "Bone regeneration" OR "Regenerative medicine" OR "Periodontal regeneration" OR "Guided tissue regeneration") AND ("Dental" OR "Dentistry"). Additional records were identified through a manual search of the references lists. The search was limited to articles in the English language and had no restriction on the time frame of publication year.

2.2. Study Selection

The initial screening of the identified studies was conducted based on the information in the titles and abstracts by two independent reviewers (N.M. and M.R.). In addition, the full text of potentially eligible studies was retrieved for further screening of their suitability determined by inclusion and exclusion criteria. Any disagreement between reviewers on study selection was resolved by a third reviewer (N.H.A.K.) through discussion.

The inclusion criteria for the included studies were defined based on the Participant/Population (P): cell-laden 3D-bioprinted construct; Concept (C): intervention to regenerate dental tissue using bioink that incorporates living cells or also in combination with biomaterial and/or growth factors before or during printing; Context (C): application of 3D bioprinting tissue-engineered in the dental field. However, studies were excluded if they were case reports, review papers or conference abstracts. Articles that reported cell seeding of the scaffolds after printing and were not related to the dental application were also excluded.

2.3. Data Extraction and Analysis

Extraction and synthesis of information from the included studies were summarized and presented into a table of evidence by the first reviewer (N.M.) and verified by the second reviewer (M.R.) to ensure that they were aligned with the research questions. The extracted data of the included studies were publication details (first author, year of publication and country of study), study design (in vitro and in vivo), 3D bioprinting strategy (type of 3D bioprinter and parameters of 3D printing technique), materials, type of cells, animal models characteristics (animal species, gender, age, weight and defect size), and application in dental field and outcomes of the 3D bioprinting.

3. Results
3.1. Study Selection and Characteristics

This revised search strategy generated 548 records from four databases: Ovid ($n = 185$), PubMed ($n = 171$), EBSCOhost ($n = 97$) and Web of Science ($n = 95$) through May 2022. In addition to electronic databases, a manual search of reference lists was carried out through primary sources and additional eligible studies were added ($n = 16$). Out of these, a total of 148 duplicates were excluded and 334 records were assessed based on their titles and abstracts. This was performed by using the online literature review application, Rayyan software (http://rayyan.qcri.org (accessed on 9 September 2022)) [40]. Moreover, full texts of the 82 articles were retrieved for eligibility based on the inclusion and exclusion criteria. Out of those, 51 were further excluded because the articles were not for dental application ($n = 15$), scaffolds seeded with cells after printing ($n = 14$), no cells involved ($n = 9$), wrong study design ($n = 7$), materials are not 3D printed ($n = 4$) and wrong printing technique ($n = 2$). Finally, there were 31 articles included in this review, as recorded in Figure 4.

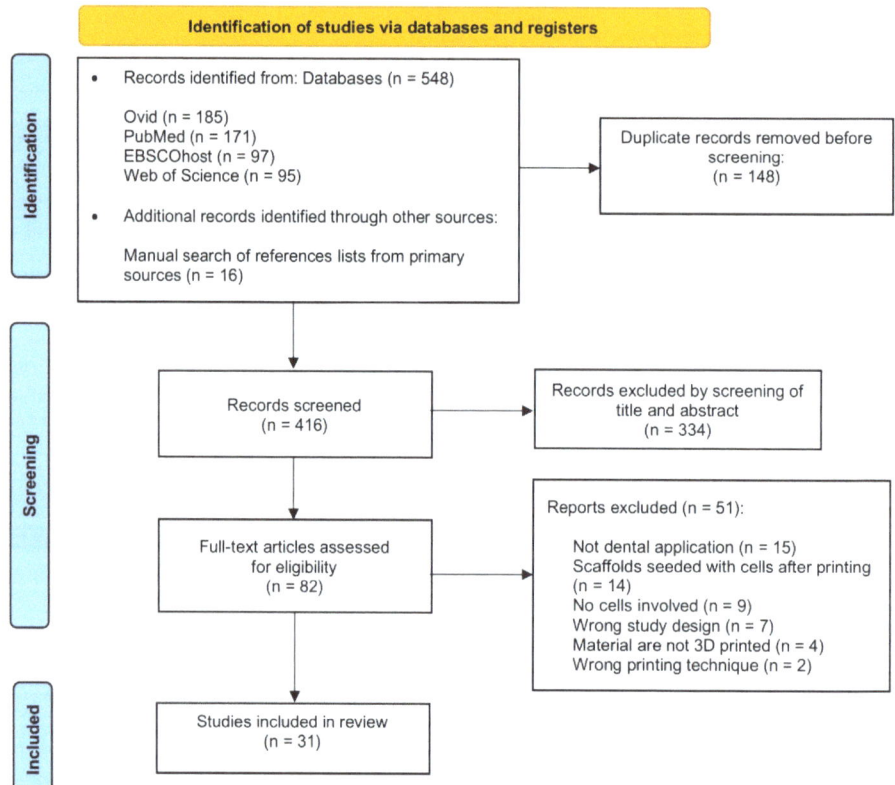

Figure 4. PRISMA flow diagram depicting the results of the search strategy.

3.2. Characteristics of Included Studies

A third of the included articles were conducted in the USA ($n = 10$) [41–50]. It was followed by Korea ($n = 5$) [51–55], France ($n = 4$) [56–59], Germany ($n = 3$) [60–62], China ($n = 3$) [63–65], Taiwan ($n = 2$) [66,67], Canada ($n = 1$) [68], Australia ($n = 1$) [69], Sweden ($n = 1$) [70] and Japan ($n = 1$) [71]. The frequency of publications showed a steady rise from 2015 to the present time, thereby reflecting a growing interest in the 3D bioprinting technology in the dental field. The main characteristics of the included studies are described in Table 1.

Table 1. Summary of the included studies based on cell-laden bioinks.

Author	Cell-Laden Bioink	Other Biomaterial/ Growth Factor	Cell Types	Bioprinting Strategy	Study Design	Application
Lee et al., 2021 [53]	Collagen	FGF-2	hPDLSCs	Extrusion	In vitro and in vivo	PDL regeneration
Wang et al., 2021 [66]	Collagen	SrCS	Human gingiva fibroblasts	Extrusion	In vitro and in vivo	Periodontal regeneration
Kérourédan et al., 2018 [57]	Collagen type 1	-	SCAPs	LAB	In vitro and in vivo	Bone regeneration
Kérourédan et al., 2019 [58]	Collagen type 1	VEGF	SCAPs and HUVECs	LAB	In vivo	Bone regeneration
Duarte Campos et al., 2020 [60]	Collagen type 1 + agarose	-	DPSCs and HUVECs	Inkjet	In vitro and ex vivo	Dental pulp regeneration

Table 1. Cont.

Author	Cell-Laden Bioink	Other Biomaterial/ Growth Factor	Cell Types	Bioprinting Strategy	Study Design	Application
Keriquel et al., 2017 [56]	Collagen type 1 + nHAp	-	Mouse bone marrow stromal precursor D1 cell line	LAB	In vitro and in vivo	Bone regeneration
Moncal et al., 2021 [49]	Collagen + chitosan + β-glycerophosphate + nHAp	rhBMP-2	Rat BMSCs	Extrusion	In vitro	Bone regeneration
Moncal et al., 2022 [50]	Collagen + chitosan + β-glycerophosphate + nHAp	PDGF and BMP-2	Rat BMSCs	Extrusion	In vitro	Bone regeneration
Touya et al., 2022 [59]	Collagen type 1 + TCP (BioRoot RCS®, Septodont, Saint-Maur-des-Fossés, France)	-	SCAPs	LAB	In vitro and in vivo	Bone regeneration
Kim et al., 2022 [55]	Collagen type 1 or dECMs + β-TCP	-	DPSCs	Extrusion	In vitro and in vivo	Dental tissue regeneration
Kang et al., 2016 [41]	Gelatin + fibrinogen + HA + glycerol	PCL/TCP	hAFSCs	Extrusion	In vitro and in vivo	Alveolar bone/bone regeneration
Han et al., 2019 [51]	Gelatin + fibrinogen + HA + glycerol	-	DPSCs	Extrusion	In vitro	Dentin/dental pulp regeneration
Han et al., 2021 [52]	Demineralized dentin matrix particles + fibrinogen + gelatin	-	DPSCs	Extrusion	In vitro	Dental tissue regeneration
Kort-Mascort et al., 2021 [68]	Alginate + gelatin + dECMs	-	Human SCC (Cell lines: UM-SCC-12 and UM-SCC-38)	Extrusion	In vitro	Head and neck cancer in vitro model
Tian et al., 2021 [65]	Sodium alginate + gelatin + nHAp	-	hPDLSCs	Extrusion	In vitro	Bone regeneration
Park et al., 2020 [47]	Gelatin + GelMA + HA + glycerol	BMP-mimetic peptide	DPSCs	Extrusion	In vitro	Dental tissue regeneration
Amler et al., 2021 [62]	GelMA	-	Bone-derived MPC/Bone marrow MPC/Periosteal MPC	Stereolithography	In vitro	Bone regeneration
Raveendran et al., 2019 [69]	GelMA	-	hPDLSCs	Extrusion	In vitro	Periodontal regeneration
Kuss et al., 2017 [42]	MeHA + GelMA + HA	PCL/HAp	Porcine stromal vascular fraction from adipose tissue	Extrusion	In vitro	Alveolar bone/bone regeneration
Ma et al., 2015 [63]	GelMA + PEGDA	-	hPDLSCs	Inkjet	In vitro	Periodontal regeneration
Ma et al., 2017 [64]	GelMA + PEGDA	-	Rat PDLSCs	Inkjet	In vitro and in vivo	Alveolar bone regeneration
Amler et al., 2021 [61]	GelMA + PEGDA3400	-	JHOBs and HUVECs	Stereolithography	In vitro	Alveolar bone in vitro model
Lin et al., 2021 [67]	Calcium silicate + GelMA	-	DPSCs	Extrusion	In vitro	Dentin regeneration
Chimene et al., 2020 [46]	GelMA + kCA + nSi (NICE bioink)	-	Human primary bone marrow-derived MSCs	Extrusion	In vitro	Alveolar bone regeneration
Athirasala et al., 2018 [43]	Alginate + dentin matrix	-	SCAPs	Extrusion	In vitro	Dentin/dental pulp regeneration
Walladbegi et al., 2020 [70]	Nanofibrillated cellulose + alginate (CELLINK AB, Gothenburg, Sweden)	β-TCP	hADSCs	Extrusion	In vitro	Bone regeneration
Dubey et al., 2020 [48]	ECM + AMP	-	DPSCs	Extrusion	In vitro	Bone regeneration

Table 1. Cont.

Author	Cell-Laden Bioink	Other Biomaterial/ Growth Factor	Cell Types	Bioprinting Strategy	Study Design	Application
Dutta et al., 2021 [54]	Poloxamer-407	-	SCAPs	Extrusion	In vitro	Dental tissue regeneration
Aguilar et al., 2019 [44]	-	-	Mice bone marrow stromal cells	Scaffold-free (Kenzan method)	In vitro	Bone regeneration
Aguilar et al., 2019 [45]	-	-	Mice bone marrow stromal cells	Scaffold-free (Kenzan method)	In vitro	Bone regeneration
Ono et al., 2021 [71]	-	-	Human PDL cell line 1-17	Scaffold-free (Needle array)	In vitro	PDL regeneration

LAB, laser-assisted bioprinting; GelMA, gelatin methacryloyl; PEGDA, poly(ethylene glycol) dimethacrylate; HA, hyaluronic acid; PCL, poly (ε-caprolactone); TCP, tricalcium phosphate; MeHA, methacrylated hyaluronic acid; kCA, kappa-carrageenan; HAp, hydroxyapatite; nHAp, nano-hydroxyapatite; AMP, amorphous magnesium phosphates; nSi, nanosilicates; Poloxamer-407, synthetic copolymer of poly(ethylene glycol) and poly(propylene glycol); ECM, extracellular matrix; dECM, decellularized extracellular matrix; SrCS, strontium-doped calcium silicate; hPDLSCs, human periodontal ligament stem cells; hAFSCs, human amniotic fluid-derived stem cells; SCAPs, human stem cells from apical papilla; DPSCs, human dental pulp stem cells; HUVECs, human umbilical vein endothelial cells; MSCs, mesenchymal stem cells; BMSCs, bone marrow mesenchymal stem cells; hADSCs, human adipose tissue-derived mesenchymal stem cells; JHOBs, jawbone-derived human osteoblasts; MPC, human mesenchymal progenitor cells; SCC, squamous cell carcinoma; VEGF, vascular endothelial growth factor; BMP, bone morphogenetic protein; rhBMP, recombinant bone morphogenetic protein; FGF, fibroblast growth factor; PDGF, platelet-derived growth factor.

3.3. Three-Dimensional Bioprinting Strategy for Dental Application

Nearly two-thirds of the research reported in this review used extrusion-based 3D bioprinting technique to fabricate scaffolds. This technique was used in eight studies for bone regeneration application [41,42,46,48–50,65,70], four studies used for general dental tissue regeneration [47,52,54,55], another three for periodontal ligament [53,66,69] and followed by dentin and dental pulp regeneration [43,51,67]. Apart from regeneration application, extrusion-based technique has also been used to explore the usage of scaffolds for head and neck cancer in vitro models [68]. For laser-assisted bioprinting, all the studies utilized this technology for bone regeneration [56–59]. However, for inkjet-based technique, there was various usage for regeneration of periodontal ligament [63], dental pulp [60] and bone [64]. Meanwhile, the other technique, stereolithography, has been used for bone regeneration [62] and alveolar bone in vitro modeling [61]. Another 3D bioprinting technique, which is a scaffold-free method, 3D tissue spheroids (cell aggregates) bioinks were developed by skewering individual cellular spheroids into a predetermined design onto a needle-array platform without any supporting hydrogel or matrix. This technique has been employed for periodontal ligament [71] and bone regeneration [44,45]. Overall, half of the studies used 3D bioprinting for alveolar bone/bone regeneration for dental tissue engineering application. Figure 5 shows 3D bioprinting in dental applications. The other information, such as the type of bioprinters and 3D bioprinting, is presented in Table 2.

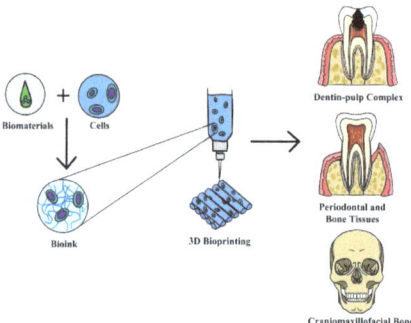

Figure 5. Three-dimensional bioprinting strategy for dental application such as regeneration of dentin–pulp complex, periodontal, alveolar bone tissues and craniomaxillofacial bone.

Table 2. Characteristics of the 3D bioprinting techniques.

Author	Cell-Laden Bioink	Type of Polymer	3D Bioprinter	3D Bioprinting Technique	Nozzle Size	Printing Speed	Printing Pressure	Crosslinking Method	Study Outcomes
Lee et al., 2021 [53]	Collagen	Natural	3DX Printer, T and R Biofab Co., Ltd., Siheung, Korea	Extrusion	400 μm ~22G	-	-	Thermal	Connective tissues interface between 3D-printed implants and calvaria bone has periodontal ligament characteristics; however, FGF-2 did not play a role in periodontal regeneration
Wang et al., 2021 [66]	Collagen	Natural	BioScaffolder 3.1, GeSiM, Großerkmannsdorf, Germany	Extrusion	400 μm ~22G	1.5–2 mm/s	10–20 kPa	Physical	Novel bilayer 3D printed SrCS with collagen bioink upregulate angiogenic- and osteogenic-related proteins and factors, and enhanced bone regeneration in vivo
Kérourédan et al., 2018 [57]	Collagen type 1	Natural	LAB workstation (U1026, Inserm, Bordeaux, France)	LAB	-	-	-	-	Potential use of magnetic resonance imaging and bioprinted micron superparamagnetic iron oxide-labeled cells to track cell patterns in vitro and calvarium defect model in mouse
Kérourédan et al., 2019 [58]	Collagen type 1	Natural	LAB workstation (U1026, Inserm, Bordeaux, France)	LAB	-	-	-	-	In situ printing of HUVECs enhance vascularization and bone regeneration in calvarial defects
Duarte Campos et al., 2020 [60]	Collagen type 1 + agarose	Natural	Hand-held bioprinter (Drop-Gun, BlackDrop Biodrucker GmbH, Aachen, Germany)	Inkjet	300 μm ~23G	-	25–250 kPa	Thermal	Handheld in situ bioprinting of cell-loaded collagen-based bioinks demonstrated successful vasculogenesis
Keriquel et al., 2017 [56]	Collagen type 1 + nHAp	Natural	LAB workstation (U1026, Inserm, Bordeaux, France)	LAB	-	250 μm/s	-	-	3D printed disk form of nHAp-collagen and D1 cells (bone marrow stromal precursor cells) showed the formation of mature bone in a calvarial defect model
Moncal et al., 2021 [49]	Collagen + chitosan + β-glycerophosphate + nHAp	Natural	In-house developed MultiArm Bioprinter, Iowa City, IA, USA	Extrusion	22G–410 μm	400 mm/min	80–140 kPa	Thermal and physical	Hybrid intra-operative bioprinting induced bone regeneration with nearly 80% regenerated critical size calvarial bone defect
Moncal et al., 2022 [50]	Collagen + chitosan + β-glycerophosphate + nHAp	Natural	In-house developed MultiArm Bioprinter, Iowa City, IA, USA	Extrusion	22G–410 μm	400 mm/min	80–140 kPa	Thermal and physical	Bioprinted bone constructs with the controlled co-delivery release of growth factors resulted in bone regeneration in critical-sized calvarial defects

Table 2. Cont.

Author	Cell-Laden Bioink	Type of Polymer	3D Bioprinter	3D Bioprinting Technique	Nozzle Size	Printing Speed	Printing Pressure	Crosslinking Method	Study Outcomes
Touya et al., 2022 [59]	Collagen type 1 + TCP (BioRoot RCS®, Septodont, France)	Natural	LAB workstation (U1026, Inserm, Bordeaux, France)	LAB	-	-	-	-	TCP-based ink demonstrated positive significance upon cell motility, and early osteogenic differentiation in vitro. However, the bioink was not successful in regenerating critical size cranial bone defects in vivo
Kim et al., 2022 [55]	Collagen type 1 or dECMs + β-TCP	Natural	DTR3-2210 T-SG; DASA Robot, Bucheon, Korea	Extrusion	250 μm ~25G	10 mm/s	17–22 kPa	Genipin	The hDPSC-laden bone-derived dECM biocomposite enhanced both osteogenic and odontogenic differentiation in vitro and in vivo
Kang et al., 2016 [41]	Gelatin + fibrinogen + HA + glycerol	Natural	Integrated tissue-organ printing system	Extrusion	300 μm ~23 G	-	50–80 kPa	Thrombin	3D tissue construct provides a favorable microenvironment for osteogenic differentiation of hAFSCs in vitro and showed the formation of mature, vascularized bone tissues in the calvarial bone defect model
Han et al., 2019 [51]	Gelatin + fibrinogen + HA + glycerol	Natural	Integrated tissue-organ printing system	Extrusion	250 μm ~25G	50–90 mm/min	-	Thrombin	Fibrin-based cell-laden bioink demonstrated spatial regulation of DPSC differentiation for the construction of 3D dentin-pulp complexes
Han et al., 2021 [52]	Demineralized dentin matrix particles + fibrinogen + gelatin	Natural	Homemade 3D bioprinter, Ulsan, Korea	Extrusion	300 μm ~23G	50 mm/min	200 kPa	Thrombin	DDMp bioink can be used to fabricate 3D cellular dental constructs and showed significantly improvement in odontogenic differentiation of DPSCs
Kort-Mascort et al., 2021 [68]	Alginate + gelatin + dECMs	Natural	BioScaffolder 3.1, GeSiM, Großerkmannsdorf, Germany	Extrusion	22G ~400 μm	10 ± 2 mm/s	45 ± 10 kPa	Calcium chloride	Cell-laden dECM-based bioink demonstrated tumor spheroids development by squamous cell carcinoma cells with high cell viability and proliferation
Tian et al., 2021 [65]	Sodium alginate + gelatin + nHAp	Natural	3D Bioplotter (EnvisionTEC GmbH, Gladbeck, Germany)	Extrusion	400 μm ~22G	6 mm/s	200 kPa	Calcium chloride	The hPDLSCs-laden bioink demonstrated good biocompatibility, stimulation of cell survival, proliferation and osteoblast
Park et al., 2020 [47]	Gelatin + GelMA + HA + glycerol	Natural	Integrated tissue-organ printing system	Extrusion	330 μm ~23G	150 mm/min	130–160 kPa	Photopolymerization	Novel BMP-GelMA bioink showed high viability, proliferation and odontogenic differentiation of hDPSC
Amler et al., 2021 [62]	GelMA	Natural	Cellbricks GmbH, Berlin, Germany	Stereolithography	-	-	-	Photopolymerization	Periosteum-derived cells showed higher mineralization of print matrix and superior osteogenic potential for 3D bone constructs

Table 2. Cont.

Author	Cell-Laden Bioink	Type of Polymer	3D Bioprinter	3D Bioprinting Technique	Nozzle Size	Printing Speed	Printing Pressure	Crosslinking Method	Study Outcomes
Ravendran et al., 2019 [69]	GelMA	Natural	BioScaffolder 3.1, GeSiM, Großerkmannsdorf, Germany	Extrusion	~220 μm 25G	10–12 mm/s	135 kPa	Photopolymerization	The best 3D bioprinting outcome of the periodontal ligament was obtained using 12.5% GelMA concentration with 0.05% LAP extruded through a 25G needle at 135kPa and crosslinking with UV-irradiation
Kuss et al., 2017 [42]	MeHA + GelMA + HA	Natural	3D Bioplotter (EnvisionTEC GmbH, Gladbeck, Germany)	Extrusion	~400 μm 22G	1.8–2.2 mm/s	-	Photopolymerization	Short-term hypoxia (up to 7 days) promoted microvessel formation of SVFC-laden constructs without significantly affecting the cell viability compared to long-term hypoxia (more than 14 days)
Ma et al., 2015 [63]	GelMA + PEGDA	Natural and synthetic	Customer-designed pressure-assisted valve-based bioprinting system	Inkjet	150 μm ~30G	-	40–60 kPa	Photopolymerization	Volume ratios of GelMA to PEG bioink have an impact on cell viability and spreading of hPDLSCs. The increasing ratio of PEG leads to a decrease in hPDLSCs viability and spreading area
Ma et al., 2017 [64]	GelMA + PEGDA	Natural and synthetic	Customer-designed pressure-assisted valve-based bioprinting system	Inkjet	150 μm ~30G	-	50 kPa	Photopolymerization	An increase in the volume ratio of 3D GelMA-PEGDA in vitro resulted in an increase in cell proliferation, spreading and osteogenic differentiation of PDLSCs. New bone formation was observed in the alveolar defect treated with 3D bioprinted PDLSC hydrogel in a rat model
Amler et al., 2021 [61]	GelMA + PEGDA3400	Natural and synthetic	Cellbricks GmbH, Berlin, Germany	Stereolithography	-	-	-	Photopolymerization	3D bioprinted constructs containing primary JHOBs with vasculature-like channel structures comprising endothelial cells demonstrated the survival of both cells and mineralization of the bone matrix
Lin et al., 2021 [67]	Calcium silicate + GelMA	Natural	BioX, CELLINK, Gothenburg, Sweden	Extrusion	30G–150 μm	20 mm/s	180 kPa	Photopolymerization	Calcium silicate/GelMA scaffolds enhanced mechanical properties and odontogenesis of hDPSCs
Chimene et al., 2020 [46]	GelMA + kCA + nSi (NICE bioink)	Natural	Modified ANET A8 3D printer, Shenzhen, China	Extrusion	400 μm ~22G	15 mm/s	-	Photopolymerization	3D NICE cell-laden bioink demonstrated the ability to form osteo-related mineralized ECM without the growth factor
Athirasala et al., 2018 [43]	Alginate + dentin matrix	Natural	Hyrel 3D, Norcross, GA, USA	Extrusion	Coaxial: 26–19G	-	-	Calcium chloride	Cell-laden alginate and dentin matrix enhances odontogenic differentiation of SCAPs

Table 2. Cont.

Author	Cell-Laden Bioink	Type of Polymer	3D Bioprinter	3D Bioprinting Technique	Nozzle Size	Printing Speed	Printing Pressure	Crosslinking Method	Study Outcomes
Walladbegi et al., 2020 [70]	Nanofibrillated cellulose + alginate (CELLINK AB, Gothenburg, Sweden)	Natural	Inkredible, CELLINK AB, Gothenburg, Sweden	Extrusion	Coaxial: 22–16G	-	75 kPa and 85 kPa	Calcium chloride	A coaxial needle enables the printing of a stable scaffold with viable hADSCs
Dubey et al., 2020 [48]	ECM + AMP	Natural	3DDiscovery, regenHU, Villaz-St-Pierre, Switzerland	Extrusion	-	15–20 mm/s	30–50 kPa	Physical	ECM/AMP-bioprinted constructs demonstrated osteogenic differentiation of DPSCs without the need for chemical inducers
Dutta et al., 2021 [54]	Poloxamer-407	Synthetic	CELLINK BIO-X 3D printer, Gothenburg, Sweden	Extrusion	27G	5 mm/s	35 kPa	Photopolymerization	3D bioprinted poloxamer hydrogels with low voltage–frequency electromagnetic fields stimulation (5V-1 Hz, 0.62 mT) enhance the SCAPs viability and osteogenic potential
Aguilar et al., 2019 [44]	-	-	Regenova Bio 3D Printer, Cyfuse K.K, Tokyo, Japan	Scaffold-free (Kenzan method)	-	-	-	-	Centrifugation cell method generated tighter BMSC spheroid formation with the optimal technique of 40k cells aggregate under 150-300G
Aguilar et al., 2019 [45]	-	-	Regenova Bio 3D Printer, Cyfuse K.K, Tokyo, Japan	Scaffold-free (Kenzan method)	-	-	-	-	Optimization of scaffold-free bioprinting resulted in a reduction in print times, the use of bioprinting nozzles and fabrication of more robust constructs
Ono et al., 2021 [71]	-	-	Regenova Bio 3D Printer, Cyfuse K.K, Tokyo, Japan	Scaffold-free (Needle array)	240 μm ~26G	-	-	-	3D bioprinted tubular structures and hydroxyapatite core materials exhibited high cell viability, collagen fibers and strongly expressed factors associated with periodontal ligament tissues

3D, three-dimensional; LAB, laser-assisted bioprinting; USA, United States of America; GelMA, gelatin methacryloyl; PEG, poly(ethylene glycol); PEGDA, poly(ethylene glycol) dimethacrylate; HA, hyaluronic acid; TCP, tricalcium phosphate; MeHA, methacrylated hyaluronic acid; kCA, kappa-carrageenan; nHAp, nano-hydroxyapatite; AMP, amorphous magnesium phosphates; nSi, nanosilicates; Poloxamer-407, synthetic copolymer of poly(ethylene glycol) and poly(propylene glycol); ECM, extracellular matrix; dECM, decellularized extracellular matrix; LAP, lithium phenyl-2,4,6-trimethylbenzoylphosphinate; DDMp, demineralized dentin matrix particles; SrCS, strontium-doped calcium silicate; SVFC, stromal vascular fraction derived cells; hPDLSCs, human periodontal ligament stem cells; hAFSCs, human amniotic fluid-derived stem cells; SCAPs, human stem cells from apical papilla; DPSCs, human dental pulp stem cells; HUVECs, human umbilical vein endothelial cells; MSCs, mesenchymal stem cells; BMSCs, bone marrow mesenchymal stem cells; hADSCs, human adipose tissue-derived mesenchymal stem cells; JHOBs, jawbone-derived human osteoblasts; FGF, fibroblast growth factor; UV, ultraviolet.

3.4. Bioinks for 3D Bioprinting

In this review, the majority of cell-laden bioinks consist of combinations of two to four polymers and/or biomaterials for 3D bioprinting applications. The commonly used materials for the fabrication of bioinks were natural polymers (collagen, gelatin, fibrin, alginate, hyaluronic acid (HA), chitosan, agarose and glycerol). Naturally derived polymers with chemical modifications such as gelatin methacryloyl (GelMA) and methacrylated hyaluronic acid (MeHA) also have been used as bioinks. Only one study used synthetic polymer alone, Poloxamer-407, a synthetic copolymer of poly(ethylene glycol) and poly(propylene glycol) [54]. Meanwhile, three studies used hybrid materials that are the combination of GelMA and poly(ethylene glycol) dimethacrylate (PEGDA) [61,63,64].

Decellularized extracellular matrix (dECM)-based, also termed tissue-specific bioink, was used by two studies [52,55]. In addition, some studies added bioceramics materials such as nano-hydroxyapatite [49,50,56,65], calcium phosphate [55] and calcium silicate [59,67] with composite bioinks. Bone morphogenetic protein (BMP) was the most commonly used growth factor reported in this review [47,49]. Other growth factors such as vascular endothelial growth factor (VEGF) [58] and fibroblast growth factors (FGF) [53] have also been investigated within 3D bioprinted constructs. Meanwhile, one study utilized gene-based growth factors using a nonviral gene delivery method, which was the combination of platelet-derived growth factor-B encoded plasmid DNA (pPDGF-B) and bone morphogenetic protein-2 encoded plasmid DNA (pBMP2) [50].

In 3D bioprinting, the crosslinking approach is an important aspect to achieve the biomechanical stability of 3D constructs. Herein, the collagen-based bioinks were crosslinked either using temperature [53,60] or physical [66], or a combination of both [49,50], or genipin [55]. Eight studies used GelMA, the modified naturally derived polymer, which was crosslinked by photopolymerization [46,47,54,61–64,67,69]. Synthetic polymer, Poloxamer-407 also uses UV light for photocrosslinking [54]. Apart from that, alginate bioink used calcium chloride as its crosslinker [43,65,68,70]. Fibrin-based bioink can be made from fibrinogen by enzymatic reaction of thrombin [41,51,52].

3.5. Cells for 3D Bioprinting

Types of cells for 3D bioprinting reported in this review were mesenchymal stem cells and cell lines. Stems cells isolated from the human oral cavity have been used, such as periodontal ligament stem cells (PDLSCs) [53,63,65,69], dental pulp stem cells (DPSCs) [47,48,51,52,55,60,67] and stem cells from apical papilla (SCAPs) [43,54,57–59]. Meanwhile, one study used gingival fibroblast in the cell-laden bioink [66]. In this review, human dental stem cells were isolated from third molar teeth of young healthy patients with an age range of 18–28 years old. Only one study isolated nonhuman periodontal ligament stem cells from rats [64].

As reported in this review, other main sources of cells used were nondental-origin stem cells from bone marrow [44–46,49,50,62] and adipose tissue [42,70]. Apart from this, some studies used extracted cells derived from bone [61,62], periosteum [62], amniotic fluid [41] and umbilical vein [58,60,61]. These MSCs sources were from humans and various animals such as rats, mice and porcine. Furthermore, two studies implemented a co-culture approach using SCAPs and human umbilical vein endothelial cells (HUVECs) [58], DSPCs and HUVECS [60] in their research.

Other types of cells that have been used were human squamous cell carcinoma lines from cancer larynx (UM-SCC-12) and tonsillar pillar (UM-SCC-38) [68], multipotent clonal human PDL cell line (line 1–17) [71] and mouse bone marrow stromal precursor D1 cell line [56]. Herein, 3D bioprinting produces high cell viability after printing in the range of 70% to greater than 95%. The details of the type of cells used in 3D bioprinting are presented in Table 3.

Table 3. Characteristics of cell types in 3D bioprinting application.

Author	Cell Type	Cell Densities	Max Cell Viability (%)	3D Bioprinting Technique	Targeted Tissue
Han et al., 2019 [51]	DPSCs	3×10^6 cells/mL	>90	Extrusion	Dentin/dental pulp
Park et al., 2020 [47]	DPSCs	-	>90	Extrusion	Dental tissue
Dubey et al., 2020 [48]	DPSCs	1×10^6 cells/mL	>90	Extrusion	Bone
Han et al., 2021 [52]	DPSCs	3×10^6 cells/mL	>95	Extrusion	Dental tissue
Lin et al., 2021 [67]	DPSCs	5×10^6 cells/mL	-	Extrusion	Dentin/pulp
Kim et al., 2022 [55]	DPSCs	1×10^7 cells/mL	>95	Extrusion	Dental tissue
Duarte Campos et al., 2020 [60]	DPSCs and HUVECs	3×10^6 cells/mL (both type of cells)	-	Inkjet	Dental pulp
Ma et al. 2015 [63]	hPDLSCs	1×10^6 cells/mL	82.4 ± 4.7	Inkjet	Periodontal ligament
Raveendran et al., 2019 [69]	hPDLSCs	2.0×10^6 cells/mL	>70	Extrusion	Periodontal ligament
Lee et al., 2021 [53]	hPDLSCs	1×10^7 cells/mL	-	Extrusion	Periodontal ligament
Tian et al., 2021 [65]	hPDLSCs	-	-	Extrusion	Bone
Ma et al., 2017 [64]	Rat PDLSCs	1×10^6 cells/mL	~90	Inkjet	Bone
Athirasala et al., 2018 [43]	SCAPs	0.8×10^6 cells/mL	>90%	Extrusion	Dentin/dental pulp
Kérourédan et al., 2018 [57]	SCAPs	7×10^7 cells/mL	-	LAB	Bone
Dutta et al., 2021 [54]	SCAPs	2.5×10^4 cells/mL	-	Extrusion	Dental tissue
Touya et al., 2022 [59]	SCAPs	2×10^3 cells/mL	-	LAB	Bone
Kérourédan et al., 2019 [58]	SCAPs and HUVECs	7×10^7 cells/mL	-	LAB	Bone
Wang et al., 2021 [66]	Human gingiva fibroblasts	5×10^5 cells/mL	-	Extrusion	Periodontal ligament/Bone
Ono et al., 2021 [71]	Human PDL cell line 1–17	2.5×10^4 cells/mL	-	Scaffold-free (Kenzan method)	Periodontal ligament
Kort-Mascort et al., 2021 [68]	Human SCC (Cell lines: UM-SCC-12 and UM-SCC-38)	1×10^6 cells/mL	>95	Extrusion	Dental tissue
Chimene et al., 2020 [46]	Human primary bone marrow-derived MSCs	-	-	Extrusion	Bone
Amler et al., 2021 [62]	Bone-derived MPC/Bone marrow MPC/Periosteal MPC	20×10^6 cells/mL	-	Stereolithography	Bone
Moncal et al., 2021 [49]	Rat BMSCs	5×10^6 cells/mL	>95	Extrusion	Bone
Moncal et al., 2022 [50]	Rat BMSCs	8×10^5 cells/mL	>95	Extrusion	Bone
Aguilar et al., 2019 [44]	Mice bone marrow stromal cells	-	-	Scaffold-free (Kenzan method)	Bone
Aguilar et al., 2019 [45]	Mice bone marrow stromal cells	-	-	Scaffold-free (Kenzan method)	Bone
Keriquel et al., 2017 [56]	Mouse bone marrow stromal precursor D1 cell line	120×10^6 cells/mL	-	LAB	Bone
Amler et al., 2021 [61]	JHOBs and HUVECs	20×10^6 cells/mL	-	Stereolithography	Bone
Walladbegi et al., 2020 [70]	hADSCs	4×10^6 cells/mL	~80	Extrusion	Bone
Kuss et al., 2017 [42]	Porcine stromal vascular fraction from adipose tissue	4×10^6 cells/mL	-	Extrusion	Bone
Kang et al., 2016 [41]	hAFSCs	5×10^6 cells/mL	91 ± 2	Extrusion	Bone

LAB, laser-assisted bioprinting; hPDLSCs, human periodontal ligament stem cells; hAFSCs, human amniotic fluid-derived stem cells; SCAPs, human stem cells from apical papilla; DPSCs, human dental pulp stem cells; HUVECs, human umbilical vein endothelial cells; MSCs, mesenchymal stem cells; BMSCs, bone marrow mesenchymal stem cells; hADSCs, human adipose tissue-derived mesenchymal stem cells; JHOBs, jawbone-derived human osteoblasts; MPC, human mesenchymal progenitor cells; SCC, squamous cell carcinoma.

3.6. In Vivo Application in Dental Tissue Engineering

Out of 31 studies, a total of 11 studies reported in vivo applications on animal models. However, only nine studies used cell-based scaffolds and the other three were cell-free bioprinted constructs implanted in vivo using the extrusion-based technique. Therefore, in this review, only nine studies were reported for in vivo evaluation, which involve implantation of the 3D bioprinted constructs into calvarium [41,53,56–59,66], alveolar bone [64] and subcutaneous area [55]. The calvarial bone defects were surgically created without penetration into the dura with a diameter ranging from 3.3 to 8 mm. In addition, the alveolar defect was created with a dimension of 4 mm length × 3 mm width × 2 mm height. One study reported implantation of bioprinted constructs (8 × 8 × 4 mm^3) on dorsal subcutaneous pockets. Meanwhile, for animal models in this review, only one article used rabbits as osteoporotic models in their study [66], whereas the others used immunodeficient rats or mice (either athymic, balb/c, NOG or NSG mice) as their animal models [41,53,55,57–59,64].

Moreover, four studies reported performing in situ or intra-operative bioprinting of the 3D constructs during surgical intervention on the cranial bony defects using laser-assisted bioprinting, as shown in Figure 6 [56–59]. After implantation of the 3D printed constructs, the animals were euthanized at time points ranging from 3 to 20 weeks to harvest implanted specimens. The characteristics of the animal models are summarized in Table 4.

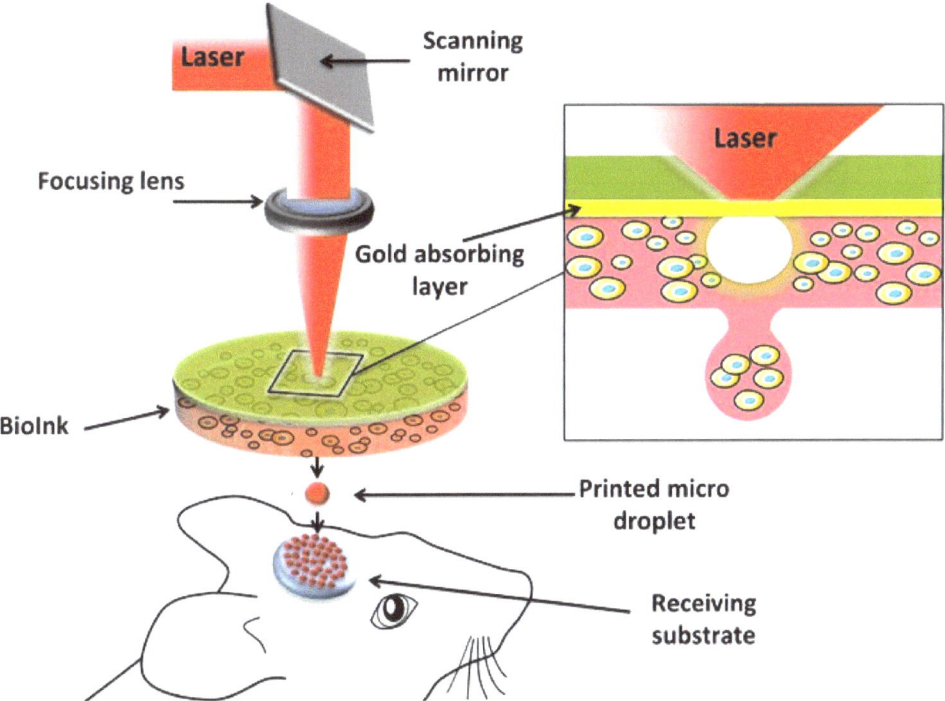

Figure 6. Intra-operative bioprinting (IOB) using laser-assisted bioprinting (LAB) approach in vivo application. LAB setup comprises a pulsed laser beam, a ribbon (transparent glass slide coated with a laser-absorbing layer of metal) and a receiving substrate. Reproduced with permission [56]. Copyright 2017 SpringerNature publishing under a Creative Commons Attribution 4.0 International (CC BY 4.0). (https://creativecommons.org/licenses/by/4.0/ (accessed on 21 August 2022)).

Table 4. Summary of animal model characteristics.

Author	Animal Model	Sex	Age	Weight	Defect Area	Defect Size	In Situ Printing	Time of Sacrifice
Keriquel et al., 2017 [56]	Balb/c mice	Female	12 weeks	19–20 g	Calvarium	3.3 mm diameter	Yes	8 weeks
Kérourédan et al., 2018 [57]	NOG mice	Female	10 weeks	25–26 g	Calvarium	3.3 mm diameter	Yes	-
Kérourédan et al., 2019 [58]	NSG mice	Female	10 weeks	25–26 g	Calvarium	3.3 mm diameter	Yes	4 or 8 weeks
Touya et al., 2022 [59]	NSG mice	Female	8 weeks	-	Calvarium	3.3 mm diameter	Yes	4 weeks or 8 weeks
Kang et al., 2016 [41]	Sprague Dawley rats	-	-	250–300 g	Calvarium	8 mm diameter, 1.2 mm depth	No	20 weeks
Lee et al., 2021 [53]	Athymic rats	Male	9 weeks	-	Calvarium	8 mm diameter, 1.5 mm depth	No	6 weeks
Wang et al., 2021 [66]	New Zealand white rabbit	Female	-	2 kg	Calvarium	7 mm diameter, 8 mm depth	No	12 weeks
Ma et al., 2017 [64]	Sprague Dawley rats	-	33 months	230–250 g	Alveolar bone	4 mm length × 3 mm width × 2 mm height	No	3 and 6 weeks
Kim et al., 2022 [55]	Athymic nude mice	-	-	-	Dorsal subcutaneous	-	No	8 weeks

4. Discussion

Three-dimensional bioprinting has become an advanced tissue engineering approach to create dental tissue constructs to address the need for regenerative dentistry. The studies included in this review showed a wide range of heterogeneity in terms of different types of novel bioinks, 3D bioprinting techniques, type of cells used and applications of 3D bioprinting in dentistry.

In addition, recent 3D bioprinting development provides multiple approaches for the biofabrication of tissue constructs within scaffolds or scaffold-free environments. This approach could produce 3D structures with spatial organization of cells that facilitates the control of the shape of regenerated tissues. However, 3D bioprinting still faces significant challenges as compared to the nonbiological printing approach in terms of more complex architectural fabrication and the stability of cell behavior. In this review, the extrusion-based technique is the most common 3D bioprinting method for dental application. This technique is widely used because it is cost-effective and able to replicate complex tissue structures using a wide variety of biomaterials and cell types [19,20,72]. Moreover, the extrusion-based techniques can produce cell-laden bioinks in the form of continuous strands or fibers, which enable fabricating of large-scale 3D scaffold constructs [15,73]. Furthermore, printing parameters such as printing speed, pressure, resolution, temperature, nozzle inner diameter, scaffold design and viscosity of the bioink are important factors in determining the uniformity of continuous strands deposition of the bioprinted scaffolds [74].

Bioink is also an important component of 3D bioprinting. The ideal bioink formulation should satisfy certain biomaterial and biological requirements. Biomaterial properties include printing compatibility, mechanical properties, biodegradation, modifiable functional groups on the surface and post-printing maturation, whereas the biological requirements mainly include biocompatibility, cytocompatibility, and bioactivity of cells after printing to support and maintain cellular viability and function [36]. Therefore, the treatment outcome of the tissue regeneration depends on the bioinks used. Nonetheless, at present there is a lack of ideal 3D printable bioinks focused on dental tissue regeneration.

Natural polymers are the most common type of polymer used as bioink because they have a similar native composition as the ECM, biocompatibility and biodegradation properties, together with established interactions between natural polymers and cells [75]. Collagen type I is a hydrogel of choice for tissue engineering, which agrees with the research reported in this review. In addition, it is the most abundant component of the native ECM and provides an encouraging environment for cell adhesion and proliferation [76]. Crosslinking collagen matrices play an important role in the strength and stability of the structure. In comparison to noncrosslinked collagen, there is an increase in tensile strength and viscoelastic properties when using a crosslinker [77,78]. The crosslinked collagen constructs demonstrated different stiffness strengths based on types of oral tissue engineering. However, for dental pulp tissue application, the combination of collagen and agarose showed a storage modulus of approximately 0.03–0.3 kPa [60]. A study by Moncal et al. showed that in calvarial bone repair, the storage modulus of the collagen-based bioink was 8.2 ± 1.4 kPa [49]. In another study for dental tissue engineering application, collagen/β-TCP 20 wt% showed 27.9 ± 2.2 kPa modulus, which was higher than collagen alone because of the added bioceramics in the bioink [55]. The balance between mechanical strength and cell viability of the 3D constructs is crucial to maintaining cell structure and promoting cell growth. The natural polymer can be combined either with synthetic or another type of natural polymer to produce a more stable construct with enhanced function and properties. Another hydrogel-based bioink that shows potential in 3D bioprinting is GelMA because of its superior biocompatibility and photocrosslinking properties [79]. Herein, various GelMA-based bioinks have been developed to fabricate tissue structures for application in periodontal ligament [63,69], dentin [67], bone [42,46,62,64] and dental tissue regeneration [47], along with in vitro modeling of alveolar bone [61].

Synthetic polymers can be manufactured in large quantities and have longer shelf life as compared to natural polymers [80]. The photocrosslinking ability and controllability of mechanical properties, degradation rate, pH and temperature are among the advantages of using the polymers. However, most synthetic polymers lack the ability to promote cellular adhesion and recognition, and have limited biodegradability and biocompatibility, which restrict their usage in clinical applications [81]. Poly(ethylene glycol) (PEG) is one of the most popular synthetic polymers in tissue engineering [82]. PEG-based bioink can be modified using diacrylate (DA) or methcrylate (MA) groups to improve mechanical strength. In addition, the combination of PEGDA/GelMA has been used for periodontal ligament and bone regeneration application [63,64] and for in vitro alveolar bone models [61]. Moreover, a combination of natural and synthetic polymers can be a promising bioink material for fabricating biomimetic tissues because of their combined properties [83]. Another bioink, dECM, has been frequently used as a bioink in 3D bioprinting because of its good inductive property that can promote cell proliferation and differentiation together with the interaction between cells to cells and cells to ECM [84,85]. Herein, the various types of novel bioinks demonstrated high printability and cell viability, which have the potential in dental tissue regeneration applications. However, a few studies showed that novel bioinks need formulation adjustment for oral tissue engineering: (i) collagen-based with TCP (BioRoot RCS®, Septodont, France) bioink did not demonstrate regenerative potential in a calvaria critical bone defect model [59], (ii) combination of collagen-based with β-TCP reduced the capability of osteogenic differentiation, mineralization and vascularization compared to dECMs with β-TCP [55] and (iii) addition of FGF-2 to the collagen bioink did not play a role in periodontal ligament regeneration [53].

The use of growth factors in 3D bioprinting is not prevalent in dental applications because of the additional complexities that may arise. In general, the strategies in utilizing the growth factor in tissue engineering are still unclear mainly because of the uncertainties of the delivered dosage in vivo by the constructs [86], the effects of multiple uses of growth factors [87], and no standardization and arbitrariness of growth factor dosage from the broad range of concentrations available [88].

Three-dimensional bioprinting technology with the support of stem-cell-containing scaffolds has emerged as an alternative treatment strategy to address the critical need for dental tissue regeneration [37]. This is because 3D bioprinting of the cell-laden hydrogel combines physical and biological properties to attain a 3D composite construct with homogenous cell distribution, proliferation and differentiation [89]. Adult stem cells are currently the most common cells used in the field of bone tissue engineering. The advantage of stem cells derived from dental tissues is that they are easily accessible and have interesting proliferation and differentiation abilities. Healthy tissues and young patients contain a large number of normal stem cells as compared to inflamed or traumatized tissues and aging patients, which can affect the potential for tissue repair [90].

In addition, dental pulp is highly vascularized; thus, it poses a major challenge in regenerating dental pulp tissues. DPSCs are a promising source for odontogenesis because of their excellent clonogenic efficiency [91] and proangiogenic capacity [92]. A study by Duarte Campos et al. has shown evidence of successful vascular tube formation using printable bioink that contains co-cultures of human umbilical vein endothelial cells (HUVEC) with DPSCs [60]. These co-cultures not only can enhance angiogenesis but also stabilize the capillary-like structures [93]. Another study also showed promising results with DPSCs, demonstrating spatial regulation of odontogenic differentiation for 3D dentin–pulp complex formation [51]. Apart from DPSCs, SCAPs isolated from immature apical papilla could enhance odontogenic differentiation, which in the future could engineer dentin–pulp tissues [43].

Periodontium is a complex structure consisting of the periodontal ligament, cementum, gingiva and alveolar bone. Designing a scaffold for periodontal regeneration would require multilayer cementum–periodontal ligament–alveolar bone components to achieve both hard and soft tissue regeneration. The biomaterials should have a combination of polymers (i.e., collagen and gelatin) and inorganic components (i.e., hydroxyapatite, calcium phosphates and bioactive glass), given that they have different mechanical strengths [94]. However, only one study in this review used a bilayered scaffold, which consisted of collagen and strontium-doped calcium silicate for periodontal regeneration [66]. Meanwhile, the others used GelMA-based PDLSCs as their bioinks for periodontal ligament regeneration application [53,63,69]. Furthermore, PDLSCs can facilitate the formation of new alveolar bone and functional ligaments in damaged periodontal tissue under proper stimulation [95–97].

In craniomaxillofacial reconstruction, the patient-specific shape is the key factor for clinical application as there are no similar defects in terms of size and shape. Hence, achieving facial symmetry is a crucial outcome to prevent problems such as aesthetics, articulation and mastication. Thus, 3D bioprinting is favorable in fabricating specific dimensions of 3D constructs with targeted regeneration of complex tissue architectures to address the reconstructive challenges [98]. Meanwhile, in dental applications for bone regeneration, stem cells from dental origin are popular cell sources in this review. DPSCs have shown to have higher osteogenic potential than bone marrow stem cells (BMSCs), and can also produce vessel-integrated bone tissue structures which are imperative for large bone defect reconstruction [48]. The third molar is the best source for DPSCs and it can proliferate and differentiate into osteoblast and odontoblast lineages to form dentin and bone [99,100]. Other cell types that have been used are PDLSCs, which have shown multidirectional differentiation to form alveolar bone and cementum for bone tissue regeneration [101].

For the research reported in this review, bone marrow stem cells that have been used were mostly sourced from rats and mice. If human-sourced bone marrow were to be used for clinical translation for oral and craniofacial defect regeneration, it presents a few disadvantages, such as painful harvesting of bone marrow procedure and the issue of harvest yield [102]. Hence, human adipose tissue presents a desirable choice for tissue regeneration considering the simple harvesting process as compared to the traditional method. It also causes less morbidity in the patient and provides an abundant amount of adipose stem cells [103,104]. Another advantage is that the cells are capable to differentiate into osteoblastic lineage [103].

Furthermore, a stable printed scaffold with viable cells which can withstand the load-bearing force is one of the contributing factors to the predictable outcome of reconstructing oral and craniofacial defects. Therefore, in the research reported in this review, the crosslinking mechanism has been used to increase the stability of materials such as photocrosslinking of GelMA bioinks [42,46,62,64]. Another strategy is by combining bioceramic materials such as nano-hydroxyapatite, calcium phosphate and calcium silicate to gain improved mechanical properties of the constructs [105]. Given that hydroxyapatite exhibits the same function and composition as bones and teeth [106], the addition of hydroxyapatite or tricalcium phosphate to form 3D osteogenic structures has been widely explored in this field because the materials mimic the inorganic component of bone tissue [76,106].

In addition, scaffold-free tissue engineering is another 3D bioprinting technology to fabricate tissue construction. As reported in this review, this approach has been utilized for periodontal ligament [71] and bone regeneration application [44,45]. This technique does not use exogenous scaffolds for support but relies on generating constructs from cell spheroids fusion because of the cell-to-cell contact behavior [107]. Moreover, it eliminates the degradation time factor of scaffold materials, which can affect the viability of the encapsulated cells caused by byproducts of fast degradation scaffolds, whereas the slow degradation time may hinder the matrix formation [108,109]. Hence, using the scaffold-free method, cells would secrete the extracellular matrix required to provide structure. Therefore, the cells are within a biologically optimized extracellular matrix (ECM) environment to which they are suited. The utilization of cell-secreted ECM also eliminates the need to rely on the degradation of synthetic scaffold materials [45].

Meanwhile, for in vivo utilization, the studies used immunodeficient rats or mice as their animal models because these models are excellent recipients for the engraftment of human cells [58]. Small animal models are a popular selection for in vivo studies because of their ease of handling and lower cost to manage [110]. The prominent dissimilarity to the human bone [111] and the healing after implantation in small tissue defects in small animals [9] indicates that the results should be interpreted with caution, and thus, it plays a small role in translating the findings into human clinical applications [112–114]. The critical-sized calvarial bone defect has been widely used to study the interaction between cells and biomaterial on bone regeneration [115]. In addition, in situ bioprinting or intra-operative bioprinting is an advanced technology that has been performed to repair the defect via the bioprinting process on a live subject during the surgical intervention [15,116]. This approach can eliminate the change in the morphology of the prefabricated 3D bioprinted constructs during in vitro construction process, transport during surgery or manipulation of the bioprinted scaffolds to conform to the defect shape [117]. Therefore, in situ bioprinting offers immediate printing of the bioink to the defect site in an anatomically accurate and personalized reconstruction for successful restoration of the tissues [118]. Moreover, it provides an interesting perspective for clinical practice considering that it could eliminate need for the in vitro fabrication phase, which may delay the implantation procedure. In this review, all in situ bioprinting was carried out on calvarial defects using the laser-assisted bioprinting technique. LAB was used to print bioinks containing SCAPs for bone regeneration application. Even though LAB produces high printing resolution and high throughput, this approach is currently not able to fabricate large-scale tissue constructs because of the relatively slow printing speed [18]. However, this technique could be suitable for in situ bioprinting for small defects and relatively flat bones [119].

Therefore, to summarize the current perspectives of advanced research in 3D bioprinting for dental application based on the included studies, some limitations need to be addressed. However, we must acknowledge this is a novel approach and very much in the early stage of development. Firstly, various novel bioinks report promising outcomes on the advancement of customized specific constructs. Nonetheless, there is a wide heterogeneity in bioink composition (type of biomaterials and cells), printing parameters and application in dental tissue engineering which presents a challenge in deciding which bioink is compatible with the best standard of care and restoring the physiological function of the teeth. Secondly, the current research is mostly in vitro studies, hence, they are still in preliminary steps and not yet possible to prove its effectiveness in vivo. In addition, the results from in vivo studies need to be interpreted with great caution considering that the surgically created defects are small. Therefore, fabrication of large 3D printed tissue constructs and implanted into large animal models such as dogs or monkeys would be an optimal study design to better investigate the outcomes of the clinically relevant size and architecture of regenerated tissues. Finally, the ideal research models developed should be able to simulate the dentoalveolar environment since the defect created on the calvarium might not give a true reflection of more complex conditions in the oral cavity. The future prospects of 3D bioprinting are highly promising, and the progress toward the potential development of 3D printed tissues for an individual patient using the patient's cells needs to be considered for clinical translation. Nevertheless, the implantation of 3D bioprinted tissues in humans, which include living cells and biomaterials, will face regulatory challenges given that the long-term effects such as safety and efficacy in humans are still unknown. Therefore, the ethical, technical and legal issues need to be addressed and regulated by national guidelines to protect the health and well-being of patients before adopting the 3D bioprinting technology into human clinical applications.

5. Conclusions

Three-dimensional bioprinted novel bioinks based on natural and synthetic polymers, dECM, cell aggregates and spheroids have shown promising results in dental applications, particularly for periodontal ligament, dentin, dental pulp and bone regeneration. The increasing use of stem cells derived from dental origin can offer a good cell source in oral tissue engineering. In addition, 3D bioprinting brings significant potential in translating advanced tissue engineering into the clinical application by creating regenerative scaffolds tailored to patient-specific requirements. It is hoped that continuous research and advancement in 3D bioprinting, particularly in the techniques and materials used in dental applications, would reach a level of refinement and standard that can be fully integrated into the management and practice in addressing oral healthcare problems.

Author Contributions: Conceptualization, N.M., M.R. and M.J.G.; methodology, N.M.; validation, N.M., M.R. and N.H.A.K.; formal analysis, N.M. and M.R.; data curation, N.M.; writing—original draft preparation, N.M. and M.R.; writing—review and editing, N.M., M.R., M.J.G. and N.H.A.K.; supervision, M.R., M.J.G. and N.H.A.K.; funding acquisition, M.R. All authors have read and agreed to the published version of the manuscript.

Funding: The work is part of a project supported by CREST (Collaborative Research in Engineering, Science and Technology) (T05C2-20), Malaysia.

Conflicts of Interest: The authors declare no conflict of interest.

References

1. Kassebaum, N.J.; Bernabe, E.; Dahiya, M.; Bhandari, B.; Murray, C.J.L.; Marcenes, W. Global Burden of Severe Periodontitis in 1990–2010: A systematic review and meta-regression. *J. Dent. Res.* **2014**, *93*, 1045–1053. [CrossRef] [PubMed]
2. Marcenes, W.; Kassebaum, N.J.; Bernabe, E.; Flaxman, A.; Naghavi, M.; Lopez, A.D.; Murray, C. Global Burden of Oral Conditions in 1990–2010: A systematic analysis. *J. Dent. Res.* **2013**, *92*, 592–597. [CrossRef] [PubMed]
3. Chen, F.-M.; Zhang, J.; Zhang, M.; An, Y.; Chen, F.; Wu, Z.-F. A review on endogenous regenerative technology in periodontal regenerative medicine. *Biomaterials* **2010**, *31*, 7892–7927. [CrossRef] [PubMed]
4. Nkenke, E.; Weisbach, V.; Winckler, E.; Kessler, P.; Schultze-Mosgau, S.; Wiltfang, J.; Neukam, F.W. Morbidity of harvesting of bone grafts from the iliac crest for preprosthetic augmentation procedures: A prospective study. *Int. J. Oral Maxillofac. Surg.* **2004**, *33*, 157–163. [CrossRef] [PubMed]
5. Liu, J.; Kerns, D.G. Mechanisms of Guided Bone Regeneration: A Review. *Open Dent. J.* **2014**, *8*, 56–65. [CrossRef] [PubMed]
6. Damien, C.J.; Parsons, J.R. Bone graft and bone graft substitutes: A review of current technology and applications. *J. Appl. Biomater.* **1991**, *2*, 187–208. [CrossRef] [PubMed]
7. Giannoudis, P.V.; Dinopoulos, H.; Tsiridis, E. Bone substitutes: An update. *Injury* **2005**, *36* (Suppl. S3), S20–S27. [CrossRef]
8. Young, C.; Terada, S.; Vacanti, J.; Honda, M.; Bartlett, J.; Yelick, P. Tissue Engineering of Complex Tooth Structures on Biodegradable Polymer Scaffolds. *J. Dent. Res.* **2002**, *81*, 695–700. [CrossRef]
9. Sigaux, N.; Pourchet, L.; Breton, P.; Brosset, S.; Louvrier, A.; Marquette, C. 3D Bioprinting:principles, fantasies and prospects. *J. Stomatol. Oral Maxillofac. Surg.* **2019**, *120*, 128–132. [CrossRef]
10. Jammalamadaka, U.; Tappa, K. Recent Advances in Biomaterials for 3D Printing and Tissue Engineering. *J. Funct. Biomater.* **2018**, *9*, 22. [CrossRef]
11. Murphy, S.V.; Atala, A. 3D bioprinting of tissues and organs. *Nat. Biotechnol.* **2014**, *32*, 773–785. [CrossRef] [PubMed]
12. Hölzl, K.; Lin, S.; Tytgat, L.; Van Vlierberghe, S.; Gu, L.; Ovsianikov, A. Bioink properties before, during and after 3D bioprinting. *Biofabrication* **2016**, *8*, 032002. [CrossRef] [PubMed]

13. Moroni, L.; Burdick, J.A.; Highley, C.; Lee, S.J.; Morimoto, Y.; Takeuchi, S.; Yoo, J.J. Biofabrication strategies for 3D in vitro models and regenerative medicine. *Nat. Rev. Mater.* **2018**, *3*, 21–37. [CrossRef]
14. Yu, J.; Park, S.A.; Kim, W.D.; Ha, T.; Xin, Y.-Z.; Lee, J.; Lee, D. Current Advances in 3D Bioprinting Technology and Its Applications for Tissue Engineering. *Polymers* **2020**, *12*, 2958. [CrossRef]
15. Ozbolat, I.T.; Hospodiuk, M. Current advances and future perspectives in extrusion-based bioprinting. *Biomaterials* **2016**, *76*, 321–343. [CrossRef] [PubMed]
16. Askari, M.; Naniz, M.A.; Kouhi, M.; Saberi, A.; Zolfagharian, A.; Bodaghi, M. Recent progress in extrusion 3D bioprinting of hydrogel biomaterials for tissue regeneration: A comprehensive review with focus on advanced fabrication techniques. *Biomater. Sci.* **2021**, *9*, 535–573. [CrossRef]
17. Gudapati, H.; Dey, M.; Ozbolat, I. A comprehensive review on droplet-based bioprinting: Past, present and future. *Biomaterials* **2016**, *102*, 20–42. [CrossRef]
18. Dou, C.; Perez, V.; Qu, J.; Tsin, A.; Xu, B.; Li, J. A State-of-the-Art Review of Laser-Assisted Bioprinting and its Future Research Trends. *ChemBioEng Rev.* **2021**, *8*, 517–534. [CrossRef]
19. Unagolla, J.M.; Jayasuriya, A.C. Hydrogel-based 3D bioprinting: A comprehensive review on cell-laden hydrogels, bioink formulations, and future perspectives. *Appl. Mater. Today* **2020**, *18*, 100479. [CrossRef]
20. Chen, Y.-S.; Chang, S.-S.; Ng, H.Y.; Huang, Y.-X.; Chen, C.-C.; Shie, M.-Y. Additive Manufacturing of Astragaloside-Containing Polyurethane Nerve Conduits Influenced Schwann Cell Inflammation and Regeneration. *Processes* **2021**, *9*, 353. [CrossRef]
21. Ning, L.; Chen, X. A brief review of extrusion-based tissue scaffold bio-printing. *Biotechnol. J.* **2017**, *12*, 1600671. [CrossRef] [PubMed]
22. Derakhshanfar, S.; Mbeleck, R.; Xu, K.; Zhang, X.; Zhong, W.; Xing, M. 3D bioprinting for biomedical devices and tissue engineering: A review of recent trends and advances. *Bioact. Mater.* **2018**, *3*, 144–156. [CrossRef] [PubMed]
23. Mandrycky, C.; Wang, Z.; Kim, K.; Kim, D.-H. 3D bioprinting for engineering complex tissues. *Biotechnol. Adv.* **2016**, *34*, 422–434. [CrossRef] [PubMed]
24. Xie, Z.; Gao, M.; Lobo, A.O.; Webster, T.J. 3D Bioprinting in Tissue Engineering for Medical Applications: The Classic and the Hybrid. *Polymers* **2020**, *12*, 1717. [CrossRef]
25. Groll, J.; Burdick, J.A.; Cho, D.-W.; Derby, B.; Gelinsky, M.; Heilshorn, S.C.; Jüngst, T.; Malda, J.; Mironov, V.A.; Nakayama, K.; et al. A definition of bioinks and their distinction from biomaterial inks. *Biofabrication* **2018**, *11*, 013001. [CrossRef]
26. Park, J.Y.; Choi, Y.-J.; Shim, J.-H.; Park, J.H.; Cho, D.-W. Development of a 3D cell printed structure as an alternative to autologs cartilage for auricular reconstruction. *J. Biomed. Mater. Res. Part B Appl. Biomater.* **2017**, *105*, 1016–1028. [CrossRef]
27. Han, Y.; Li, X.; Zhang, Y.; Han, Y.; Chang, F.; Ding, J. Mesenchymal Stem Cells for Regenerative Medicine. *Cells* **2019**, *8*, 886. [CrossRef]
28. Zhai, Q.; Dong, Z.; Wang, W.; Li, B.; Jin, Y. Dental stem cell and dental tissue regeneration. *Front. Med.* **2019**, *13*, 152–159. [CrossRef]
29. Hernández-Monjaraz, B.; Santiago-Osorio, E.; Monroy-García, A.; Ledesma-Martínez, E.; Mendoza-Núñez, V.M. Mesenchymal Stem Cells of Dental Origin for Inducing Tissue Regeneration in Periodontitis: A Mini-Review. *Int. J. Mol. Sci.* **2018**, *19*, 944. [CrossRef]
30. Keating, A. Mesenchymal Stromal Cells: New Directions. *Cell Stem Cell* **2012**, *10*, 709–716. [CrossRef]
31. Jones, E.; Yang, X. Mesenchymal stem cells and bone regeneration: Current status. *Injury* **2011**, *42*, 562–568. [CrossRef]
32. Kyburz, K.A.; Anseth, K.S. Synthetic Mimics of the Extracellular Matrix: How Simple is Complex Enough? *Ann. Biomed. Eng.* **2015**, *43*, 489–500. [CrossRef] [PubMed]
33. Li, L.; Yu, F.; Zheng, L.; Wang, R.; Yan, W.; Wang, Z.; Xu, J.; Wu, J.; Shi, D.; Zhu, L.; et al. Natural hydrogels for cartilage regeneration: Modification, preparation and application. *J. Orthop. Transl.* **2019**, *17*, 26–41. [CrossRef] [PubMed]
34. Chung, J.H.Y.; Naficy, S.; Yue, Z.; Kapsa, R.; Quigley, A.; Moulton, S.E.; Wallace, G.G. Bio-ink properties and printability for extrusion printing living cells. *Biomater. Sci.* **2013**, *1*, 763–773. [CrossRef] [PubMed]
35. Busra, M.F.M. Recent Development in the Fabrication of Collagen Scaffolds for Tissue Engineering Applications: A Review. *Curr. Pharm. Biotechnol.* **2019**, *20*, 992–1003. [CrossRef]
36. Gopinathan, J.; Noh, I. Recent trends in bioinks for 3D printing. *Biomater. Res.* **2018**, *22*, 11. [CrossRef]
37. Obregon, F.; Vaquette, C.; Ivanovski, S.; Hutmacher, D.W.; Bertassoni, L. Three-Dimensional Bioprinting for Regenerative Dentistry and Craniofacial Tissue Engineering. *J. Dent. Res.* **2015**, *94*, 143S–152S. [CrossRef]
38. Peters, M.D.; Marnie, C.; Tricco, A.C.; Pollock, D.; Munn, Z.; Alexander, L.; McInerney, P.; Godfrey, C.M.; Khalil, H. Updated methodological guidance for the conduct of scoping reviews. *JBI Évid. Synth.* **2020**, *18*, 2119–2126. [CrossRef]
39. Tricco, A.C.; Lillie, E.; Zarin, W.; O'Brien, K.K.; Colquhoun, H.; Levac, D.; Moher, D.; Peters, M.D.J.; Horsley, T.; Weeks, L.; et al. PRISMA Extension for Scoping Reviews (PRISMA-ScR): Checklist and Explanation. *Ann. Intern. Med.* **2018**, *169*, 467–473. [CrossRef]
40. Ouzzani, M.; Hammady, H.; Fedorowicz, Z.; Elmagarmid, A. Rayyan—A web and mobile app for systematic reviews. *Syst. Rev.* **2016**, *5*, 210. [CrossRef]
41. Kang, H.-W.; Lee, S.J.; Ko, I.K.; Kengla, C.; Yoo, J.J.; Atala, A. A 3D bioprinting system to produce human-scale tissue constructs with structural integrity. *Nat. Biotechnol.* **2016**, *34*, 312–319. [CrossRef] [PubMed]

42. Kuss, M.A.; Harms, R.; Wu, S.; Wang, Y.; Untrauer, J.B.; Carlson, M.A.; Duan, B. Short-term hypoxic preconditioning promotes prevascularization in 3D bioprinted bone constructs with stromal vascular fraction derived cells. *RSC Adv.* **2017**, *7*, 29312–29320. [CrossRef]
43. Athirasala, A.; Tahayeri, A.; Thrivikraman, G.; Franca, C.M.; Monteiro, N.; Tran, V.; Ferracane, J.; Bertassoni, L.E. A dentin-derived hydrogel bioink for 3D bioprinting of cell laden scaffolds for regenerative dentistry. *Biofabrication* **2018**, *10*, 024101. [CrossRef] [PubMed]
44. Aguilar, I.N.; Smith, L.J.; Olivos, D.J., 3rd; Chu, T.-M.G.; Kacena, M.A.; Wagner, D.R. Scaffold-free bioprinting of mesenchymal stem cells with the regenova printer: Optimization of printing parameters. *Bioprinting* **2019**, *15*, e00048. [CrossRef] [PubMed]
45. Aguilar, I.N.; Olivos, D.J.; Brinker, A.; Alvarez, M.B.; Smith, L.J.; Chu, T.-M.G.; Kacena, M.A.; Wagner, D.R. Scaffold-free bioprinting of mesenchymal stem cells using the Regenova printer: Spheroid characterization and osteogenic differentiation. *Bioprinting* **2019**, *15*, e00050. [CrossRef]
46. Chimene, D.; Miller, L.; Cross, L.M.; Jaiswal, M.K.; Singh, I.; Gaharwar, A.K. Nanoengineered Osteoinductive Bioink for 3D Bioprinting Bone Tissue. *ACS Appl. Mater. Interfaces* **2020**, *12*, 15976–15988. [CrossRef]
47. Park, J.H.; Gillispie, G.J.; Copus, J.S.; Zhang, W.; Atala, A.; Yoo, J.J.; Yelick, P.C.; Lee, S.J. The effect of BMP-mimetic peptide tethering bioinks on the differentiation of dental pulp stem cells (DPSCs) in 3D bioprinted dental constructs. *Biofabrication* **2020**, *12*, 035029. [CrossRef]
48. Dubey, N.; Ferreira, J.A.; Malda, J.; Bhaduri, S.B.; Bottino, M.C. Extracellular Matrix/Amorphous Magnesium Phosphate Bioink for 3D Bioprinting of Craniomaxillofacial Bone Tissue. *ACS Appl. Mater. Interfaces* **2020**, *12*, 23752–23763. [CrossRef]
49. Moncal, K.K.; Gudapati, H.; Godzik, K.P.; Heo, D.N.; Kang, Y.; Rizk, E.; Ravnic, D.J.; Wee, H.; Pepley, D.F.; Ozbolat, V.; et al. Intra-Operative Bioprinting of Hard, Soft, and Hard/Soft Composite Tissues for Craniomaxillofacial Reconstruction. *Adv. Funct. Mater.* **2021**, *31*, 2010858. [CrossRef]
50. Moncal, K.K.; Aydın, R.S.T.; Godzik, K.P.; Acri, T.M.; Heo, D.N.; Rizk, E.; Wee, H.; Lewis, G.S.; Salem, A.K.; Ozbolat, I.T. Controlled Co-delivery of pPDGF-B and pBMP-2 from intraoperatively bioprinted bone constructs improves the repair of calvarial defects in rats. *Biomaterials* **2022**, *281*, 121333. [CrossRef]
51. Han, J.; Kim, D.S.; Jang, H., II; Kim, H.-R.; Kang, H.-W. Bioprinting of three-dimensional dentin–pulp complex with local differentiation of human dental pulp stem cells. *J. Tissue Eng.* **2019**, *10*, 2041731419845849. [CrossRef] [PubMed]
52. Han, J.; Jeong, W.; Kim, M.-K.; Nam, S.-H.; Park, E.-K.; Kang, H.-W. Demineralized Dentin Matrix Particle-Based Bio-Ink for Patient-Specific Shaped 3D Dental Tissue Regeneration. *Polymers* **2021**, *13*, 1294. [CrossRef] [PubMed]
53. Lee, U.-L.; Yun, S.; Cao, H.-L.; Ahn, G.; Shim, J.-H.; Woo, S.-H.; Choung, P.-H. Bioprinting on 3D Printed Titanium Scaffolds for Periodontal Ligament Regeneration. *Cells* **2021**, *10*, 1337. [CrossRef] [PubMed]
54. Dutta, S.D.; Bin, J.; Ganguly, K.; Patel, D.K.; Lim, K.-T. Electromagnetic field-assisted cell-laden 3D printed poloxamer-407 hydrogel for enhanced osteogenesis. *RSC Adv.* **2021**, *11*, 20342–20354. [CrossRef]
55. Kim, D.; Lee, H.; Lee, G.; Hoang, T.; Kim, H.; Kim, G.H. Fabrication of Bone-derived decellularized extracellular matrix/Ceramic-based Biocomposites and Their Osteo/Odontogenic Differentiation Ability for Dentin Regeneration. *Bioeng. Transl. Med.* **2022**, *7*, e10317. [CrossRef]
56. Keriquel, V.; Oliveira, H.; Rémy, M.; Ziane, S.; Delmond, S.; Rousseau, B.; Rey, S.; Catros, S.; Amédée, J.; Guillemot, F.; et al. In situ printing of mesenchymal stromal cells, by laser-assisted bioprinting, for in vivo bone regeneration applications. *Sci. Rep.* **2017**, *7*, 1778. [CrossRef]
57. Kérourédan, O.; Ribot, E.J.; Fricain, J.-C.; Devillard, R.; Miraux, S. Magnetic Resonance Imaging for tracking cellular patterns obtained by Laser-Assisted Bioprinting. *Sci. Rep.* **2018**, *8*, 15777. [CrossRef]
58. Kérourédan, O.; Hakobyan, D.; Rémy, M.; Ziane, S.; Dusserre, N.; Fricain, J.-C.; Delmond, S.; Thébaud, N.B.; Devillard, R. In situ prevascularization designed by laser-assisted bioprinting: Effect on bone regeneration. *Biofabrication* **2019**, *11*, 045002. [CrossRef]
59. Touya, N.; Devun, M.; Handschin, C.; Casenave, S.; Omar, N.A.; Gaubert, A.; Dusserre, N.; De Oliveira, H.; Kérourédan, O.; Devillard, R. In vitro and in vivo characterization of a novel tricalcium silicate-based ink for bone regeneration using laser-assisted bioprinting. *Biofabrication* **2022**, *14*, 024104. [CrossRef]
60. Campos, D.F.D.; Zhang, S.; Kreimendahl, F.; Köpf, M.; Fischer, H.; Vogt, M.; Blaeser, A.; Apel, C.; Esteves-Oliveira, M. Hand-held bioprinting for de novo vascular formation applicable to dental pulp regeneration. *Connect. Tissue Res.* **2020**, *61*, 205–215. [CrossRef]
61. Amler, A.-K.; Thomas, A.; Tüzüner, S.; Lam, T.; Geiger, M.-A.; Kreuder, A.-E.; Palmer, C.; Nahles, S.; Lauster, R.; Kloke, L. 3D bioprinting of tissue-specific osteoblasts and endothelial cells to model the human jawbone. *Sci. Rep.* **2021**, *11*, 4876. [CrossRef] [PubMed]
62. Amler, A.-K.; Dinkelborg, P.; Schlauch, D.; Spinnen, J.; Stich, S.; Lauster, R.; Sittinger, M.; Nahles, S.; Heiland, M.; Kloke, L.; et al. Comparison of the Translational Potential of Human Mesenchymal Progenitor Cells from Different Bone Entities for Autologous 3D Bioprinted Bone Grafts. *Int. J. Mol. Sci.* **2021**, *22*, 796. [CrossRef] [PubMed]
63. Ma, Y.; Ji, Y.; Huang, G.; Ling, K.; Zhang, X.; Xu, F. Bioprinting 3D cell-laden hydrogel microarray for screening human periodontal ligament stem cell response to extracellular matrix. *Biofabrication* **2015**, *7*, 044105. [CrossRef] [PubMed]
64. Ma, Y.; Ji, Y.; Zhong, T.; Wan, W.; Yang, Q.; Li, A.; Zhang, X.; Lin, M. Bioprinting-Based PDLSC-ECM Screening for in Vivo Repair of Alveolar Bone Defect Using Cell-Laden, Injectable and Photocrosslinkable Hydrogels. *ACS Biomater. Sci. Eng.* **2017**, *3*, 3534–3545. [CrossRef]

65. Tian, Y.; Liu, M.; Liu, Y.; Shi, C.; Wang, Y.; Liu, T.; Huang, Y.; Zhong, P.; Dai, J.; Liu, X. The performance of 3D bioscaffolding based on a human periodontal ligament stem cell printing technique. *J. Biomed. Mater. Res. Part A* **2021**, *109*, 1209–1219. [CrossRef]
66. Wang, C.-Y.; Chiu, Y.-C.; Lee, A.K.-X.; Lin, Y.-A.; Lin, P.-Y.; Shie, M.-Y. Biofabrication of Gingival Fibroblast Cell-Laden Collagen/Strontium-Doped Calcium Silicate 3D-Printed Bi-Layered Scaffold for Osteoporotic Periodontal Regeneration. *Biomedicines* **2021**, *9*, 431. [CrossRef]
67. Lin, Y.-T.; Hsu, T.-T.; Liu, Y.-W.; Kao, C.-T.; Huang, T.-H. Bidirectional Differentiation of Human-Derived Stem Cells Induced by Biomimetic Calcium Silicate-Reinforced Gelatin Methacrylate Bioink for Odontogenic Regeneration. *Biomedicines* **2021**, *9*, 929. [CrossRef]
68. Kort-Mascort, J.; Bao, G.; Elkashty, O.; Flores-Torres, S.; Munguia-Lopez, J.G.; Jiang, T.; Ehrlicher, A.J.; Mongeau, L.; Tran, S.D.; Kinsella, J.M. Decellularized Extracellular Matrix Composite Hydrogel Bioinks for the Development of 3D Bioprinted Head and Neck in Vitro Tumor Models. *ACS Biomater. Sci. Eng.* **2021**, *7*, 5288–5300. [CrossRef]
69. Raveendran, N.T.; Vaquette, C.; Meinert, C.; Ipe, D.S.; Ivanovski, S. Optimization of 3D bioprinting of periodontal ligament cells. *Dent. Mater.* **2019**, *35*, 1683–1694. [CrossRef]
70. Walladbegi, J.; Schaefer, C.; Pernevik, E.; Sämfors, S.; Kjeller, G.; Gatenholm, P.; Sándor, G.K.; Rasmusson, L. Three-dimensional bioprinting using a coaxial needle with viscous inks in bone tissue engineering—An In vitro study. *Ann. Maxillofac. Surg.* **2020**, *10*, 370–376. [CrossRef]
71. Ono, T.; Tomokiyo, A.; Ipposhi, K.; Yamashita, K.; Alhasan, M.A.; Miyazaki, Y.; Kunitomi, Y.; Tsuchiya, A.; Ishikawa, K.; Maeda, H. Generation of biohybrid implants using a multipotent human periodontal ligament cell line and bioactive core materials. *J. Cell. Physiol.* **2021**, *236*, 6742–6753. [CrossRef] [PubMed]
72. Matai, I.; Kaur, G.; Seyedsalehi, A.; McClinton, A.; Laurencin, C.T. Progress in 3D bioprinting technology for tissue/organ regenerative engineering. *Biomaterials* **2020**, *226*, 119536. [CrossRef] [PubMed]
73. Jang, J.; Yi, H.-G.; Cho, D.-W. 3D Printed Tissue Models: Present and Future. *ACS Biomater. Sci. Eng.* **2016**, *2*, 1722–1731. [CrossRef]
74. Billiet, T.; Gevaert, E.; De Schryver, T.; Cornelissen, M.; Dubruel, P. The 3D printing of gelatin methacrylamide cell-laden tissue-engineered constructs with high cell viability. *Biomaterials* **2014**, *35*, 49–62. [CrossRef] [PubMed]
75. Zorlutuna, P.; Vrana, N.E.; Khademhosseini, A. The Expanding World of Tissue Engineering: The Building Blocks and New Applications of Tissue Engineered Constructs. *IEEE Rev. Biomed. Eng.* **2013**, *6*, 47–62. [CrossRef]
76. Walters, B.; Stegemann, J. Strategies for directing the structure and function of three-dimensional collagen biomaterials across length scales. *Acta Biomater.* **2014**, *10*, 1488–1501. [CrossRef]
77. Mori, H.; Shimizu, K.; Hara, M. Dynamic viscoelastic properties of collagen gels with high mechanical strength. *Mater. Sci. Eng. C* **2013**, *33*, 3230–3236. [CrossRef]
78. Ferreira, A.M.; Gentile, P.; Chiono, V.; Ciardelli, G. Collagen for bone tissue regeneration. *Acta Biomater.* **2012**, *8*, 3191–3200. [CrossRef]
79. Daly, A.; Critchley, S.E.; Rencsok, E.M.; Kelly, D.J. A comparison of different bioinks for 3D bioprinting of fibrocartilage and hyaline cartilage. *Biofabrication* **2016**, *8*, 045002. [CrossRef]
80. Sheikh, Z.; Najeeb, S.; Khurshid, Z.; Verma, V.; Rashid, H.; Glogauer, M. Biodegradable Materials for Bone Repair and Tissue Engineering Applications. *Materials* **2015**, *8*, 5744–5794. [CrossRef]
81. Tavelli, L.; McGuire, M.K.; Zucchelli, G.; Rasperini, G.; Feinberg, S.E.; Wang, H.; Giannobile, W.V. Extracellular matrix-based scaffolding technologies for periodontal and peri-implant soft tissue regeneration. *J. Periodontol.* **2020**, *91*, 17–25. [CrossRef] [PubMed]
82. Yang, X.; Sarvestani, S.K.; Moeinzadeh, S.; He, X.; Jabbari, E. Three-Dimensional-Engineered Matrix to Study Cancer Stem Cells and Tumorsphere Formation: Effect of Matrix Modulus. *Tissue Eng. Part A* **2013**, *19*, 669–684. [CrossRef] [PubMed]
83. Kumar, S.; Tharayil, A.; Thomas, S. 3D Bioprinting of Nature-Inspired Hydrogel Inks Based on Synthetic Polymers. *ACS Appl. Polym. Mater.* **2021**, *3*, 3685–3701. [CrossRef]
84. Skardal, A.; Devarasetty, M.; Kang, H.-W.; Mead, I.; Bishop, C.; Shupe, T.; Lee, S.J.; Jackson, J.; Yoo, J.; Soker, S.; et al. A hydrogel bioink toolkit for mimicking native tissue biochemical and mechanical properties in bioprinted tissue constructs. *Acta Biomater.* **2015**, *25*, 24–34. [CrossRef] [PubMed]
85. Pizzo, A.M.; Kokini, K.; Vaughn, L.C.; Waisner, B.Z.; Voytik-Harbin, S.L. Extracellular matrix (ECM) microstructural composition regulates local cell-ECM biomechanics and fundamental fibroblast behavior: A multidimensional perspective. *J. Appl. Physiol.* **2005**, *98*, 1909–1921. [CrossRef] [PubMed]
86. Santo, V.E.; Gomes, M.E.; Mano, J.F.; Reis, R.L. Controlled Release Strategies for Bone, Cartilage, and Osteochondral Engineering—Part II: Challenges on the Evolution from Single to Multiple Bioactive Factor Delivery. *Tissue Eng. Part B Rev.* **2013**, *19*, 327–352. [CrossRef]
87. Kuhn, L.T.; Ou, G.; Charles, L.; Hurley, M.M.; Rodner, C.M.; Gronowicz, G. Fibroblast Growth Factor-2 and Bone Morphogenetic Protein-2 Have a Synergistic Stimulatory Effect on Bone Formation in Cell Cultures from Elderly Mouse and Human Bone. *J. Gerontol. Ser. A* **2013**, *68*, 1170–1180. [CrossRef] [PubMed]
88. Gothard, D.; Smith, E.; Kanczler, J.; Rashidi, H.; Qutachi, O.; Henstock, J.; Rotherham, M.; El Haj, A.; Shakesheff, K.; Oreffo, R. Tissue engineered bone using select growth factors: A comprehensive review of animal studies and clinical translation studies in man. *Eur. Cells Mater.* **2014**, *28*, 166–208. [CrossRef]

89. Ng, W.L.; Lee, J.M.; Yeong, W.Y.; Naing, M.W. Microvalve-based bioprinting—process, bio-inks and applications. *Biomater. Sci.* **2017**, *5*, 632–647. [CrossRef]
90. Liu, Y.; Liu, W.; Hu, C.; Xue, Z.; Wang, G.; Ding, B.; Luo, H.; Tang, L.; Kong, X.; Chen, X.; et al. MiR-17 Modulates Osteogenic Differentiation Through a Coherent Feed-Forward Loop in Mesenchymal Stem Cells Isolated from Periodontal Ligaments of Patients with Periodontitis. *Stem Cells* **2011**, *29*, 1804–1816. [CrossRef]
91. Gronthos, S.; Brahim, J.; Li, W.; Fisher, L.W.; Cherman, N.; Boyde, A.; DenBesten, P.; Robey, P.G.; Shi, S. Stem Cell Properties of Human Dental Pulp Stem Cells. *J. Dent. Res.* **2002**, *81*, 531–535. [CrossRef] [PubMed]
92. Dissanayaka, W.; Zhang, C. The Role of Vasculature Engineering in Dental Pulp Regeneration. *J. Endod.* **2017**, *43*, S102–S106. [CrossRef] [PubMed]
93. Dissanayaka, W.; Zhan, X.; Zhang, C.; Hargreaves, K.M.; Jin, L.; Tong, E.H. Coculture of Dental Pulp Stem Cells with Endothelial Cells Enhances Osteo-/Odontogenic and Angiogenic Potential In Vitro. *J. Endod.* **2012**, *38*, 454–463. [CrossRef]
94. Liang, Y.; Luan, X.; Liu, X. Recent advances in periodontal regeneration: A biomaterial perspective. *Bioact. Mater.* **2020**, *5*, 297–308. [CrossRef] [PubMed]
95. Wang, L.; Shen, H.; Zheng, W.; Tang, L.; Yang, Z.; Gao, Y.; Yang, Q.; Wang, C.; Duan, Y.; Jin, Y. Characterization of Stem Cells from Alveolar Periodontal Ligament. *Tissue Eng. Part A* **2011**, *17*, 1015–1026. [CrossRef]
96. Park, J.-Y.; Jeon, S.H.; Choung, P.-H. Efficacy of Periodontal Stem Cell Transplantation in the Treatment of Advanced Periodontitis. *Cell Transplant.* **2011**, *20*, 271–286. [CrossRef]
97. Lei, M.; Li, K.; Li, B.; Gao, L.-N.; Chen, F.-M.; Jin, Y. Mesenchymal stem cell characteristics of dental pulp and periodontal ligament stem cells after In Vivo transplantation. *Biomaterials* **2014**, *35*, 6332–6343. [CrossRef]
98. Tarafder, S.; Koch, A.; Jun, Y.; Chou, C.; Awadallah, M.R.; Lee, C.H. Micro-precise spatiotemporal delivery system embedded in 3D printing for complex tissue regeneration. *Biofabrication* **2016**, *8*, 025003. [CrossRef]
99. Gronthos, S.; Mankani, M.; Brahim, J.; Robey, P.G.; Shi, S. Postnatal human dental pulp stem cells (DPSCs) in vitro and in vivo. *Proc. Natl. Acad. Sci. USA* **2000**, *97*, 13625–13630. [CrossRef]
100. D'Aquino, R.; Graziano, A.; Sampaolesi, M.; Laino, G.; Pirozzi, G.; De Rosa, A.; Papaccio, G. Human postnatal dental pulp cells co-differentiate into osteoblasts and endotheliocytes: A pivotal synergy leading to adult bone tissue formation. *Cell Death Differ.* **2007**, *14*, 1162–1171. [CrossRef]
101. Seo, B.-M.; Miura, M.; Gronthos, S.; Bartold, P.M.; Batouli, S.; Brahim, J.; Young, M.; Robey, P.G.; Wang, C.Y.; Shi, S. Investigation of multipotent postnatal stem cells from human periodontal ligament. *Lancet* **2004**, *364*, 149–155. [CrossRef]
102. Oryan, A.; Kamali, A.; Moshiri, A.; Eslaminejad, M.B. Role of Mesenchymal Stem Cells in Bone Regenerative Medicine: What Is the Evidence? *Cells Tissues Organs* **2017**, *204*, 59–83. [CrossRef] [PubMed]
103. Gimble, J.M.; Zvonic, S.; Floyd, E.; Kassem, M.; Nuttall, M.E. Playing with bone and fat. *J. Cell. Biochem.* **2006**, *98*, 251–266. [CrossRef] [PubMed]
104. Chamberlain, G.; Fox, J.; Ashton, B.; Middleton, J. Concise Review: Mesenchymal Stem Cells: Their Phenotype, Differentiation Capacity, Immunological Features, and Potential for Homing. *Stem Cells* **2007**, *25*, 2739–2749. [CrossRef] [PubMed]
105. Hassan, M.N.; Yassin, M.A.; Suliman, S.; Lie, S.A.; Gjengedal, H.; Mustafa, K. The bone regeneration capacity of 3D-printed templates in calvarial defect models: A systematic review and meta-analysis. *Acta Biomater.* **2019**, *91*, 1–23. [CrossRef] [PubMed]
106. Mohd, N.; Razali, M.; Ghazali, M.J.; Abu Kasim, N.H. 3D-Printed Hydroxyapatite and Tricalcium Phosphates-Based Scaffolds for Alveolar Bone Regeneration in Animal Models: A Scoping Review. *Materials* **2022**, *15*, 2621. [CrossRef] [PubMed]
107. Mironov, V.; Visconti, R.P.; Kasyanov, V.; Forgacs, G.; Drake, C.J.; Markwald, R.R. Organ printing: Tissue spheroids as building blocks. *Biomaterials* **2009**, *30*, 2164–2174. [CrossRef]
108. Norotte, C.; Marga, F.S.; Niklason, L.E.; Forgacs, G. Scaffold-free vascular tissue engineering using bioprinting. *Biomaterials* **2009**, *30*, 5910–5917. [CrossRef]
109. Ozbolat, I.T. Scaffold-Based or Scaffold-Free Bioprinting: Competing or Complementing Approaches? *J. Nanotechnol. Eng. Med.* **2015**, *6*, 024701. [CrossRef]
110. Omar, N.I.; Baharin, B.; Lau, S.F.; Ibrahim, N.; Mohd, N.; Fauzi, A.A.; Muhammad, N.; Fernandez, N.M. The Influence of Ficus deltoidea in Preserving Alveolar Bone in Ovariectomized Rats. *Veter.-Med. Int.* **2020**, *2020*, 8862489. [CrossRef]
111. Pearce, A.I.; Richards, R.G.; Milz, S.; Schneider, E.; Pearce, S.G. Animal models for implant biomaterial research in bone: A review. *Eur. Cells Mater.* **2007**, *13*, 1–10. [CrossRef] [PubMed]
112. Prabhakar, S. Translational Research Challenges: Finding the right animal models. *J. Investig. Med.* **2012**, *60*, 1141–1146. [CrossRef] [PubMed]
113. Lorbach, O.; Baums, M.H.; Kostuj, T.; Pauly, S.; Scheibel, M.; Carr, A.; Zargar, N.; Saccomanno, M.F.; Milano, G. Advances in biology and mechanics of rotator cuff repair. *Knee Surg. Sports Traumatol. Arthrosc.* **2015**, *23*, 530–541. [CrossRef] [PubMed]
114. Shamsuddin, S.A.; Ramli, R.; Razali, M.; Baharin, B.; Sulaiman, S.; Hwei Ng, M.; Low, C.K.; Jabar, M.N.A.; Nordin, R.; Yahaya, N. Guided bone regeneration using autologous plasma, bone marrow cells and β-TCP/HA granules for experimental alveolar ridge reconstruction in Macaca fascicularis. *J. Biomater. Tissue Eng.* **2017**, *7*, 111–118. [CrossRef]
115. Hollinger, J.O.; Kleinschmidt, J.C. The Critical Size Defect as an Experimental Model to Test Bone Repair Materials. *J. Craniofacial Surg.* **1990**, *1*, 60–68. [CrossRef] [PubMed]

116. Albanna, M.; Binder, K.W.; Murphy, S.V.; Kim, J.; Qasem, S.A.; Zhao, W.; Tan, J.; El-Amin, I.B.; Dice, D.D.; Marco, J.; et al. In Situ Bioprinting of Autologous Skin Cells Accelerates Wound Healing of Extensive Excisional Full-Thickness Wounds. *Sci. Rep.* **2019**, *9*, 1856. [CrossRef]
117. Wu, Y.; Ravnic, D.J.; Ozbolat, I.T. Intraoperative Bioprinting: Repairing Tissues and Organs in a Surgical Setting. *Trends Biotechnol.* **2020**, *38*, 594–605. [CrossRef]
118. Ozbolat, I.T. Bioprinting scale-up tissue and organ constructs for transplantation. *Trends Biotechnol.* **2015**, *33*, 395–400. [CrossRef]
119. Keriquel, V.; Guillemot, F.; Arnault, I.; Guillotin, B.; Miraux, S.; Amédée, J.; Fricain, J.-C.; Catros, S. In Vivo bioprinting for computer- and robotic-assisted medical intervention: Preliminary study in mice. *Biofabrication* **2010**, *2*, 014101. [CrossRef]

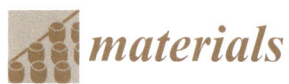

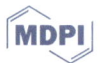

Article

Comparison of Tensile Bond Strength of Fixed-Fixed Versus Cantilever Single- and Double-Abutted Resin-Bonded Bridges Dental Prosthesis

Shweta Narwani [1], Naveen S. Yadav [1], Puja Hazari [1], Vrinda Saxena [2], Abdulrahman H. Alzahrani [3], Ahmed Alamoudi [4], Bassam Zidane [5], Nasreen Hassan Mohammed Albar [6], Ali Robaian [7], Sushil Kishnani [8], Kirti Somkuwar [1], Shilpa Bhandi [6], Kumar Chandan Srivastava [9,*], Deepti Shrivastava [10,*] and Shankargouda Patil [11,*]

1. Department of Prosthodontics and Crown & Bridge and Implantology, Peoples Dental Academy, Peoples University, Bhopal 462037, India
2. Department of Public Health Dentistry, Government Dental College, Indore 452001, India
3. Department of Prosthodontics, Faculty of Dentistry, Taif University, Taif 21944, Saudi Arabia
4. Department of Oral Biology, King Abdulaziz University, Jeddah 80200, Saudi Arabia
5. Department of Restorative Dentistry, King Abdulaziz University, Jeddah 22254, Saudi Arabia
6. Department of Restorative Dentistry, Jazan University, Jazan 45142, Saudi Arabia
7. Department of Conservative Dental Sciences, College of Dentistry, Prince Sattam bin Abdulaziz University, Al-Kharj 16278, Saudi Arabia
8. Department of Conservative Dentistry & Endodontics, Peoples College of Dental Sciences, Peoples University, Bhopal 462037, India
9. Department of Oral & Maxillofacial Surgery & Diagnostic Sciences, College of Dentistry, Jouf University, Sakaka 72388, Saudi Arabia
10. Department of Preventive Dentistry, College of Dentistry, Jouf University, Sakaka 72388, Saudi Arabia
11. Department of Maxillofacial Surgery and Diagnostic Sciences, Division of Oral Pathology, College of Dentistry, Jazan University, Jazan 45142, Saudi Arabia
* Correspondence: drkcs.omr@gmail.com (K.C.S.); sdeepti20@gmail.com (D.S.); dr.ravipatil@gmail.com (S.P.)

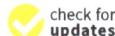

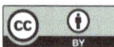

Abstract: Resin-bonded fixed dental prostheses (RBFDP) are minimally invasive alternatives to traditional full-coverage fixed partial dentures as they rely on resin cements for retention. This study compared and evaluated the tensile bond strength of three different resin-bonded bridge designs, namely, three-unit fixed-fixed, two-unit cantilever single abutment, and three-unit cantilever double-abutted resin-bonded bridge. Furthermore, the study attempted to compare the tensile bond strengths of the Maryland and Rochette types of resin-bonded bridges. Based on the inclusion and exclusion criteria, a total of seventy-five extracted maxillary incisors were collected and later were mounted on the acrylic blocks. Three distinct resin-bonded metal frameworks were designed: three-unit fixed-fixed (n = 30), two-unit cantilever single abutment (n = 30), and a three-unit cantilever double abutment (n = 30). The main groups were further divided into two subgroups based on the retainer design such as Rochette and Maryland. The different prosthesis designs were cemented to the prepared teeth. Later, abutment preparations were made on all specimens keeping the preparation as minimally invasive and esthetic oriented. Impression of the preparations were made using polyvinyl siloxane impression material, followed by pouring cast using die stone. A U-shaped handle of 1.5 mm diameter sprue wax with a 3 mm hole in between was attached to the occlusal surface of each pattern. The wax patterns were sprued and cast in a cobalt–chromium alloy. The castings were cleaned by sandblasting, followed by finishing and polishing. Lastly, based on the study group, specimens for Rochette bridge were perforated to provide mechanical retention between resin cement and metal, whereas the remaining 15 specimens were sandblasted on the palatal side to provide mechanical retention (Maryland bridge). In order to evaluate the tensile bond strength, the specimens were subjected to tensile forces on a universal testing machine with a uniform crosshead speed. The fixed-fixed partial prosthesis proved superior to both cantilever designs, whereas the single abutment cantilever design showed the lowest tensile bond strength. Maryland bridges uniformly showed higher bond strengths across all framework designs. Within the limitations of this study, the three-unit fixed-fixed design and Maryland bridges had greater bond strengths, implying that they may demonstrate lower clinical failure than cantilever designs and Rochette bridges.

Keywords: properties; bond strength; debonding; dental prosthesis; resin-bonded; fixed prosthesis; cantilever; fixed-fixed; Maryland bridge; Rochette bridge

1. Introduction

Loss of teeth is generally an unpleasant outcome for patients, and it can be considered as a reflection of the patient's history of dental conditions and treatments. According to the estimates from the Global Burden of Disease, more than half of the world's population experience single or partial tooth loss [1]. A person's quality of life in terms of oral health might have a negative impact due to tooth loss [2]. The field of prosthetic rehabilitation has changed drastically as a result of advancements in high-strength ceramics and digital dentistry. Conventional procedures for the replacement of missing teeth comprises full veneer fixed partial dentures for which the preparation of abutment teeth often involves major removal of the tooth structure. Significant advancements in material sciences have made it possible to use adhesive techniques that need less invasive tooth preparation. Resin-bonded bridges (also known as resin-bonded permanent dental prostheses or resin-retained bridges) are a less intrusive treatment option than single implants. As a result, it is implied that fewer dentinal tubules are opened, which is advantageous for the long-term health and vitality of teeth [3]. Additionally, patients may choose resin-bonded fixed dental prostheses because of cost considerations and a desire to avoid extensive tooth preparation or surgery for dental implants [4]. The endurance of resin-bonded bridges has been demonstrated by long-term clinical data [5]. They are effective and considered as a reasonably priced therapeutic option for replacing teeth.

Resin-bonded bridges (RBBs) are a type of fixed dental prostheses used to replace missing teeth. They are held in place by adhesive composite resin and are supported by abutments [6]. The Rochette bridge was the RBB's original design, and it relied on the macromechanical nature of retention through metal retaining wings [7]. The resin rivet holding the prosthesis to the acid-etched enamel would be created by the luting cement that flows through the tapered pinholes. However, Rochette-type RBBs had a short lifespan. In order to enable micromechanical retention, Maryland bridges were created [8]. They had a metal surface that had been electrochemically etched, which allowed for improved resin bonding and higher survival rates [9].

The lifespan of resin-bonded fixed dental prosthesis (RBFDP) has been the focus of discussion since its conception [10]. According to the research on RBFDP retention, numerous factors can affect its clinical performance, including choosing the right patient, choosing the right occlusal contacts, and designing the framework. The quantity of abutments that are connected to the pontic is another element that affects the clinical retention [11].

Fixed partial dentures' durability may be influenced by the prosthesis design [12]. For resin-bonded fixed partial dentures (RBFDP), two-unit cantilevered or three-unit fixed-fixed designs are the two common options. One of the most recommended and effective tooth replacement procedures in the past was the three-unit fixed-fixed design [13].

The usefulness of fixed-fixed bridges is constrained by complex clinical settings. As a result, there are many designs that take into account the patient's needs, anatomical constraints, and biomechanics [14]. A cantilevered single-abutment fixed partial prosthesis can be used to treat patients with distal extension edentulous space [15]. They have several benefits such as better oral hygiene, low maintenance, and a lower propensity for dental cavities. The preservation of the tooth anatomy, ease of preparation, and fabrication are just a few additional benefits [16].

In RBFDPs, minor and varied tooth motions are inevitable [17]. A troublesome issue with cantilevered structures is unilateral debonding [18], which might be a consequence of flexible cross-section and strong peeling forces under stress. In the past, it was considered that FPDs should have two firm abutment ends [19], and thus the abutment teeth were subjected to greater demands for tooth preparation. Recent studies have refuted the conventional dogma by demonstrating that two-unit fixed cantilevered RBFDPs have comparable clinical and patient-reported outcomes to double-abutted designs [15,20]. This might be a result of complicated inter-abutment strains from the older designs.

The resin-bonded bridge's retainer edges are placed supragingivally, which makes these prostheses more pleasing to the periodontium, eases the impression-making and finishing procedure, and makes them easier for the patient to clean. They also offer a shorter chair time, which makes them appealing to both the patient and the dentist [21]. Patients experience less dental anxiety and worry because the preparations are mainly limited to enamel and can be performed without local anesthesia [10].

Several clinical studies and systematic reviews have reported on the survivability of RBFDPs [22,23]. RBBs have a survival rate of 87.7% at five years and 64.9% at ten years [23,24]. The most frequent complication noted was debonding such as loss of retention [23,24].

On the other hand, the heterogeneous designs of the resin-bonded dental prosthesis are not scrutinized and are evaluated as a monolith. This makes it impossible to evaluate the performance of a specific design. The connection between the framework and the resin is still the most susceptible part of a resin-retained prosthesis. As a result, the primary goal of this study was to determine whether RBFDP design, Maryland or Rochette, and which type of abutment support will give the highest retention.

In summary, most of the earlier studies performed in relation to this topic are clinical trials, the results of which may be influenced by various patients' dependent variables due to which the results may not be applicable to a wider population. So, in order to increase the authenticity, the current study was performed with an in vitro design where the variables can be standardized to find out the effect of the number of abutments and the prosthesis design on the strength of the prostheses specifically.

This study aimed to compare and evaluate the tensile bond strength of three different resin-bonded bridge designs, namely, a three-unit fixed-fixed, two-unit cantilever single abutment, and a three-unit cantilever double-abutted resin-bonded bridge. The study further compared the tensile bond strengths of the Maryland and Rochette types of resin-bonded bridges. The null hypothesis considered was that the tensile bond strength of the cantilever designs is comparable to fixed-fixed designs, and the tensile bond strength of the prosthesis will not be affected by number of abutments and design of the prosthesis.

2. Materials and Methods

This in vitro experimental study was conducted in the Department of Prosthodontics, Crown, and Bridge and Implantology at People's Dental Academy, Bhopal, India, with supporting technical assistance from the Central Institute of Plastics Engineering and Technology, Bhopal, India. Prior to the study, ethical approval from the Institutional Ethics Review Board (2014/IEC/300/19) was obtained.

The specimens were divided into three groups based on support provided at the end of the prostheses. These were further allocated into two subcategories based on the design of the retainer. The resin-bonded frameworks with different prosthesis designs were cemented to the prepared teeth, and the cemented frameworks were subjected to tensile forces on a universal testing machine with a uniform crosshead speed.

2.1. Specimen Preparation

2.1.1. Mounting of Extracted Teeth on the Acrylic Block

The inclusion criteria considered was recently extracted healthy teeth, whereas carious, unrestorable, fractured, and hypoplastic teeth were excluded from the study. A total of seventy-five sound maxillary incisors were collected after extraction from the patients with rapidly progressive periodontitis. A prior informed consent was acquired from all subjects.

Initially, the extracted teeth were stored in 10% formalin. Later, they were mounted on acrylic molds such that the roots were embedded in acrylic, whereas the crown portion above the cementoenamel junction was left exposed. The incisors were mounted in the following three different forms based on the support provided at the end of the prostheses:

(a) Fixed-fixed bridge—Two incisors were mounted such that space for a pontic was left between the two teeth. A total of 30 teeth were mounted to make 15 fixed-fixed bridge specimens.
(b) Cantilever single-abutted bridge—A single incisor was mounted in acrylic which could be used as the abutment. A total of 15 incisors were mounted in this manner to create 15 similar cantilever single-abutment bridge specimens.
(c) Cantilever double-abutted bridge—Two central incisors were placed at adjacent positions to be used as abutments. In total, 30 teeth were mounted to build 15 cantilever double-abutted bridge specimens.

These main groups were further divided into two subgroups based on the design of the retainer (Figure 1), such as the Rochette and Maryland types. In summary, a total of 90 prostheses were made, where 30 prostheses were made for each main group, of which 15 were kept for the Rochette type and 15 were kept for the Maryland type.

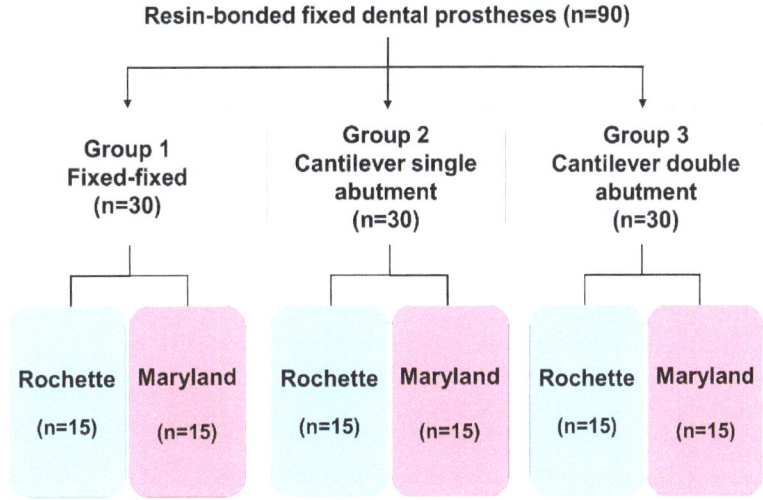

Figure 1. Sample Distribution.

2.1.2. Preparation of Incisors for the Prosthesis

The abutment teeth were prepared to adapt the retainers within the initial tooth outline keeping in mind the concern of satisfactory appearance. On the proximal aspect, the tooth preparation included axial trimming and guide planes, slightly extending onto the facial aspect to attain a facio-lingual lock. The preparation encompassed at least 180° of the teeth to augment the resistance of the retainer. The finish line of the incisor was kept 2 mm short of the incisal edge so as to prevent the incisal edge translucency from being esthetically impaired. Additionally, the lingual aspect was trimmed to produce a lingual clearance of 0.5 mm. The gingival finish line was kept 1 mm supragingival to maintain the preparation in enamel in order to ensure optimal bonding. Interproximally, the preparation was extended to the center of the contact area which maximized wraparound and at the same time minimized the visibility of metal from the facial aspect. The proximal surfaces were kept as parallel as possible to increase the retention form. Proximal grooves were added to compensate for any lack of proximal wraparound and to increase the retention form.

2.1.3. Laboratory Procedures

After tooth preparation, impressions of the preparation were made with polyvinyl siloxane impression material (3M ESPE, MN, USA). Stone dies (Die stone class IV, Kalrock, Kalabhai Dental, India) were constructed from each impression followed by wax pattern fabrication. A U-shaped handle of 1.5 mm diameter sprue wax with a 3 mm hole in between was attached to the occlusal surface of each pattern to facilitate seating and removal during subsequent stages. It also assisted in pulling the specimen with the help of fixtures during tensile bond strength testing in a universal testing machine. The wax patterns were sprued and cast in a cobalt–chromium alloy (Wironium plus, Bego). The castings were cleaned by sandblasting, followed by finishing and polishing. Fifteen frameworks from each group were perforated to provide mechanical retention between resin cement and metal (Rochette bridge) (Figure 2). The remaining 15 specimens were sandblasted on the palatal side using 50–250 µm aluminum oxide to provide mechanical retention (Maryland bridge) (Figure 3).

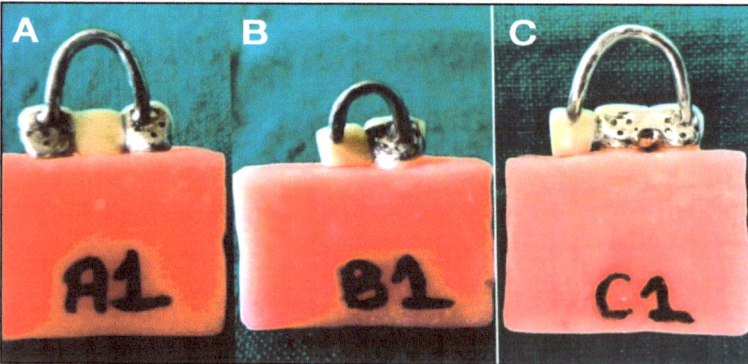

Figure 2. Specimens of Rochette-type resin-bonded fixed dental prostheses for (**A**) fixed-fixed, (**B**) cantilever single abutment, and (**C**) cantilever double abutted.

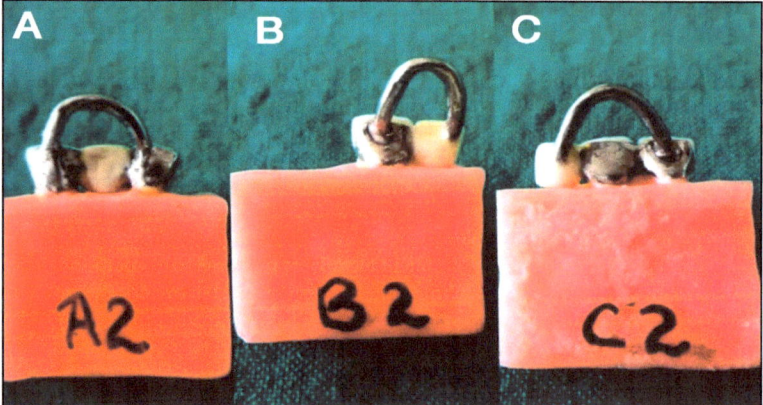

Figure 3. Specimens of Maryland-type resin-bonded fixed dental prostheses for (**A**) fixed-fixed, (**B**) cantilever single abutment, and (**C**) cantilever double abutted.

2.1.4. Cementation and Testing of the Specimens

The frameworks were cemented using resin cement (Rely X U200 resin cement, 3M, India). Each cemented specimen was placed in a lower holder such that the tooth die was oriented with its longitudinal axis parallel to the detaching force and a hook was placed in the upper holder of the universal testing machine. This hook was entangled in the U-shaped holder attached to the casted specimen. They were subjected to tensile force on the universal testing machine (Instron-3382, Instron, MA, USA) with a crosshead speed of 1 mm/min. The maximum load required to remove the crown was measured on the universal testing machine and compared with specimens of the other study group. Each mounted specimen was cemented with a Rochette bridge, which was subjected to tensile force. This was followed by cementation of the Maryland bridge on the same specimen, and the specimen was subjected to debonding force. This procedure for tensile bond assessment was carried out on all fifteen samples of each main group, with each sample being subjected twice to the debonding force: once for the Rochette type and once for the Maryland type.

2.2. Statistical Analysis

The data were statistically analyzed using the Statistical Package of Social Science (SPSS software v.20; IBM Corp., Armonk, NY, USA). Kruskal–Wallis and Mann–Whitney 'U' tests were applied for comparing data between the study groups. The significance level was set at $p < 0.05$.

3. Results

According to the results obtained, the fixed-fixed design resin-bonded fixed dental prosthesis (RBFDP) showed the greatest tensile bond strength, followed by the cantilever double abutment design (Figure 4). The cantilever single abutment design had the least tensile bond strength (Table 1). The mean tensile bond strength of fixed-fixed partial prosthesis (Group 1) was 127.23 N with a standard deviation (SD) of 21.91 N, whereas the mean tensile bond strength of cantilever single- (Group 2) and double-abutted FPD (Group 3) was 69.99 N and 106.90 N, respectively, with an SD of 30.06 N and 29.92 N (Table 1).

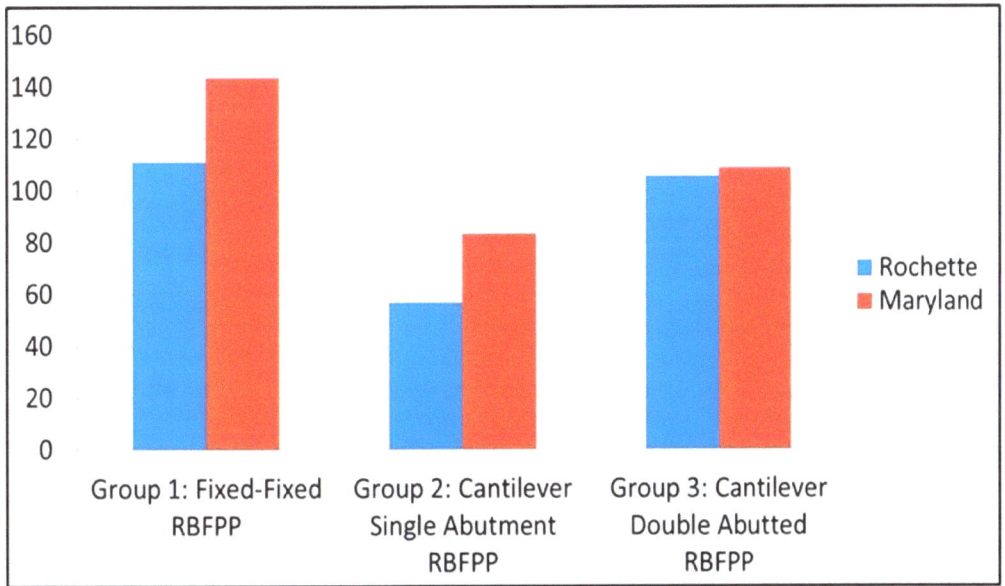

Figure 4. Comparison of Tensile Bond Strength (N) between Rochette and Maryland Type of Fixed-Fixed Denture, Cantilever Single and Double Abutted Resin Bonded Fixed Partial Prosthesis.

Table 1. Comparative evaluation of tensile bond strength (N) between the different resin-bonded fixed dental prosthesis.

Study Groups	Sample Size	Tensile Bond Strength			p Value
		Mean	SD	Median	
Group 1: Fixed-fixed denture	30	127.23	21.91	117.76	
Group 2: Cantilever single abutment	30	69.99	30.06	64.26	0.001
Group 3: Cantilever double abutment	30	106.90	29.92	114.13	

Note: Result expressed in mean; $p < 0.01$—Highly significant.

The Maryland design of resin-bonded fixed dental prosthesis (RBFDP) had greater tensile bond strength than the older Rochette bridge (Table 2) in two groups, i.e., fixed-fixed and cantilever single abutment RBFDP. In Group 3, i.e., cantilever double-abutted RBFDP, the Maryland type had greater tensile bond strength than the Rochette type, but the difference was non-significant. The Maryland type had a tensile strength of 143.32 ± 19.60 N compared to 111.13 ± 7.44 N in the Rochette type in fixed-fixed designs of RBFDP.

Table 2. Tensile bond strength (in N) of Rochette and Maryland types of resin-bonded fixed dental prosthesis (RBFDP).

		Group 1 Fixed-Fixed		Group 2 Cantilever Single Abutment		Group 3 Cantilever Double-Abutted	
		Rochette (N = 15)	Maryland (N = 15)	Rochette (N = 15)	Maryland (N = 15)	Rochette (N = 15)	Maryland (N = 15)
Tensile Bond Strength	Mean	111.13	143.32	56.59	83.38	105.27	108.52
	SD	7.44	19.60	15.30	35.41	33.48	26.98
	Median	109.56	145.56	58.27	86.59	112.21	119.30
Mann–Whitney 'U' Test Value		14.00		62.00		111.00	
p value		0.001 (HS)		0.036 (S)		0.950 (NS)	

Note: Result expressed in mean; $p > 0.05$—Not Significant; $p < 0.05$—Significant.

In the cantilever single-abutted RBFDP group, the Maryland type had a bond strength of 83.38 ± 35.41 compared to 56.59 ± 15.30 for the Rochette type (Table 2).

4. Discussion

For decades, resin-bonded bridges have been used to rehabilitate the edentulous spaces. They have a number of advantages over the traditional full-coverage fixed partial dentures, including lower costs and higher patient satisfaction [25,26], although, due to debonding, resin-bonded fixed dental prostheses (RBFDP) are more likely to fail than traditional fixed prostheses. However, the failures are often less catastrophic [27], and they do not include apical disease, migration, or cavities, which can lead to abutment loss [28,29]. The current study aimed to evaluate and compare the tensile bond strength of three desired designs of resin-bonded fixed dental prostheses based on the framework design and the number of abutments.

We found that fixed-fixed RBFDPs had the highest tensile bond strength compared to cantilever single-abutment and cantilever double-abutment RBFDPs. This suggests that fixed-fixed RBFDPs have a higher survival rate and better retention than cantilever designs. These findings are contrary to data obtained by Chai et al., who reported that two-unit RBFDPs had a better prognosis at 48–60 months with a survival rate of 81% compared to three-unit RBFDPs with a survival rate of 63% [16]. Our results are also inconsistent with findings of Wong and Botelho et al., who reported that bond strengths of the fixed-fixed group were lowered by fatigue loading. They concluded that three-unit fixed-fixed RBFDPs have a lower bond strength than two-unit cantilevered prostheses [11]. The discrepancies in outcomes may be due to the study design. Wong and Botelho et al. investigated the bond strength of framework designs bonded to stainless steel tooth dies, whereas, in the current study, the bond strength of frameworks bonded to extracted teeth were evaluated. Debonding may be connected to inter-abutment stress, functional loads, and framework biomechanics. Debonding and failure may also be caused by the framework's substance. Metal–ceramic RBFDPs generally fail due to debonding, whereas all-ceramic RBFDPs fracture [28]. According to a thorough review by Wei et al., RBFDP longevity is dependent on the resin bond and the operator technique [30].

Our findings differ from those of Botelho et al. [31], who found that two-unit cantilevered RBFDP (CL2) designs performed much better than three-unit fixed-fixed designs (FF3). Only 50% of FF3 designs survived, but 100% of CL2 designs performed well. The greater failure rate of FF3 designs is related to differential abutment tooth motions, which cause stress at the bonding interface and debonding. The CL2 designs are not concerned with such inter-abutment stress [18]. Cantilever designs have lower biological costs and are simpler to produce, resulting in fewer difficulties than fixed-fixed structures [30].

The higher bond strength of fixed-fixed RBFDPs and cantilever double-abutted RBFDPs can be attributed to their design. Both frameworks have increased surface area due to the involvement of two abutments compared to a cantilever single abutment design. Fixed-fixed RBFDPs show greater bond strength due to their bilateral support. In cantilever double-abutment RBFDPs there is unilateral support, which may lead to stress concentration on one side only. This may lead to a greater risk of debonding with this design.

We found that cantilevered single-abutment frameworks had the lowest tensile strength. Our finding differs from a majority of previous literature that describes single-abutment cantilever designs as having a low risk of failure and greater longevity [32–34]. Alraheam et al. also reported that although the dental implants seem to have provided reliable support for dental restorations in recent decades, the RBFDPs can serve as a promising alternative because the estimated 5-year clinical performance of RBFDPs was similar to that of FDPs and implant-supported crowns; thus, they concluded that clinicians should consider using RBFDPs frequently [35]. In their review, Mine et al. stated that cantilever RBFDPs were found to have better prognosis as compared to two retainer RBFDPs. The explanation given by them for the inferior clinical outcome of two retainer RBFDPs was because of their two major disadvantages. Firstly, the difference in the mobility of the two abutment teeth often leads to torquing and shear forces on abutment teeth resulting in debonding of the retainer from the tooth having lesser mobility. Secondly, the differential mobility can result in unrecognized debonding, increasing their predisposition to caries [36]. The contrary results of our study could be due to the design differences. A majority of information is based on longitudinal studies, which have been poorly controlled [23]. In the in vivo study design, it may be difficult to control a single variable and several factors can influence the outcomes such as the oral environment during cementation, operator technique, and prosthesis site. The use of different cements and preparation techniques leads to heterogeneity in study designs, making it difficult to isolate factors affecting the outcome [6].

In all three configurations, we discovered that the Maryland bridge design had stronger bond strength than the Rochette bridge design. We chose air particle abrasion over standard electrochemical etching because it improves retention of metal-framework RBFDPs [37]. Our findings substantially support the findings of Berekally and Smales, who stated that the failure rate of Rochette bridges (75%) was significantly higher than that of Maryland bridges (42%). Debonding was the primary cause of their failure [38]. Similarly, Creugers et al. showed that at 7.5 years, Rochette bridges had a poor survival rate of only 28% [39].

The results were comparable to those reported by Brady et al. in 1985, when the etched discs could sustain more than four times the breaking load of the perforated discs [40]. Creugers et al. demonstrated that micromechanical retainers retained more than macromechanical retainers [41]. According to Creugers et al., the survival rates for etched metal RBBs and perforated RBBs were 78 and 63 percent, respectively [42].

The Rochette design was the first resin-bonded permanent dental prosthesis design framework. They had a significant failure rate, necessitating the Maryland bridges' developed design. Surface treatment can alter the lifespan of resin-bonded bridges, according to el-Mowafy et al. [43]. Priest observed that chemical or electrolytic etching produces favorable long-term results, suggesting the superiority of Maryland bridges [44].

Several variables could explain why Rochette bridges performed poorly in our investigation. The retention area in RBFDPs based on macromechanical retention is limited to the perforated apertures and is not distributed evenly across the metal surface [41]. In RBFDPs based on macromechanical retention, the luting agent is introduced to the oral cavity. This allows for abrasion, fluid leakage between the metal and resin interfaces, and resin fluid absorption [41].

Our study is limited by its in vitro design. It may have failed to replicate the nuances of the oral cavity which may affect bond strength. The extracted teeth used may have had morphological differences that may contribute to variability.

Overall, our study found that fixed-fixed designs were superior to single and double abutment cantilever designs. Maryland bridges had higher bond strengths than Rochette bridges. Further research is necessary to confirm and validate these findings. Future studies may better demonstrate the clinical efficacy of resin-bonded fixed dental prostheses by including multiple operators across several prosthesis sites.

5. Conclusions

Replacement of missing teeth with a resin-bonded fixed dental prosthesis (RBFDP) is a conservative alternative to conventional fixed partial dentures. Various research performed in relation to RBFDP has shown that the long-term prognosis of RBFDP depends upon physical, chemical, and biological factors [45]. Within the limitations of this in vitro study, the fixed-fixed framework showed the greatest tensile bond strength. The cantilever single abutment RBFDP had the least bond strength. The Maryland bridge design of prosthesis was superior to the Rochette bridge in all three designs. Careful case selection and meticulous treatment planning are central to achieving the long-term survival of the prosthesis. Further research is needed to understand the effects of various prognostic factors.

Author Contributions: Conceptualization, S.N., N.S.Y., P.H. and V.S.; methodology, S.N., N.S.Y., V.S. and K.S.; software, A.H.A., A.A., B.Z. and N.H.M.A.; validation, A.H.A., A.A., B.Z., N.H.M.A., A.R. and S.K.; formal analysis, K.C.S., D.S. and S.P.; investigation, S.N., N.S.Y., P.H. and V.S.; resources, S.N. and N.S.Y.; writing—original draft preparation, S.N., N.S.Y., K.C.S., D.S. and S.P.; writing—review and editing, S.N., N.S.Y., P.H., V.S., A.H.A., A.A., B.Z., N.H.M.A., A.R., S.K., K.S., S.B., K.C.S., D.S. and S.P.; supervision, N.S.Y., K.C.S. and S.P.; funding acquisition, A.H.A., A.A., B.Z., N.H.M.A., A.R., S.K. and S.P. All authors have read and agreed to the published version of the manuscript.

Funding: This research received no external funding.

Institutional Review Board Statement: The study was conducted in accordance with the Declaration of Helsinki and approved by the Institutional Review Board of People's Dental Academy, Bhopal, Madhya Pradesh, India (2014/IEC/300/19).

Informed Consent Statement: Not applicable.

Data Availability Statement: The datasets will be available and accessible from the corresponding author on reasonable request.

Conflicts of Interest: The authors declare no conflict of interest.

References

1. Global Burden of Disease Study 2019 (GBD 2019) Reference Life Table | GHDx. Available online: https://ghdx.healthdata.org/record/ihme-data/global-burden-disease-study-2019-gbd-2019-reference-life-table (accessed on 10 April 2022).
2. Tan, H.; Peres, K.G.; Peres, M.A. Retention of Teeth and Oral Health-Related Quality of Life. *J. Dent. Res.* **2016**, *95*, 1350–1357. [CrossRef] [PubMed]
3. Kern, M. *RBFDPs Resin-Bonded Fixed Dental Prostheses Minimally Invasive–Esthetic–Reliable*; Quintessence Pub Co.: Chicago, IL, USA, 2017; ISBN 978-1-78698-020-5.

4. Morton, D.; Gallucci, G.; Lin, W.-S.; Pjetursson, B.; Polido, W.; Roehling, S.; Sailer, I.; Aghaloo, T.; Albera, H.; Bohner, L.; et al. Group 2 ITI Consensus Report: Prosthodontics and Implant Dentistry. *Clin. Oral Implants Res.* **2018**, *29* (Suppl. S16), 215–223. [CrossRef] [PubMed]
5. Abuzar, M.; Locke, J.; Burt, G.; Clausen, G.; Escobar, K. Longevity of Anterior Resin-Bonded Bridges: Survival Rates of Two Tooth Preparation Designs. *Aust. Dent. J.* **2018**, *63*, 279–284. [CrossRef] [PubMed]
6. Durey, K.A.; Nixon, P.J.; Robinson, S.; Chan, M.-Y. Resin Bonded Bridges: Techniques for Success. *Br. Dent. J.* **2011**, *211*, 113–118. [CrossRef] [PubMed]
7. Mourshed, B.; Samran, A.; Alfagih, A.; Samran, A.; Abdulrab, S.; Kern, M. Anterior cantilever resin-bonded fixed dental prostheses: A review of the literature. *J. Prosthodont.* **2018**, *27*, 266–275. [CrossRef]
8. St George, G.; Hemmings, K.; Patel, K. Resin-Retained Bridges Re-Visited. Part 1. History and Indications. *Prim. Dent. Care* **2002**, *9*, 87–91. [CrossRef]
9. Kimura, O. Fifteen-year survival of resin-bonded vs. full-coverage fixed dental prostheses. *J. Prosthodont. Res.* **2019**, *63*, 374–382.
10. Botelho, M.G.; Dyson, J.E. Long-Span, Fixed-Movable, Resin-Bonded Fixed Partial Dentures: A Retrospective, Preliminary Clinical Investigation. *Int. J. Prosthodont.* **2005**, *18*, 371–376.
11. Wong, T.L.; Botelho, M.G. The Fatigue Bond Strength of Fixed-Fixed versus Cantilever Resin-Bonded Partial Fixed Dental Prostheses. *J. Prosthet. Dent.* **2014**, *111*, 136–141. [CrossRef]
12. Botelho, M. Design Principles for Cantilevered Resin-Bonded Fixed Partial Dentures. *Quintessence Int.* **2000**, *31*, 613–619.
13. Christensen, G.J. Three-Unit Fixed Prostheses versus Implant-Supported Single Crowns. *J. Am. Dent. Assoc.* **2008**, *139*, 191–194. [CrossRef] [PubMed]
14. Madhok, S.; Madhok, S. Evolutionary Changes in Bridges Designs. *IOSR J. Dent. Med. Sci.* **2014**, *13*, 50–56. [CrossRef]
15. Botelho, M.G.; Yon, M.J.Y.; Mak, K.C.K.; Lam, W.Y.H. A Randomised Controlled Trial of Two-Unit Cantilevered or Three-Unit Fixed-Movable Resin-Bonded Fixed Partial Dentures Replacing Missing Molars. *J. Dent.* **2020**, *103*, 103519. [CrossRef]
16. Chai, J.; Chu, F.C.S.; Newsome, P.R.H.; Chow, T.W. Retrospective Survival Analysis of 3-unit Fixed-fixed and 2-unit Cantilevered Fixed Partial Dentures. *J. Oral Rehabil.* **2005**, *32*, 759–765. [CrossRef]
17. Mendes, J.M.; Bentata, A.L.; de Sá, J.; Silva, A.S. Survival Rates of Anterior-Region Resin-Bonded Fixed Dental Prostheses: An Integrative Review. *Eur. J. Dent.* **2021**, *15*, 788–797. [CrossRef] [PubMed]
18. Botelho, M.G.; Chan, A.W.K.; Leung, N.C.H.; Lam, W.Y.H. Long-Term Evaluation of Cantilevered versus Fixed–Fixed Resin-Bonded Fixed Partial Dentures for Missing Maxillary Incisors. *J. Dent.* **2016**, *45*, 59–66. [CrossRef]
19. Shen, J. *Advanced Ceramics for Dentistry*; Butterworth-Heinemann: Oxford, UK, 2013; ISBN 0123948363.
20. Kern, M.; Sasse, M. Ten-Year Survival of Anterior All-Ceramic Resin-Bonded Fixed Dental Prostheses. *J. Adhes. Dent.* **2011**, *13*, 407–410. [CrossRef]
21. Izgi, A.D.; Kale, E.; Eskimez, S. A Prospective Cohort Study on Cast-Metal Slot-Retained Resin-Bonded Fixed Dental Prostheses in Single Missing First Molar Cases: Results after up to 7.5 Years. *J. Adhes. Dent.* **2013**, *15*, 73–84.
22. Thoma, D.S.; Sailer, I.; Ioannidis, A.; Zwahlen, M.; Makarov, N.; Pjetursson, B.E. A Systematic Review of the Survival and Complication Rates of Resin-Bonded Fixed Dental Prostheses after a Mean Observation Period of at Least 5 Years. *Clin. Oral Implants Res.* **2017**, *28*, 1421–1432. [CrossRef]
23. Pjetursson, B.E.; Tan, W.C.; Tan, K.; Brägger, U.; Zwahlen, M.; Lang, N.P. A Systematic Review of the Survival and Complication Rates of Resin-Bonded Bridges after an Observation Period of at Least 5 Years. *Clin. Oral Implants Res.* **2008**, *19*, 131–141. [CrossRef]
24. Balasubramaniam, G.R. Predictability of Resin Bonded Bridges—A Systematic Review. *Br. Dent. J.* **2017**, *222*, 849–858. [CrossRef] [PubMed]
25. Burke, F.J.T. Resin-Retained Bridges: Fiber-Reinforced versus Metal. *Dent. Update* **2008**, *35*, 521–522. [CrossRef]
26. Creugers, N.H.; De Kanter, R.J. Patients' Satisfaction in Two Long-Term Clinical Studies on Resin-Bonded Bridges. *J. Oral Rehabil.* **2000**, *27*, 602–607. [CrossRef] [PubMed]
27. Di Fiore, A.; Stellini, E.; Savio, G.; Rosso, S.; Graiff, L.; Granata, S.; Monaco, C.; Meneghello, R. Assessment of the different types of failure on anterior cantilever resin-bonded fixed dental prostheses fabricated with three different materials: An in vitro study. *Appl. Sci.* **2020**, *10*, 4151. [CrossRef]
28. Miettinen, M.; Millar, B.J. A Review of the Success and Failure Characteristics of Resin-Bonded Bridges. *Br. Dent. J.* **2013**, *215*, E3. [CrossRef]
29. Barber, M.W.; Preston, A.J. An Update on Resin-Bonded Bridges. *Eur. J. Prosthodont. Restor. Dent.* **2008**, *16*, 2–9.
30. Wei, A.Y.; Qin, X.W. Clinical Performance of Anterior Resin-Bonded Fixed Dental Prostheses with Different Framework Designs: A Systematic Review and Meta-Analysis. *J. Dent.* **2016**, *47*, 1–7. [CrossRef]
31. Botelho, M.G.; Nor, L.C.; Kwong, H.W.; Kuen, B.S. Two-Unit Cantilevered Resin-Bonded Fixed Partial Dentures—A Retrospective, Preliminary Clinical Investigation. *Int. J. Prosthodont.* **2000**, *13*, 25–28.
32. Djemal, S.; Setchell, D.; King, P.; Wickens, J. Long-Term Survival Characteristics of 832 Resin-Retained Bridges and Splints Provided in a Post-Graduate Teaching Hospital between 1978 and 1993. *J. Oral Rehabil.* **1999**, *26*, 302–320. [CrossRef]
33. Kern, M. Clinical Long-Term Survival of Two-Retainer and Single-Retainer All-Ceramic Resin-Bonded Fixed Partial Dentures. *Quintessence Int.* **2005**, *36*, 141–147.

34. van Dalen, A.; Feilzer, A.J.; Kleverlaan, C.J. A Literature Review of Two-Unit Cantilevered FPDs. *Int. J. Prosthodont.* **2004**, *17*, 281–284. [PubMed]
35. Alraheam, I.A.; Ngoc, C.N.; Wiesen, C.A.; Donovan, T.E. Five-year success rate of resin-bonded fixed partial dentures: A systematic review. *J. Esthet. Restor. Dent.* **2019**, *31*, 40–50. [CrossRef] [PubMed]
36. Mine, A.; Fujisawa, M.; Miura, S.; Yumitate, M.; Ban, S.; Yamanaka, A.; Ishida, M.; Takebe, J.; Yatani, H. Critical review about two myths in fixed dental prostheses: Full-Coverage vs. Resin-Bonded, non-Cantilever vs. Cantilever. *Jpn. Dent. Sci. Rev.* **2021**, *57*, 33–38. [CrossRef] [PubMed]
37. Creugers, N.H.; De Kanter, R.J.; Verzijden, C.W.; Van't Hof, M.A. Risk Factors and Multiple Failures in Posterior Resin-Bonded Bridges in a 5-Year Multi-Practice Clinical Trial. *J. Dent.* **1998**, *26*, 397–402. [CrossRef]
38. Berekally, T.L.; Smales, R.J. A Retrospective Clinical Evaluation of Resin-bonded Bridges Inserted at the Adelaide Dental Hospital. *Aust. Dent. J.* **1993**, *38*, 85–96. [CrossRef]
39. Creugers, N.H.; Käyser, A.F.; Van't Hof, M.A. A Seven-and-a-Half-Year Survival Study of Resin-Bonded Bridges. *J. Dent. Res.* **1992**, *71*, 1822–1825. [CrossRef]
40. Brady, T.; Doukoudakis, A.; Rasmussen, S.T. Experimental Comparison between Perforated and Etched-Metal Resin-Bonded Retainers. *J. Prosthet. Dent.* **1985**, *54*, 361–365. [CrossRef]
41. Creugers, N.H.J.; van't Hof, M.A.; Vrijhoef, M.M.A. A Clinical Comparison of Three Types of Resin-Retained Cast Metal Prostheses. *J. Prosthet. Dent.* **1986**, *56*, 297–300. [CrossRef]
42. Creugers, N.H.J.; Snoek, P.A.; Van't Hof, M.A.; KÄUYSER, A.F. Clinical Performance of Resin-bonded Bridges: A 5-year Prospective Study. Part III: Failure Characteristics and Survival after Rebonding. *J. Oral Rehabil.* **1990**, *17*, 179–186. [CrossRef]
43. El-Mowafy, O.; Rubo, M.H.M. Resin-Bonded Fixed Partial Dentures—A Literature Review with Presentation of a Novel Approach. *Int. J. Prosthodont.* **2000**, *13*, 460–467.
44. Priest, G. An 11-Year Reevaluation of Resin-Bonded Fixed Partial Dentures. *Int. J. Periodontics Restor. Dent.* **1995**, *15*, 238–247.
45. Tanoue, N. Longevity of resin-bonded fixed partial dental prostheses made with metal alloys. *Clin. Oral Investig.* **2016**, *20*, 1329–1336. [CrossRef] [PubMed]

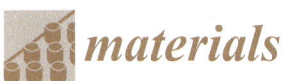

Article

Marginal and Internal Gap of Metal Copings Fabricated Using Three Types of Resin Patterns with Subtractive and Additive Technology: An In Vitro Comparison

Hemavardhini Addugala [1,2], Vidyashree Nandini Venugopal [1,*], Surya Rengasamy [1], Pradeep Kumar Yadalam [3], Nassreen H. Albar [4], Ahmed Alamoudi [5], Sarah Ahmed Bahammam [6], Bassam Zidane [7], Hammam Ahmed Bahammam [8], Shilpa Bhandi [4,9], Deepti Shrivastava [10,*], Kumar Chandan Srivastava [11] and Shankargouda Patil [12,13,*]

[1] Department of Prosthodontics and Implantology, SRM Kattankulathur Dental College and Hospital, SRM Institute of Science and Technology, SRM Nagar, Chennai 603203, India
[2] Independent Researcher, Chennai 603203, India
[3] Department of Periodontics, Saveetha Dental College and Hospitals, Saveetha Institute of Medical and Technical Sciences, Saveetha University, Chennai 602117, India
[4] Department of Restorative Dental Sciences, Division of Operative Dentistry, College of Dentistry, Jazan University, Jazan 45142, Saudi Arabia
[5] Department of Oral Biology, King Abdulaziz University, P.O. Box 80209, Jeddah 21589, Saudi Arabia
[6] Department of Pediatric Dentistry and Orthodontics, College of Dentistry, Taibah University, P.O. Box 344, Medina 42353, Saudi Arabia
[7] Department of Restorative Dentistry, King Abdulaziz University, P.O. Box 80209, Jeddah 21589, Saudi Arabia
[8] Department of Pediatric Dentistry, College of Dentistry, King Abdulaziz University, P.O. Box 80209, Jeddah 21589, Saudi Arabia
[9] Department of Cariology, Saveetha Dental College & Hospitals, Saveetha Institute of Medical and Technical Sciences, Saveetha University, Chennai 600077, India
[10] Department of Preventive Dentistry, College of Dentistry, Jouf University, Sakaka 72388, Saudi Arabia
[11] Department of Oral & Maxillofacial Surgery & Diagnostic Sciences, College of Dentistry, Jouf University, Sakaka 72345, Saudi Arabia
[12] Department of Maxillofacial Surgery and Diagnostic Science, Division of Oral Pathology, College of Dentistry, Jazan University, Jazan 45142, Saudi Arabia
[13] Centre of Molecular Medicine and Diagnostics (COMManD), Saveetha Dental College & Hospitals, Saveetha Institute of Medical and Technical Sciences, Saveetha University, Chennai 600077, India
* Correspondence: vidyashv@srmist.edu.in (V.N.V.); sdeepti20@gmail.com (D.S.); dr.ravipatil@gmail.com (S.P.)

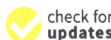

Citation: Addugala, H.; Venugopal, V.N.; Rengasamy, S.; Yadalam, P.K.; Albar, N.H.; Alamoudi, A.; Bahammam, S.A.; Zidane, B.; Bahammam, H.A.; Bhandi, S.; et al. Marginal and Internal Gap of Metal Copings Fabricated Using Three Types of Resin Patterns with Subtractive and Additive Technology: An In Vitro Comparison. *Materials* 2022, *15*, 6397. https://doi.org/10.3390/ma15186397

Academic Editors: Laura-Cristina Rusu and Lavinia Cosmina Ardelean

Received: 9 July 2022
Accepted: 12 September 2022
Published: 15 September 2022

Publisher's Note: MDPI stays neutral with regard to jurisdictional claims in published maps and institutional affiliations.

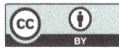

Copyright: © 2022 by the authors. Licensee MDPI, Basel, Switzerland. This article is an open access article distributed under the terms and conditions of the Creative Commons Attribution (CC BY) license (https://creativecommons.org/licenses/by/4.0/).

Abstract: This study analyzes the evidence of the marginal discrepancy and internal adaptation of copings fabricated using three types of resin patterns with subtractive (milling) and additive technology (3D printing), as it is not widely reported. Working casts (n = 15) were scanned and patterns were completed using computer-aided designing (CAD). Resin patterns were fabricated using the designed data and divided into three groups according to the method of fabrication of patterns: subtractive technology–CAD milled polymethyl methacrylate resin (Group-PMMA), additive technology [digital light processing (DLP) technique]–acrylonitrile–butadiene–styrene (ABS) patterns (Group-ABS), and polylactic acid (PLA) patterns (Group-PLA). Resin patterns were casted with Cobalt–Chromium (Co–Cr) alloy (lost wax technique). Internal and marginal gaps of the metal copings were analyzed with the replica technique under optical microscope. The Kruskal–Wallis test was used to compare values among the groups, and post hoc multiple tests confirmed the specific differences within the groups. The median marginal gap was least for CAD milled resin patterns, followed by PLA printed resin patterns and ABS printed resin patterns. There were significant differences between Group-PMMA and Group-PLA and Group-ABS (p = 0.0001). There was no significant difference between Group-PLA and Group-ABS (p = 0.899). The median internal gap was least for metal copings fabricated from Group-PLA, followed by Group-ABS and Group-PMMA. The differences were not statistically significant (p = 0.638) for the internal gap. Full metal Co–Cr copings fabricated from the milled PMMA group had a better marginal fit, followed by the PLA and ABS printed groups. Copings fabricated with the PLA printed group had the best internal fit, though the values were statistically insignificant between the groups.

Keywords: computer-aided manufacturing; internal gap; marginal gap; 3D printing; replica technique

1. Introduction

The precise seating of restoration is essential in dental restorations to fulfill biological, physical, and esthetic requirements. The occurrence of any marginal discrepancy causes dissolution of cement, micro-leakage, and plaque retention, which in turn leads to the accumulation of bacteria, inflammation, and secondary caries.

Laboratory and clinical factors impact internal and marginal gaps in restorations to a great extent. Laboratory factors include the incompatibility of dental materials such as die stone, pattern materials, die spacer, casting investments, and casting techniques [1,2]. Clinical factors are tooth preparation geometry, degree of taper, type of finish line, and impression materials used for the restoration in a dental office [3,4].

Despite the importance of marginal fidelity, there is no consensus on margin opening or misfit that is considered clinically acceptable. Previous studies have reported a wide range of acceptable marginal gap, from 50 μm to 300 μm [5–9]. Von Fraunhofer and McLean stated 120μm as acceptable for clinical use, and it is the most quoted in original research studies [10]. An acceptable pattern fabrication is an important factor influencing the internal and marginal fit of the restorations [11,12].

The evolution of digital technology has made the possibility of fabricating restorations with subtractive or additive methods. Subtractive manufacturing is the process of constructing three-dimensional objects by successively cutting away material from a solid material block. In additive technology/rapid prototyping, 3D objects are built by adding layer-upon-layer of material. The additive technologies reported in literature are selective laser sintering (SLS), digital light processing (DLP), stereo lithography (SL), polyjet, and so on [13]. The patterns obtained from these techniques can be subjected to casting procedures. The accuracy of resin patterns fabricated using the above-mentioned technologies has not been studied extensively. Utilizing technology at this stage of casting process enables the faster fabrication of patterns that can provide uniform quality in all restorations in lesser time.

However, there is limited available literature about the fabrication of restorations using resin patterns for the casting of crowns and on the fit of such restorations [14,15]. There is also a lack of studies comparing the discrepancies of the copings made using pattern resins that were fabricated by subtractive and additive technology in peer-reviewed literature.

The aim of this present study was to compare the marginal and internal gap of metal copings fabricated using three types of resin patterns with subtractive (milling) and additive (3D printing) technology. The secondary objective was to compare the internal and marginal gaps of the different walls of the preparation.

The study began with the following null hypothesis: there will be no difference in the marginal gap and internal gap of copings fabricated using subtractive and additive technology.

2. Materials and Methods

The study was approved by the Institutional Ethical Committee (Ref No.1475/IEC/2018). A Mandibular typodont was utilized as the master model (Model type: D91SHD-200, Nissin Dental products INC. Kyoto, Japan). Tooth preparation was done for a full-coverage restoration in the right second premolar region (45) following the preparation guidelines with 16^0 total occlusal convergence (TOC) [16]. Fifteen conventional impressions were made using low viscosity and putty consistency polyvinyl siloxane material (Photosil, DPI, Mumbai, India), using the double mix putty–wash technique. Each of the fifteen impressions was sprayed with a debubblizer (Unicoat, Delta, Chennai, India) and poured with Type IV Gypsum (Die stone–Ultrarock, Kalabhai Karson, Mumbai, India) using a vibrator (AX-2000, Aixin Medical Equipment Co., Ltd., Tianjin, China) to make fifteen working casts (Figure 1).

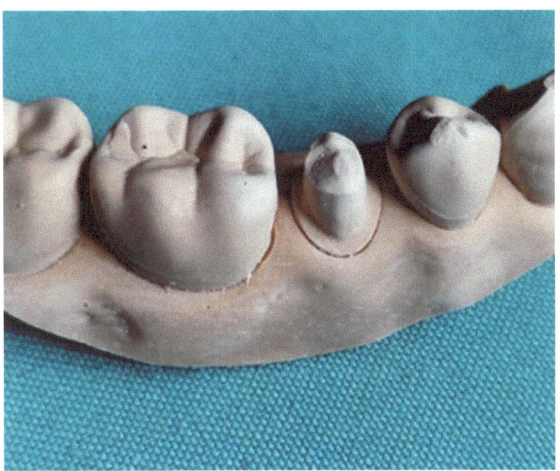

Figure 1. Working cast.

The working casts were then scanned and digitized using a model scanner (Blue light LED scanner, D900 L, 3 Shape, Copenhagen, Denmark). 3D images of casts were projected on the monitor for designing the resin patterns in the CAD software (3 Shape Dental Manager Dental System 2020 -1 88.1.9 (DS 20.1.2), Copenhagen, Denmark). Designing involves the following steps: i. determining the area of interest, ii. assessing the path of insertion with minimal undercuts, iii. outlining the margins of the patterns, and iv. designing the anatomical contour of the resin patterns (Figure 2).

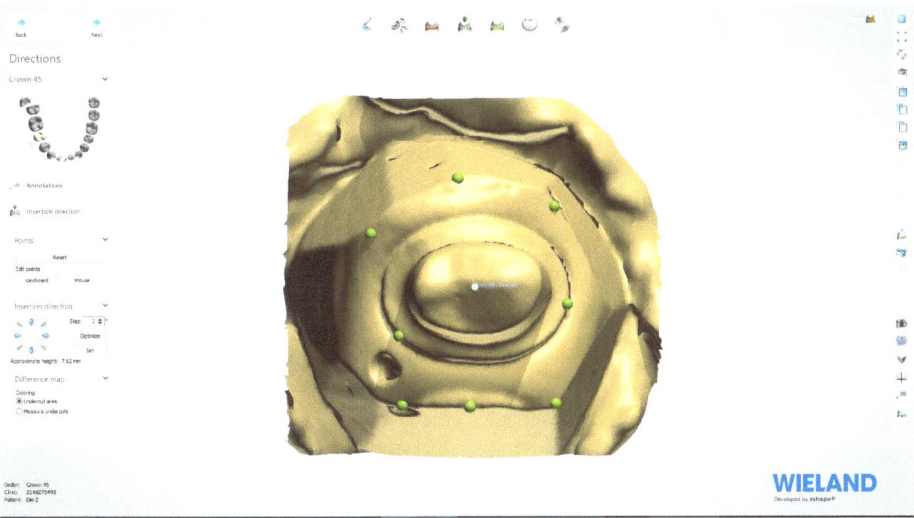

Figure 2. Designing in CAD software.

The design was saved in STL (standard tessellation language, or standard triangulation language) file format and transferred to the milling software (subtractive technology/CAD/CAM milling method), as well as to the slicing software (additive technology/3D printing additive technology), to get three types of resin patterns such as CAD milled PMMA resin patterns (Group-PMMA, n = 15), DLP printed acrylonitrile–butadiene–

styrene (ABS) resin patterns (Group-ABS, n = 15), DLP printed polylactic acid (PLA) resin pattern (Group-PLA, n = 15) (Table 1).

Table 1. Materials and techniques used for pattern fabrication.

Resin Fabrication Technology	Material–Brand Name, Model and Place of Manufacture	Materials–Composition
Milling	Aidite, 0D9, Hebei, China	Polymethyl methacrylate (PMMA) resin disc 14 mm–A2 shade
3D Printing-Digital Light Processing (DLP)	Weistek, ABS-1000-BL, China	Acrylo-nitrile butadiene styrene (ABS) resin material
3D Printing-Digital Light Processing (DLP)	e-sun, e-resin, PLAgray05A, China	Polylactic acid (PLA) resin material

2.1. Fabrication of Group-PMMA Samples

In Group-PMMA, the casts were scanned using the model scanner (Blue light LED scanner, D900 L, 3 Shape, Denmark). Designing of the scanned working cast was done using CAD software (3 Shape Dental System, Denmark). This was followed by design transfer to the milling software as STL files, and the patterns were milled in a CAD–CAM milling unit (Zenotec Hybrid Select, Wieland, Stuttgart, Germany) using a PMMA disc (Figure 3).

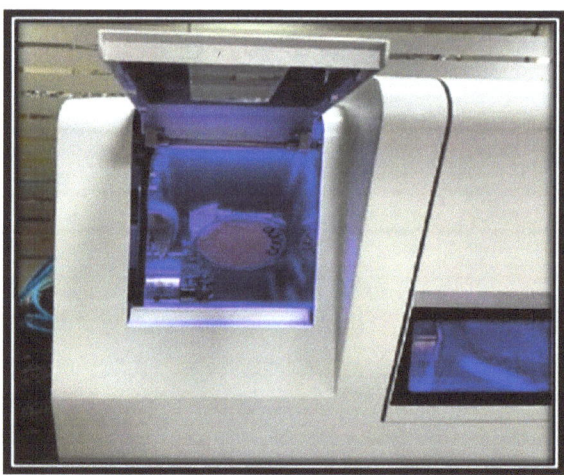

Figure 3. Milling of PMMA resin pattern.

A total of 15 resin patterns were milled and placed over their corresponding dies. Wax sprues of 3 mm length were used to join resin patterns and were invested using a phosphate-bonded investment material (Bellavest SH +Begoso, Bego, Bremen, Germany). The casting was done with Co–Cr alloy (Wirobond LFC, Bego, Bremen, Germany) using an induction casting machine (Fornax T-Bego, Bremen, Germany). The castings were sectioned from the sprues by an ultra-fine carborundum disc, and then the metal copings were finished and placed over their respective dies.

2.2. Fabrication of Group-ABS (Acrylonitrile–Butadiene–Styrene) Samples

The working casts were scanned and digitized similarly to that of Group-PMMA. The STL file was exported to a slicing software (Chitubox v1.6.4.3 Beta) to edit the layers, tooth path, temperature, color, and print speed. The software helped in slicing the model file into layers and generated a specific g-code for the 3D printer. The physical model was printed using this g-code. The 3D printer (Anycubic 3D Printer (Model no. Anycubic Photon S UV, Shenzhen, China)) works by digital light processing (DLP) technique, wherein a light source is projected to cure the photosensitive liquid resin layer-by-layer, following a specific path of the designed model. The building up of the object was done incrementally upside down on an elevating platform, where the occlusal surface was facing downwards towards the resin tank, and the cervical portion was attached to the building platform with the help of supporters. The 120° direction was defined as the orientation angle after positioning the lingual surface of the crown parallel to the build platform and rotating it 30° on the Y-axis. The crown was rotated 15° or 30° in the direction of the Y-axis until the support was placed on the buccal surface. The support was to be automatically positioned only on the surface that formed an angle of ≥30° with the Z-axis. The photopolymer used here had monomers of acrylonitrile–butadiene–styrene (ABS) to fabricate ABS resin patterns. A total of 15 resin patterns were printed (Figure 4).

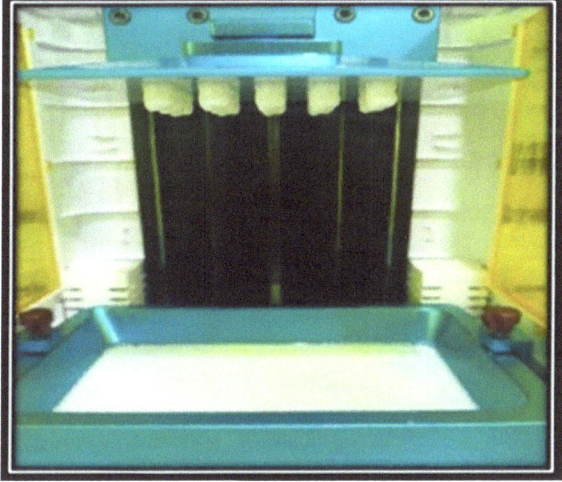

Figure 4. Printing of acrylonitrile–butadiene–styrene (ABS) resin patterns.

The patterns were submerged for 3 min and swirled around in isopropyl alcohol to remove excess resin along with the uncured layer, and also to reduce the residual stickiness. All these resin patterns were cast similarly to that of Group-PMMA to make 15 Co–Cr copings using the lost wax technique.

2.3. Fabrication of Group-PLA (Polylactic Acid) Samples

Fabrication of this type of resin pattern was similar to that of Group-ABS. Once the STL files of the fifteen working casts were transferred to a 3D printer, for this group photopolymer, polylactic acid (PLA) resin material was used to print the resin patterns. The printer and printing technique used was the same as for Group-ABS. Only the resin material used was different. All the resin patterns were subjected to the lost wax technique to fabricate 15 Co–Cr copings.

2.4. Measurement of Marginal and Internal Gaps

After the fabrication of crowns, marginal and internal gaps were analyzed by using the replica technique. Marginal and internal gaps were determined according to the terminology previously reported by Holmes [17]. The internal gap is the measurement of the internal surface of the restoration to the axial wall of the preparation in the perpendicular direction. Measurement between the axial wall and internal surface at the margin is called the marginal gap. These gaps are analyzed using the replica technique described by

Boening [18]. Using this technique, low viscosity polyvinyl siloxane (Reprosil, Dentsply, Sirona, India) was injected into each coping and placed on the corresponding cast with constant finger pressure for 10 s on the occlusal surface. Once the impression material was set, it was removed from the cast along with the coping. The thin silicon film was supported by another low-viscosity polyvinyl siloxane material (Aquasil LV, Dentsply, Konstanz, Germany) with contrasting color to merge into a single piece with the film [19]. Once the supporting low-viscosity PVS impression material hardened, each replica was removed and sectioned with sharp surgical Bard-Parker blade no.15 buccolingual and mesiodistally [18] (Figure 5). All the procedures were performed by a single operator.

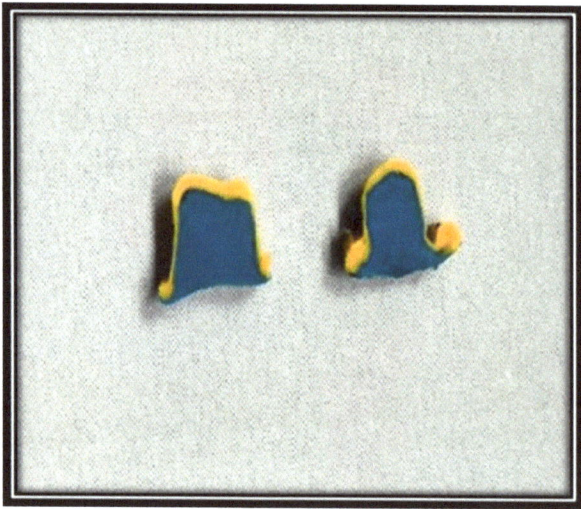

Figure 5. Buccolingual and Mesiodistal sectioned replica.

For each coping, the measurements were obtained from the buccolingual and mesiodistal sections in sixteen locations (eight in the buccolingual section and eight in the mesiodistal section): four marginal (MG-B, MG-L, MG-M, MG-D), four cervical (IG-C1, IG-C2, IG-C3, IG-C4), four axial (IG-B, IG-L, IG-M, IG-D), and four occlusal areas (IG-O1, IG-O2, IG-O3, IG-O4). The locations measured in the buccolingual section are: MG-B, IG-C1, IG-B, IG-O1, IG-O2, IG-L, IG-C2, MG-L (Figure 6A); and in mesiodistal sections are: MG-M, IG-C3, IG-M, IG-O3, IG-O4, IG-D, IG-C4, MG-D (Figure 6B).

All these measurements were recorded after stabilizing the cross-section of light body impression material with clay over the slide, held under an optical microscope (Leica DMC 2900, Leica Microsystems, Maharashtra, India). The thicknesses were measured using a software tool.

2.5. Statistical Analysis

The data obtained were subjected to normality tests, i.e., Kolmogorov–Smirnov and Shapiro–Wilk tests, which revealed that the distribution of data was non-normal. Hence, the statistical analyses performed were non-parametric tests. The Kruskal–Wallis test was conducted to compare the median values between the three groups. Post hoc Dunn's multiple comparison test was conducted to determine the significance between the groups.

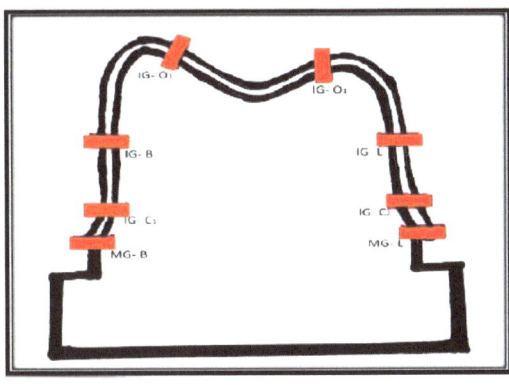
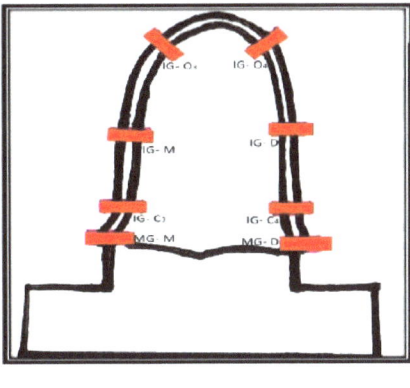

(A) (B)

Figure 6. (**A**,**B**): Line diagram showing the location of areas of measurements of the gap on (**A**). Buccolingual section, (**B**) Mesiodistal section.

3. Results

The results showed that the median marginal gap was least on the lingual wall in all the groups (PMMA milled group, 48.93 ± 14.19 μm; ABS printed group, 104.48 ± 19.58 μm; PLA printed group, 101.32 ± 19.80 μm). The median marginal gap was the least on all four walls in the resin pattern fabricated from PMMA milled group (48.93 ± 14.19 μm). The median marginal gap was highest on the buccal wall in the resin pattern fabricated from the ABS printed group (111.85 ± 23.83 μm). The median values of PMMA milled resin patterns, ABS printed resin patterns, and PLA printed resin patterns groups were within 120 μm, which happens to be the range of clinical acceptance level. The Kruskal–Wallis test was conducted to find the significance of the marginal gap values obtained using the three different resin patterns. The p-value was found to be 0.0001, which is significant as $p < 0.05$ (Table 2).

Table 2. Comparison of the marginal gap on all four walls among the three different resin patterns in micrometers.

Resin Pattern Groups (n = 15)	Buccal (MG-B)	Lingual (MG-L)	Mesial (MG-M)	Distal (MG-D)	p-Value
PMMA milled	51.18 ± 8.03	48.93 ± 14.19	69.24 ± 14.16	51.18 ± 8.38	0.307
ABS printed	111.85 ± 23.83	104.48 ± 19.58	107.89 ± 20.29	110.08 ± 18.76	0.823
PLA printed	108.75 ± 21.90	101.32 ± 19.80	106.89 ± 20.49	109.17 ± 18.94	0.642
p-value	0.0001 ¶	0.0001 ¶	0.0001 ¶	0.0001 ¶	

Note: Results are expressed in median ± standard deviation; MG-B—marginal gap on buccal side; MG-L—marginal gap on lingual side; MG-M—marginal gap on mesial side; MG-D—marginal gap on distal side; PMMA—polymethyl methacrylate resin; ABS—acrylonitrile–butadiene–styrene; PLA—polylactic acid; ¶ $p < 0.001$.

The post hoc analysis was done using Dunn's multiple comparison test between three different resin patterns. Results showed that the comparison of marginal gap values between PMMA milled resin patterns and PLA printed resin patterns, and PMMA milled resin patterns and ABS printed resin patterns, were statistically significant, showing a p-value of 0.0001. Conversely, comparison between ABS printed resin patterns and PLA printed resin patterns showed that the difference was not statistically significant ($p > 0.05$) (Table 3). Therefore, from the analysis, we can infer that PMMA milled resin patterns have a marginal gap, followed by PLA printed resin patterns and ABS printed resin patterns.

Table 3. Post-hoc Dunn's multiple comparison test to compare the marginal gap on the four different walls within the groups.

Groups	Walls	Difference in Rank Sum	p-Value
PMMA & PLA	Buccal	−66.87	<0.0001 ¶
	Lingual	−85.4	<0.0001 ¶
	Mesial	−70.07	<0.05 ¶
	Distal	−95.67	<0.0001 ¶
PMMA & ABS	Buccal	−97.07	<0.0001 ¶
	Distal	−107.3	<0.0001 ¶
	Lingual	−97.13	<0.0001 ¶
	Mesial	−69.27	<0.0001 ¶
ABS & PLA	Buccal	30.2	ns
	Lingual	11.73	ns
	Mesial	−0.8	ns
	Distal	11.67	ns

Note: PMMA—polymethyl methacrylate resin; ABS—acrylonitrile–butadiene–styrene; PLA—polylactic acid; ¶ $p < 0.001$, statistical significance; ns—no significance ($p > 0.05$).

A comparison of the median internal gap values in the buccolingual cross-section in four different locations revealed that the ABS printed resin patterns group had the highest median internal gap on the occlusal surface (118.31 ± 7.44 μm). the least internal gap was seen in the PLA resin pattern group (107.84 ± 9.43 μm). The median values of PMMA milled resin patterns, ABS printed resin patterns, and PLA printed resin patterns groups were within the range of clinical acceptance (120 μm). However, Kruskal–Wallis analysis showed no statistical significance ($p > 0.05$) (Table 4).

Table 4. Comparison of the internal gap on all six locations among the three different resin patterns in buccolingual cross-section in micrometers.

Resin Pattern Groups (n = 15)	Cervical (1) (IG-C1)	Buccal (IG-B)	Occlusal (1) (IG-O1)	Occlusal (2) (IG-O2)	Lingual (IG-L)	Cervical (2) (IG-C2)	p-Value
PMMA milled	112.52 ± 12.11	108.39 ± 10.99	117.59 ± 9.27	119.44 ± 9.16	111.11 ± 11.77	116.09 ± 9.04	0.732
ABS printed	108.71 ± 9.77	108.00 ± 9.01	116.50 ± 7.95	118.31 ± 7.44	110.64 ± 7.29	115.42 ± 8.15	0.428
PLA printed	108.10 ± 8.17	106.81 ± 8.67	115.36 ± 7.01	113.81 ± 6.48	107.84 ± 9.43	113.29 ± 9.45	0.503
p-value	0.528	0.896	0.687	0.108	0.638	0.753	

Note: Results are expressed in median ± standard deviation; IG-C1—internal gap on cervical side 1; IG-B—internal gap on buccal side; IG-O1—internal gap on occlusal side 1; IG-O2—internal gap on occlusal side 2; IG-L—internal gap on lingual side; IG-C2—internal gap on cervical side 2; PMMA—polymethyl methacrylate resin; ABS—acrylonitrile–butadiene–styrene; PLA—polylactic acid.

The median internal gap values in the mesiodistal cross-section in four different locations revealed that the PMMA resin pattern group had the highest median internal gap (119.78 ± 8.66 μm). The median values of all the groups were within the range of clinical acceptance (120 μm). Further Kruskal–Wallis analysis showed no statistical significance ($p > 0.05$) (Table 5).

Table 5. Comparison of the internal gap on all six locations among the three different resin patterns in mesiodistal cross-section using Kruskal–Wallis test.

Resin Pattern Groups (n = 15)	Cervical (3) (IG-C3)	Mesial (IG-M)	Occlusal (3) (IG-O1)	Occlusal (4) (IG-O2)	Distal (IG-D)	Cervical (4) (IG-C4)	p-Value
PMMA milled	113.50 ± 11.93	111.05 ± 13.59	119.78 ± 8.66	118.81 ± 10.28	112.43 ± 8.86	117.24 ± 11.17	0.427
ABS printed	111.21 ± 7.41	108.37 ± 10.51	116.75 ± 7.33	116.52 ± 7.55	111.87 ± 5.08	115.72 ± 7.00	0.322
PLA printed	110.41 ± 10.05	107.05 ± 10.71	115.89 ± 7.33	116.19 ± 6.96	110.16 ± 8.79	114.57 ± 7.58	0.765
p-value	0.673	0.649	0.360	0.654	0.694	0.639	

Note: Results are expressed in median ± standard deviation; IG-C3—internal gap on cervical side 3; IG-M—internal gap on mesial side; IG-O1—internal gap on occlusal side 1; IG-O2—internal gap on occlusal side 2; IG-D—internal gap on distal side; IG-C4—internal gap on cervical side 4; PMMA—polymethyl methacrylate resin; ABS—acrylonitrilo-butadiene-styrene; PLA—polylactic acid.

4. Discussion

The lost wax technique advocated by Taggart is the widely used method for the fabrication of indirect cast restorations [20]. Traditional casting techniques involve the fabrication of patterns. In this casting technique, wax is usually utilized as the pattern-forming material. One of the disadvantages of the conventional wax pattern is its dimensional inaccuracy. To overcome this drawback, resin pattern material has been introduced. The advantages of the resin materials are rigidity, adequate strength, low polymerization shrinkage, ease of use, lesser chair time, good dimensional stability, and no residue on burnout. An acceptable pattern fabrication is an important factor that influences the internal and marginal fit of the restoration. Fabrication of patterns with wax/resin leads to varied results, as the skill of the person at work determines the outcome. With the increasing influence of digital technology, we have additive and subtractive technologies available to us at affordable costs. The present study compared the marginal gap and internal gap of metal copings fabricated using three different types of pattern resin materials using two different technologies, namely subtractive (milling) and additive (3D printing) technology.

There are several methods for analyzing the internal and marginal gap, such as the cross-sectional method (CSM), silicone replica technique (SRT), triple scan method (TSM), micro-computed tomography (MCT), and optical coherence tomography (OCT). The replica technique is used in many studies since it is a simple, precise, and non-destructive method. In the present study, the replica technique was used to determine the marginal gap and internal gap. This technique has an advantage over other techniques, as it doesn't require the sectioning of the crown. Possible negative changes might be due to the shrinkage of polyvinyl siloxane, but this technique has been found to be reliable and used in internal gap measurement. Each replica was carefully segmented buccolingually and mesiodistally. Mesiodistal and buccolingual cross-sections were analyzed at sixteen points (eight in the buccolingual section and eight in the mesiodistal section). The replica was measured under an optical microscope at 5× magnification. The thicknesses were measured using a software tool. The results showed that there were significant differences between the three different resin patterns ($p < 0.05$). Hence, post hoc multiple tests were carried out to find if the difference between the groups were significant. Post hoc multiple tests revealed that the marginal gap of the PMMA milled patterns group had statistical significance when compared to ABS and PLA printed patterns groups ($p = 0.0001$). This could be because, in additive processing, parameters that might have the greatest effect on the results are the axes (z-axis) of build directions, where the z-axis movement is responsible for moving layers at a pre-defined height set in the 3D slicer [21]. The stair-stepping effects may have affected the dimensional accuracy of the pattern.

In the additive technique, each slice or layer is placed on top of the preceding one, resulting in the creation of the model. The thickness of the slices used to manufacture the model can bring about an effect called stepping error, layering error, or staircase effect. The extent of this staircase effect depends on the layer thickness [22]. The staircase error increases with the layer thickness. Distortion of pattern parts can occur during the polymerizing process in additive technique, as it is combined with a lot of heat, thus influencing the interlayer binding. There is a possibility of damage while removing the supporting material after the print is completed. This can increase the marginal gap. Similar results were obtained in the study conducted by Kim et al., and they found that the least marginal and internal gap was seen in crowns fabricated by milling when compared to crowns fabricated using selective laser melting [23]. None of the earlier studies compared the three different resin patterns fabricated using additive and subtractive technology that was cast using the lost wax process; in this way, the current study provides new insights into the available digital technology.

The results of the measured internal gaps showed that the PLA printed resin patterns group had a better internal fit (least internal gap), followed by the ABS printed resin patterns group and the PMMA milled resin patterns group, though the differences were not statistically significant ($p = 0.638$). The mean internal gap obtained from PMMA milled resin patterns, ABS printed resin patterns, and PLA printed resin patterns groups were within the clinically acceptable level of 120 µm. One of the reasons could have been the wear and tear of the milling burs. This can be compensated if the burs are changed often to reduce their decreasing diameter. Milling device vibrations can also be another reason. Similar results were obtained in the study conducted by Elfar M et al. [24]. For each coping, the data were obtained from measurements on sixteen locations in the buccolingual and mesiodistal sections: four marginal, four cervical, four axial, and four occlusal measurements. Though the values were not statistically significant, among all the measured locations, in both techniques, occlusal surfaces showed higher discrepancies, followed by the cervical, marginal, and axial surfaces. This is because the error-prone areas are the curved surfaces, compared to the vertical surfaces affecting the accuracy of the crowns [25]. The occlusal surfaces with larger grooves and fossa make the morphology more complex to print without discrepancies.

The limitations of the present in vitro study include errors during impression making. Procedures of scanning and software alignment in crown fabrication can also influence results. In the present study, marginal and internal gaps were evaluated using a two-dimensional method. The same can also be studied using the three-dimensional method. The replica technique has the disadvantage of the tearing of the silicone layer replica and errors that occur while sectioning in different planes. For making the replica, the copings were filled with low-viscosity polyvinyl siloxane and seated on the master die using finger pressure. Though this method simulates the clinical situation, the use of finger pressure can result in variability. This study assessed only the copings; future studies can be done with full-contour crowns. Further studies with a long-span fixed dental prosthesis can also be taken up. Clinical trials can validate the study results further.

5. Conclusions

The marginal fit was found to be better in milled resin patterns (subtractive technology) than in 3D printed resin patterns (additive technology). The mean marginal gap was found to be maximum in ABS printed resin patterns, followed by PLA printed resin patterns and then in PMMA milled resin patterns. PLA printed resin patterns had a better internal fit, followed by ABS printed resin patterns and then milled resin patterns. The mean marginal and internal gap of metal copings obtained from 3D printed resin patterns (additive technology) and milled PMMA resin patterns (subtractive technology) were within the clinically acceptable range. Digital technologies, both subtractive and additive techniques, showed an increased gap (least fit) on the occlusal surface when compared to the marginal, cervical, and axial surfaces.

Author Contributions: Conceptualization, V.N.V., S.R. and H.A.; methodology, N.H.A., S.B. and S.R.; software, A.A., S.A.B. and P.K.Y.; validation, K.C.S., D.S., H.A. and S.B.; formal analysis, N.H.A. and H.A.B.; investigation, A.A., P.K.Y. and B.Z.; resources, S.A.B., S.B. and H.A.; data curation,

V.N.V. and S.P.; writing—original draft preparation V.N.V., S.R., P.K.Y., H.A., N.H.A., K.C.S. and D.S.; writing—review and editing, S.B., A.A., S.A.B., B.Z., H.A.B., K.C.S., D.S. and S.P.; visualization, H.A.B., B.Z., K.C.S., D.S. and S.B.; supervision, A.A. and S.A.B.; project administration, V.N.V. and S.P. All authors have read and agreed to the published version of the manuscript.

Funding: This research received no external funding.

Institutional Review Board Statement: Not applicable.

Informed Consent Statement: Not applicable.

Data Availability Statement: Not applicable.

Conflicts of Interest: The authors declare no conflict of interest.

References

1. Blackman, R.; Baez, R.; Barghi, N. Marginal accuracy and geometry of cast titanium copings. *J. Prosthet. Dent.* **1992**, *67*, 435–440. [CrossRef]
2. Marsaw, F.A.; de Rijk, W.G.; Hesby, R.A.; Hinman, R.W.; Pelleu, G.B. Internal volumetric expansion of casting investments. *J. Prosthet. Dent.* **1984**, *52*, 361–366. [CrossRef]
3. Rai, R.; Kumar Sa Prabhu, R.; Govindan, R.; Tanveer, F. Evaluation of marginal and internal gaps of metal ceramic crowns obtained from conventional impressions and casting techniques with those obtained from digital techniques. *Indian J. Dent. Res.* **2017**, *28*, 291. [CrossRef] [PubMed]
4. Schwartz, I.S. A review of methods and techniques to improve the fit of cast restorations. *J. Prosthet. Dent.* **1986**, *56*, 279–283. [CrossRef]
5. Hung, S.H.; Hung, K.-S.; Eick, J.D.; Chappell, R.P. Marginal fit of porcelain-fused-to-metal and two types of ceramic crown. *J. Prosthet. Dent.* **1990**, *63*, 26–31. [CrossRef]
6. Sulaiman, F.; Chai, J.; Jameson, L.M.; Wozniak, W.T. A comparison of the marginal fit of In-Ceram, IPS Empress, and Procera crowns. *Int. J. Prosthodont.* **1997**, *10*, 478–484.
7. Moldovan, O.; Rudolph, H.; Quaas, S.; Bornemann, G.; Luthardt, R.G. Internal and external fit of CAM-made zirconia bridge frameworks—A pilot study. *Dtsch. Zahnarztl. Z.* **2006**, *61*, 38–42.
8. Quante, K.; Ludwig, K.; Kern, M. Marginal and internal fit of metal-ceramic crowns fabricated with a new laser melting technology. *Dent. Mater.* **2008**, *24*, 1311–1315. [CrossRef]
9. Ucar, Y.; Akova, T.; Akyil, M.S.; Brantley, W.A. Internal fit evaluation of crowns prepared using a new dental crown fabrication technique: Laser-sintered Co-Cr crowns. *J. Prosthet. Dent.* **2009**, *102*, 253–259. [CrossRef]
10. McLean, J.W.; Von, F. The estimation of cement film thickness by an in vivo technique. *Br. Dent. J.* **1971**, *131*, 107–111. [CrossRef]
11. Ushiwata, O.; de Moraes, J.V.; Bottino, M.A.; da Silva, E.G. Marginal fit of nickel-chromium copings before and after internal adjustments with duplicated stone dies and disclosing agent. *J. Prosthet. Dent.* **2000**, *83*, 634–643. [CrossRef] [PubMed]
12. Milan, F.M.; Consani, S.; Correr Sobrinho, L.; Sinhoreti, M.A.C.; Sousa-Neto, M.D.; Knowles, J.C. Influence of casting methods on marginal and internal discrepancies of complete cast crowns. *Braz. Dent. J.* **2004**, *15*, 127–132. [CrossRef] [PubMed]
13. Jain, R.; Takkar, R.; Jain, G.; Takkar, R.; Deora, N. CAD-CAM the future of digital dentistry: A review. *Ann. Prosthodont. Restor. Dent.* **2016**, *2*, 33–36.
14. White, S.N.; Yu, Z.; Tom, J.F.M.D.; Sangsurasak, S. In vivo marginal adaptation of cast crowns luted with different cements. *J. Prosthet. Dent.* **1995**, *74*, 25–32. [CrossRef]
15. Ushiwata, O.; de Moraes, J.V. Method for marginal measurements of restorations: Accessory device for Toolmakers microscope. *J. Prosthet. Dent.* **2000**, *83*, 362–366. [CrossRef]
16. Örtorp, A.; Jönsson, D.; Mouhsen, A.; Vult von Steyern, P. The fit of cobalt–chromium three-unit fixed dental prostheses fabricated with four different techniques: A comparative in vitro study. *Dent. Mater.* **2011**, *27*, 356–363. [CrossRef]
17. Holmes, J.R.; Bayne, S.C.; Holland, G.A.; Sulik, W.D. Considerations in measurement of marginal fit. *J. Prosthet. Dent.* **1989**, *62*, 405–408. [CrossRef]
18. Boening, K.W.; Wolf, B.H.; Schmidt, A.E.; Kästner, K.; Walter, M.H. Clinical fit of Procera AllCeram crowns. *J. Prosthet. Dent.* **2000**, *84*, 419–424. [CrossRef]
19. Trifkovic, B.; Budak, I.; Todorovic, A.; Hodolic, J.; Puskar, T.; Jevremovic, D.; Vukelić, Đ. Application of Replica Technique and SEM in Accuracy Measurement of Ceramic Crowns. *Meas. Sci. Rev.* **2012**, *12*, 90–97. [CrossRef]
20. Lombardas, P.; Carbunaru, A.; McAlarney, M.E.; Toothaker, R.W. Dimensional accuracy of castings produced with ringless and metal ring investment systems. *J. Prosthet. Dent.* **2000**, *84*, 27–31. [CrossRef]
21. Park, G.-S.; Kim, S.-K.; Heo, S.-J.; Koak, J.-Y.; Seo, D.-G. Effects of Printing Parameters on the Fit of Implant-Supported 3D Printing Resin Prosthetics. *Materials* **2019**, *12*, 2533. [CrossRef] [PubMed]
22. Yasa, E.; Poyraz, O.; Solakoglu, E.U.; Akbulut, G.; Oren, S. A Study on the Stair Stepping Effect in Direct Metal Laser Sintering of a Nickel-based Superalloy. *Procedia CIRP* **2016**, *45*, 175–178. [CrossRef]

23. Kim, D.-Y.; Kim, J.-H.; Kim, H.-Y.; Kim, W.-C. Comparison and evaluation of marginal and internal gaps in cobalt–chromium alloy copings fabricated using subtractive and additive manufacturing. *J. Prosthodont. Res.* **2018**, *62*, 56–64. [CrossRef] [PubMed]
24. Elfar, M.; Korsel, A.; Kamel, M. Marginal fit of heat pressed lithium disilicate crowns fabricated by three-dimensional printed and subtractive CAD/CAM wax patterns. *Tanta Dent. J.* **2018**, *15*, 199. [CrossRef]
25. Wang, W.; Yu, H.; Liu, Y.; Jiang, X.; Gao, B. Trueness analysis of zirconia crowns fabricated with 3-dimensional printing. *J. Prosthet. Dent.* **2019**, *121*, 285–291. [CrossRef] [PubMed]

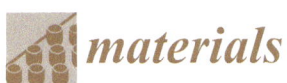

Review

Biofilm Formation on Hybrid, Resin-Based CAD/CAM Materials for Indirect Restorations: A Comprehensive Review

Konstantinos Tzimas, Christos Rahiotis * and Eftychia Pappa

Department of Operative Dentistry, National and Kapodistrian University of Athens, 11527 Athens, Greece; kwstastzimas@dent.uoa.gr (K.T.); effiepappa@dent.uoa.gr (E.P.)
* Correspondence: craxioti@dent.uoa.gr

Abstract: Hybrid materials are a recent addition in the field of restorative dentistry for computer-aided design/computer-aided manufacturing (CAD/CAM) indirect restorations. The long-term clinical success of modern dental restorative materials is influenced by multiple factors. Among the characteristics affecting the longevity of a restoration, the mechanical properties and physicochemical interactions are of utmost importance. While numerous researchers constantly evaluate mechanical properties, the biological background of resin-based CAD/CAM biomaterials is scarcely investigated and, therefore, less described in the literature. This review aims to analyze biofilm formation on the surfaces of novel, hybrid, resin-based CAD/CAM materials and evaluate the methodological protocols followed to assess microbial growth. It is demonstrated that the surface structure, the composition and the finishing and polishing procedures on the surface of a dental restorative material influence initial bacterial adhesion; however, most studies focus on in vitro protocols, and in vivo and/or in situ research of microbiomics in CAD/CAM restorative materials is lacking, obstructing an accurate understanding of the bioadhesion phenomenon in the oral cavity.

Keywords: CAD/CAM; biofilm; resin-based biomaterials; dental materials

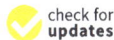

Citation: Tzimas, K.; Rahiotis, C.; Pappa, E. Biofilm Formation on Hybrid, Resin-Based CAD/CAM Materials for Indirect Restorations: A Comprehensive Review. *Materials* 2024, 17, 1474. https://doi.org/10.3390/ma17071474

Academic Editors: Lavinia Cosmina Ardelean and Laura-Cristina Rusu

Received: 5 March 2024
Revised: 14 March 2024
Accepted: 21 March 2024
Published: 23 March 2024

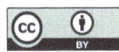

Copyright: © 2024 by the authors. Licensee MDPI, Basel, Switzerland. This article is an open access article distributed under the terms and conditions of the Creative Commons Attribution (CC BY) license (https:// creativecommons.org/licenses/by/ 4.0/).

1. Introduction

Significant advances in the field of restorative dentistry have led to the transition from older metallic dental materials for direct restorations, such as the dental amalgam, to more esthetic, tooth-colored and "tooth-friendly" counterparts, namely composite resin materials. The polymerization process is the critical drawback concerning using these restorative materials for direct intraoral applications. Residual monomers and polymerization shrinkage reduce their clinical success [1]. Further disadvantages of direct resin-based restorations include inferior mechanical strengths, rapid occlusal and proximal wear, marginal discoloration, loss of integrity, a low fracture toughness and postoperative sensitivity [2]. The limitations of this direct, sensitive approach have been partially overcome by the development of nano-filled and nano-hybrid direct composite resins and by the application of indirect laboratory methods [3–6].

Furthermore, indirect restorations, either by using resin-based materials or ceramics, have proven to be a viable alternative therapeutic modality [7]. Due to the fact that ceramics have long been characterized as expensive, brittle materials that induce wear to the opposing dentition and are not repairable after fracture, indirect resin-based restorations are continuously gaining attention [8,9]. The everlasting need for more conservative, minimally invasive, and, at the same time, predictable procedures that maximize patients' comfort has led to the incorporation of digital means in the fabrication of dental restorations. The introduction of computer-aided design/computer-aided manufacturing (CAD/CAM) appliances followed the rising demand for digital dentistry, and, subsequently, the dental market was overrun with new dental biomaterials for several types of restorations (inlays, onlays, endocrowns, etc.) [10–12]. The first subtractive manufacturing materials used were feldspar ceramic blocks [13]. Although they are strong, ceramics are brittle materials with a low fracture toughness and a high susceptibility to failure in the presence of flaws [9]. Therefore, using "hybrid ceramic" or resin-based CAD/CAM restorative materials has proven an ideal alternative. Their main benefit is based on adequate factory polymerization, involving high-heat and high-pressure techniques, eliminating polymerization defects and monomer release in this way. Simultaneously, incorporating a more significant amount of filler particles and altering the polymer matrix enhance their mechanical properties. The hybridity of these newly introduced CAD/CAM blocks depends on the common goal of combining the positive effects of ceramic and resin-based components [14]. Since the flexural strength of hybrid resin-based CAD/CAM blocks is higher than that of recently developed nano-filled composite resins and their elastic modulus is similar to that of dentin, a more uniform stress distribution during loading may be anticipated [15].

Through the years, researchers have constantly evaluated the mechanical properties of hybrid, ceramic, resin-based CAD/CAM blocks. The flexural strength, Vickers hardness and elastic modulus are of utmost importance for excellent clinical performance. Surface properties, such as the surface roughness and surface topography, have also been investigated, but to a lesser extent compared to mechanical properties [15–25]. Unfortunately, scarce evidence exists concerning bacterial attachment and subsequent biofilm formation on hybrid ceramic, resin-based CAD/CAM blocks for permanent, indirect restorations, meaning that this is a field that needs further investigation. Biofilm formation is a potential causative factor facilitating restoration failure since it promotes the appearance of secondary caries on the restoration's margins and provokes biodegradation, thus altering the restorative material's surface characteristics [26,27]. To the best of our knowledge, until recently, no critical reviews of the existing literature focusing on bacterial formation on CAD/CAM dental materials for indirect restorations have been published, and a comprehensive evaluation of the methodology, observations and results of current research protocols is lacking. Therefore, the aims of this review are, firstly, to introduce the resin-based CAD/CAM materials used for single indirect restorations and to present the recent data concerning biofilm formation on their surfaces, and secondly, to shed light on the methodological patterns used, as well as their limitations. Furthermore, future directions in microbiome analysis will be highlighted. A visualization of the structure of this comprehensive review is presented in Figure 1.

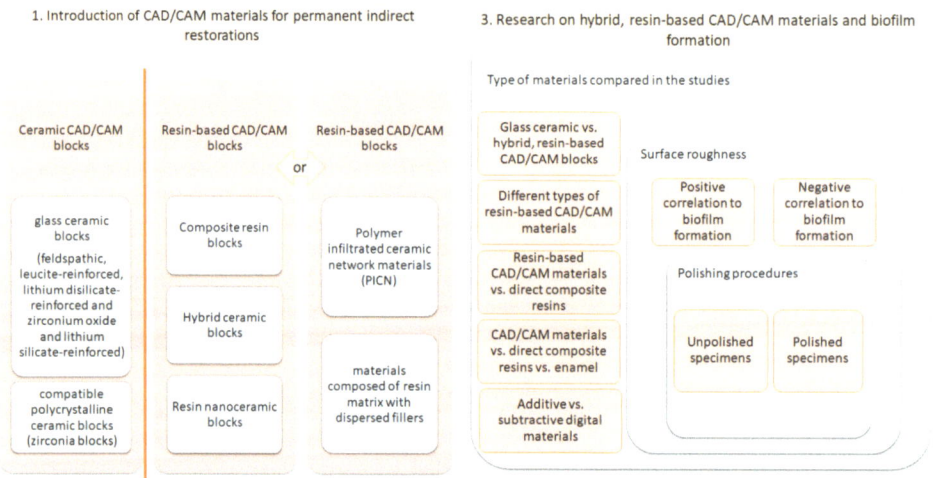

Figure 1. *Cont.*

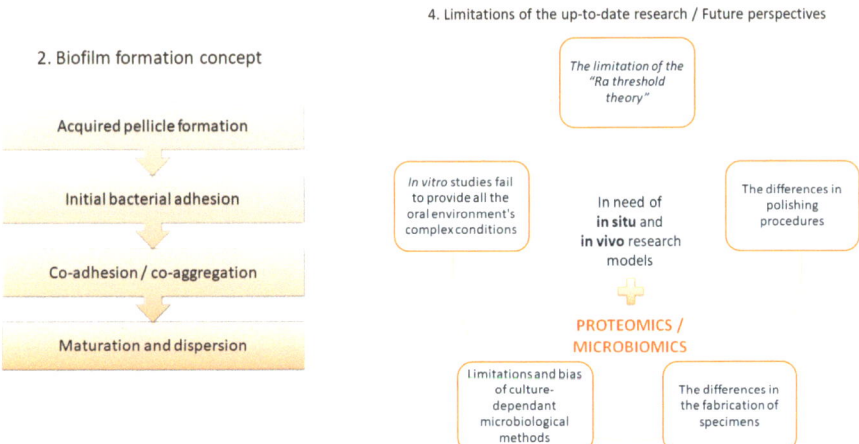

Figure 1. Succinct description of the sections of this review.

2. "Hybrid", Resin-Based Materials in the Digital Dentistry Era

There are a lot of different classification systems regarding CAD/CAM blocks and their application in contemporary restorative dentistry. The raw classes of CAD/CAM blocks fabricated for single, permanent indirect restorations are *ceramic CAD/CAM blocks* and *resin-based CAD CAM blocks*. According to their composition and microstructure, ceramic CAD/CAM blocks can be further divided into *glass ceramics*, subcategorized into feldspathic, leucite-reinforced, lithium-disilicate-reinforced and zirconium-oxide- and lithium-silicate-reinforced ceramic blocks, and *compatible polycrystalline ceramics*, namely zirconia CAD/CAM blocks [12]. The CAD/CAM blocks that incorporate a resin-based organic matrix can be subcategorized as follows: *polymer-infiltrated ceramic network materials* and *materials composed of a resin matrix with dispersed fillers* [28,29]. Other resin-based CAD/CAM block classes include *composite resin* CAD/CAM blocks, *hybrid ceramic* CAD/CAM blocks and *resin nanoceramic* CAD/CAM blocks [12,14,30]. The latter refers to polymeric networks that are reinforced with ceramic fillers (ceramics, glass ceramics, glasses, ultrafine glass particles, nanohybrid fillers, etc.). The term "hybrid" is often misinterpreted and should only be used to describe a CAD/CAM block that consists of a polymer-infiltrated ceramic network (PICN). This CAD/CAM block (VitaEnamic, VITA Zahnfabrik, Bad Säckingen, Germany) presents a double network hybrid structure composed of a porous, pre-sintered ceramic network, conditioned by a coupling agent and infiltrated with a polymer via capillary action [31–33]. Caution is required, since the misclassification of CAD/CAM materials in the dental literature is significant and might lead to misuse and incorrect clinical identification of CAD/CAM materials [34]. Although resin-based, hybrid ceramic, nanoceramic CAD/CAM materials exhibit inferior optical properties, their advantages compared to traditional glass ceramics are summarized as follows: they are not stiff, brittle materials; they mimic the structure of natural tooth components; they present direct composite repairability; and they are more easily and quickly fabricated [9]. Moreover, resin-based materials may be less susceptible to chipping during the milling procedure [35]. Occlusal and proximal adjustments (polishing procedures) are much more easily accomplished [14,36].

The most used resin-based CAD/CAM blocks are summarized in Table 1.

Table 1. Commonly used hybrid, resin-based CAD/CAM materials in the dental market.

Hybrid, Resin-Based CAD/CAM Material	Description	Manufacturer	Composition
Vita Enamic	Polymer-infiltrated ceramic network material (PICN) Hybrid ceramic block	VITA Zahnfabrik, Bad Säckingen, Germany	86% by weight inorganic fillers (mainly silicon dioxide and aluminum oxide) 14% organic matrix by weight: UDMA and TEGDMA
Lava Ultimate	Resin nanoceramic block	3M ESPE, St. Paul, MN, USA	80% by weight inorganic fillers (nanomers of silica and zirconia and zirconia and silica nanoclusters of 0.6–10 µm) 20% organic matrix: Bis-GMA, UDMA, Bis-EMA and TEGDMA
Shofu Block HC	Hybrid ceramic block	Shofu Inc., Kyoto, Japan	61% inorganic fillers (silica powder, zirconium silicate, and microfumed silica) Organic matrix: UDMA and TEGDMA
Cerasmart	Force-absorbing hybrid ceramic block	GC Corporation, Tokyo, Japan	71% by weight inorganic fillers (silica (20 nm) and barium glass (300 nm)) Organic matrix: Bis-MEPP, UDMA, DMA
Grandio Bloc	Nanoceramic hybrid block	VOCO GmbH, Cuxhaven, Germany	86% by weight inorganic fillers Organic matrix: UDMA and DMA
Brilliant Crios	Reinforced composite block	Coltene Whaledent AG, Altstätten, Switzerland	70.7% by weight inorganic fillers (barium glass and amorphous silica) Organic matrix: Cross-Bis, GMA, Bis-EMA and TEGDMA
Katana Avencia Block	Hybrid ceramic composite resin CAD/CAM block	Kuraray Noritake Dental, Tokyo, Japan	82% by weight inorganic fillers (colloidal silica and aluminum oxide) Organic matrix: UDMA and other methacrylate monomers)
Tetric CAD	Composite block	Ivoclar Vivadent AG, Schaan, Lichtenstein	71% by weight barium glass (<1 µm) and silicon dioxide fillers Organic matrix: cross-linked methacrylates, (Bis-GMA, Bis-EMA, TEGDMA, UDMA)

According to the manufacturer, the polymer-infiltrated ceramic network material (Vita Enamic, VITA Zahnfabrik, Bad Säckingen, Germany) consists of 86% filler by weight and 14% UDMA and TEGDMA polymer network by weight. More precisely, the inorganic fillers are primarily silicon dioxide and aluminum oxide and secondarily sodium, potassium, and calcium oxide, as well as boron trioxide and zirconia [37–39]. One commonly used resin nanoceramic CAD/CAM material is Lava Ultimate (3M ESPE, St. Paul, MN, USA). Nanomers of 20 nm in diameter made from silica and 4–11 nm in diameter made from zirconia, as well as zirconia and silica nanoclusters of 0.6–10 µm, comprise the approximately 80% by weight inorganic filler content, which is placed in an organic matrix of Bis-GMA, UDMA, Bis-EMA, and TEGDMA [28,40]. Shofu Block HC (Shofu Inc., Kyoto, Japan) is described as a ceramic-based restorative material, consisting of 61% silica powder, zirconium silicate and microfumed silica in a UDMA and TEGDMA organic matrix [28,41]. Cerasmart (GC Corporation, Tokyo, Japan) is now off the market and has been replaced by Cerasmart 270, which is described as a force-absorbing hybrid ceramic CAD/CAM block. Its predecessor's composition included Bis-MEPP, UDMA, DMA, silica (20 nm) and barium glass (300 nm). Its inorganic filler load was 71% by weight [28,42]. Grandio Block (VOCO GmbH, Cuxhaven, Germany) is described as a nano-hybrid CAD/CAM block of 86% by weight nanoceramic filler particles in a UDMA and DMA organic matrix [43]. Another often used resin-based material is Brilliant Crios (Coltene Whaledent AG, Altstätten,

Switzerland), described by the manufacturer as a reinforced composite block for permanent restorations. It consists of a cross-linked methacrylate resin matrix (Cross-Bis-GMA, Bis-EMA and TEGDMA) and 70.7% by weight dental glass (barium glass < 1.0 µm) and amorphous silica (<20 nm) [44]. Katana Avencia Block (Kuraray Noritake Dental, Tokyo, Japan) consists of UDMA, other methacrylate monomers and mixed fillers of colloidal silica and aluminum oxide and was launched as a hybrid, ceramic, composite resin CAD/CAM block [45]. Lastly, Tetric CAD (Ivoclar Vivadent AG, Schaan, Lichtenstein) is composed of cross-linked methacrylates, such as Bis-GMA, Bis-EMA, TEGDMA and UDMA, and 71% by weight barium glass (<1 µm) and silicon dioxide fillers [46]. As observed, resin-based CAD/CAM materials have almost the same microstructures, but in different proportions.

3. The Concept of Biofilm Formation

The oral microbiome, hosting approximately 700 different species of bacteria, represents the second largest microbiota environment, following the gut microbiome [47]. The oral cavity is a complex host with unique anatomical structures, including hard (natural teeth and restorative materials) and soft tissues (oral mucosa). The oral microbiome is the sum of the oral microbes, their genetic information, and the oral environment in which all components interact [48]. The so-called "climax community", consisting of dietary habits, environmental conditions, host genetics and early microbial exposure, plays a pivotal role in the oral microbiota composition [49]. Biofilms are formed on every existing surface (soft and hard tissues, dental materials, etc.) in the oral cavity. The presence of biofilms is not necessarily malicious per se, since under normal circumstances, pathogenic and physiological microorganisms exhibit a phenomenon called symbiosis, which leads to the maintenance of oral health [50]. Several factors may disrupt this sensitive balance and result in dysbiosis (imbalance of the microbiome). Inadequate oral health conditions and dietary habits rich in low-molecular-weight carbohydrates, as well as inflammatory and autoimmune disorders, create the ideal environment for the establishment of pathological processes, such as the demineralization of tooth structures, tooth decay, secondary caries at the margins of restorative materials, gingivitis–periodontitis–peri-implantitis, tooth loss and/or stomatitis [51,52]. Biofilm formation (dental plaque) is a multiple-stage process [53]. When a dental biomaterial, in our case a resin-based CAD/CAM material, is adhered to a tooth structure and starts functioning in the oral cavity, it is immediately coated by saliva, and an acquired pellicle is formed [54]. After the first stage of acquired pellicle formation, the initial bacterial adhesion commences, and the formation of the dental plaque biofilm continues with the adhesion and coagulation of further microorganisms. Maturation, followed by dispersion, leads to the final dental plaque composition [55]. More precisely, the acquired pellicle is a noncellular, micellar structure that is composed of salivary glycoproteins, phosphoproteins, lipids and components of gingival crevice fluids, plus microbial products (glycosyltrasferases and glycans). The acquired pellicle modifies the surface properties of the dental biomaterial and alters the interactions between the biomaterial and the host response [56,57]. The salivary molecules activate receptors, which interact with adhesins on the surfaces of bacteria [58]. The bacterial conjunction is divided into three categories, depending on the distance between bacteria and the dental surface. If the distance is greater than 100nm, the initial bacteria are transported to the point of interest via natural salivary flow, Brownian motion (fluid dynamics) and chemotaxis (chemical signaling).

When the distance between the bacteria and the surface is 20 to 100 nm, van der Waals forces and electrostatic interactions are of utmost importance for cell attachment. Lastly, when the distance is short (<20 nm), biofilm attachment due to nonspecific and specific bonding mechanisms is observed. Signaling transactions, as well as activation of specific transmembrane receptors, are examples of specific bonding mechanisms. After the arrival of microorganisms, bacterial attachment commences and pioneer colonizers are established [59]. The initial binding is reversible due to the weak physicochemical interactions (van der Waals and electrostatic forces). The next step is the irreversible phase, where strong stereochemical interactions between microbial adhesins and receptors on the acquired pellicle occur. Adhesins expressed by secondary colonizers recognize receptors on the surfaces of pioneer colonizers, and the co-aggregation or co-adhesion phase takes place. Microbial succession, meaning the gradual replacement of initial colonizers by other bacterial species through the initial bacteria's metabolic process, follows, and mature dental plaque is built [49,60]. Figure 2 briefly describes the dental plaque formation stages.

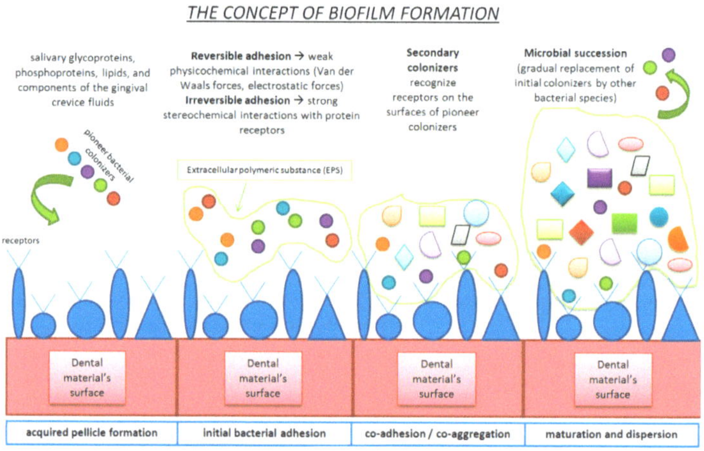

Figure 2. Schematic representation of biofilm formation.

All in all, bacterial colonization, especially at its early stage, is contingent upon detachment shear forces and the surface energetic state of the substrate. The decisive role of surface roughness, surface free energy, surface wettability, surface topography and surface chemical composition on biofilm formation is scientifically documented, mainly by in vitro studies [61–64]. An increased surface roughness promotes greater bacterial attachment due to the greater surface contact area available for adhesion, the presence of stagnation points and the shielding of microbial cells from shear forces. Bacteria adhere easily to a surface with a high surface energy (hydrophilic), rather than to a substrate with a low surface energy [65,66]. However, since a plethora of factors has been proven to be responsible for the alterations at the interface between the substratum and biofilms, a cautious interpretation of the literature and further investigations into the correlation of surface characteristics and biofilm formation are necessary. Furthermore, it should not be forgotten that the properties of a dental material have a significant effect on the biofilm and that the biofilm may conversely affect and alter the material properties [67,68].

4. Research on Biofilm Formation on Resin-Based, Hybrid CAD/CAM Materials

Research focusing on biofilm formation on resin-based CAD/CAM materials for permanent indirect restorations predominantly originates from in vitro studies. An overall overview demonstrates a possible correlation between biofilm formation and surface characteristics (mainly surface roughness), as well as a strong association between bacterial growth, surface roughness and surface modification techniques (polishing procedures).

More precisely, after a thorough investigation of the recent literature concerning biofilm formation on resin-based CAD/CAM blocks for permanent indirect restorations, a total of eleven research articles were found [69–79]. These studies investigated one or more hybrid, resin-based CAD/CAM materials with regard to biofilm attachment and growth. They evaluated either the biofilm formation as an independent variable or biofilm formation in association with surface characteristics, such as surface roughness and surface free energy. The materials investigated in each study differed. Some researchers solely examined resin-based CAD/CAM blocks [70,76–78]. Others compared resin-based CAD/CAM blocks to conventional composite resins [74], whereas some in vitro research incorporated direct composite resins, indirect CAD/CAM blocks and human enamel [72,73]. Moreover, other studies focused on ceramic CAD/CAM materials and hybrid resin-based CAD/CAM materials [69,71]. Lastly, a newly conducted in vitro study compared CAD/CAM-manufactured resin-based materials for indirect restorations with 3D-printed resin-based materials [79]. Other researchers investigated the potential correlation between the surface modification procedures on CAD/CAM resin-based materials and increased or decreased biofilm formation. In this kind of research, control groups were not subjected to further surface treatments, in contrast to the experimental groups, where finishing and polishing procedures with specific grinding and polishing protocols established by each researcher took place. Most in vitro studies used *Streptococcus mutans* (*S. mutans*) as the monospecies for bacterial adherence to the tested materials. Other bacterial strains used were *Candida albicans* (*C. albicans*), *Streptococcus sanguis* (*S. sanguis*), *Streptococcus gordonii* (*S. gordonii*) and *Lactobacillus* species. Only two in situ studies, which tried to identify the biofilm formed on smooth restorative materials, integrated hybrid resin-based CAD/CAM materials into their experimental groups [72,75].

The methods used for the evaluation of surface properties and the assessment of biofilm formation are scientifically documented by former researchers. Using a stylus profilometer or a 3D optical profilometer in contact or non-contact mode is the gold standard in the assessment of surface roughness [27,80]. Most researchers measuring surface roughness record and compare the Sa value (arithmetical mean height, expressing, as an absolute value, the difference in height of each point compared to the arithmetical mean of the surface). Scanning electron microscopy (SEM) provides qualitative information on the surface structure of a dental material [81]. Furthermore, the use of attenuated total reflectance, Fourier transform infrared spectrometry (ATR–FT–IR spectrometry) and energy-dispersive X-ray microanalysis (EDX microanalysis) enriches protocols with information concerning the molecular composition and elemental analysis of the surfaces tested (surface topography and chemical composition assessment) [82–84]. The sessile drop method calculates the surface free energy using contact angle measurements and customized optical goniometers [85]. For the microbiological analysis of the tested specimens, various diverse methods (direct as well as indirect) have been introduced. Still, the most commonly used method is the application of a bioreactor followed by colony-forming unit counting (CFU/mL). Scanning electron microscopy (SEM) and confocal scanning laser microscopy (CSLM) are supplementary qualitative methods for biofilm evaluation [86].

The objectives, the experimental methods and the results of these studies are analyzed on a large scale in Table 2.

Table 2. Research focusing on bacterial adhesion on hybrid resin-based CAD/CAM materials for indirect restorations.

Objective	Type of Specimens/Type of Control Group	Tests	Conclusion	Study/Year
Evaluation of surface roughness and biofilm formation on CAD/CAM materials before and after polishing	(1) Vita Enamic, Vita Zahnfabrik (2) Lava Ultimate, 3M ESPE (3) Vitablocs Mark II, VITA Zahnfabrik, Bad Säckingen, Germany (4) Wieland Reflex Veneering porcelain, Wieland Dental, Pforzheim, Germany POLISHING PROCEDURES Unpolished specimens (control group) Uniformly polished specimens with diamond burs, finishing burs and extrafine porcelain burs (experimental group)	(1) SEM, CLSM, crystal violet assay for microbial analysis of *S. grodonii* (2) 3D Slicer software for surface roughness evaluation	More irregular surface topography in polished specimens compared to controls Greater surface roughness (*Ra*) values in polished CAD/CAM blocks compared to controls. Greater biofilm growth on polished specimens compared to controls	Kim et al., 2017 [69]

Table 2. Cont.

Objective	Type of Specimens/Type of Control Group	Tests	Conclusion	Study/Year
Evaluation of the surface topography and bacterial adhesion CAD/CAM blocks after different surface finishing procedures	(1) Vita Enamic, Vita Zahnfabrik (2) Lava Ultimate, 3M ESPE POLISHING PROCEDURES (1) No surface finish (control group) (2) Diamond bur surface finish (3) Polishing system for hybrid ceramics (4) Polishing system for ceramics	(1) Stylus profilometer for surface roughness evaluation (Ra, Rz, Rq height parameters) (2) Spectrophotometry, CFU/mL, SEM and CSLM for microbial analysis of *S. mutans*	Surface roughness and bacterial adhesion are lower for Vita Enamic compared to Lava Ultimate, regardless of the finishing procedures The type of material and the finishing techniques have an effect on surface roughness and bacterial adhesion	Hammerschnitt et al., 2018 [70]
Comparison of biofilm formation on CAD/CAM materials in accordance with their roughness	(1) Vita Enamic, Vita Zahnfabrik (2) IPS Empress, Ivoclar Vivadent AG, Schaan, Lichtenstein (3) IPS Empress Multi, Ivoclar Vivadent AG, Schaan, Lichtenstein (4) IPS emax, Ivoclar Vivadent AG, Schaan, Lichtenstein, before and after sintering POLISHING PROCEDURES Unpolished specimens (control group) were uniformly polished with 800–1200 grit sandpaper discs (experimental group)	(1) Powder X-ray diffraction pattern (XRPD) and (ATR–FT–IR) for surface topography evaluation (2) Contact angle measurement for wettability evaluation (3) Fluorescence microscopy and CFU/mL counting for microbial analysis of *S. mutans*, *C. albicans* and *Lactobacillus rhamnosus*	Non-polished surfaces are more susceptible to biofilm adhesion compared to their polished counterparts The degree of biofilm formation depends on the tested microbial species	Dobrzynski et al., 2019 [71]
Identification and comparison of the oral microbiome on resin-based materials in vivo and in vitro	(1) Grandio flow, VOCO GmbH, Cuxhaven, Germany (conventional flowable composite resin) (2) Grandio Bloc, Voco GmbH Cuxhaven, Germany (resin-based CAD/CAM material) (3) Bovine enamel (control group)	For the in situ project: 15 volunteers wore oral splints with slabs of resin-based materials and bovine enamel for 48 h, and Ilumina Miseq Next Generation Sequencing of 16S ribosomal RNA (V1–V2 regions) for bacterial identification followed	No significant differences in bacterial colonization for the different dental composites and the control group in vivo	Conrads et al., 2019 [72]
Differences in biofilm formation between indirect CAD/CAM resin-based composites and their direct resin-based counterparts	(1) Grandio Bloc, VOCO GmbH (2) Lava Ultimate, 3M ESPE (3) Katana Avencia, Kuraray Corp. (4) Vita Enamic, Vita Zahnfabrik (5) Grandio SO, VOCO GmbH, Cuxhaven, Germany (6) Filtek Supreme XTE, 3M ESPE, St. Paul, MN, USA (7) Ionostar Plus, VOCO GmbH, Cuxhaven, Germany (positive control) (8) Human enamel (negative control) POLISHING PROCEDURES All specimens were uniformly finished and polished with silica–alumina grinding papers (600–4000 grit) and stored in artificial saliva	(1) Profilometry in contact mode for surface roughness evaluation (Ra height parameter) (2) SEM/EDX analysis and X-ray diffraction (XRD analysis) for molecular, elemental and structural analysis of the specimens. (3) Thermogravimetric analysis (TG) and differential scanning calorimetry (DSC) for quantification of filler content of the specimens. (4) Static, orbital shaking, continuous flow and mixed-plaque formation bioreactors for microbial investigation of *S. mutans* and mixed plaque biofilm	CAD/CAM blocks yielded lower *S. mutans* and mixed plaque biofilm formation compared to direct resin-based materials No strong correlation between biofilm formation and surface roughness Stronger corellation between biofilm formation, manufacturing techniques and curing processes	Ionescu et al., 2020 [73]

Table 2. Cont.

Objective	Type of Specimens/Type of Control Group	Tests	Conclusion	Study/Year
Evaluation of biofilm formation on different dental restorative materials	(1) IPS Emax Press, Ivoclar Vivadent (2) IPS Emax CAD, Ivoclar Vivadent (3) Lava Ultimate, 3M ESPE (4) Vita Enamic, Vita Zahnfabrik (5) Two conventional composite resins POLISHING PROCEDURES CAD/CAM specimens subjected to sandblasting, polished by sandpaper discs (180–2000 grit), Sof–Lex discs, green stone and rubber points. Composite resins polished with polishing brushes, Sof–Lex discs, diamond paste and cotton tassel	(1) Atomic force microscopy for surface roughness evaluation (Ra, Rmax, Rz height parameters) (2) Dynamic bioreactor, CLSM analysis and arbitary fluorescence unit counting (AFU) for microbial analysis of S. mutans	Positive correlation between surface roughness and biofilm formation on ceramic CAD/CAM blocks and composite resins	Contreras-Guererro et al., 2020 [74]
Comparison of biofilm adhesion and formation on different smooth dental restorative materials with human enamel	(1) Ceram X, Dentsply-Sirona, Konstanz, Germany (2) IPS emax Press, Ivoclar Vivadent (3) Lava Plus, 3M ESPE (4) Vita Enamic, Vita Zahnfabrik (5) metal alloy (CoCrMo) (6) human enamel (control group) POLISHING PROCEDURES Finished and polished according to the manufacturers' instructions	(1) 3D optical profilometer for surface roughness evaluation (Sa height parameter) (2) SEM analysis and CFU/mL counting for microbiological analysis (3) Mass spectrometry for species identification	Biofilm maturation on specific restorative materials is influenced by surface properties and material composition Microbiological analysis showed that bacterial strains differed between the materials	Engel et al., 2020 [75]
Evaluation of surface roughness, biofilm formation, cytotoxicity and genotoxicity of three resin-based CAD/CAM materials	(1) Vita Enamic, Vita Zahnfabrik (2) Cerasmart, GC (3) Brilliant Crios, Coltene Whaledent AG POLISHING PROCEDURES All specimens were uniformly polished with silicone carbide paper discs up to 1200 grit, diamond grit polishing discs and a diamond polishing paste	(1) Non-contact optical profilometer + SEM for surface roughness evaluation (2) CFU/mL counting for microbial analysis of S. mutans and Lactobacilli	Brilliant Crios showed the highest biofilm formation values No statistically significant differences in surface roughness values between groups No statistically significant correlation between surface roughness and bacterial adhesion for all groups	Hassan et al., 2022 [76]
Comparison of physicomechanical properties and biofilm formation between resin-based hybrid materials	(1) Grandio Blocs, VOCO GmbH (2) Lava Untimate, 3M ESPE POLISHING PROCEDURES Materials were polished according to the manufacturer's instructions	(1) Stylus profilometer for surface roughness evaluation (Ra height parameter) (2) SEM analysis and CFU/mL counting for microbial analysis of S. mutans	Grandio Blocs showed significantly lower roughness and bacterial adhesion when compared to Lava Ultimate Positive correlation between surface roughness and bacterial adherence for both resin-based CAD/CAM materials.	Mokhtar et al., 2022 [77]
Effect of different polishing techniques on surface properties and bacterial adhesion on resin-based CAD/CAM materials	(1) Vita Enamic, Vita Zahnfabrik (2) Lava Ultimate, 3M ESPE (3) Cerasmart, GC POLISHING PROCEDURES (1) Non-polished (control group) (2) Manually polished (3) Glazed	(1) Profilometer in contact mode for surface roughness evaluation (Ra height parameter) (2) Contact angle measurement for surface free energy evaluation (3) SEM/EDS analysis for elemental and topographical evaluation (4) CFU/mL counting and SEM analysis for microbial evaluation of S. mutans	Non-polished CAD/CAM controls showed the highest surface roughness values Non-polished CAD/CAM controls showed higher bacterial adhesion Positive correlation between polishing procedures, surface properties and bacterial adhesion	Ozarslan et al., 2022 [78]

Table 2. *Cont.*

Objective	Type of Specimens/Type of Control Group	Tests	Conclusion	Study/Year
Evaluation of surface roughness, surface wettability and biofilm formation on CAD/CAM and 3D-printed materials for permanent restorations	(1) Vita Enamic, Vita Zahnfabrik (2) Cerasmart, GC Corp. (3) Lava Unltimate, 3M ESPE (4) Varseo Smile Crown Plus, BEGO, Bremen, Germany (5) Saremco Print Crowntech, Saremco dental AG, Rebstein, Switzerland (6) Formlabs 3D Permanent Crown, Formlabs, Somerville, MA, USA POLISHING PROCEDURES Equally polished with 600–800-grit-sized silicon carbide discs and aluminum oxide-coated discs (coarse, medium, fine and extrafine discs)	(1) Profilometer in contact mode for surface roughness evaluation (Ra height parameter) (2) Contact angle measurement for surface wettability (3) CFU/mL counting and SEM analysis for microbiological analysis of *S. mutans* and *S. sanguis*	Different digital manufacturing techniques and material compositions affect surface roughness No statistically signifcant diference between the groups in contact angle values Microbial adhesion varies regarding the bacterial species tested No correlation between surface roughness and bacterial adhesion	Ozer et al., 2023 [79]

5. Limitations of the Current Research

Delving deeper into the aforementioned research, a cautious interpretation of their ambiguous results should be accomplished.

On the one hand, when evaluating resin-based CAD/CAM materials, a group of researchers demonstrate a definite association between biofilm formation and surface roughness or surface modification procedures [69–71,74,75,77,78], whereas, on the other hand, no correlation between these factors is found in research studies conducted by other groups of investigators [73,76,79]. These discrepancies are also present in previously conducted in vitro studies assessing surface roughness, different polishing techniques and their impact on biofilm formation for laboratory-fabricated indirect and direct resin-based restorative materials [27,87–96].

This divergence may rely on the following factors:

1. The Ra threshold theory of 0.2 μm.

In several studies that incorporate CAD/CAM samples in their protocols, with initial Sa values of samples greater than 0.2 μm, a positive correlation between surface roughness and bacterial attachment has been found [69,70,77]. Additionally, it is further demonstrated that surface roughness has an insignificant effect on bacterial adhesion when the Sa values of the tested specimens are below this threshold [97]. In the research protocol of Ionescu et al. in 2020, where surface roughness values (Sa) were less than 0.2 μm, no strong correlation between Sa and bacterial adhesion was present [73]. Interestingly, in some research protocols with Sa values greater than the 0.2 μm threshold, no correlation between the two investigated factors has been observed [76,79], and in other research where the Sa values were lower than the established threshold, a strong correlation between surface roughness and biofilm adhesion has been demonstrated [74,78]. This fact highlights the potential influence of additional factors, such as polishing procedures, chemical composition and topography, on the outcomes of bacterial adhesion. Moreover, a systematic review by Duetra et al. in 2018 [98] concluded that the impact of roughness on bacterial adhesion is not related to a roughness threshold but rather to a range of surface roughness, which is wide and material-dependent. The majority of in vitro studies evaluating either the surface roughness as a single parameter or the relationship between surface roughness and bacterial colonization use only the Sa value, which is a single height parameter of a surface. Additional spatial, functional or hybrid (e.g., developed interfacial area ratio, Sdr) parameters, may give a greater insight into surface texture and bacterial colonization.

2. The polishing procedure may affect bacterial adhesion on resin-based CAD/CAM materials for indirect restorations.

CAD/CAM materials directly after their milling procedure present an insufficient smoothness, which may be adjusted by additional polishing protocols [99]. Although no standard protocol for polishing CAD/CAM restorations has been established [100], each company manufacturing CAD/CAM resin-based materials fabricates and promotes its finishing and polishing sets to achieve optimal surface characteristics in the final restoration. According to the literature, finishing and polishing protocols affect the surface roughness of dental materials and promote a heterogeneous impact on bacterial adhesion [98]. Comparing polished resin-based CAD/CAM blocks to unpolished control groups, statistically significant differences were found concerning the decreased amount of bacterial adhesion on polished specimens [70,71,74,78]. It is evident that different polishing techniques remove the superficial layers of the tested materials, resulting in a physically as well as chemically altered surface compared to the unpolished control group and in a subsequently reduced surface roughness [101,102]. Meanwhile, significant differences in surface roughness values were obtained while using the same polishing protocols for different resin-based CAD/CAM materials. This may be attributed to the third factor that generates variance in the results of the studies mentioned above, namely the elemental composition and the microstructure of resin-based CAD/CAM materials.

3. The chemical and topographical microstructure of hybrid, resin-based CAD/CAM materials.

More precisely, a different structural composition is present in lithium disilicate glass ceramic CAD/CAM blocks compared to polymer-infiltrated ceramic network materials, nano-ceramic filler-infiltrated polymer networks or direct resin-based materials, leading subsequently to different surface roughness and biofilm adherence values. Furthermore, biofilm formation is positively linked to the amount of the resin matrix rather than the amount of filler particles. It is scientifically proven that some released monomers stimulate bacterial growth [90]. This may explain the fact that in the research of Hassan et al. in 2022 [76], Brilliant Crios blocks exhibited more outstanding bacterial adhesion compared to Vita Enamic and Cerasmart blocks, since the former contain a greater proportion of resin matrix (29%wt). It should not be forgotten that CAD/CAM blocks are produced under a high pressure and a high temperature, improving their properties. This should be counted as an additional factor explaining the reduced biofilm formation on these materials compared to conventional composite resins [9,19].

All in all, the type of resin-based CAD/CAM material and the surface finishing and polishing techniques are significantly related to surface roughness and biofilm adherence.

4. The lack of standardization in the fabrication of specimens.

The results of the research protocols of Contreras-Guererro et al. in 2020 [74] are opposed to other similar in vitro studies evaluating biofilm formation on ceramic CAD/CAM, hybrid resin-based CAD/CAM and composite resin specimens, since they demonstrate greater surface roughness and biofilm formation values for the hybridized resin-based CAD/CAM blocks compared to conventional composite resins. Kim et al. in 2017 [69] also demonstrated that simulated intraoral adjustment and polishing procedures have a negative effect on surface roughness and on biofilm formation in hybrid resin-based materials, leucite-reinforced glass ceramics and nanoleucite-glass ceramics compared to their unpolished counterparts. Such discrepancies may be justified by the disparities in the preparation of the specimens between different research protocols. For the fabrication of conventional composite resin specimens, a universal approach has been proposed using molds with specific dimensions, glass slides, and acetate strips. On the other hand, for the fabrication of CAD/CAM samples, several approaches have been used. Some researchers generated CAD/CAM samples by the use of a diamond bur or a trepan bur under a constant water flow [73,75], whereas some others used diamond discs attached to low-speed straight handpieces [69]. In two research protocols, CAD/CAM samples were fabricated by the use of a milling unit [72,74]. Most researchers used a low-speed precision cutting machine and a diamond blade under flowing water [70,76–79]. All these different fabrication methods may result in different study outcomes.

Furthermore, in some studies, finishing and polishing were accomplished by the use of grinding and polishing devices under a constant water flow combined with silicone carbide grinding papers of different grit sizes, and the specimens were additionally polished by polishing sets of different manufacturers, whereas some others used several polishing systems on the fabricated (by the use of rotary instruments) specimens directly. These variations in the methodology of experimental protocols result in divergent outcomes in the research. All we need is the standardization of the procedures and the establishment of ideal conditions that can mimic, to the greatest extent, the intraoral environment. In vitro studies fail to provide all the oral environment's complex conditions, and future research should focus on in situ and in vivo protocols.

5. The biofilm assessment method

Referring to intraoral conditions, another factor affecting the results of biofilm formation on resin-based CAD/CAM materials is the method of biofilm assessment. Most in vitro studies use one microbial strain (monospecies colony), mainly *S. mutans*, since it is a well-known predominant cariogenic species [79]. A plethora of artificial systems try to mimic the intraoral environmental conditions for biofilm development on the surface of a dental material; these systems are called bioreactors. They are used for in vitro biofilm growth and are categorized either as static or dynamic bioreactors. They can be made of artificial oral microcosms, single species or defined consortia of a few species growing together [103,104]. Most in vitro studies assessing biofilm formation on resin-based CAD/CAM surfaces use a single species, since this is a simple, controlled, inexpensive, highly reproducible technique [105]. Attempting to imitate oral conditions, most in vitro studies incorporate in their microbiological protocol the immersion of samples in mucin containing artificial saliva or whole mouth saliva, secreted from a volunteer, to form the acquired pellicle. Colony-forming unit counting (CFU/mL), combined with SEM investigations and confocal laser scanning microscopy (CLSM), is used to perform qualitative and quantitative evaluations of bacterial formation [106]. SEM and CLSM have limitations, including the high cost and complexity of their protocols, the inability of CLSM to discriminate strains, the inability of SEM to discriminate live and dead bacteria, and the fact that only a specific selected area of the substrate may be evaluated [107].

Furthermore, bacterial adhesion on the surface of a substratum is not only influenced by the surface characteristics of the materials tested but also by the selected bacterial strain, the growth medium used and the specific adhesion mechanisms of the selected monospecies. Only one in vitro study by Ionescu et al. in 2020 [74] used four models of bioreactors for microbial investigations (static, orbital shaking, continuous flow and mixed-plaque formation bioreactors) to assess biofilm formation on resin-based CAD/CAM materials, concluding that, when bioreactors with shear forces or bioreactors where multi plaque formation takes place are used, lower *S. mutans* formation on resin-based CAD/CAM blocks was observed compared to conventional composite resin specimens. Unfortunately, in vitro biofilm formation has only been investigated via culture-dependent, close-ended molecular methods with a great risk of bias which do not coincide with real in vivo conditions.

Until recently, only two in situ studies that evaluated biofilm adhesion and formation on different dental restorative materials used a resin-based CAD/CAM material in their experimental groups [72,75], meaning that this is a field that nowadays attracts the interest of a lot of researchers.

Lastly, it should not be forgotten that under clinical conditions, surfaces are immediately coated by saliva and the composition, the flow and the volume of saliva differ based on neural control system signaling, as well as on physical, environmental and/or pathological factors, which include circadian rhythm, age, gender, physical exercise, oral hygiene, food consumption (diet), medication and systematic diseases [108]. It is almost impossible to mimic all these above-mentioned conditions in in vitro protocols; therefore, in vivo studies incorporating parts of these factors in their study design should be conducted.

6. Conclusions

Newly introduced CAD/CAM restorative materials are gaining attention due to their more than satisfactory mechanical properties. The biological background of the tested dental materials proves to be a significant factor in dental science since bacterial adhesion is inextricably linked to secondary caries on the margins of a restoration and subsequently to the good or the poor clinical performance of a restoration. Bacterial adhesion on CAD/CAM resin-based materials is primarily investigated in in vitro studies that, unfortunately, do not represent the exact conditions of the oral environment. The current literature demonstrates a possible interaction between biofilm formation and the surface of the substratum. Surface roughness, surface free energy, surface topography and elemental and chemical composition may have a crucial impact on biofilm growth, mainly in the early stages of bacterial adherence. Further studies should be conducted in order to shed light on the unknown phenomenon of bioadhesion.

7. Future Perspectives

When conducting an in vitro study, caution should be exercised concerning the standardization of the applied procedures. Since in vitro studies present, inter alia, culturing bias, the scientific interest of most researchers focuses on the use of culture-independent methods for the identification of the total bacterial community in the oral environment. To do so, open-ended genome sequencing technologies, such as next-generation sequencers (NGSs), as well as proteomic and metaproteomic techniques that may identify the host and the microbial proteome, are gradually being incorporated in the microbiological armamentarium. The conduction of in situ and/or in vivo studies using resin-based CAD/CAM restorative materials as experimental groups and human enamel and conventional composite resins as control groups, incorporated on oral splints worn by volunteers, may provide an insight into how surface characteristics, saliva, acquired pellicles and the oral microbiome interact. Interestingly, via 16S ribosomal RNA gene sequencing, the whole microbiome present in biofilms may be identified [109]. Furthermore, mass spectrometry (MS) devices may provide information concerning the proteomic profile of a tested material. Utilizing specific databases of bioinformatics, bacterial species adhered to a surface may be recognized using MS (metaproteomics). The "-Omics" era focuses on the principle that the whole organism works in synergy, and each bacterium is dependent on the other species present. Since biofilms are described as conglomerates, a more holistic, ecological approach to controlling dental biofilms is necessary.

Author Contributions: Conceptualization, K.T. and E.P.; methodology, K.T.; validation, K.T., C.R. and E.P.; formal analysis, K.T.; investigation, K.T.; data curation, K.T.; writing—original draft preparation, K.T.; writing—review and editing, C.R. and E.P.; visualization, K.T.; supervision, C.R. and E.P.; project administration, K.T., C.R. and E.P. All authors have read and agreed to the published version of the manuscript.

Funding: This research received no external funding.

Institutional Review Board Statement: Not applicable.

Informed Consent Statement: Not applicable.

Data Availability Statement: Not applicable.

Conflicts of Interest: The authors declare no conflicts of interest.

References

1. Watts, D.C.; Marouf, A.S.; Al-Hindi, A.M. Photo-polymerization shrinkage-stress kinetics in resin-composites: Methods development. *Dent. Mater.* **2003**, *19*, 1–11. [CrossRef] [PubMed]
2. Azeem, R.A.; Sureshbabu, N.M. Clinical performance of direct versus indirect composite restorations in posterior teeth: A systematic review. *J. Conserv. Dent.* **2018**, *21*, 2–9. [CrossRef] [PubMed]
3. Mitra, S.B.; Wu, D.; Holmes, B.N. An application of nanotechnology in advanced dental materials. *J. Am. Dent. Assoc.* **2003**, *134*, 1382–1390. [CrossRef] [PubMed]

4. Alzraikat, H.; Burrow, M.F.; Maghaireh, G.A.; Taha, N.A. Nanofilled Resin Composite Properties and Clinical Performance: A Review. *Oper. Dent.* **2018**, *43*, 173–190. [CrossRef]
5. Dejak, B.; Młotkowski, A.A. Comparison of stresses in molar teeth restored with inlays and direct restorations, including polymerization shrinkage of composite resin and tooth loading during mastication. *Dent. Mater.* **2015**, *31*, 77–87. [CrossRef] [PubMed]
6. Nandini, S. Indirect resin composites. *J. Conserv. Dent.* **2010**, *13*, 184–194. [CrossRef] [PubMed]
7. Peutzfeldt, A. Indirect Resin and Ceramic Systems. *Oper. Dent.* **2001**, *200*, 1153–1176.
8. Burke, E.J.; Qualtrough, A.J. Aesthetic inlays: Composite or ceramic? *Br. Dent. J.* **1994**, *176*, 53–60. [CrossRef]
9. Ruse, N.D.; Sadoun, M.J. Resin-composite blocks for dental CAD/CAM applications. *J. Dent. Res.* **2014**, *93*, 1232–1234. [CrossRef]
10. van Noort, R. The future of dental devices is digital. *Dent. Mater.* **2012**, *28*, 3–12. [CrossRef]
11. Fasbinder, D.J. Materials for chairside CAD/CAM restorations. *Compend. Contin. Educ. Dent.* **2010**, *31*, 702–709.
12. Lambert, H.; Durand, J.C.; Jacquot, B.; Fages, M. Dental biomaterials for chairside CAD/CAM: State of the art. *J. Adv. Prosthodont.* **2017**, *9*, 486–495. [CrossRef]
13. Mörmann, W.H. The evolution of the CEREC system. *J. Am. Dent. Assoc.* **2006**, *137*, 7–13. [CrossRef]
14. Horvath, S.D. Key Parameters of Hybrid Materials for CAD/CAM-Based Restorative Dentistry. *Compend. Contin. Educ. Dent.* **2016**, *37*, 638–643.
15. Palacios, T.; Tarancón, S.; Pastor, J.Y. On the Mechanical Properties of Hybrid Dental Materials for CAD/CAM Restorations. *Polymers* **2022**, *14*, 3252. [CrossRef] [PubMed]
16. Papathanasiou, I.; Kamposiora, P.; Dimitriadis, K.; Papavasiliou, G.; Zinelis, S. In vitro evaluation of CAD/CAM composite materials. *J. Dent.* **2023**, *136*, 104623. [CrossRef] [PubMed]
17. Koenig, A.; Schmidtke, J.; Schmohl, L.; Schneider-Feyrer, S.; Rosentritt, M.; Hoelzig, H.; Kloess, G.; Vejjasilpa, K.; Schulz-Siegmund, M.; Fuchs, F.; et al. Characterisation of the Filler Fraction in CAD/CAM Resin-Based Composites. *Materials* **2021**, *14*, 1986. [CrossRef] [PubMed]
18. Rexhepi, I.; Santilli, M.; D'Addazio, G.; Tafuri, G.; Manciocchi, E.; Caputi, S.; Sinjari, B. Clinical Applications and Mechanical Properties of CAD-CAM Materials in Restorative and Prosthetic Dentistry: A Systematic Review. *J. Funct. Biomater.* **2023**, *14*, 431. [CrossRef] [PubMed]
19. Goujat, A.; Abouelleil, H.; Colon, P.; Jeannin, C.; Pradelle, N.; Seux, D.; Grosgogeat, B. Mechanical properties and internal fit of 4 CAD-CAM block materials. *J. Prosthet. Dent.* **2018**, *119*, 384–389. [CrossRef] [PubMed]
20. Stockl, C.; Hampe, R.; Stawarczyk, B.; Haerst, M.; Roos, M. Macro- and microtopographical examination and quantification of CAD-CAM composite resin 2- and 3-body wear. *J. Prosthet. Dent.* **2018**, *120*, 537–545. [CrossRef]
21. Papathanasiou, I.; Zinelis, S.; Papavasiliou, G.; Kamposiora, P. Effect of aging on color, gloss and surface roughness of CAD/CAM composite materials. *J. Dent.* **2023**, *130*, 104423. [CrossRef]
22. Furtado de Mendonca, A.; Shahmoradi, M.; Gouvea, C.V.D.; De Souza, G.M.; Ellakwa, A. Microstructural and mechanical characterization of CAD/CAM materials for monolithic dental restorations. *J. Prosthodont.* **2019**, *28*, 587–594. [CrossRef] [PubMed]
23. Stawarczyk, B.; Liebermann, A.; Eichberger, M.; Güth, J.F. Evaluation of mechanical and optical behavior of current esthetic dental restorative CAD/CAM composites. *J. Mech. Behav. Biomed. Mater.* **2015**, *55*, 1–11. [CrossRef] [PubMed]
24. Lauvahutanon, S.; Takahashi, H.; Shiozawa, M.; Iwasaki, N.; Asakawa, Y.; Oki, M.; Finger, W.J.; Arksornnukit, M. Mechanical properties of composite resin blocks for CAD/CAM. *Dent. Mater. J.* **2014**, *33*, 705–710. [CrossRef] [PubMed]
25. Sonmez, N.; Gultekin, P.; Turp, V.; Akgungor, G.; Sen, D.; Mijiritsky, E. Evaluation of five CAD/CAM materials by microstructural characterization and mechanical tests: A comparative in vitro study. *BMC Oral Health* **2018**, *18*, 5. [CrossRef] [PubMed]
26. Kramer, N.; Kunzelmann, K.H.; Garcia-Godoy, F.; Haberlein, I.; Meier, B.; Frankenberger, R. Determination of caries risk at resin composite margins. *Am. J. Dent.* **2007**, *20*, 59–64.
27. Cazzaniga, G.; Ottobelli, M.; Ionescu, A.; Garcia-Godoy, F.; Brambilla, E. Surface properties of resin-based composite materials and biofilm formation: A review of the current literature. *Am. J. Dent.* **2015**, *28*, 311–320. [PubMed]
28. Mainjot, A.K.; Dupont, N.M.; Oudkerk, J.C.; Dewael, T.Y.; Sadoun, M.J. From Artisanal to CAD-CAM Blocks: State of the Art of Indirect Composites. *J. Dent. Res.* **2016**, *95*, 487–495. [CrossRef]
29. Della Bona, A.; Corazza, P.H.; Zhang, Y. Characterization of a polymer-infiltrated ceramic-network material. *Dent. Mater.* **2014**, *30*, 564–569. [CrossRef]
30. Marchesi, G.; Camurri Piloni, A.; Nicolin, V.; Turco, G.; Di Lenarda, R. Chairside CAD/CAM Materials: Current Trends of Clinical Uses. *Biology* **2021**, *10*, 1170. [CrossRef]
31. Skorulska, A.; Piszko, P.; Rybak, Z.; Szymonowicz, M.; Dobrzyński, M. Review on Polymer, Ceramic and Composite Materials for CAD/CAM Indirect Restorations in Dentistry-Application, Mechanical Characteristics and Comparison. *Materials* **2021**, *14*, 1592. [CrossRef]
32. Blatz, M.B.; Conejo, J. The Current State of Chairside Digital Dentistry and Materials. *Dent. Clin. N. Am.* **2019**, *63*, 175–197. [CrossRef]
33. Xie, C.; Zhang, J.F.; Li, S. Polymer Infiltrated Ceramic Hybrid Composites as Dental Materials. *Oral Health Dent. Stud.* **2018**, *1*, 2. [CrossRef]

34. Rocha, M.G.; Oliveira, D.; Sinhoreti, M.A.C.; Roulet, J.F.; Zoidis, P.; Duncan, W. Assessment of CAD/CAM composites classification in abstracts using machine learning. *Dent. Mater.* **2023**, *39*, 60–61. [CrossRef]
35. Tsitrou, E.A.; Northeast, S.E.; van Noort, R. Brittleness index of machinable dental materials and its relation to the marginal chipping factor. *J. Dent.* **2007**, *35*, 897–902. [CrossRef] [PubMed]
36. Fasbinder, D.J.; Neiva, G.F. Surface evaluation of polishing techniques for new resilient CAD/CAM restorative materials. *J. Esthet. Restor. Dent.* **2016**, *28*, 56–66. [CrossRef] [PubMed]
37. Coldea, A.; Swain, M.V.; Thiel, N. Mechanical properties of polymer-infiltrated-ceramic-network materials. *Dent. Mater.* **2013**, *29*, 419–426. [CrossRef] [PubMed]
38. Nguyen, J.F.; Migonney, V.; Ruse, N.D.; Sadoun, M. Resin composite blocks via high-pressure high-temperature polymerization. *Dent. Mater.* **2012**, *28*, 529–534. [CrossRef] [PubMed]
39. Vita Enamic®. Technical and Scientific Documentation. Available online: https://www.vita-zahnfabrik.com/en/VITA-ENAMIC-24970.html (accessed on 3 March 2024).
40. Lava™ Ultimate CAD/CAM Restorative for E4D. Available online: https://multimedia.3m.com/mws/media/756863O/3m-lava-ultimate-cad-cam-restorative-for-e4d-the-edge-you-need.pdf (accessed on 2 March 2024).
41. SHOFU Block & Disk HC: Instructions for Use. Available online: https://www.shofu.com/wp-content/uploads/SHOFU-Block-HC-IFU-US.pdf (accessed on 2 March 2024).
42. CERASMART GC Dental Product Technical Product Profile. Available online: www.gcamerica.com (accessed on 7 July 2022).
43. Grandio Blocs/Grandio Disc—Nano-Ceramic Hybrid CAD/CAM Material: Instructions for Use. Available online: https://www.voco.dental/en/portaldata/1/resources/products/instructions-for-use/e1/grandio-blocs_ifu_e1.pdf (accessed on 2 March 2024).
44. Brilliant Crios: Instructions for Use. Available online: https://products.coltene.com/EN/AG/media/DOC_IFU_30003998-12-22-IFU-BRILLIANT-Crios_IND.pdf?sprache=EN (accessed on 2 March 2024).
45. Katana Avencia Blocks SDS. Available online: https://katanaavencia.com/wp-content/uploads/KATANA_AVENCIA_Block_SDS_US.pdf (accessed on 2 March 2024).
46. Tetric CAD Instructions for Use. Available online: https://www.ivoclar.com/en_li/eifu?brand=Tetric+CAD (accessed on 2 March 2024).
47. Deo, P.N.; Deshmukh, R. Oral microbiome: Unveiling the fundamentals. *J. Oral Maxillofac. Pathol.* **2019**, *23*, 122–128. [CrossRef]
48. Kilian, M.; Chapple, I.L.; Hannig, M.; Marsh, P.D.; Meuric, V.; Pedersen, A.M.; Tonetti, M.S.; Wade, W.G.; Zaura, E. The oral microbiome—An update for oral healthcare professionals. *Br. Dent. J.* **2016**, *221*, 657–666. [CrossRef]
49. Samaranayake, L.; Bandara, N.; Pesee, S. Oral Biofilms: What Are They? In *Oral Biofilms and Modern Dental Materials*, 1st ed.; Ionescu, A.C., Hahnel, S., Eds.; Springer Nature: Cham, Switzerland, 2021; pp. 1–7. [CrossRef]
50. Ptasiewicz, M.; Grywalska, E.; Mertowska, P.; Korona-Głowniak, I.; Poniewierska-Baran, A.; Niedźwiedzka-Rystwej, P.; Chałas, R. Armed to the Teeth-The Oral Mucosa Immunity System and Microbiota. *Int. J. Mol. Sci.* **2022**, *23*, 882. [CrossRef]
51. Lin, N.J. Biofilm over teeth and restorations: What do we need to know? *Dent. Mater.* **2017**, *33*, 667–680. [CrossRef]
52. Sterzenbach, T.; Helbig, R.; Hannig, C.; Hannig, M. Bioadhesion in the oral cavity and approaches for biofilm management by surface modifications. *Clin. Oral Investig.* **2020**, *24*, 4237–4260. [CrossRef]
53. Kreth, J.; Herzberg, M.C. Molecular principles of adhesion and biofilm formation. In *The Root Canal Biofilm*, 1st ed.; Chávez de Paz, L.E., Sedgley, C.M., Kishen, A., Eds.; Springer Nature: Berlin, Germany, 2015; pp. 23–54. [CrossRef]
54. Enax, J.; Ganss, B.; Amaechi, B.T.; Schulze Zur Wiesche, E.; Meyer, F. The composition of the dental pellicle: An updated literature review. *Front. Oral Health* **2023**, *4*, 1260442. [CrossRef]
55. Kreth, J.; Merritt, J.; Pfeifer, C.S.; Khajotia, S.; Ferracane, J.L. Interaction between the Oral Microbiome and Dental Composite Biomaterials: Where We Are and Where We Should Go. *J. Dent. Res.* **2020**, *99*, 1140–1149. [CrossRef]
56. Lindh, L.; Aroonsang, W.; Sotres, J.; Arnebrant, T. Salivary pellicles. *Monogr. Oral Sci.* **2014**, *24*, 30–39. [CrossRef]
57. Fischer, N.G.; Aparicio, C. The salivary pellicle on dental biomaterials. *Colloids Surf. B Biointerfaces* **2021**, *200*, 111570. [CrossRef]
58. Chawhuaveang, D.D.; Yu, O.Y.; Yin, I.X.; Lam, W.Y.; Mei, M.L.; Chu, C.H. Acquired salivary pellicle and oral diseases: A literature review. *J. Dent. Sci.* **2021**, *16*, 523–529. [CrossRef]
59. Eliades, G.; Eliades, T.; Vavuranakis, M. General aspects of biomaterial surface alterations following exposure to biologic fluids. In *Dental Materials In Vivo: Aging and Related Phenomena*, 1st ed.; Eliades, G., Eliades, T., Brantley, W.A., Walts, D.C., Eds.; Quintessence Publishing Co.: Chicago, IL, USA, 2003; pp. 3–23.
60. Sbordone, L.; Bortolaia, C. Oral microbial biofilms and plaque-related diseases: Microbial communities and their role in the shift from oral health to disease. *Clin. Oral Investig.* **2003**, *7*, 181–188. [CrossRef]
61. Song, F.; Koo, H.; Ren, D. Effects of Material Properties on Bacterial Adhesion and Biofilm Formation. *J. Dent. Res.* **2015**, *94*, 1027–1034. [CrossRef]
62. Schmalz, G.; Cieplik, F. Biofilms on Restorative Materials. *Monogr. Oral Sci.* **2021**, *29*, 155–194. [CrossRef]
63. Teughels, W.; Van Assche, N.; Sliepen, I.; Quirynen, M. Effect of material characteristics and/or surface topography on biofilm development. *Clin. Oral Implants Res.* **2006**, *17*, 68–81. [CrossRef]
64. Bürgers, R.; Krohn, S.; Wassmann, T. Surface Properties of Dental Materials and Biofilm Formation. In *Oral Biofilms and Modern Dental Materials*, 1st ed.; Ionescu, A.C., Hahnel, S., Eds.; Springer Nature: Cham, Switzerland, 2021; pp. 55–70. [CrossRef]

65. Quirynen, M.; Bollen, C.M. The influence of surface roughness and surface-free energy on supra- and subgingival plaque formation in man. A review of the literature. *J. Clin. Periodontol.* **1995**, *22*, 1–14. [CrossRef]
66. Zheng, S.; Bawazir, M.; Dhall, A.; Kim, H.E.; He, L.; Heo, J.; Hwang, G. Implication of Surface Properties, Bacterial Motility, and Hydrodynamic Conditions on Bacterial Surface Sensing and Their Initial Adhesion. *Front. Bioeng. Biotechnol.* **2021**, *9*, 643722. [CrossRef]
67. Auschill, T.M.; Arweiler, N.B.; Brecx, M.; Reich, E.; Sculean, A.; Netuschil, L. The effect of dental restorative materials on dental biofilm. *Eur. J. Oral Sci.* **2002**, *110*, 48–53. [CrossRef]
68. Padovani, G.; Fúcio, S.; Ambrosano, G.; Sinhoreti, M.; Puppin-Rontani, R. In situ surface biodegradation of restorative materials. *Oper. Dent.* **2014**, *39*, 349–360. [CrossRef]
69. Kim, K.H.; Loch, C.; Waddell, J.N.; Tompkins, G.; Schwass, D. Surface Characteristics and Biofilm Development on Selected Dental Ceramic Materials. *Int. J. Dent.* **2017**, *2017*, 7627945. [CrossRef]
70. Hamerschmitt, R.M.; Tomazinho, P.H.; Camporês, K.L.; Gonzaga, C.C.; da Cunha, L.F.; Correr, G.M. Surface topography and bacterial adhesion of CAD/CAM resin based materials after application of different surface finishing techniques. *Braz. J. Oral Sci.* **2018**, *17*, e18135. [CrossRef]
71. Dobrzynski, M.; Pajaczkowska, M.; Nowicka, J.; Jaworski, A.; Kosior, P.; Szymonowicz, M.; Kuropka, P.; Rybak, Z.; Bogucki, Z.A.; Filipiak, J.; et al. Study of Surface Structure Changes for Selected Ceramics Used in the CAD/CAM System on the Degree of Microbial Colonization, In Vitro Tests. *Biomed. Res. Int.* **2019**, *12*, 9130806. [CrossRef]
72. Conrads, G.; Wendt, L.K.; Hetrodt, F.; Deng, Z.L.; Pieper, D.; Abdelbary, M.M.H.; Barg, A.; Wagner-Döbler, I.; Apel, C. Deep sequencing of biofilm microbiomes on dental composite materials. *J. Oral Microbiol.* **2019**, *11*, 1617013. [CrossRef]
73. Ionescu, A.C.; Hahnel, S.; König, A.; Brambilla, E. Resin composite blocks for dental CAD/CAM applications reduce biofilm formation in vitro. *Dent. Mater.* **2020**, *36*, 603–616. [CrossRef]
74. Contreras-Guerrero, P.; Ortiz-Magdaleno, M.; Urcuyo-Alvarado, M.S.; Cepeda-Bravo, J.A.; Leyva-Del Rio, D.; Pérez-López, J.E.; Romo-Ramírez, G.F.; Sánchez-Vargas, L.O. Effect of dental restorative materials surface roughness on the in vitro biofilm formation of *Streptococcus mutans* biofilm. *Am. J. Dent.* **2020**, *33*, 59–63.
75. Engel, A.S.; Kranz, H.T.; Schneider, M.; Tietze, J.P.; Piwowarcyk, A.; Kuzius, T.; Arnold, W.; Naumova, E.A. Biofilm formation on different dental restorative materials in the oral cavity. *BMC Oral Health* **2020**, *20*, 162. [CrossRef]
76. Hassan, S.A.; Beleidy, M.; El-Din, Y.A. Biocompatibility and Surface Roughness of Different Sustainable Dental Composite Blocks: Comprehensive In Vitro Study. *ACS Omega* **2022**, *7*, 34258–34267. [CrossRef]
77. Mokhtar, M.M.; Farahat, D.S.; Eldars, W.; Osman, M.F. Physico-mechanical properties and bacterial adhesion of resin composite CAD/CAM blocks: An in-vitro study. *J. Clin. Exp. Dent.* **2022**, *14*, 413–419. [CrossRef]
78. Ozarslan, M.; Bilgili Can, D.; Avcioglu, N.H.; Çalışkan, S. Effect of different polishing techniques on surface properties and bacterial adhesion on resin-ceramic CAD/CAM materials. *Clin. Oral Investig.* **2022**, *26*, 5289–5299. [CrossRef]
79. Ozer, N.E.; Sahin, Z.; Yikici, C.; Duyan, S.; Kilicarslan, M.A. Bacterial adhesion to composite resins produced by additive and subtractive manufacturing. *Odontology* **2023**, *112*, 460–471. [CrossRef]
80. Gadelmawla, E.S.; Koura, M.M.; Maksoud, T.M.A.; Elewa, I.M.; Soliman, H.H. Roughness parameters. *J. Mater. Res. Technol.* **2002**, *123*, 133–145. [CrossRef]
81. Van Meerbeek, B.; Vargas, M.; Inoue, S.; Yoshida, Y.; Perdigão, J.; Lambrechts, P.; Vanherle, G. Microscopy investigations. Techniques, results, limitations. *Am. J. Dent.* **2000**, *13*, 3–18.
82. Kaczmarek, K.; Leniart, A.; Lapinska, B.; Skrzypek, S.; Lukomska-Szymanska, M. Selected Spectroscopic Techniques for Surface Analysis of Dental Materials: A Narrative Review. *Materials* **2021**, *14*, 2624. [CrossRef]
83. Kaczmarek, K.; Konieczny, B.; Siarkiewicz, P.; Leniart, A.; Lukomska-Szymanska, M.; Skrzypek, S.; Lapinska, B. Surface Characterization of Current Dental Ceramics Using Scanning Electron Microscopic and Atomic Force Microscopic Techniques. *Coatings* **2022**, *12*, 1122. [CrossRef]
84. Sacher, E.; França, R. Surface Analysis Techniques for Dental Materials. *Dent. Biomater.* **2018**, *2*, 1–31. [CrossRef]
85. Liber-Kneć, A.; Łagan, S. Surface Testing of Dental Biomaterials-Determination of Contact Angle and Surface Free Energy. *Materials* **2021**, *14*, 2716. [CrossRef]
86. Wilson, C.; Lukowicz, R.; Merchant, S.; Valquier-Flynn, H.; Caballero, J.; Sandoval, J.; Okuom, M.; Huber, C.; Brooks, T.D.; Wilson, E.; et al. Quantitative and Qualitative Assessment Methods for Biofilm Growth: A mini-review. *Res. Rev. J. Eng. Technol.* **2017**, *6*, 1–42.
87. Ionescu, A.; Wutscher, E.; Brambilla, E.; Schneider-Feyrer, S.; Giessibl, F.J.; Hahnel, S. Influence of surface properties of resin-based composites on in vitro *Streptococcus mutans* biofilm development. *Eur. J. Oral Sci.* **2012**, *120*, 458–465. [CrossRef]
88. Aykent, F.; Yondem, I.; Ozyesil, A.G.; Gunal, S.K.; Avunduk, M.C.; Ozkan, S. Effect of different finishing techniques for restorative materials on surface roughness and bacterial adhesion. *J. Prosthet. Dent.* **2010**, *103*, 221–227. [CrossRef]
89. Ikeda, M.; Matin, K.; Nikaido, T.; Foxton, R.M.; Tagami, J. Effect of surface characteristics on adherence of S. mutans biofilms to indirect resin composites. *Dent. Mater. J.* **2007**, *26*, 915–923. [CrossRef]
90. Ionescu, A.; Brambilla, E.; Wastl, D.S.; Giessibl, F.J.; Cazzaniga, G.; Schneider Feyrer, S.; Hahnel, S. Influence of matrix and filler fraction on biofilm formation on the surface of experimental resin-based composites. *J. Mater. Sci. Mater. Med.* **2015**, *26*, 5372. [CrossRef]

91. Buergers, R.; Schneider-Brachert, W.; Hahnel, S.; Rosentritt, M.; Handel, G. Streptococcal adhesion to novel low-shrink silorane-based restorative. *Dent. Mater.* **2009**, *25*, 269–275. [CrossRef]
92. Pereira, C.A.; Eskelson, E.; Cavalli, V.; Liporoni, P.C.S.; Jorge, A.O.; do Rego, M.A. Streptococcus mutans biofilm adhesion on composite resin surfaces after different finishing and polishing techniques. *Oper. Dent.* **2011**, *36*, 311–317. [CrossRef]
93. Yuan, C.X.; Wang, X.; Gao, F.; Chen, X.; Liang, D.; Li, D. Effects of surface properties of polymer-based restorative materials on early adhesion of *Streptococcus mutans* in vitro. *J. Dent.* **2016**, *54*, 33–40. [CrossRef]
94. Cazzaniga, G.; Ottobelli, M.; Ionescu, A.C.; Paolone, G.; Gherlone, E.; Ferracane, J.L.; Brambilla, E. In vitro biofilm formation on resin-based composites after different finishing and polishing procedures. *J. Dent.* **2017**, *67*, 43–52. [CrossRef]
95. Bilgili, D.; Dündar, A.; Barutçugil, Ç.; Tayfun, D.; Özyurt, Ö.K. Surface properties and bacterial adhesion of bulk-fll composite resins. *J. Dent.* **2020**, *95*, 103317. [CrossRef] [PubMed]
96. Hahnel, S.; Ionescu, A.C.; Cazzaniga, G.; Ottobelli, M.; Brambilla, E. Biofilm formation and release of fluoride from dental restorative materials in relation to their surface properties. *J. Dent.* **2017**, *60*, 14–24. [CrossRef]
97. Bollen, C.M.; Lambrechts, P.; Quirynen, M. Comparison of surface roughness of oral hard materials to the threshold surface roughness for bacterial plaque retention: A review of the literature. *Dent. Mater.* **1997**, *13*, 258–269. [CrossRef]
98. Dutra, D.; Pereira, G.; Kantorski, K.Z.; Valandro, L.F.; Zanatta, F.B. Does Finishing and Polishing of Restorative Materials Affect Bacterial Adhesion and Biofilm Formation? A Systematic Review. *Oper. Dent.* **2018**, *43*, 37–52. [CrossRef] [PubMed]
99. Kara, D.; Tekçe, N.; Fidan, S.; Demirci, M.; Tuncer, S.; Balcı, S. The efects of various polishing procedures on surface topography of CAD/CAM resin restoratives. *J. Prosthodont.* **2021**, *30*, 481–489. [CrossRef] [PubMed]
100. da Silva, T.M.; Salvia, A.C.R.D.; Carvalho, R.F.; Pagani, C.; Rocha, D.M.; da Silva, E.G. Polishing for glass ceramics: Which protocol? *J. Prosthodont. Res.* **2014**, *58*, 160–170. [CrossRef]
101. de Oliveira, A.L.B.M.; Domingos, P.A.D.S.; Palma-Dibb, R.G.; Garcia, P.P.N.S. Chemical and morphological features of nanofilled composite resin: Influence of finishing and polishing procedures and fluoride solutions. *Microsc. Res. Tech.* **2012**, *75*, 212–219. [CrossRef]
102. Kurt, A.; Cilingir, A.; Bilmenoglu, C.; Topcuoglu, N.; Kulekci, G. Effect of different polishing techniques for composite resin materials on surface properties and bacterial biofilm formation. *J. Dent.* **2019**, *90*, 103199. [CrossRef]
103. Ionescu, A.C.; Brambilla, E. Bioreactors: How to Study Biofilms In Vitro. In *Oral Biofilms and Modern Dental Materials*, 1st ed.; Ionescu, A.C., Hahnel, S., Eds.; Springer Nature: Cham, Switzerland, 2021; pp. 37–54. [CrossRef]
104. Cieplik, F.; Aparicio, C.; Kreth, J.; Schmalz, G. Development of standard protocols for biofilm-biomaterial interface testing. *JADA Found. Sci.* **2022**, *1*, 100008. [CrossRef]
105. Brown, J.L.; Johnston, W.; Delaney, C.; Short, B.; Butcher, M.C.; Young, T.; Butcher, J.; Riggio, M.; Culshaw, S.; Ramage, G. Polymicrobial oral biofilm models: Simplifying the complex. *J. Med. Microbiol.* **2019**, *68*, 1573–1584. [CrossRef] [PubMed]
106. Ramachandra, S.S.; Wright, P.; Han, P.; Abdal-Hay, A.; Lee, R.S.B.; Ivanovski, S. Evaluating models and assessment techniques for understanding oral biofilm complexity. *MicrobiologyOpen* **2023**, *12*, 1377. [CrossRef] [PubMed]
107. Darrene, L.N.; Cecile, B. Experimental Models of Oral Biofilms Developed on Inert Substrates: A Review of the Literature. *Biomed. Res. Int.* **2016**, *2016*, 7461047. [CrossRef]
108. Helmerhorst, E.J.; Dawes, C.; Oppenheim, F.G. The complexity of oral physiology and its impact on salivary diagnostics. *Oral Dis.* **2018**, *24*, 363–371. [CrossRef]
109. Verma, D.; Garg, P.K.; Dubey, A.K. Insights into the human oral microbiome. *Arch. Microbiol.* **2018**, *200*, 525–540. [CrossRef]

Disclaimer/Publisher's Note: The statements, opinions and data contained in all publications are solely those of the individual author(s) and contributor(s) and not of MDPI and/or the editor(s). MDPI and/or the editor(s) disclaim responsibility for any injury to people or property resulting from any ideas, methods, instructions or products referred to in the content.

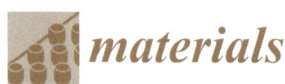 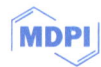

Article

The Effect of Restoration Thickness on the Fracture Resistance of 5 mol% Yttria-Containing Zirconia Crowns

Po-Hsu Chen [1], Esra Elamin [1], Akram Sayed Ahmed [2], Daniel A. Givan [1], Chin-Chuan Fu [1] and Nathaniel C. Lawson [1,*]

[1] Division of Prosthodontics, University of Alabama at Birmingham School of Dentistry, Birmingham, AL 35209, USA; pohsu@uab.edu (P.-H.C.); esra@uab.edu (E.E.); dgivan@uab.edu (D.A.G.); ccfu@uab.edu (C.-C.F.)
[2] Faculty of Dentistry, Department of Dental Biomaterials, Tanta University, Tanta 31527, Egypt; akram_gad@dent.tanta.edu.eg
* Correspondence: nlawson@uab.edu; Tel.: +1-205-975-8302

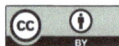

Citation: Chen, P.-H.; Elamin, E.; Sayed Ahmed, A.; Givan, D.A.; Fu, C.-C.; Lawson, N.C. The Effect of Restoration Thickness on the Fracture Resistance of 5 mol% Yttria-Containing Zirconia Crowns. *Materials* 2024, 17, 365. https://doi.org/10.3390/ma17020365

Academic Editors: Lavinia Cosmina Ardelean and Laura-Cristina Rusu

Received: 18 December 2023
Revised: 4 January 2024
Accepted: 8 January 2024
Published: 11 January 2024

Copyright: © 2024 by the authors. Licensee MDPI, Basel, Switzerland. This article is an open access article distributed under the terms and conditions of the Creative Commons Attribution (CC BY) license (https:// creativecommons.org/licenses/by/ 4.0/).

Abstract: Background: To determine what thickness of 5 mol% yttria zirconia (5Y-Z) translucent crowns cemented with different cements and surface treatments would have equivalent fracture resistance as 3 mol% yttria (3Y-Z) crowns. Methods: The study included 0.8 mm, 1.0 mm, and 1.2 mm thickness 5Y-Z (Katana UTML) crowns and 0.5 and 1.0 mm thickness 3Y-Z (Katana HT) crowns as controls. The 5Y-Z crowns were divided among three treatment subgroups ($n = 10$/subgroup): (1) cemented using RMGIC (Rely X Luting Cement), (2) alumina particle-abraded then luted with the same cement, (3) alumina particle-abraded and cemented using a resin cement (Panavia SA Cement Universal). The 3Y-Z controls were alumina particle-abraded then cemented with RMGIC. The specimens were then loaded in compression at 30° until failure. Results: All 5Y-Z crowns (regardless of thickness or surface treatment) had a similar to or higher fracture force than the 0.5 mm 3Y-Z crowns. Only the 1.2 mm 5Y-Z crowns with resin cement showed significantly similar fracture force to the 1 mm 3Y-Z crowns. Conclusion: In order to achieve a similar fracture resistance to 0.5 mm 3Y-Z crowns cemented with RMGIC, 5Y-Z crowns may be as thin as 0.8 mm. To achieve a similar fracture resistance to 1.0 mm 3Y-Z crowns cemented with RMGIC, 5Y-Z crowns must be 1.2 mm and bonded with resin cement.

Keywords: zirconia; cementation; crown fracture

1. Introduction

The use of all-ceramic dental restorations has increased in the past decade due to their cost, esthetic appearance, advances in adhesive dentistry, and improvements in dental ceramic materials [1]. Compared with other high-strength ceramic materials, 3 mol% yttria-stabilized zirconia (3Y-Z) has a higher flexural strength and fracture toughness, allows a more conservative dental preparation, minimizes wear on its antagonist, and lacks the unwanted complication of chipping when used as a monolithic restoration [2,3]. Due to the inferior translucency of 3Y-Z relative to glass ceramics, more translucent zirconia has been developed [4]. Crystal structure modifications induced by an increased yttrium oxide content from 3 to 5 mol% led to the development of translucent 5 mol% yttria-stabilized zirconia polycrystal (5Y-Z). This zirconia contains a cubic crystal content of approximately 50% of the structure, which allows improved light transmission [5–7]. In contrast, the higher proportion of cubic crystals in 5Y-Z also contributes to its weaker flexural strength and fracture toughness due to the lack of transformation toughening that occurs in 3Y-Z [8,9].

The present ubiquity of dental zirconia necessitates clear preparation guidelines for its use. The manufacturer's recommended minimum thickness for 3Y-Z is 0.5 mm and for 5Y-Z is 1.0 mm [10]. These proposed minimum material thicknesses are presumably based on laboratory strength testing of these materials relative to clinically proven materials.

Unfortunately, the source of justification for the manufacturer's minimum thickness values is not provided. A previous study examined the strength of 3Y-Z at different thicknesses and recommended 1.0 mm thickness to achieve an equivalent fracture resistance to a 1.5 mm metal ceramic crown [11]. To date, there has not been a previous study to verify the minimum thickness of 5Y-Z relative to a more clinically validated material, such as a 3Y-Z control.

One previous study examined the strength of 3Y-Z and 5Y-Z crowns at different thicknesses. Adabo et al. tested 1.0 and 1.5 mm thick premolar crowns fabricated from 3Y-Z and 5Y-Z that were bonded to metal dies with resin cement and fatigue-loaded with step-wise load increases [12]. The characteristic strength of the 5Y-Z crowns at both 1 and 1.5 mm was less than that of the 1 mm 3Y-Z crowns.

Several other studies examined 3Y-Z and 5Y-Z discs at different thicknesses. Alraheam et al. fatigue-loaded 0.7 and 1.2 mm thick 3Y and 5Y zirconia discs for 1.2 million cycles and 110 N of load [13]. After fatigue testing, none of the 3Y zirconia specimens of either thickness fractured, whereas 80% of the 0.7 mm thick 5Y-Z specimens and 30% of the 1.2 mm thick 5Y-Z specimens fractured. Longhini et al. studied 0.5, 1, and 1.5 mm 3Y-Z and 5Y-Z discs bonded to G10 epoxy discs with resin cement and tested them using a biaxial flexural strength apparatus [14]. The strength of the 0.5 mm thick 3Y-Z and 5Y-Z discs was statistically similar; although no statistical comparison was performed, the strength after bonding was similar between the 1.0 mm thick 3Y-Z discs and the 1.5 mm thick 5Y-Z discs. Machry et al. studied 0.7 and 1.0 mm thick discs of 3Y-Z and 5Y-Z bonded to epoxy resin, resin composite, or metal dies and fatigue-loaded with step-wise load increases [15]. The 0.7 mm 3Y-Z discs produced higher fracture resistance than the 0.7 and 1.0 mm 5Y-Z discs on the epoxy resin and resin composite dies.

Aside from the thickness of a crown, its fracture resistance may also be affected by the cement used and its surface preparation. The use of resin cement has been shown to improve the fracture resistance of both 3Y-Z and 5Y-Z crowns [16–18]. Regardless, resin-modified glass ionomer cement (RMGIC) is the most commonly used cement for zirconia crowns [19]. Therefore, this study employed 3Y-Z controls cemented with RMGIC and tested 5Y-Z crowns with both RMGIC and resin cement to determine the ability of resin cement to compensate for the reduced material strength of 5Y-Z.

Bonding to zirconia requires air particle abrasion and the use of a primer or resin cement containing 10-methacryloyloxydecyl dihydrogen phosphate (10-MDP) monomers [20,21]. Without air particle abrasion, the bond strength to both 3Y-Z and 5Y-Z decreases significantly [22–24]. The flexural strength of 3Y-Z is not negatively affected by air particle abrasion; however, 5Y-Z can be weakened following air particle abrasion [22,25,26]. With the use of RMGIC on zirconia crowns, air particle abrasion has not been shown to improve the bond as it has with resin cement [27]. Therefore air particle abrasion would not be necessary for 5Y-Z when used with RMGIC. Regardless, there may be some laboratories and clinicians who routinely air particle-abrade 5Y-Z crowns, even if RMGIC will be used for cementation [28]. Additionally, instructions for the use of some RMGICs recommend air particle abrasion on the internal surface of zirconia crowns [29]. In the current study, the recommended protocol for bonding 5Y-Z (air particle abrasion and resin cement), the recommended protocol for the conventional cementation of 5Y-Z (air particle abrasion and RMGIC), and an alternative protocol for conventional cementation (no air particle abrasion and RMGIC) were evaluated.

There are different testing methodologies to study the effect of restoration material thickness and surface treatment on the strength of dental ceramics. The International Standards Organization (ISO) standard for dental ceramic materials (ISO 6872:2015 [30]) describes three methods for the calculation of strength: three-point flexural, four-point flexure, and biaxial flexure (piston-on-three-ball). Three- and four-point tests utilize a bar supported on two ends and loaded across its center at one or two points, respectively. Biaxial flexural testing employs a disc specimen supported near its periphery and loaded in the center. Ceramics fail when the weakest flaw within the material propagates a critical crack. For this reason, four-point flexural testing leads to lower strength values than three-point flexural testing because there is a greater area subjected to the maximum bending moment (between the loading points), and there is a higher probability that a critical flaw will be present in this area [31]. Biaxial flexural testing will provide higher strength than three- or four-point flexural testing as the specimens are not loaded on their edges, where they are susceptible to failure due to flaws introduced in their fabrication process [31]. The advantage of using standardized geometry for specimens when testing the strength of materials is that specimens are consistent between testing sites, and loading may be applied such that stresses are determined by known calculations.

Another method of testing strength is the use of the crown fracture test, which utilizes a crown form cemented to a tooth preparation die that is loaded on its occlusal/lingual surface to failure. The advantages of crown fracture tests include the following. First, flaws or stress risers introduced into the crowns that result from their fabrication process can be factored into their measured strength. The method of fabrication of different ceramics may lead to specimens with different surface flaws that are more representative of actual clinical conditions than a flat bar [32]. Treating the specimens similarly to how they are used clinically ensures that testing is representative of clinical situations rather than selecting specimen preparation that is convenient for laboratory testing [33]. Despite the standardization offered by ISO testing, the ISO standard is not specific in the methods required to polish flexural strength specimens, which has led to different laboratories reporting 50% lower strength values of the same dental ceramic in round robin testing [34].

Second, the presence of a supporting structure may affect the strength of one material more than another [35]. Some materials may bond better to their substructure die, which more efficiently allows stress transfer [36]. Also, the different mismatch in elastic modulus between the crown and the substructure die may allow some materials to fare better than others [15,37]. Previous studies have reported that rankings of materials with crown fracture load testing do not correlate with flexural strength testing [38].

The objective of this study was to investigate the fracture resistance of 5Y-Z crowns at 0.8 mm, 1.0 mm, and 1.2 mm thickness that were bonded with resin cement (with air particle abrasion) or cemented with RMGIC (with and without air particle abrasion) using a crown fracture test. The values were compared to 3Y-Z cemented with its most common cement (RMGIC) at the manufacturer's recommended thickness (0.5 mm) and a thickness which has been shown to be equivalent to a metal ceramic crown (1.0 mm). The purpose of the study is to provide clinical guidance for the preparation of 5Y-Z crowns. The two null hypotheses are that there would be no difference in the fracture resistance of any of the 5Y-Z crowns tested relative to the 0.5 mm 3Y-Z control or the 1.0 mm 3Y-Z control.

2. Materials and Methods

An acrylic maxillary premolar on an artificial dentiform was used to form a standardized tooth preparation of minimum height 4 mm and 1 mm margin width. A coarse diamond tapered rotary cutting bur (6856.31.016 FG Coarse Round-End Taper Diamond, Brasseler, Savannah, GA, USA) was secured on the high-speed handpiece and kept parallel to the vertical axis of the tooth to create a standardized angle of convergence (6–10°). The shape of the diamond rotary formed a modified chamfer finish line. Occlusal, anatomical reduction of 1 mm was accomplished with the same bur. The prepared tooth was scanned with a lab scanner (E3 Scanner, 3Shape Inc., Copenhagen, Denmark); then, subsequent design and model construction were accomplished through computer-aided design (CAD) software (Dental System 2020, 3Shape Inc.) for both digital die and crown fabrication (Figure 1). Crowns were fabricated using a uniform coping design with a thickness of either 0.5, 0.8, 1.0, or 1.2 mm and a 20 μm die spacer.

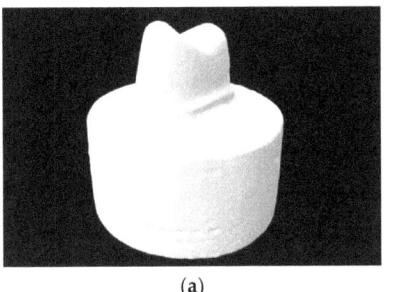
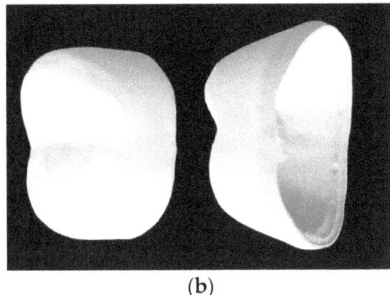

(a) (b)

Figure 1. (a) Standardized tooth preparation; (b) representative zirconia crown design.

The uniform crowns were milled from either a 5Y-Z disk (Katana UTML, Kuraray Noritake, Tokyo, Japan) for the 0.8, 1.0, and 1.2 mm groups or the 3Y-Z disk (Katana HT, Kuraray Noritake) for the 0.5 and 1.0 mm control groups (Table 1). Milling was performed using a 5-axis milling machine (DWX-52D, Roland DGA, Irvine, CA, USA) and computer-aided manufacturing software (Millbox 2020, CIM System, Padova, Italy). After the milling procedure, final sintering of zirconia was performed according to manufacturers' instructions.

Table 1. Materials used in this study.

Material	Manufacturer	Composition
Katana UTML	Kuraray Noritake	5Y-Z
Katana HT	Kuraray Noritake	3Y-Z
Rely X Luting Cement	3M	RMGIC
Panavia SA Cement Universal	Kuraray Noritake	Resin cement

Resin dies were fabricated using a dental 3D-printer (Pro S Dental 3D Printer, SprintRay Inc., Los Angeles, CA, USA) with a micro-filled hybrid composite resin (NextDent C&B MFH, NextDent B.V., Soesterberg, The Netherlands) with elastic modulus of 2.1 GPa [39]. After printing, the dies were cleaned in 91% alcohol and post-cured with a curing machine (SprintRay Procure 2, SprintRay Inc.).

Specimens were further divided into 3 subgroups to evaluate the cements and surface treatments utilized. The first subgroup of crowns (5Y-Z crowns only) was cemented on the resin dies using self-curing resin-modified glass ionomer cement (RMGIC; Rely X Luting Cement, 3M, St Paul, MN, USA) without surface treatment. The second subgroup of crowns (3Y-Z and 5Y-Z crowns) was air particle-abraded using 50 µm particles of Al_2O_3 (Cobra, Renfert, Hilzingen, Germany) at 0.2 MPa for 15 s, at a distance of 10 mm on intaglio surfaces at 30-degree incidence using a laboratory sandblaster (Basic Master, Renfert). Crowns were then cleaned ultrasonically in a distilled water bath for 10 min and dried using oil-free air, then cemented using the same RMGIC. The third subgroup of crowns (5Y-Z crowns only) was air particle-abraded and cleaned using the protocol above. Crowns were then bonded using a self-adhesive resin cement which contained the monomer 10-MDP (Panavia SA Cement Universal, Kuraray Noritake). For each group, a 10 N load was applied on the occlusal surface of all crowns, and the cement margin was tack-cured for 3–5 s per side. The excess cement was removed, and the crowns were allowed to self-cure for 7 (RMGIC) or 5 (resin cement) minutes. Specimens were stored in water at 37 °C for 7 days.

Specimens were inserted into a custom fixture in a universal testing machine (Instron 5583, Instron Inc., Canton, MA, USA) that allowed the long axis of the tooth to be positioned at a 30° angle to the indenter (Figure 2). A 3.5 mm diameter stainless steel indenter was centered in the occlusal groove of the crowns such that the crowns were loaded on their buccal cusp (Figure 2). A rubber sheet was inserted between the indenter and the crowns to account for any irregularities in the surface of the indenter. A load was applied at a crosshead speed of 0.5 mm/min until fracture. Fracture was defined as a 30% reduction in the applied load. After each test, specimens were examined to ensure that either a complete fracture or crack was present in the specimen. Fracture force was recorded as the highest load prior to fracture.

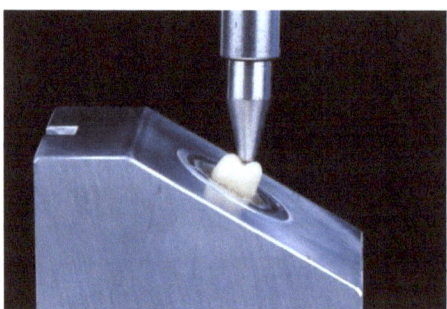

Figure 2. Loading of crowns at 30° off axis by 3.5 mm diameter steel indenter.

Normality of data was examined using histograms and confirmed with Shapiro–Wilk test. A one-way Analysis of Variance (ANOVA) test was employed to determine if statistical differences existed between 5Y-Z crown fracture values and the 0.5 mm 3Y-Z control using analytics software (SAS 9.4, SAS Institute, Nashville, TN, USA). A separate 1-way ANOVA was performed to determine if statistical differences existed between 5Y-Z crown fracture values and the 1 mm 3Y-Z control. Subsequent Dunnett post hoc tests were performed to determine which groups of the 5Y-Z crowns were statistically less than each control. A p value of less than 0.05 was considered significant.

3. Results

A post hoc power analysis was completed using an effect size = 0.4, a = 0.05, number of groups = 11, and sample size = 110. The G-power calculation determined a power of 80% [40]. The results of the crown fracture testing are presented in Table 2 and Figure 3. The one-way ANOVA tests determined significant differences between groups with both the 0.5 mm control (F = 33.177, $p < 0.001$) and 1.0 mm control (F = 33.250, $p < 0.001$). The Dunnett post hoc test determined that none of the 5Y-Z crown groups had a significantly lower fracture strength than the 0.5 mm 3Y-Z control. A second Dunnett post hoc test determined that all of the 5Y-Z crown groups had significantly lower fracture strength than the 1.0 mm 3Y-Z control other than the 1.2 mm 5Y-Z crowns bonded with resin cement.

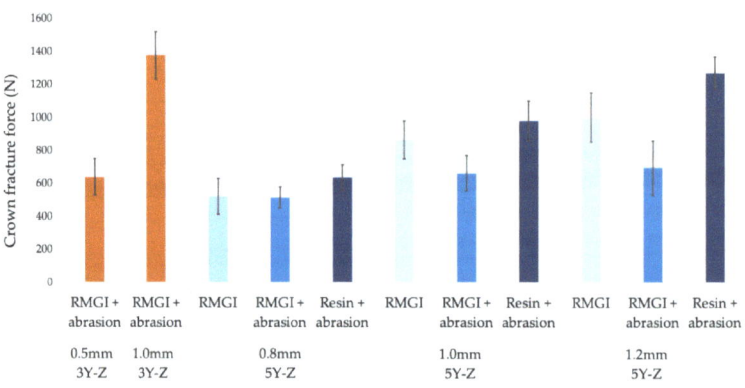

Figure 3. Crown fracture force (mean ± standard deviation).

Table 2. Crown fracture force (mean ± standard deviation).

Zirconia	Thickness (mm)	Particle Abrasion	Cement	Crown Fracture Force (N)
3Y-Z	0.5	Yes	RMGI	639.30 ± 111.77
	1.0	Yes	RMGI	1378.10 ± 143.22
5Y-Z	0.8	No	RMGI	522.67 ± 108.57 *
		Yes	RMGI	516.86 ± 63.32 *
		Yes	Resin	635.89 ± 78.00 *
	1.0	No	RMGI	865.30 ± 116.39 *
		Yes	RMGI	663.78 ± 106.80 *
		Yes	Resin	980.10 ± 123.50 *
	1.2	No	RMGI	1002.56 ± 149.58 *
		Yes	RMGI	696.30 ± 165.72 *
		Yes	Resin	1272.44 ± 97.78

* groups with a * were determined to be significantly lower than the 1.0 mm 3Y-Z control group. None of the groups were statistically lower than the 0.5 mm 3Y-Z control group.

Observation of failed specimens reveals that crowns fractured into two major pieces. The location of the fracture on the external aspect of the crowns was between the area of indenter contact and the occlusal groove of the crown. The crowns fractured either with or with die fracture (Figure 4a,b).

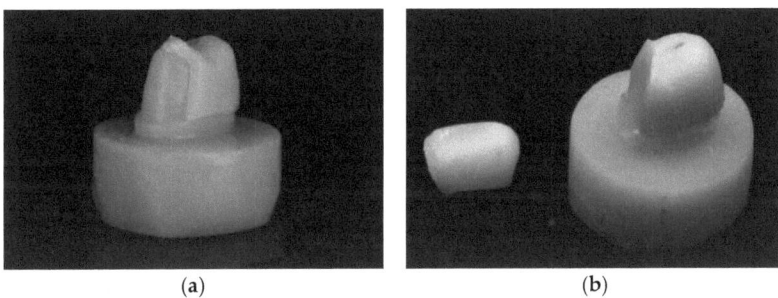

(a) (b)

Figure 4. (a) Fracture of die alone; (b) fracture of die and crown.

4. Discussion

The first aim of this study was to examine what thickness and cementation condition of 5Y-Z would produce a crown with similar fracture resistance to a 0.5 mm thick 3Y-Z cemented with RMGIC. This reference chosen as 0.5 mm is the manufacturer's recommended thickness for 3Y-Z, and most zirconia crowns are cemented with RMGIC [11,16]. All thicknesses of 5Y-Z tested (0.8, 1.0, and 1.2 mm) achieved a similar fracture force to this reference regardless of cement type or surface treatment.

The second aim of this study was to examine what thickness and cementation condition of 5Y-Z would produce a crown with similar fracture resistance to a 1.0 mm thick 3Y-Z cemented with RMGIC. This reference chosen as 1.0 mm thickness of 3Y-Z was reported to have a similar fracture resistance as metal ceramic crowns [10]. The results of the study demonstrated that all 5Y-Z crowns (0.8, 1.0, and 1.2 mm thickness) with all cementation conditions had significantly lower fracture resistance than 1.0 mm thick 3Y-Z crowns cemented with RMGIC aside from 1.2 mm 5Y-Z crowns bonded with resin cement.

Only one previous study also compared the strength of 3Y-Z and 5Y-Z crowns at different thicknesses. The study from Adabo et al. of particle-abraded crowns bonded to metallic dies reported that 1.5 mm 5Y-Z premolar crowns had a lower characteristic strength than 1.0 mm 3Y-Z crowns [12]. In the current study, 1.2 mm bonded premolar 5Y-Z crowns had a similar strength to 1.0 mm 3Y-Z cemented crowns. The difference in the results is because a resin cement was used for all groups in their study, whereas the 3Y-Z control groups were cemented with RMGIC in the current study.

In a study by Alraheam et al., 30% of 1.2 mm 5Y-Z discs failed in fatigue, whereas 0% of the 0.7 mm 3Y-Z discs failed in fatigue [12]. Another study by Machry et al. of bonded, particle-abraded discs reported that 1.0 mm discs of 5Y-Z bonded to epoxy resin had a lower fracture resistance than 0.7 mm discs of 3Y-Z bonded to epoxy dies [15]. These studies suggest that a 1.0 mm thickness of 5Y-Z is not as strong as 0.7 mm of 3Y-Z. As a result, a thickness greater than 1.0 mm was suggested for 5Y-Z. These results vary slightly from the current study in which 0.8 mm thick 5Y-Z was equivalent to 0.5 mm 3Y-Z controls. The current study differs from these previous studies as crowns were used rather than discs, RMGIC was used for 3Y-Z controls, and the 3Y-Z was used at its manufacturer's recommended minimum thickness of 0.5 mm.

A study from Longhini et al. reported a similar fracture resistance of 0.5 mm particle-abraded and resin-bonded discs of 5Y-Z and 3Y-Z [14]. Additionally, the 1.5 mm bonded 5Y-Z discs had a similar strength to the 1.0 mm 3Y-Z bonded discs. The conclusions of their study vary from the current study due to the use of resin cement for the 3Y-Z control group.

The manufacturer's recommended thickness for 5Y-Z is 1 mm, and no cementation type is specified [11]. Although the present study suggests that 5Y-Z can be used at 0.8 mm with RMGIC, it is prudent to follow the manufacturer's instructions of a 1 mm minimum thickness. In order to achieve a fracture resistance equivalent to a 1 mm 3Y-Z crown (and a 1.5 mm metal ceramic crown), 5Y-Z would need to be 1.2 mm and bonded with resin cement.

Air particle abrasion is recommended for the preparation of zirconia crowns in the instructions for use of both the resin and RMGI cements used in this study [29]. In a previous study, air particle abrasion did not significantly decrease the fracture resistance of 5Y-Z crowns cemented with RMGIC [18]. These results are in contrast with studies which report that air particle abrasion reduces the strength of 5Y-Z discs [22,25,26]. As air particle abrasion has not been shown to impact the bond strength with RMGIC, it is at the clinicians' and laboratories' discretion if 5Y-Z crowns are routinely air particle-abraded [27].

To substitute for tooth structure, this study used a 3D-printed resin die material similar to the frequently used epoxy resin in previous studies. The modulus and strength of printed resin dies (elastic modulus = 2.1 GPa, flexural strength = 97.1 MPa) are lower than dentin (elastic modulus = 19.64 GPa, flexural strength = 164.3 MPa), and their appropriateness as a die substitute could be questioned [38,40]. Pilot testing in our laboratory revealed that the fracture force of zirconia crowns on dentin dies was similar to the 3D-printed resin composite used in this study. The advantage of using 3D-printed dies rather than natural tooth dies is that the same geometry could be used for all specimens, whereas natural tooth specimens would vary in size and preparation design. A previous study revealed that zirconia crown fracture resistance testing was more discerning between groups with the use of resin dies rather than metal dies [15]. Another study comparing the fracture strength of zirconia crowns reported that crowns fractured on resin dies produced a similar strength to enamel dies, whereas metal dies produced a significantly higher strength [35].

The loading configuration used in the current study employs a rounded sphere loading a single cusp at 30° off the axis of the tooth (Figure 2). Likely load was transferred to the occlusal groove in some specimens as evidenced by the observation of the fracture surfaces of the crowns near the occlusal groove (Figure 4). A previous finite element analysis of crowns indented by a sphere reported that loading on steeper cusps transfers stress to the occlusal groove, whereas loading a flatter cusp concentrates stress below the indenter [38].

Several limitations could be observed in the present study. The results of this study are specific to the materials tested; differences in the composition of other brands of cement and ceramic materials may have significant effects on the results of the study. This study did not examine a group of 5Y-Z that was bonded with resin cement without air particle abrasion. That decision was made as the elimination of particle abrasion would significantly decrease the bond between 5Y-Z and resin cement and, therefore, eliminate the clinical advantage of the use of resin cement [22].

A blatant limitation of the current study is that crowns were tested in static load-to-failure testing rather than fatigue. High static loads applied by blunt spherical indenters produce Hertzian cone cracks located at the contact surface just outside the contact area. When lower stresses are applied cyclically, a single crack may be initiated on the cement surface which is driven towards the contact surface until fracture occurs. The latter form of fracture is more representative of clinical failures [33]. Fatigue studies may also incorporate a horizontal slide, which may transfer forces to the cement, leading to gaps [41]. Fatigue studies have limitations, including the technical challenge of discerning true failure when using a crown geometry and the large number of specimens and time required to generate an S-N curve. A future study might validate the relevant groups from the current study using fatigue cycling.

5. Conclusions

Based on the findings of this in vitro study and for the materials included in this study, the following conclusions were drawn:

- 5Y-Z crowns as thin as 0.8 mm (regardless of the cement or surface treatment) have a similar fracture resistance to 0.5 mm thick 3Y-Z cemented with RMGIC. Despite this finding, manufacturers' recommendations should be followed regarding the minimum restoration thickness.
- 5Y-Z crowns with 1.2 mm thickness that are bonded with resin cement have a similar fracture resistance to 1.0 mm thick 3Y-Z cemented with RMGIC.

Author Contributions: Conceptualization, N.C.L., C.-C.F. and D.A.G.; methodology, N.C.L.; formal analysis, N.C.L.; investigation, E.E. and A.S.A.; resources, D.A.G.; data curation, E.E. and A.S.A.; writing—original draft preparation, E.E., P.-H.C. and N.C.L.; writing—review and editing, D.A.G. and C.-C.F.; supervision, P.-H.C. and N.C.L.; project administration, D.A.G. and C.-C.F. All authors have read and agreed to the published version of the manuscript.

Funding: This research received no external funding.

Institutional Review Board Statement: Not applicable.

Informed Consent Statement: Not applicable.

Data Availability Statement: All source data may be obtained from the corresponding author.

Acknowledgments: The SprintRay Pro95 printer used in this study was donated by SprintRay. All zirconia was donated by Kuraray Noritake.

Conflicts of Interest: Lawson has received both a speaking honorarium and research grants from Kuraray Noritake and 3M.

References

1. Etman, M.K.; Woolford, M.; Dunne, S. Quantitative measurement of tooth and ceramic wear: In vivo study. *Int. J. Prosthodont.* **2008**, *21*, 245–252. [PubMed]
2. Kon, M.; Ishikawa, K.; Kuwayam, N. Effects of zirconia addition on fracture toughness and bending strength of dental porcelains. *Dent. Mater. J.* **1990**, *9*, 181–192. [CrossRef]
3. Kontonasaki, E.; Rigos, A.E.; Ilia, C.; Istantsos, T. Monolithic zirconia: An update to current knowledge. optical properties, wear, and clinical performance. *Dent. J.* **2019**, *7*, 90. [CrossRef]
4. da Silva, A.O.; Fiorin, L.; Faria, A.C.L.; Ribeiro, R.F.; Rodrigues, R.C.S. Translucency and mechanical behavior of partially stabilized monolithic zirconia after staining, finishing procedures and artificial aging. *Sci. Rep.* **2022**, *12*, 16094. [CrossRef] [PubMed]
5. Zhang, F.; Inokoshi, M.; Batuk, M.; Hadermann, J.; Naert, I.; Van Meerbeek, B.; Vleugels, J. Strength, toughness and aging stability of highly-translucent Y-TZP ceramics for dental restorations. *Dent. Mater.* **2016**, *32*, e327–e337. [CrossRef]
6. Zhang, Y.; Lawn, B.R. Novel zirconia materials in dentistry. *J. Dent. Res.* **2018**, *97*, 140–147. [CrossRef]
7. Qiu, H.Q.; Zhang, Y.Q.; Huang, W.W.; Chen, J.; Gao, L.; Omran, M.; Li, N.; Chen, G. Sintering properties of tetragonal zirconia nanopowder preparation of the NaCl+KCl binary system by the sol-gel-flux method. *ACS Sustain. Chem. Eng.* **2023**, *11*, 1067–1077. [CrossRef]

8. Arellano Moncayo, A.M.; Peñate, L.; Arregui, M.; Giner-Tarrida, L.; Cedeño, R. State of the art of different zirconia materials and their indications according to evidence-based clinical performance: A narrative review. *Dent. J.* **2023**, *11*, 18. [CrossRef]
9. Kim, H.K.; Yoo, K.W.; Kim, S.J.; Jung, C.H. Phase transformations and subsurface changes in three dental zirconia grades after sandblasting with various Al_2O_3 particle sizes. *Materials* **2021**, *14*, 5321. [CrossRef]
10. Katana Zirconia Technical Guideline. Available online: https://kuraraydental.com/wp-content/uploads/sds/Guides/katana_zirconia_utml_stml_tg.pdf (accessed on 3 January 2024).
11. Sun, T.; Zhou, S.; Lai, R.; Liu, R.; Ma, S.; Zhou, Z.; Longquan, S. Load-bearing capacity and the recommended thickness of dental monolithic zirconia single crowns. *J. Mech. Behav. Biomed. Mater.* **2014**, *35*, 93–101. [CrossRef]
12. Adabo, G.L.; Longhini, D.; Baldochi, M.R.; Bergamo, E.T.P.; Bonfante, E.A. Reliability and lifetime of lithium disilicate, 3Y-TZP, and 5Y-TZP zirconia crowns with different occlusal thicknesses. *Clin. Oral Investig.* **2023**, *27*, 3827–3838. [CrossRef]
13. Alraheam, I.A.; Donovan, T.; Boushell, L.; Cook, R.; Ritter, A.V.; Sulaiman, T.A. Fracture load of two thicknesses of different zirconia types after fatiguing and thermocycling. *J. Prosthet. Dent.* **2020**, *123*, 635–640. [CrossRef] [PubMed]
14. Longhini, D.; Rocha, C.; de Oliveira, L.T.; Olenscki, N.G.; Bonfante, E.A.; Adabo, G.L. Mechanical behavior of ceramic monolithic systems with different thicknesses. *Oper. Dent.* **2019**, *44*, E244–E253. [CrossRef] [PubMed]
15. Machry, R.V.; Cadore-Rodrigues, A.C.; Borges, A.L.S.; Pereira, G.K.R.; Kleverlaan, C.J.; Venturini, A.B.; Valandro, L.F. Fatigue resistance of simplified CAD-CAM restorations: Foundation material and ceramic thickness effects on the fatigue behavior of partially- and fully-stabilized zirconia. *Dent. Mater.* **2021**, *37*, 568–577. [CrossRef] [PubMed]
16. Campos, F.; Valandro, L.F.; Feitosa, S.A.; Kleverlaan, C.J.; Feilzer, A.J.; de Jager, N.; Bottino, M.A. Adhesive cementation promotes higher fatigue resistance to zirconia crowns. *Oper. Dent.* **2017**, *42*, 215–224. [CrossRef]
17. Indergård, J.A.; Skjold, A.; Schriwer, C.; Øilo, M. Effect of cementation techniques on fracture load of monolithic zirconia crowns. *Biomater. Investig. Dent.* **2021**, *8*, 160–169. [CrossRef]
18. Lawson, N.C.; Jurado, C.A.; Huang, C.T.; Morris, G.P.; Burgess, J.O.; Liu, P.R.; Kinderknecht, K.E.; Lin, C.P.; Givan, D.A. Effect of surface treatment and cement on fracture load of traditional zirconia (3Y), translucent zirconia (5Y), and lithium disilicate crowns. *J. Prosthodont.* **2019**, *28*, 659–665. [CrossRef]
19. Lawson, N.C.; Litaker, M.S.; Ferracane, J.L.; Gordan, V.V.; Atlas, A.M.; Rios, T.; Gilbert, G.H.; McCracken, M.S.; National Dental Practice-Based Research Network Collaborative Group. Choice of cement for single-unit crowns: Findings from The National Dental Practice-Based Research Network. *J. Am. Dent. Assoc.* **2019**, *150*, 522–530. [CrossRef]
20. Inokoshi, M.; De Munck, J.; Minakuchi, S.; Van Meerbeek, B. Meta-analysis of bonding effectiveness to zirconia ceramics. *J. Dent. Res.* **2014**, *93*, 329–334. [CrossRef]
21. Alammar, A.; Blatz, M.B. The resin bond to high-translucent zirconia-A systematic review. *J. Esthet. Restor. Dent.* **2022**, *34*, 117–135. [CrossRef]
22. Darkoue, Y.A.; Burgess, J.O.; Lawson, N.; McLaren, E.; Lemons, J.E.; Morris, G.P.; Givan, D.A.; Fu, C.C. Effects of particle abrasion media and pressure on flexural strength and bond strength of zirconia. *Oper. Dent.* **2023**, *48*, 59–67. [CrossRef] [PubMed]
23. Kulunk, S.; Kulunk, T.; Ural, C.; Kurt, M.; Baba, S. Effect of air abrasion particles on the bond strength of adhesive resin cement to zirconia core. *Acta Odontol. Scand.* **2011**, *69*, 88–94. [CrossRef]
24. Yoshida, K. Influence of alumina air-abrasion for highly translucent partially stabilized zirconia on flexural strength, surface properties, and bond strength of resin cement. *J. Appl. Oral Sci.* **2020**, *28*, e20190371. [CrossRef]
25. Hergeröder, C.; Wille, S.; Kern, M. Comparison of testing designs for flexural strength of 3Y-TZP and 5Y-PSZ Considering different surface treatment. *Materials* **2022**, *15*, 3915. [CrossRef]
26. AlMutairi, R.; AlNahedh, H.; Maawadh, A.; Elhejazi, A. Effects of different air particle abrasion protocols on the biaxial flexural strength and fractography of high/ultra-translucent zirconia. *Materials* **2021**, *15*, 244. [CrossRef]
27. Blatz, M.B.; Chiche, G.; Holst, S.; Sadan, A. Influence of surface treatment and simulated aging on bond strengths of luting agents to zirconia. *Quintessence Int.* **2007**, *38*, 745–753. [PubMed]
28. Lawson, N.C.; Khajotia, S.; Bedran-Russo, A.K.; Frazier, K.; Park, J.; Leme-Kraus, A.; Urquhart, O.; Council on Scientific Affairs. Bonding crowns and bridges with resin cement: An American Dental Association Clinical Evaluators Panel survey. *J. Am. Dent. Assoc.* **2020**, *151*, 796–797.e2. [CrossRef] [PubMed]
29. 3M RelyX Simple Steps Cement Guide for Labs. Available online: https://multimedia.3m.com/mws/media/1304258O/3m-relyx-simple-steps-cement-guide-for-labs.pdf (accessed on 3 January 2024).
30. ISO 6872:2015; Dentistry—Ceramic Materials. International Organization for Standardization. European Committee for Standardizatio: Geneva, Switzerland, 2015.
31. Xu, Y.; Han, J.; Lin, H.; An, L. Comparative study of flexural strength test methods on CAD/CAM Y-TZP dental ceramics. *Regen. Biomater.* **2015**, *2*, 239–244. [CrossRef]
32. Schriwer, C.; Skjold, A.; Gjerdet, N.R.; Øilo, M. Monolithic zirconia dental crowns. Internal fit, margin quality, fracture mode and load at fracture. *Dent. Mater.* **2017**, *33*, 1012–1020. [CrossRef]
33. Kelly, J.R. Clinically relevant approach to failure testing of all-ceramic restorations. *J. Prosthet. Dent.* **1999**, *81*, 652–661. [CrossRef]
34. Spintzyk, S.; Geis-Gerstorfer, J.; Bourauel, C.; Keilig, L.; Lohbauer, U.; Brune, A.; Greuling, A.; Arnold, C.; Rues, S.; Adjiski, R.; et al. Biaxial flexural strength of zirconia: A round robin test with 12 laboratories. *Dent. Mater.* **2021**, *37*, 284–295. [CrossRef]
35. Yucel, M.T.; Yondem, I.; Aykent, F.; Eraslan, O. Influence of the supporting die structures on the fracture strength of all-ceramic materials. *Clin. Oral Investig.* **2012**, *16*, 1105–1110. [CrossRef] [PubMed]

36. Rohr, N.; Märtin, S.; Fischer, J. Correlations between fracture load of zirconia implant supported single crowns and mechanical properties of restorative material and cement. *Dent. Mater. J.* **2018**, *37*, 222–228. [CrossRef]
37. Chen, Y.; Maghami, E.; Bai, X.; Huang, C.; Pow, E.H.N.; Tsoi, J.K.H. Which dentine analogue material can replace human dentine for crown fatigue test? *Dent. Mater.* **2023**, *39*, 86–100. [CrossRef] [PubMed]
38. Okada, R.; Asakura, M.; Ando, A.; Kumano, H.; Ban, S.; Kawai, T.; Takebe, J. Fracture strength testing of crowns made of CAD/CAM composite resins. *J. Prosthodont. Res.* **2018**, *62*, 287–292. [CrossRef] [PubMed]
39. Bora, P.V.; Sayed Ahmed, A.; Alford, A.; Pitttman, K.; Thomas, V.; Lawson, N.C. Characterization of materials used for 3D printing dental crowns and hybrid prostheses. *J. Esthet. Restor. Dent.* 2023, *in press*. [CrossRef]
40. Faul, F.; Erdfelder, E.; Buchner, A.; Lang, A.G. Statistical power analyses using G*Power 3.1: Tests for correlation and regression analyses. *Behav. Res. Methods* **2009**, *41*, 1149–1160. [CrossRef]
41. Comba, A.; Baldi, A.; Carossa, M.; Michelotto Tempesta, R.; Garino, E.; Llubani, X.; Rozzi, D.; Mikonis, J.; Paolone, G.; Scotti, N. Post-fatigue fracture resistance of lithium disilicate and polymer-infiltrated ceramic network indirect restorations over endodontically-treated molars with different preparation designs: An in-vitro study. *Polymers* **2022**, *14*, 5084. [CrossRef]

Disclaimer/Publisher's Note: The statements, opinions and data contained in all publications are solely those of the individual author(s) and contributor(s) and not of MDPI and/or the editor(s). MDPI and/or the editor(s) disclaim responsibility for any injury to people or property resulting from any ideas, methods, instructions or products referred to in the content.

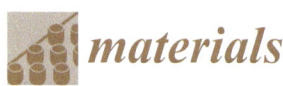

Article

The Shear Bond Strength of Resin-Based Luting Cement to Zirconia Ceramics after Different Surface Treatments

Grzegorz Sokolowski [1], Agata Szczesio-Wlodarczyk [2,*], Małgorzata Iwona Szynkowska-Jóźwik [3], Wioleta Stopa [2], Jerzy Sokolowski [4], Karolina Kopacz [5,6] and Kinga Bociong [4,*]

[1] Department of Prosthodontics, Medical University of Lodz, 251 Pomorska St., 92-213 Lodz, Poland
[2] University Laboratory of Materials Research, Medical University of Lodz, Pomorska 251, 92-213 Lodz, Poland
[3] Faculty of Chemistry, Institute of General and Ecological Chemistry, Lodz University of Technology, Zeromskiego 116, 90-543 Lodz, Poland
[4] Department of General Dentistry, Medical University of Lodz, Pomorska 251, 92-213 Lodz, Poland
[5] "DynamoLab" Academic Laboratory of Movement and Human Physical Performance, Medical University of Lodz, ul. Pomorska 251, 92-216 Lodz, Poland
[6] Warsaw Medical Academy, Ludwika Rydygiera 8, 01-793 Warszawa, Poland
* Correspondence: agata.szczesio@umed.lodz.pl (A.S.-W.); kinga.bociong@umed.lodz.pl (K.B.)

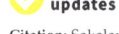

Citation: Sokolowski, G.; Szczesio-Wlodarczyk, A.; Szynkowska-Jóźwik, M.I.; Stopa, W.; Sokolowski, J.; Kopacz, K.; Bociong, K. The Shear Bond Strength of Resin-Based Luting Cement to Zirconia Ceramics after Different Surface Treatments. Materials 2023, 16, 5433. https://doi.org/10.3390/ma16155433

Academic Editors: Lavinia Cosmina Ardelean and Laura-Cristina Rusu

Received: 24 May 2023
Revised: 28 June 2023
Accepted: 30 June 2023
Published: 2 August 2023

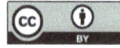

Copyright: © 2023 by the authors. Licensee MDPI, Basel, Switzerland. This article is an open access article distributed under the terms and conditions of the Creative Commons Attribution (CC BY) license (https://creativecommons.org/licenses/by/4.0/).

Abstract: Due to its unique properties, zirconia is increasingly being used in dentistry, but surface preparation for bonding is difficult because of its polycrystalline structure. This study aimed to determine the effect of a new etching technique (Zircos-E) on Ceramill Zi (Amann Girrbach). The effect of etching and the use of primers (Monobond Plus and MKZ Primer) on the bond strength of zirconia with resin cement (NX3) was assessed. Shear bond strength was evaluated after storage in water for 24 h and after thermal aging (5000 thermocycling at 5 °C/55 °C). A scanning electron microscope (Hitachi S-4700) was used to evaluate the surface structure before and after the Zircos-E system. The roughness parameters were assessed using an SJ-410 profilometer. The etched zirconia surface is more homogeneous over the entire surface, but some localized forms of erosion exist. The etching of zirconia ceramics caused changes in the surface structure of zirconia and a significant increase in the shear bond strength between zirconia and resin cement. The use of primers positively affects the adhesion between resin cement and zirconia. Aging with thermocycler significantly reduced the shear bond strength, with one exception—sandblasted samples with MKZ Primer. Standard ceramic surface preparation, involving only alumina sandblasting, does not provide a satisfactory bond. The use of etching with the Zircos-E system and primers had a positive effect on the strength of the zirconium–resin cement connection.

Keywords: zirconia; surface; treatment; Zircos-E; etching; primers; resin; cements; SBS; bond; adhesion

1. Introduction

The most popular ceramics used in dental practice are lithium disilicate, silica, alumina, leucite, and zirconia-based materials. However, zirconia is favored both in research and in the clinic. The number of research publications related to this type of ceramic nearly tripled in the years 2012–2019 compared to 2007–2011 [1]. This may be related to its remarkable mechanical strength and aesthetic properties. Some oxides, such as CaO, MgO, Y_2O_3, and CeO_2, are added to stabilize the high-temperature zirconia phase (tetragonal) at normal temperatures. Yttrium-stabilized zirconia (Y-TZP) is most often used in dentistry due to its combination of high strength and optimum optical properties [2]. Sintered Y-TZP has been shown to have superior flexural strength (900–1200 MPa), fracture resistance (>2000 N), and fracture toughness (9–10 MPa·$m^{0.5}$) in comparison with other conventional ceramics, including alumina-reinforced and lithium-disilicate-based ceramics [3,4]. Because of its high biocompatibility, corrosion resistance, and light weight, zirconia is a material that is frequently used in biomedical applications [5]. In addition, prosthetic restorations can be made using zirconia with the assistance of computer-aided design (CAD) and computer-aided manufacturing (CAM) systems in order to obtain a final product that is perfectly integrated into the physiognomy of each patient [6].

Success in prosthetic treatment is not only related to selecting the appropriate material for the reconstruction, but requires the creation of appropriate adhesion. Unfortunately, due to the crystalline structure of zirconia and the lack of a silicon dioxide (silica) phase, conventional methods of preparing dental ceramics (including etching with acidic solutions and applying silane coupling agents) do not result in sufficient bond strength in restorations [3]. Different treatments of the zirconia surface have been studied in recent years. One of the basic methods used in prosthetics is sandblasting. In this method, the sandblaster emits alumina particles (which are most often used) under a certain pressure. The energy of the ejected particles erodes the ceramic surface, increasing its roughness and wettability [7]. Of note is the fact that the air abrasion of zirconia can also lead to surface deformation, i.e., plastic deformation and/or melting of the surface, micro-cracks, gaps, driving of the abrasive grain into the surface, etc. [8]. In order to avoid damage to the zirconia surface, the sandblasting protocol with a small particle size (30 μm) at moderate pressure (2.5 bar) is recommended [9,10]. Some reports show that high-pressure (0.4 MPa) air abrasion may have a negative impact on the biaxial flexural strength of Y-TZP [11]. In addition, the presence of a monoclinic phase was reported in zirconia materials after sandblasting and etching. The content was up to 5% [12–14]. However, a meta-analysis carried out by Aurélio I. L at al. [15] indicated that the flexural strength of Y-TZP is improved by airborne-particle abrasion, regardless of the particle size, the parameters of blasting (pressure and time), and the presence of aging.

Nevertheless, the surface of zirconia should be prepared before bonding with any cement in order to promote micromechanical interlocking mechanisms. The durability and stability of the bonds between ceramics and adhesives can be improved because the physical bonds are not susceptible to the degradation caused by environmental factors, such as humidity [8]. Some authors have studied the possibility of applying zirconia surface primers (e.g., 10-methacryloyloxydecyl dihydrogen phosphate (MDP)) or silanes to promote better adhesion. Studies have shown that some primers achieved a high and durable bond strength. It is most likely that only primers containing monomers with phosphate ester groups can bond directly to metal oxides [16,17]. Considering the internal structure of yttrium-stabilized zirconia, its surface cannot be activated with traditional etching methods, for example, 9.5% hydrofluoric acid for 60 s. Various acid treatments have been proposed for zirconia. Most of the proposed acid treatments assume the use of a high concentration of acid (>30%) and prolonged action (with a minimum of several minutes) and, very often, the treatments are conducted at an elevated temperature [12,18–20]. The Zircos-E system (M & C Dental, Seoul, Republic of Korea) is a commercially available product that is dedicated to zirconia etching. It contains hydrofluoric acid (HF), hydrochloric acid (HCl), sulfuric acid (H_2SO_4), nitric acid (HNO_3), and phosphoric acid (H_3PO_4). This patented technology uses ionization to create a microporous surface, which may improve bonding strength [21]. In the literature, only limited studies use this method for zirconia surface conditioning compared with abrasion and primer treatment [22].

The first null hypothesis was that etching with the Zircos-E system or using primers (MKZ Primer or Monobond Plus) does not affect bond strength. The second was that the surface topography of Ceramill Zi (Amann Girrbach AG, Koblach, Austria) is not affected by etching with the Zircos-E system (M & C Dental, Seoul, Republic of Korea).

2. Materials and Methods

The monolithic zirconia CAD-CAM blocks (Ceramil Zi, Amann Girrbach AG, Koblach, Austria) were sectioned using a milling device (Ceramill Motion 1, Amann Girrbach AG, Koblach, Austria). Subsequently, the specimens were sintered according to the manufacturer's instructions. The samples were cylinder-shaped with a diameter of 10 mm and a height of 10 mm. The surface was ground under water coolant with 180 grit, followed by

320 and 600 grit silicon carbide paper, to unify sample surfaces. Prepared specimens were sandblasted with 50 μm Al_2O_3 particles under a pressure of 2 bar. After that, the specimens were washed under running water for 30 s and then air-dried. Half of the specimens were etched for 30 min at 30 °C using Zircos-E Etching Solution (M & C Dental, Seoul, Republic of Korea). Zircos-E Etching Solution contains hydrofluoric acid (HF), hydrochloric acid (HCl), sulfuric acid (H_2SO_4), nitric acid (HNO_3) and phosphoric acid (H_3PO_4). After the etching process, the samples were cleaned with running water for 3 min and then with steam.

According to the conducted surface preparation, the specimens were divided into 6 groups (n = 22), as follows:

- Control: No chemical treatment was conducted.
- Primer MKZ: MKZ Primer (Bredent, Senden, Germany) was applied according to the manufacturer's instructions.
- Primer Monobond Plus: Monobond Plus (Ivoclar Vivadent, Schaan, Lichtenstein) was applied according to the manufacturer's instructions.
- Etched: No additional treatment after etching was conducted.
- Etched + Primer MKZ: After etching, MKZ Primer was applied according to the manufacturer's instructions.
- Etched + Primer Monobond Plus: After etching, Monobond Plus was applied according to the manufacturer's instructions.

OptiBond Solo Plus (bonding agent) was applied according to the manufacturer's instructions on prepared samples. Next, composite cement (NX3, Kerr, Brea, CA, USA) was packed into a plastic mold with a diameter of 3 mm and a height of 3 mm and light-cured for 20 s using a light-curing unit (1200 mW/cm^2, the CURE—TC-01, Spring Health Products, Norristown, PA, USA).

Eleven samples of each group were stored at 37 °C in distilled water. After 24 h storage, the samples were shear-loaded (Figure A1, Appendix A) to fracture at 2 mm/min crosshead speed using a universal testing machine of 5 kN maximum load cell capacity (Zwick-Roell Z005, Zwick-Roell, Ulm, Germany), with a distance between the crosshead and substrate of smaller than 1 mm.

Another 11 samples of each group were subjected to thermocycling between 5 °C and 55 °C for 5000 cycles, with a 20 s dwell time (THE 1200, SD Mechatronic, Feldkirchen-Westerham, Germany). After that, the shear bond strength was evaluated.

The roughness of the control and etched samples was investigated using a compact surface roughness tester SJ-410 (Mitutoyo, Kawasaki, Japan). Surface roughness for each study group was measured five times in different directions, from which the mean values were calculated. The evaluation length was 4 mm. Six roughness profile parameters were compared: roughness average (Ra), the average maximum height of the profile (Rz), maximum profile peak height (Rp), maximum profile valley depth (Rv), mean spacing of profile irregularities (Sm), retention volume (Vo).

Control and etched materials' surface topography was investigated with a scanning electron microscope energy-dispersive spectroscopy (SEM–EDS) microscope Hitachi S-4700 (Tokyo, Japan). The images were made at a magnification of 1000×, 5000× and 15,000×.

Shear bond strength data were analyzed by the Shapiro–Wilk test to assess the normality of the distributions. Based on the results, the Kruskal–Wallis test with multiple comparisons of mean ranks was applied. Data obtained from roughness measurements were subjected to Student's t-test to compare parameters (Ra, Rz, Rp, Rv, Sm, Vo) of control and etched samples. All analyses were performed using Statistica version 13 software (StatSoft, Kraków, Poland). The value α = 0.05 was adopted as significant.

3. Results

The results of shear bond strength after 24 h in water and thermocycling are presented in Figure 1. All failures were determined to be adhesive based on visual observations.

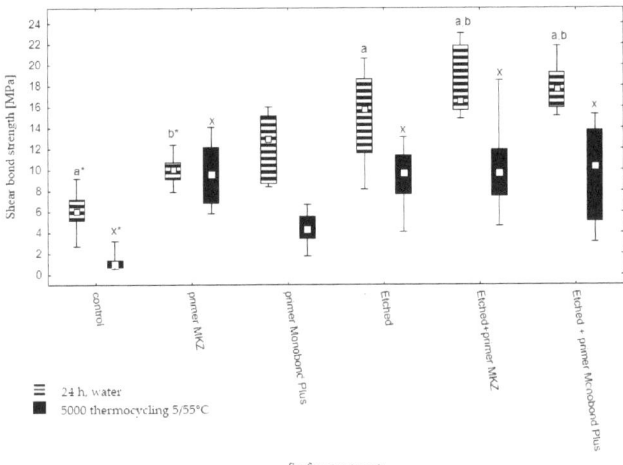

Figure 1. Box and whisker plot of shear bond strength (median values with minimum and maximum value) of resin-based luting cement to zirconia ceramics after different surface treatments. Shear bond strength was evaluated after storage in water for 24 h and after thermal aging (5000 thermocycling at 5 °C and 55 °C). a Significant difference at the level of $p \leq 0.05$ were found between results assigned with the letter with asterisk and the same letter.

The highest median value of shear bond strength evaluated after 24 h in water was 17.7 MPa (etched+ Primer Monobond Plus), and the lowest was 6.1 MPa (control) (Figure 1). The use of thermal aging (5000 thermocycles at 5 °C and 55 °C) resulted in a significant decrease in the bond strength for almost all tested groups. Based on the Kruskal–Wallis's test, a statistically significant difference was found with p-value ≤ 0.0000.

According to multiple comparisons of mean ranks for 24 h, water series, statistically significant differences were found between:

- Control vs. Etched ($p = 0.000434$);
- Control vs. Etched + primer MKZ ($p = 0.000001$);
- Control vs. Etched + primer Monobond Plus ($p = 0.000001$);
- Primer MKZ vs. (b) Etched + primer MKZ ($p = 0.003873$);
- Primer MKZ vs. Etched + primer Monobond Plus ($p = 0.004601$).

According to multiple comparisons of mean ranks for 5000 thermocycling, 5/55 °C series, statistically significant differences were found between:

- Control vs. (x) primer MKZ ($p = 0.000114$);
- Control vs. Etched ($p = 0.000069$);
- Control vs. Etched + primer MKZ ($p = 0.000059$);
- Control vs. Etched + primer Monobond Plus ($p = 0.00075$).

Results of roughness measurements are presented in Figure 2a–d.

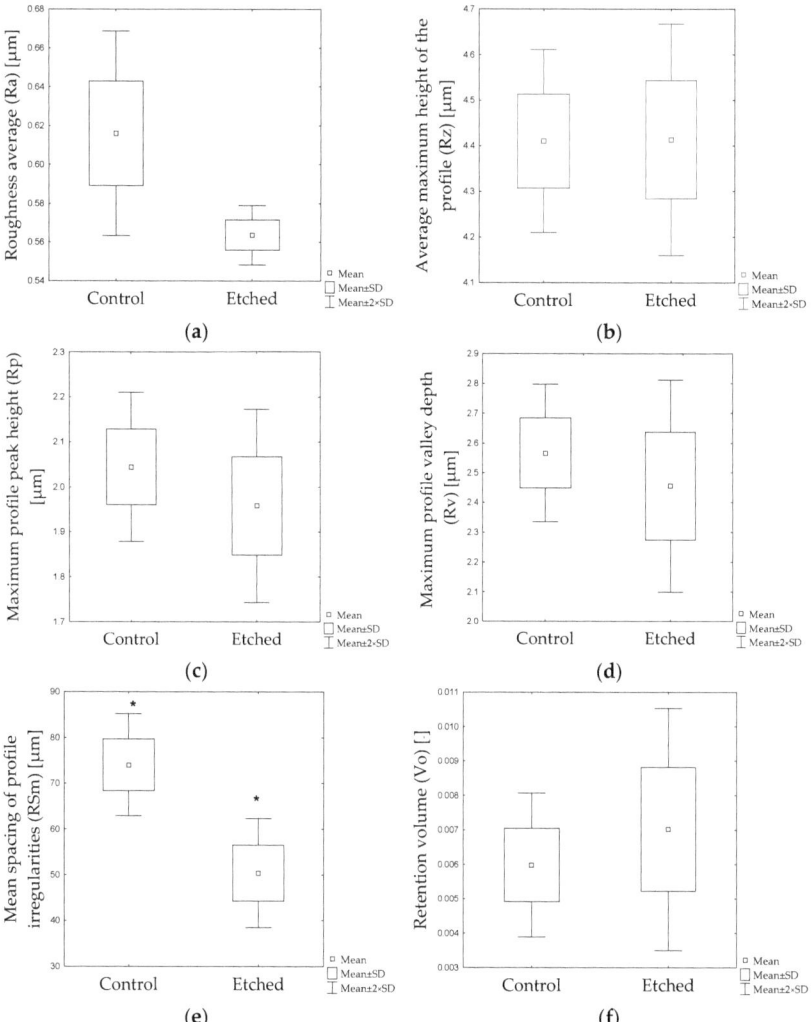

Figure 2. Roughness parameters of control and etched Ceramill Zi. (**a**) roughness average (Ra), (**b**) the average maximum height of the profile (Rz), (**c**) maximum profile peak height (Rp), (**d**) maximum profile valley depth (Rv), (**e**) mean spacing of profile irregularities (RSm), (**f**) retention volume (Vo). The results assigned with the asterisk show significant difference at the level of $p \leq 0.05$.

According to Student's *t*-test, statistically significant differences were found in the mean spacing of the profile irregularities (RSm); parameter ($p < 0.05$).

The surface topography of control and etched samples at a magnification of 1000×, 5000×, and 15,000× is presented in Figure 3a–f. A chemical composition analysis of the tested materials is given in Figure 4A,B.

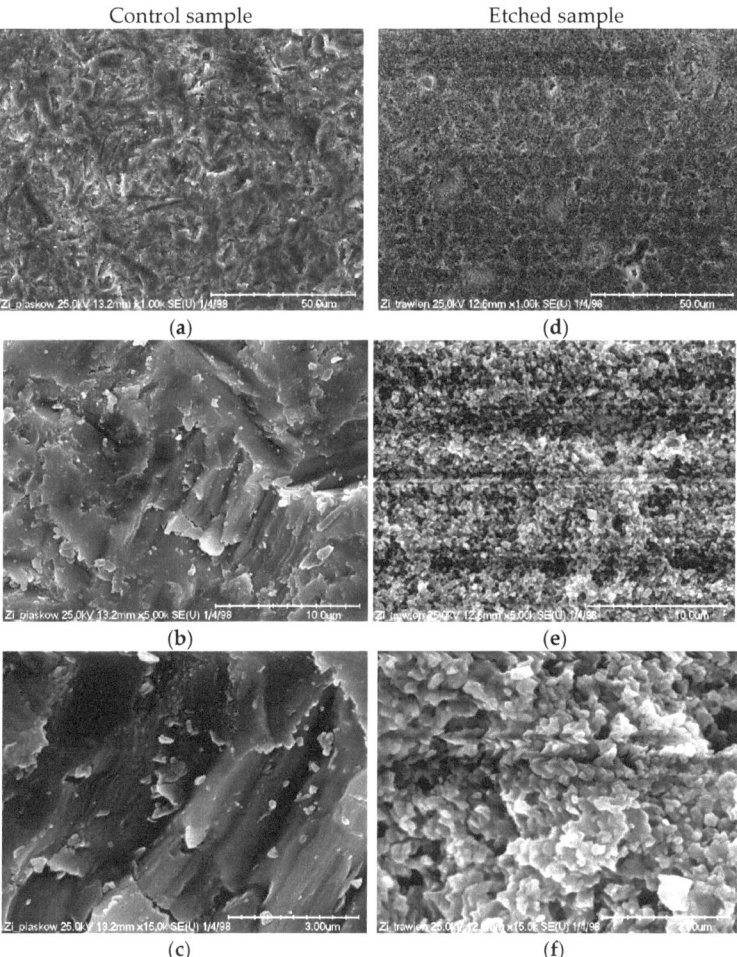

Figure 3. Scanning electron microscopy (SEM) micrographs of control ((**a–c**)—sandblasted, 50 μm Al_2O_3, 2 bar) and etched ((**d–f**)—sandblasted, 50 μm Al_2O_3, 2 bar and etched 30 min. at 30 °C using Zircos-E Etching Solution) Ceramill Zi at 1000× ((**a,d**), scale bar—50 μm), 5000× ((**b,e**), scale bar—10 μm) and 15,000× ((**c,f**), scale bar—3 μm) magnification. The figures demonstrate increased brightness.

The images obtained with the SEM evaluation show clear differences between the surface topography of the two materials. Both samples show an isotropic structure; however, the etched sample is more homogeneous, with regularly and evenly distributed crystal grains. Ceramill Zi is composed of zirconium oxide and the signals corresponding to zirconium (Zr) and oxygen (O) are mainly visible in the analyzed spectra (Figure 4A,B). The spectrum of the control sample shows a clear signal from aluminum (Al); the amount of this element in the sample subjected to etching is decreased.

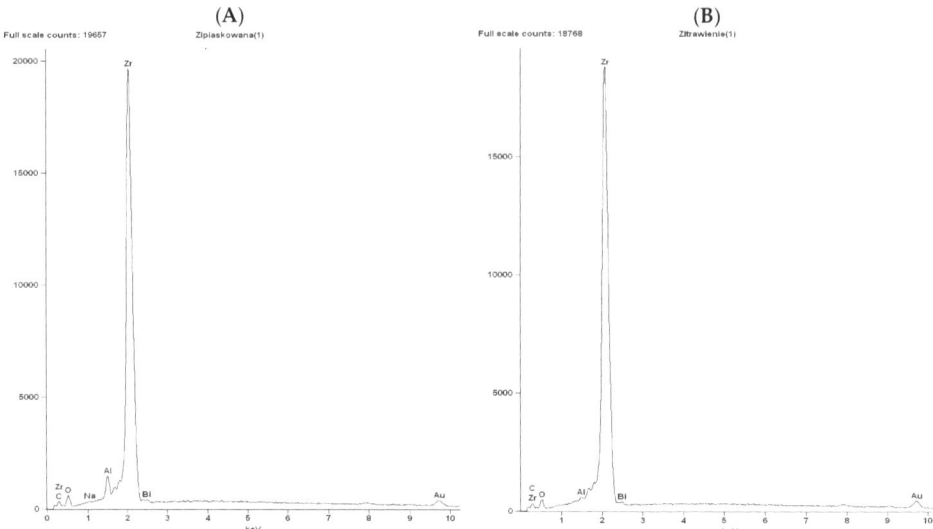

Figure 4. Chemical composition analysis of Ceramill Zi (**A**) control (sandblasted, 50 μm Al_2O_3, 2 bar), (**B**) etched (sandblasted, 50 μm Al_2O_3, 2 bar and etched 30 min. at 30 °C using Zircos-E Etching Solution). Data were obtained by energy-dispersive spectroscopy (EDS).

4. Discussion

Manufacturing a zirconia prosthetic restoration poses a challenge, as it requires the creation of an appropriate connection with resin cement. Traditional etching methods are ineffective because the material is polycrystalline and has no silica phase compared to conventional ceramic materials. Our findings, based on analyses of shear bond strength, suggest that the etching (Zircos-E system) and presence of primers (MKZ Primer or Monobond Plus) influence the adhesion of resin cement (NX3). SEM micrographs showed differences in the structure after etching. Therefore, the null hypothesis can be rejected.

All samples were first sandblasted (control sample). This treatment caused isotropic roughening and irregularities formed on the surface (Figure 3). The structure after the etching process is also irregular and resembles erosion. However, the structure after etching is more homogeneous over the entire surface. There seem to be some localized forms of erosion on the etched sample—pitting. Comparable structure observations were made by A. Sales et al. [21], who also used the Zircos-E system for their research. Similar differences between sandblasted samples and those additionally etched with a strong acid solutions were also observed in other studies [12,23,24]. Proper surface treatments may promote the micromechanical interlocking of resin cement by creating fitting roughness and increasing surface energy [11,25–27]. Profilometers are commonly used to characterize roughness. They enable the determination of certain parameters of the evaluated surface. The roughness average parameter, Ra, due to its relative repeatability and stability, is most frequently used. However, more roughness parameters should be determined to characterize material structure because Ra does not fully characterize the surface of the material [28,29]. In the present study, six parameters were analysed (Figure 2). Some changes in roughness parameters were observed. Ra for the sandblasted surface (control sample) was 0.6160 ± 0.0601 μm, whereas the value for the sandblasted and etched surface was 0.5636 ± 0.0174 μm; however, this difference was statistically insignificant. The peaks and valleys characteristics of both samples were comparable (Figure 2b–d). A significant difference was observed for the mean spacing of profile irregularities between the control (74.04 ± 12.74 μm) and etched (50.42 ± 13.62 μm) sample (Figure 2e). Smaller distances between irregularities on the surface can cause zirconia micro-retentions, resulting in increased bond strength. There are only a few studies evaluating the surface roughness after sandblasting and etching. Some reports show that the value of Ra is lower than or close to that of sandblasted samples in materials subjected to etching [30]. In contrast, in some reports, Ra values after etching are higher [20]. Compared to the untreated (polished) sample, etching causes surface roughening [19,24,31–33]. It should be noted that not every surface development is positively reflected in bond strength [34]. In addition, in the case of bond strength, not only is the height of the roughness important, but other parameters should also be considered, e.g., roughness, width, frequency and regularity. Our study confirms that etching creates a more homogenous surface structure and enlarges surface area. This surface condition more easily contributed to a higher bond strength [35]. In the present study, the shear bond strength (SBS) of zirconia with resin cement was evaluated after different surface treatments: air abrasion, air abrasion and etching, and a combination of those with two primers (MKZ Primer, Monobond Plus). SBS results showed statistical differences between control and etched samples (with or without primers) (Figure 1).

Treatment with the Zircos-E system improved the bond strength compared to the sandblasted samples. Observed changes in surface topography and smaller distances between irregularities on the surface result in the better micromechanical interlocking of resin cement. A similar dependency can be found in other studies [21]. In the mentioned study, the connection (assessed with micro-shear bond strength) of resin cement with zirconia improved when Zircos–E was used, juxtaposing this with sandblasting or a surface without any preparation (28.48 MPa vs. 22.66 MPa or 18.96 MPa for opaque zirconia and translucent 28.12 MPa vs. 25.36 MPa or 22.82 MPa, respectively) [21]. Besides, the best results were observed when the zirconia surface was both sandblasted and etched. In a study conducted by Cho et al. [22], the shear bond strength between zirconia after air-abrasion, acid etching (nitric acid–hydrofluoric acid) and tribochemical silica-coating and resin cement were measured. The bond strength in the etching group was higher compared to other studied groups but the authors did not determine how durable this connection was. In a study carried out by Sadid-Zadeh R. et al. [36], all prepared specimens (air-abraded with 50 μm Al_2O_3; etched with Zircos-E; air-abraded and then etched with Zircos-E; etched with Zircos-E and then sandblasting) were subjected to thermocycling for 1000 cycles between 5 °C and 55 °C. Similar results (around 10 MPa) were obtained regardless of the surface preparation method. The authors suggested that an additional study should be performed, nothing the potentially hazardous nature of such an acid solution [36]. In another study, the SBS (after 10,000 thermocycles) of etched zirconia surface bonded with enamel by resin cement was insignificantly lower than the connection with sandblasted zirconia, and both surface preparation methods appeared to be more effective than those observed in the control (non-prepared ultra-translucent zirconia) [37]. The authors claimed that lower bond strength observed for Zircos-E is attributed to high viscosity of resin cement which prevents flow in the irregularity of the etched surface [37].

In our study, the application of selected primers also increased bond strength. This increase was, however, statistically insignificant. MKZ primer contains 3-Methacryloyloxypropyl-trimethoxysilan and 10-Methacryloyloxydecyl dihydrogen phosphate. Monobond Plus has three different functional methacrylates—silane, phosphoric, and sulfide methacrylate. Silanes can react with hydroxyl groups of silica and the methacrylate of resin cement, creating quite a strong connection with inorganic ceramics. However, in zirconia, there is no silica phase, so this bonding cannot occur with silane substances of used primers [38,39]. However, the used primers contain some acidic monomers with a phosphate ester group that can bond directly to zirconium oxide and enhance the wettability of the ceramic surface [40,41]. In addition, sandblasting and etching not only develop a surface that is conducive to the formation of micro-retentions, but also contribute to the formation of hydroxyl groups, which may chemically react with phosphate monomers [25]. Some studies have shown that primers enhance the bond strength of resin cement to zirconia ceramics [41,42]. The important aspect are sandblasting and the type of cement used (conventional vs. self-adhesive) [43].

Long-term water storage and thermocycling are common methods of assessing bond durability [44–46]. In thermocycling aging, degradation is caused not only by the reaction of water molecules with bond interface/resin cement, but also by the contraction and expansion of the materials due to temperature variations. It is worth noting that zirconia and resin cement have different thermal coefficients, which may result in greater stress accumulation at the interface. In addition, the larger the bonding interface in clinical conditions in comparison with laboratory tests, the greater the observed degradation effect. In the present study, after 5000 thermocycles, which correspond to six months of service life as 10,000 cycles are supposed to correspond to 12 months of service [47], shear bond strengths decreased significantly in comparison with initial values (24 h, water 37 °C). This result corresponded to the results obtained in other studies showing that bonding between zirconia ceramics and resin luting agents is not as stable after thermocycling [34]. The minimum value of bond resin cement, which guarantees the safe exploitation of ceramic under clinical conditions, is about 10–13 MPa [48,49]. A similar value of the minimum bond strength of the resin-to-restoration interface (not lower than 10 MPa) was proposed by Behr M. et al. [50] for resin-bonded fixed partial dentures from the Maryland type. Except for zirconia, which was only air-abraded (control) before and after thermocycling, and when Monobond was used after thermocycling, the value of all connections with cement in our study are close to this value.

In summary, our study confirms that zirconia can be etched. It also shows an increase in shear bond strength. The observed changes in SEM images may be related to the corrosion of zirconia grains. More chemically reactive atoms around the crystal boundaries dissolve faster than those inside the crystal, which leads to the formation of irregular grooves around the crystals and grain size reductions [51]. It was shown that HF dissolves zirconium oxide and yttrium oxide but, during this process, fluoride, oxide, and hydroxide complexes are formed [52]. The resulting structure is more homogeneous compared to the sandblasted samples. Additionally, there are some porosities that can contribute to the formation of better microretentions following micromechanical interlocking with adhesive. Furthermore, it has been shown that acid contributes to the formation of -OH groups on the zirconia surface. Hydroxyl groups can be used for chemical reaction with primer components and chemically modify the zirconia surface, as well as enhancing the adhesion of resin cement [53,54]. It has also been found that there is a direct chemical connection between the phosphate ester group of adhesive monomers and zirconia oxide [55]. Not only are ionic interactions between 10-MDP and zirconia observed, hydrogen bonding can be observed too [56].

Further studies on different types of cement and variations in the etching protocol (time, temperature) would provide a more detailed insight into the effect of the Zircos-E Etching solution on zirconia to improve bond strength. A comparison of the use of silane alone would allow for an evaluation of the effectiveness of this substance in comparison with primers dedicated to zirconium (containing other monomers). Testing mechanical properties, such as hardness and flexural strength after such aggressive etching, should be evaluated in the future for zirconia ceramic. In addition, an evaluation of the effect of certain treatments on zirconia phases with the use of X-ray diffraction and FITR would be an interesting contribution to research on zirconia.

5. Conclusions

Considering the limitations of the present study, the following conclusions can be drawn:

- Use of the Zircos-E system influences the shear bond strength between zirconia and resin cement. In consequence, SBS is significantly higher than that observed in the control group (only sandblasted zirconia) and when only a primer (after sandblasting) is used.
- Etching with the Zircos-E system leads to changes in the surface structure—a lower average roughness and mean spacing of profile irregularities. Etching also reduces the amount of alumina element (from air abrasion) on the zirconia surface.

- Use of primers preceded with etching with the Zircos-E system positively affects the adhesion between resin cement and zirconia.
- Aging with thermocycler significantly reduced the shear bond strength, except for sandblasted samples with MKZ Primer, which stayed on the same level ~10 MPa, before and after aging.

Author Contributions: Conceptualization, J.S.; data curation, A.S.-W.; formal analysis, K.K.; investigation, G.S., M.I.S.-J. and W.S.; methodology, W.S. and K.B.; project administration, G.S. and A.S.-W.; resources, J.S.; supervision, K.B.; visualization, K.K.; writing—original draft, A.S.-W., M.I.S.-J., W.S., J.S. and K.K.; writing—review and editing, G.S., A.S.-W. and K.B. All authors have read and agreed to the published version of the manuscript.

Funding: This research received no external funding.

Institutional Review Board Statement: Not applicable.

Informed Consent Statement: Not applicable.

Data Availability Statement: Data are available in a publicly accessible repository Zenodo at https://zenodo.org/record/8215149 (last accessed 4 July 2023).

Acknowledgments: The authors would like to thank to Natrodent (Łódź, Poland) for carrying out the sample etching process using the Zircos-E Etching Solution.

Conflicts of Interest: The authors declare no conflict of interest.

Appendix A

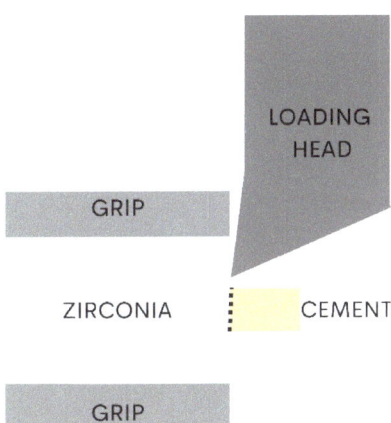

Figure A1. Illustration of the shear bond strength test.

References

1. Iftikhar, S.; Jahanzeb, N.; Saleem, M.; ur Rehman, S.; Matinlinna, J.P.; Khan, A.S. The trends of dental biomaterials research and future directions: A mapping review. *Saudi Dent. J.* **2021**, *33*, 229–238. [CrossRef]
2. Kulyk, V.; Duriagina, Z.; Kostryzhev, A.; Vasyliv, B.; Vavrukh, V.; Marenych, O. The Effect of Yttria Content on Microstructure, Strength, and Fracture Behavior of Yttria-Stabilized Zirconia. *Materials* **2022**, *15*, 5212. [CrossRef] [PubMed]
3. Özcan, M.; Bernasconi, M. Adhesion to zirconia used for dental restorations: A systematic review and meta-analysis. *J. Adhes. Dent.* **2015**, *17*, 7–26. [CrossRef] [PubMed]
4. Luthardt, R.G.; Holzhüter, M.; Sandkuhl, O.; Herold, V.; Schnapp, J.D.; Kuhlisch, E.; Walter, M. Reliability and properties of ground Y-TZP-zirconia ceramics. *J. Dent. Res.* **2002**, *81*, 487–491. [CrossRef]
5. Gautam, C.; Joyner, J.; Gautam, A.; Rao, J.; Vajtai, R. Zirconia based dental ceramics: Structure, mechanical properties, biocompatibility and applications. *Dalton Trans.* **2016**, *45*, 19194–19215. [CrossRef]
6. Nistor, L.; Grădinaru, M.; Rîcă, R.; Mărășescu, P.; Stan, M.; Manolea, H.; Ionescu, A.; Moraru, I. Zirconia Use in Dentistry—Manufacturing and Properties. *Curr. Health Sci. J.* **2019**, *45*, 28–35. [CrossRef] [PubMed]

7. Russo, D.S.; Cinelli, F.; Sarti, C.; Giachetti, L. Adhesion to zirconia: A systematic review of current conditioning methods and bonding materials. *Dent. J.* **2019**, *7*, 74. [CrossRef]
8. Hallmann, L.; Ulmer, P.; Reusser, E.; Hämmerle, C.H.F. Effect of blasting pressure, abrasive particle size and grade on phase transformation and morphological change of dental zirconia surface. *Surf. Coat. Technol.* **2012**, *206*, 4293–4302. [CrossRef]
9. Souza, R.O.A.; Valandro, L.F.; Melo, R.M.; Machado, J.P.B.; Bottino, M.A.; Özcan, M. Air-particle abrasion on zirconia ceramic using different protocols: Effects on biaxial flexural strength after cyclic loading, phase transformation and surface topography. *J. Mech. Behav. Biomed. Mater.* **2013**, *26*, 155–163. [CrossRef]
10. Ozcan, M. Air abrasion of zirconia resin-bonded fixed dental prostheses prior to adhesive cementation: Why and how? *J. Adhes. Dent.* **2013**, *15*, 394. [CrossRef]
11. Okada, M.; Taketa, H.; Torii, Y.; Irie, M.; Matsumoto, T. Optimal sandblasting conditions for conventional-type yttria-stabilized tetragonal zirconia polycrystals. *Dent. Mater.* **2019**, *35*, 169–175. [CrossRef] [PubMed]
12. Lee, Y.; Oh, K.C.; Kim, N.H.; Moon, H.S. Evaluation of zirconia surfaces after strong-acid etching and its effects on the shear bond strength of dental resin cement. *Int. J. Dent.* **2019**, *2019*, 3564275. [CrossRef]
13. Sato, H.; Yamada, K.; Pezzotti, G.; Nawa, M.; Ban, S. Mechanical properties of dental zirconia ceramics changed with sandblasting and heat treatment. *Dent. Mater. J.* **2008**, *27*, 408–414. [CrossRef] [PubMed]
14. Franco-Tabares, S.; Wardecki, D.; Nakamura, K.; Ardalani, S.; Hjalmarsson, L.; Stenport, V.F.; Johansson, C.B. Effect of airborne-particle abrasion and polishing on novel translucent zirconias: Surface morphology, phase transformation and insights into bonding. *J. Prosthodont. Res.* **2021**, *65*, 97–105. [CrossRef]
15. Aurélio, I.L.; Marchionatti, A.M.E.; Montagner, A.F.; May, L.G.; Soares, F.Z.M. Does air particle abrasion affect the flexural strength and phase transformation of Y-TZP? A systematic review and meta-analysis. *Dent. Mater.* **2016**, *32*, 827–845. [CrossRef] [PubMed]
16. Wolfart, M.; Lehmann, F.; Wolfart, S.; Kern, M. Durability of the resin bond strength to zirconia ceramic after using different surface conditioning methods. *Dent. Mater.* **2007**, *23*, 45–50. [CrossRef]
17. Kitayama, S.; Nikaido, T.; Takahashi, R.; Zhu, L.; Ikeda, M.; Foxton, R.M.; Sadr, A.; Tagami, J. Effect of primer treatment on bonding of resin cements to zirconia ceramic. *Dent. Mater.* **2010**, *26*, 426–432. [CrossRef]
18. Xie, H.; Shen, S.; Qian, M.; Zhang, F.; Chen, C.; Tay, F.R. Effects of acid treatment on dental zirconia: An in vitro study. *PLoS ONE* **2015**, *10*, e0136263. [CrossRef]
19. Lv, P.; Yang, X.; Jiang, T. Influence of hot-etching surface treatment on zirconia/resin shear bond strength. *Materials* **2015**, *8*, 8087–8096. [CrossRef]
20. Seo, S.H.; Kim, J.E.; Nam, N.E.; Moon, H.S. Effect of air abrasion, acid etching, and aging on the shear bond strength with resin cement to 3Y-TZP zirconia. *J. Mech. Behav. Biomed. Mater.* **2022**, *134*, 105348. [CrossRef]
21. Sales, A.; Rodrigues, S.J.; Mahesh, M.; Ginjupalli, K.; Shetty, T.; Pai, U.Y.; Saldanha, S.; Hegde, P.; Mukherjee, S.; Kamath, V.; et al. Effect of Different Surface Treatments on the Micro-Shear Bond Strength and Surface Characteristics of Zirconia: An In Vitro Study. *Int. J. Dent.* **2022**, *2022*, 1546802. [CrossRef] [PubMed]
22. Cho, J.H.; Kim, S.J.; Shim, J.S.; Lee, K. Effect of zirconia surface treatment using nitric acid-hydrofluoric acid on the shear bond strengths of resin cements. *J. Adv. Prosthodont.* **2017**, *9*, 77–84. [CrossRef] [PubMed]
23. Ruyter, E.I.; Vajeeston, N.; Knarvang Torbjørn, K.; Kvam, K. A novel etching technique for surface treatment of zirconia ceramics to improve adhesion of resin- based luting cements. *Acta Biomater. Odontol. Scand.* **2017**, *3*, 36–46. [CrossRef]
24. Kim, S.H.; Cho, S.C.; Lee, M.H.; Kim, H.J.; Oh, N.S. Effect of 9% Hydrofluoric Acid Gel Hot-Etching Surface Treatment on Shear Bond Strength of Resin Cements to Zirconia Ceramics. *Medicina* **2022**, *58*, 1469. [CrossRef]
25. Szawioła-Kirejczyk, M.; Chmura, K.; Gronkiewicz, K.; Gala, A.; Loster, J.E.; Ryniewicz, W. Adhesive Cementation of Zirconia Based Ceramics-Surface Modification Methods Literature Review. *Coatings* **2022**, *12*, 1067. [CrossRef]
26. Phark, J.H.; Duarte, S.; Blatz, M.; Sadan, A. An in vitro evaluation of the long-term resin bond to a new densely sintered high-purity zirconium-oxide ceramic surface. *J. Prosthet. Dent.* **2009**, *101*, 29–38. [CrossRef]
27. Shen, D.; Wang, H.; Shi, Y.; Su, Z.; Hannig, M.; Fu, B. The Effect of Surface Treatments on Zirconia Bond Strength and Durability. *J. Funct. Biomater.* **2023**, *14*, 89. [CrossRef] [PubMed]
28. Rashid, H. Evaluation of the surface roughness of a standard abraded dental porcelain following different polishing techniques. *J. Dent. Sci.* **2012**, *7*, 184–189. [CrossRef]
29. Moon, J.E.; Kim, S.H.; Lee, J.B.; Han, J.S.; Yeo, I.S.; Ha, S.R. Effects of airborne-particle abrasion protocol choice on the surface characteristics of monolithic zirconia materials and the shear bond strength of resin cement. *Ceram. Int.* **2016**, *42*, 1552–1562. [CrossRef]
30. Flores-Ferreyra, B.I.; Cougall-Vilchis, R.J.S.; Velazquez-Enriquez, U.; Garcia-Contreras, R.; Aguillon-Sol, L.; Olea-Mejia, O.F. Effect of airborne-particle abrasion and, acid and alkaline treatments on shear bond strength of dental zirconia. *Dent. Mater. J.* **2019**, *38*, 182–188. [CrossRef]
31. Abdulateef, M.R.; Nayif, M.M. Surface Roughness Assessment of the Sandblasted and Acid-Etched Zirconia Ceramic. *Al–Rafidain Dent. J.* **2021**, *21*, 146–157. [CrossRef]
32. Fayaz, A.; Bali, S.K.; Bhat, M.M.; Bashir, A. Effect of 37% Phosphoric Acid Etchant on Surface Topography of Zirconia Crowns—An In Vitro Study. *Ann. Int. Med. Dent. Res.* **2020**, *6*, 4–7.
33. Smielak, B.; Klimek, L. Effect of hydrofluoric acid concentration and etching duration on select surface roughness parameters for zirconia. *J. Prosthet. Dent.* **2015**, *113*, 596–602. [CrossRef]

34. Tsuo, Y.; Yoshida, K.; Atsuta, M. Effects of alumina-blasting and adhesive primers on bonding between resin luting agent and zirconia ceramics. *Dent. Mater. J.* **2006**, *25*, 669–674. [CrossRef] [PubMed]
35. Zhang, Q.; Yao, C.; Yuan, C.; Zhang, H.; Liu, L.; Zhang, Y.; Bai, J.; Tang, C. Evaluation of surface properties and shear bond strength of zirconia substructure after sandblasting and acid etching. *Mater. Res. Express* **2020**, *7*, 095403. [CrossRef]
36. Sadid-zadeh, R.; Strazzella, A.; Li, R.; Makwoka, S. Effect of zirconia etching solution on the shear bond strength between zirconia and resin cement. *J. Prosthet. Dent.* **2021**, *126*, 693–697. [CrossRef] [PubMed]
37. Nasr, D.M.; Koheil, S.A.; Mahy, W.A. El Effect of different surface treatments on bonding of ultra-translucent zirconia. *Alex. Dent. J.* **2020**, *46*, 84–91. [CrossRef]
38. Thompson, J.Y.; Stoner, B.R.; Piascik, J.R.; Smith, R. Adhesion/cementation to zirconia and other non-silicate ceramics: Where are we now? *Dent. Mater.* **2011**, *27*, 71–82. [CrossRef] [PubMed]
39. Murakami, T.; Takemoto, S.; Nishiyama, N.; Aida, M. Zirconia surface modification by a novel zirconia bonding system and its adhesion mechanism. *Dent. Mater.* **2017**, *33*, 1371–1380. [CrossRef]
40. Oba, Y.; Koizumi, H.; Nakayama, D.; Ishii, T.; Akazawa, N.; Matsumura, H. Effect of silane and phosphate primers on the adhesive performance of a tri-n-butylborane initiated luting agent bonded to zirconia. *Dent. Mater. J.* **2014**, *33*, 226–232. [CrossRef]
41. Attia, A.; Lehmann, F.; Kern, M. Influence of surface conditioning and cleaning methods on resin bonding to zirconia ceramic. *Dent. Mater.* **2010**, *27*, 207–213. [CrossRef]
42. Attia, A.; Kern, M. Long-term resin bonding to zirconia ceramic with a new universal primer. *J. Prosthet. Dent.* **2010**, *106*, 319–327. [CrossRef] [PubMed]
43. Thammajaruk, P.; Inokoshi, M.; Chong, S.; Guazzato, M. Bonding of composite cements to zirconia: A systematic review and meta-analysis of in vitro studies. *J. Mech. Behav. Biomed. Mater.* **2018**, *80*, 258–268. [CrossRef] [PubMed]
44. Keui, C.; Liebermann, A.; Roos, M.; Uhrenbacher, J.; Stawarczyk, B. The effect of ceramic primer on shear bond strength of resin composite cement to zirconia. A function of water storage and thermal cycling. *J. Am. Dent. Assoc.* **2013**, *144*, 1261–1271. [CrossRef]
45. Heikkinen, T.T.; Lassila, L.V.J.; Matinlinna, J.P.; Vallittu, P.K. Thermocycling effects on resin bond to silicatized and silanized zirconia. *J. Adhes. Sci. Technol.* **2009**, *23*, 1043–1051. [CrossRef]
46. Kern, M.; Wegner, S.M. Bonding to zirconia ceramic: Adhesion methods and their durability. *Dent. Mater.* **1998**, *14*, 64–71. [CrossRef]
47. Gale, M.S.; Darvell, B.W. Thermal cycling procedures for laboratory testing of dental restorations. *J. Dent.* **1999**, *27*, 89–99. [CrossRef]
48. Thurmond, J.W.; Barkmeier, W.; Wilwerding, T.M. Effect of porcelain treatmens on bond strengths of composite resin bonded to porcelain. *J. Prosthet. Dent.* **1994**, *72*, 359. [CrossRef]
49. Luthy, H.; Olivier, L.; Christoph, H.F.; Hammerlea, H. Effect of thermocycling on bond strength of luting cements to zirconia ceramic. *Dent. Mater.* **2006**, *2*, 195–200. [CrossRef]
50. Behr, M.; Proff, P.; Kolbeck, C.; Langrieger, S.; Kunze, J.; Handel, G.; Rosentritt, M. The bond strength of the resin-to-zirconia interface using different bonding concepts. *J. Mech. Behav. Biomed. Mater.* **2011**, *4*, 2–8. [CrossRef]
51. Sriamporn, T.; Thamrongananskul, N.; Busabok, C.; Poolthong, S.; Uo, M. Dental zirconia can be etched by hydrofluoric acid. *Dent. Mater. J.* **2014**, *33*, 79–85. [CrossRef] [PubMed]
52. Flamant, Q.; García Marro, F.; Roa Rovira, J.J.; Anglada, M. Hydrofluoric acid etching of dental zirconia. Part 1: Etching mechanism and surface characterization. *J. Eur. Ceram. Soc.* **2016**, *36*, 121–134. [CrossRef]
53. Lohbauer, U.; Zipperle, M.; Rischka, K.; Petschelt, A.; Müller, F.A. Hydroxylation of dental zirconia surfaces: Characterization and bonding potential. *J. Biomed. Mater. Res. Part B Appl. Biomater.* **2008**, *87*, 461–467. [CrossRef] [PubMed]
54. Lung, C.Y.K.; Kukk, E.; Hägerth, T.; Matinlinna, J.P. Surface modification of silica-coated zirconia by chemical treatments. *Appl. Surf. Sci.* **2010**, *257*, 1228–1235. [CrossRef]
55. Chen, L.; Suh, B.; Brown, D.; Chen, X. Bonding of primed zirconia ceramics: Evidence of chemical bonding and improved bond strengths. *Am. J. Dent.* **2012**, *25*, 103–108.
56. Nagaoka, N.; Yoshihara, K.; Feitosa, V.P.; Tamada, Y.; Irie, M.; Yoshida, Y.; Van Meerbeek, B.; Hayakawa, S. Chemical interaction mechanism of 10-MDP with zirconia. *Sci. Rep.* **2017**, *7*, 45563. [CrossRef]

Disclaimer/Publisher's Note: The statements, opinions and data contained in all publications are solely those of the individual author(s) and contributor(s) and not of MDPI and/or the editor(s). MDPI and/or the editor(s) disclaim responsibility for any injury to people or property resulting from any ideas, methods, instructions or products referred to in the content.

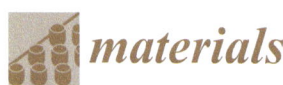

Article

Expression of Interleukin-1β and Histological Changes of the Three-Dimensional Oral Mucosal Model in Response to Yttria-Stabilized Nanozirconia

Naziratul Adirah Nasarudin [1], Masfueh Razali [1,*], Victor Goh [1], Wen Lin Chai [2] and Andanastuti Muchtar [3]

1 Department of Restorative Dentistry, Faculty of Dentistry, Universiti Kebangsaan Malaysia, Kuala Lumpur 50300, Malaysia
2 Department of Restorative Dentistry, Faculty of Dentistry, University of Malaya, Kuala Lumpur 50603, Malaysia
3 Department of Mechanical and Manufacturing Engineering, Faculty of Engineering and Built Environment, Universiti Kebangsaan Malaysia, Bangi 43600, Malaysia
* Correspondence: masfuah@ukm.edu.my; Tel.: +60-392897745

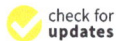

Citation: Nasarudin, N.A.; Razali, M.; Goh, V.; Chai, W.L.; Muchtar, A. Expression of Interleukin-1β and Histological Changes of the Three-Dimensional Oral Mucosal Model in Response to Yttria-Stabilized Nanozirconia. *Materials* 2023, 16, 2027. https://doi.org/10.3390/ma16052027

Academic Editors: Laura-Cristina Rusu and Lavinia Cosmina Ardelean

Received: 30 December 2022
Revised: 19 February 2023
Accepted: 24 February 2023
Published: 1 March 2023

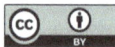

Copyright: © 2023 by the authors. Licensee MDPI, Basel, Switzerland. This article is an open access article distributed under the terms and conditions of the Creative Commons Attribution (CC BY) license (https://creativecommons.org/licenses/by/4.0/).

Abstract: Over the years, advancement in ceramic-based dental restorative materials has led to the development of monolithic zirconia with increased translucency. The monolithic zirconia fabricated from nano-sized zirconia powders is shown to be superior in physical properties and more translucent for anterior dental restorations. Most in vitro studies on monolithic zirconia have focused mainly on the effect of surface treatment or the wear of the material, while the nanotoxicity of this material is yet to be explored. Hence, this research aimed to assess the biocompatibility of yttria-stabilized nanozirconia (3-YZP) on the three-dimensional oral mucosal models (3D-OMM). The 3D-OMMs were constructed using human gingival fibroblast (HGF) and immortalized human oral keratinocyte cell line (OKF6/TERT-2), co-cultured on an acellular dermal matrix. On day 12, the tissue models were exposed to 3-YZP (test) and inCoris TZI (IC) (reference material). The growth media were collected at 24 and 48 h of exposure to materials and assessed for IL-1β released. The 3D-OMMs were fixed with 10% formalin for the histopathological assessments. The concentration of the IL-1β was not statistically different between the two materials for 24 and 48 h of exposure ($p = 0.892$). Histologically, stratification of epithelial cells was formed without evidence of cytotoxic damage and the epithelial thickness measured was the same for all model tissues. The excellent biocompatibility of nanozirconia, as evidenced by the multiple endpoint analyses of the 3D-OMM, may indicate the potential of its clinical application as a restorative material.

Keywords: biocompatibility; interleukin-1; nanozirconia; pro-inflammatory cytokines; three-dimensional oral mucosal model

1. Introduction

Over the past few decades, zirconia ceramic has been used extensively in dentistry due to its aesthetic property and superior mechanical strength. In clinical applications, 3 mol % yttria-stabilized tetragonal zirconia polycrystals (3Y-TZP) are widely utilized. This is because the yttria-partially stabilized tetragonal zirconia polycrystalline (Y-TZP) showed better mechanical properties and superior resistance to fracture than other conventional dental ceramics [1]. The Y-TZP has a high fracture toughness, from 5 to 10 MPa m$^{1/2}$, and a flexural strength of 900–1400 MPa [2]. The bonding of translucent veneering material to zirconia core materials is usually carried out to cover their opaqueness. However, the most frequently reported complication of zirconia restoration is the chipping or fracture of the veneer ceramic [3]. Henceforward, monolithic zirconia restoration is preferred to overcome such complications.

Nanoparticles can exist between 1 and 100 nm [4,5], and evidence shows that these nanosized particles have a higher surface area-to-volume ratio [6,7]. Hence, this corresponds to the increased particles' surface energy [8]. Consecutively, nanoparticles have enhanced physical properties compared to their larger-scale counterparts [9]. Due to these exceptionally superior physical properties, nanomaterial applications in dentistry have expanded from caries prevention to restorative dentistry [8,10]. The zirconia dental blocks processed from the nanosized powder have higher translucency than conventional zirconia [11].

So far, toxicological studies on zirconia nanoparticles are limited, and the results are controversial. A study by Laiteerapong et al. [12] reported that zirconia nanoparticles did not have a genotoxic effect on the human gingival fibroblast (HGF). However, evidence from other studies suggested that a reduction in cell viability occurred in a concentration- or time-dependent manner [13,14]. The reduced cell viability was correlated with an increase in the production of reactive oxygen species (ROS), cell death, and significant deoxyribonuclease acid (DNA) damage in the human skin epithelial cells exposed to more than 30 μg/mL yttria stabilized zirconia nanoparticles for 48 h [15]. Zirconia nanoparticles could also induce a toxic effect on osteoblast cells. The cell proliferation assay demonstrated a decrease in the cell's viability, with the highest harmful effect at a concentration of 150 μg/mL for 48 h. Additionally, the shape of the osteoblast cells changed, and pyknotic nuclei were observed [16].

Apart from the cytotoxicity testing, it is also essential to investigate the immunogenic potentials of dental materials. Dental materials may provoke local inflammatory reactions of the native gingiva with the induction of pro-inflammatory cytokines. Cytokines are small-sized proteins, normally present in a minimal quantity in body fluids. However, the concentrations can amount to 1000-fold when associated with trauma or inflammation [17]. Cytokines that aggravate inflammation are known as pro-inflammatory cytokines. interleukin-1β (IL-1β) is synthesized by macrophages, monocytes, fibroblast, epithelial and dendritic cells when stimulated by stress or inflammation [18]. Interleukin-1β causes an increased production of cyclooxygenase-2 (COX-2) and phospholipase A2 (PLA2). The increased production, in turn, will activate the prostaglandin E2 (PGE2), leukotrienes, and emigration of neutrophils to the gingiva [19]. As such, increased concentration of interleukin-1β has been implicated in gingival inflammation and bone resorption in periodontal disease [18,20].

The effects of zirconia nanoparticles on the inflammatory response of the human gingival mesenchymal stromal cells (hG-MSCs) were investigated by Nemec et al [21]. They discovered that the addition of zirconia nanoparticles with a size of 100 nm greatly increased the expression of interleukin-6 (IL-6) and interleukin-8 (IL-8) in hG-MSCs. Conversely, no upregulation of IL-6 or IL-1β released by monocytes (THP-1) was observed upon stimulation with zirconia nanoparticles with a diameter of 2–75 μm [22].

With the exponentially increasing clinical use of nanoparticles [23], there is a need to identify the risks concerning human health and the environmental implications of manufactured nanoparticles [16]. Even though studies regarding the toxicity of nanoparticles are rapidly growing, knowledge of the toxic effects of these nanoparticles is limited. Most have agreed that physicochemical characteristics such as shape, surface charge and size play vital roles in nanotoxicity [23,24]. More specifically, grinding activities and wear and tear of the dental restorative materials during function pose a concern that these nanoparticles may leach and cause detrimental effects to the oral cavity and the gingiva.

Nanosized zirconia powders in this study were processed through a combined consolidation method, colloidal slip casting and cold isostatic pressing (CIP) to form zirconia dental blocks [5]. Considering the limited information about cell behaviour with this nanomaterial, utilizing the biological endpoint of 3D-OMMs, this study aimed to assess the biocompatibility of the 3-YZP and to compare it with similar commercially available zirconia.

2. Materials and Methods

2.1. Preparations of Specimens

Two types of 3 mol% yttria-stabilized tetragonal zirconia were used in this experiment: (1) Sirona inCoris TZI (IC) (Sirona Dental Systems GmbH, Bensheim, Germany), which acted as control; (2) newly developed nanozirconia (3-YZP), prepared from tetragonal zirconia polycrystalline (Y-TZP) nano powder partially stabilized with 3 mol% of Y_2O_3 (US Research Nanomaterials Inc., Houston, TX, USA). The primary particle size of the nanopowder was approximated at 20 nm. Briefly, The Y-TZP nanopowder suspension was subjected to the slip-cast method followed by a cold isostatic pressing (CIP) method to produce the green bodies. Subsequently, the green bodies were pre-sintered at 1200 °C to produce the 3-YZP [5]. Both zirconia specimens were trimmed into a disc-shaped form with a dimension of 10 mm diameter and 2 mm thickness. Next, 3-YZP and IC were trimmed to produce a disc-shaped specimen using the high-speed handpiece and straight fissure diamond bur. The zirconia specimens were later polished with sandpaper grit 60, 120, 140, 400, 800, 1200, 1500 and 2000. After final sintering the tested material at 1500 °C, the final dimensions of all samples were approximately 9 mm in diameter and 2 mm in height. Meanwhile, the IC was prepared according to the manufacturer's instructions.

The surface roughness of the materials was evaluated using the atomic force microscope (AFM) (Park NX-10, Park System, Suwon, South Korea) in contact mode. Six samples were used to determine the surface roughness of the materials. In brief, five random points were chosen in each sample, and these values were averaged.

Before the experiments, all specimens were cleaned with an acetone solution for 20 min in an ultrasonic bath and immersed in the ascending concentrations of ethyl alcohol (10%, 50%, 75% and 100%) each for 5 min. The zirconia specimens were also sterilized on both surfaces under ultraviolet radiation for 20 min (NU-430, LabGard, Class II, Type B2 Biological safety cabinets, NuAire Inc.®, Plymouth, MA, USA).

2.2. Human Oral Epithelial Cell Line and Human Gingival Fibroblast Cells Culture and Maintenance

The human epithelial cells (OKF6/TERT-2) and human gingival fibroblast cells (HGF) (passage 4–5) used in this study were courtesy of Professor Dr Chai Wen Lin under her research grant supported by the Ministry of Higher Education High Impact Research Grant (UM.C/625/HIR/MOHE/DENT/05). This study received approval from the Research and Ethics Committee, Secretariat of Research and Innovation, Faculty of Medicine, Universiti Kebangsaan Malaysia (UKM PPI/111/8/JEP-2020-618).

The OKF6/TERT-2 cell is an immortalized epithelial cell line processed by the forced expression of the telomerase. This cell line was chosen because it has been proven to resemble the primary oral keratinocytes [25]. The cells were grown in the keratinocyte serum-free media (K-SFM) (Thermo Fisher Scientific Inc., Waltham, MA, USA) with bovine pituitary extract and epithelial growth factor.

The primary human gingival fibroblast cells were isolated from healthy gingival tissues obtained from the crown lengthening surgery. The primary cell was extracted from the gingival tissue using an explant technique. The Dispase® (Gibco™ Thermo Fisher Scientific Inc., Waltham, MA, USA) was added to the tissue, to separate the connective tissue from the epithelium. The separated tissues were minced into small pieces of 1 mm × 1 mm in size using a scalpel blade in separate Petri dishes and transferred to culture flasks. The growth media in the flasks were changed every 2 days and subcultured once they had attained 70% confluency.

2.3. Fabrication of the 3D-OMM

The 3D-OMM was developed based on the modification from the protocols developed by Chai et al. [26]. A mixture of 5×10^5 HGFs and 5×10^5 OKF6/TERT-2 was co-cultured onto the basement membrane side of the rehydrated acellular dermal membrane (Puros® Dermis Allograft Tissue Matrix, Zimmer Biomet, Warsaw, IN, USA).

Prior to cell seeding, the membrane was cut into a round shape with a 12 mm diameter to fit into a 12 mm ring insert (Corning® Costar® Snapwell™ Insert, Corning Life Sciences, Corning, NY, USA). The membrane was rehydrated in a 5 mL Dulbecco's phosphate buffer saline (Thermo Fisher Scientific Inc., Waltham, MA, USA) for 30 s and then immersed in a 5 mL DMEM for 15 min. The 3D-OMMs were fabricated inside 12 mm diameter inserts with a 0.4 µm pore size and a 1×10^8 pore density/cm² in a six-well plate. The seeded membrane was submerged in 3 mL of K-SFM and incubated for five days. On the sixth day, the tissues were raised at the air-liquid interface (ALI) to promote epithelial differentiation. The cells were allowed to be stratified further for up to seven days in the incubator, with the media changed every two days. On day 12, the samples (3-YZP and IC) were placed on top of the models.

2.4. Expression of Interleukin-1β

The expression of pro-inflammatory cytokine (IL-1β) from cell culture supernatants of unexposed, 3-YZP-exposed and IC-exposed models were measured using an ELISA kit. Human IL-1β ELISA kit from Abcam PLC, Cambridge, UK (Catalogue Number. ab214025) was used. The cell culture media were collected at 2 time points, after 24 h and 48 h of exposure.

For the assay procedure, all the reagents, controls and samples were prepared based on the manufacturer's instructions. The optical density was measured using a multi-plate reader (Thermo Scientific™ Multiskan™ Go Microplate Spectrophotometer, Thermo Fisher Scientific, MA, USA) at 450 nm and correction at 570 nm. The concentration of IL-1β was expressed as pg/mL and compared with a standard curve provided by the manufacturer.

2.5. Histology Preparation

Histological analyses of the 3D-OMMs were performed after 72 h of contact. The models were fixed in a 10% formalin solution for 24 h, processed for histological sections via dehydration in a graded series of ethanol concentrations (70–100%) and embedded in a paraffin block. Vertical sections of 5 µm thickness were cut and stained with hematoxylin and eosin staining (H&E staining).

The resultant histology sections were evaluated for evidence of cytotoxic epithelial damage using the inverted microscope (IX51 Olympus, Olympus Corporation, Shinjuku, Japan) at 20× and 40× magnification. The damage was manifested as the loss of the normal cell's morphology, such as the separation of the epithelium from a scaffold and the presence of the pyknotic nuclei. Two examiners were assigned to examine the histological appearance of the models.

The thickness of the epithelial layers of all models was measured using the imaging software (Cell^B, Olympus Soft Imaging Solutions GmbH, Imaging Software, Muenster, Germany) at 20× magnification. A linear scale was placed perpendicular to the histology image. The distance was taken from the basement membrane's basal surface to the epithelium's uppermost keratinized layer. Measurements were taken at five random points per section, and these values were averaged.

2.6. Statistical Analyses

All experiments were conducted in triplicate. The thickness of epithelial layers and the concentration of IL-1β were expressed as mean data and standard deviations. The data were analyzed with IBM SPSS version 25. The Shapiro–Wilk normality test was used to determine normally distributed data with p-values > 0.05. Levene's test and Box's M test were used to test the assumption of homogeneity of variance and covariances. A two-way mixed ANOVA and post hoc test were used to analyse the mean concentration of IL-1β expression, the difference between and within the models. While a one-way Welch ANOVA and post hoc test were used to assess the differences in models' epithelial thickness. The hypothesis of no difference was accepted when p-values > 0.05.

3. Results

3.1. Surface Roughness of the Materials

The individual components of each sample and the surface roughness values of two zirconia discs are tabulated in Table 1. All materials surfaces were categorized within the range of smooth surface values (Ra 0.0–0.5 µm). There was no statistically significant difference ($p > 0.05$) between the two types of zirconia. Figure 1 shows the topographic surface profile of each material used in this study, as scanned by AFM.

Table 1. The composition and surface roughness of each material.

Materials	Components and Composition by Weight %	Mean Surface Roughness ± (SD) (Ra) (nm)	p-Value
Nanozirconia (3-YZP)	$ZrO_2/Y_2O_3/HfO_2$ 95%/<5%/<1	93.8 ± 52.5	0.794 *
inCoris TZI (IC)	$ZrO_2/Al_2O_3/Y_2O_3$	85.9 ± 49.5	

* Both Ra values of 3-YZP and IC were not statistically significant. SD = standard deviation; ZrO_2 = zirconium oxide; Y_2O_3 = yttrium oxide; HfO_2 = hafnium dioxide; Al_2O_3 = aluminum oxide.

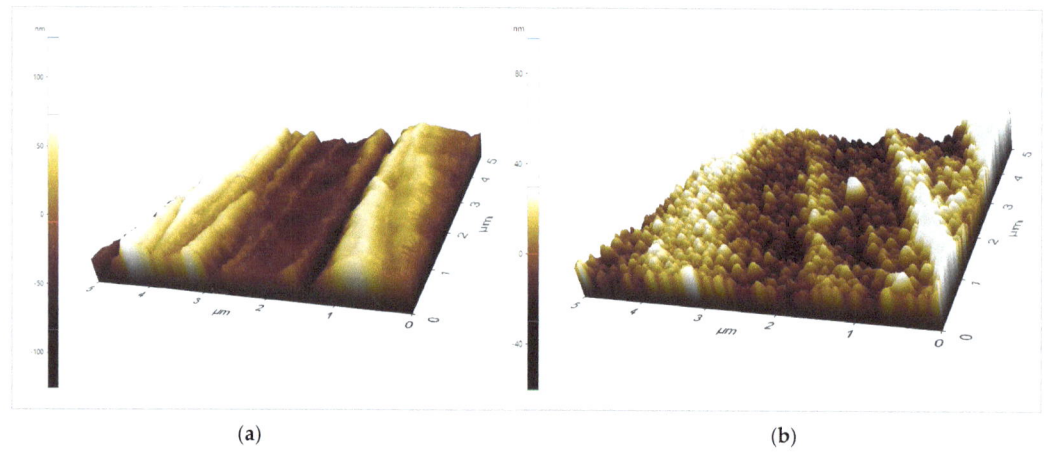

(a) (b)

Figure 1. The surface topography of (a) 3−YZP and (b) IC surfaces., areas of 5 μm × 5 μm were captured. The z scale bar (a) −100–100 nm; (b) −40–80 nm.

3.2. Expression of the Interleukin-1β following Exposure to 3-YZP

Figure 2 shows the concentration of IL-1β expressed when in contact with 3-YZP and IC. For 24 h of contact, the unexposed model released a statistically significantly lowered amount of IL-1β (19.59 ± 3.88 pg/mL) compared to both 3-YZP-exposed (44.09 ± 3.65 pg/mL) and IC-exposed (43.52 ± 4.14 pg/mL) oral mucosal models. The difference was also significant for 48 h of contact compared to the blank model. The concentration of IL-1β measured after 48 h on contact was 23.38 ± 4.17 pg/mL, 43.74 ± 4.45 pg/mL and 45.85 ± 4.47 pg/mL for the unexposed model, 3-YZP-exposed and IC-exposed oral mucosal model, respectively. However, the IL-Iβ expression between 3-YZP and IC was not statistically significant (0.77, 95% CI (−3.5 to 5.07), p = 0.892). It is interesting to note that from this chart (Figure 2), the prolonged contact with 3-YZP did not increase the amount of IL-1β released.

3.3. Histological Sections of 3D-OMMs

This study fabricated the full-thickness model that contained both types of cells. The acellular dermal membrane used in this study allowed the migration of the fibroblasts (indicated by black arrows in Figure 3) within the membrane and the fibroblasts played an important role in modulating epithelial cell differentiation, thus mimicking the intra-oral situation in which the cells interact with materials. The resultant histology sections were evaluated for evidence of cytotoxic epithelial damage using a light microscope at 40× magnification. Histologically, the epithelium continuity was preserved in all models. The absence of pyknotic nuclei was observed, and the integrity of the connective tissue layer was intact. The epithelial layers of 3D-OMMs were inconsistent, while the HGFs were not homogenized after seeding into the acellular dermal scaffolds. All hematoxylin and eosin staining results of 3D-OMM are shown in Figure 3.

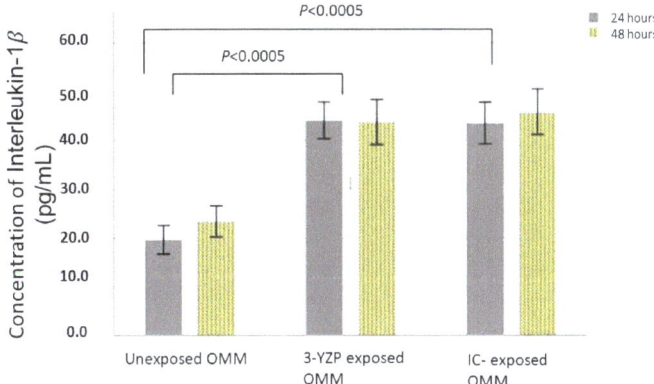

Figure 2. IL-1β released after exposure of the 3-D oral mucosal model to 3-YZP and IC, after 24 and 48 h. Error bars represent standard deviation.

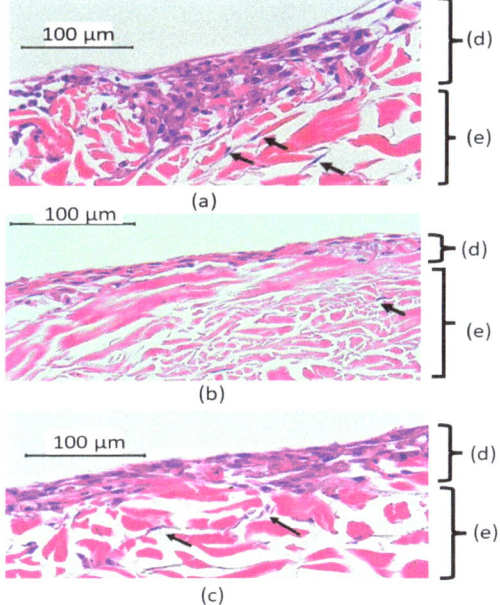

Figure 3. Histological appearance of 3D-OMMs, unexposed (**a**), after 72 h exposed to 3-YZP (**b**) IC (**c**). Black arrows indicate that the HGFs migrated into connective tissue and were occasionally present inside the stroma (**e**). The epithelial layers (**d**) were inconsistent. (Original magnification, 40×).

The epithelial thickness was highest in the unexposed group (120 ± 19.8), followed by 3-YZP-exposed (115.34 ± 41) and IC-exposed (102.84 ± 41.2). The differences between these groups were not statistically significant, Welch's $F_{(2,14.0)} = 0.68$, $p = 0.523$. Figure 4 shows the epithelial thickness of the unexposed model, 3-YZP, and IC-exposed models.

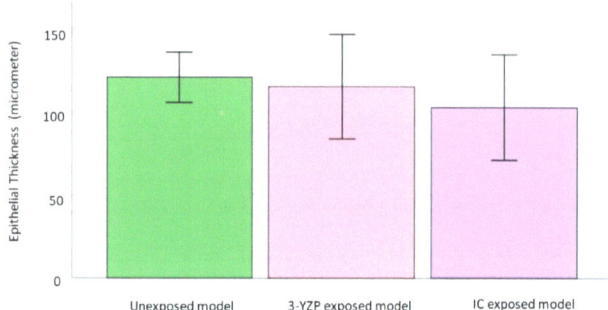

Figure 4. Graph reported on the epithelial thickness of unexposed model, 3-YZP and IC-exposed model. Error bars indicate standard deviation (SD).

4. Discussion

Surface roughness typically plays an essential role in cell attachment and proliferation [27,28]. In our study, the surface roughness was standardized via the polishing method to reduce a possible confounding factor in cell attachment. Additionally, surface roughness promoted biofilm formation. Others have shown that the surface of an abutment should have a moderate smoothness to hamper plaque formation and permit cell adhesion. With that being said, an optimal surface roughness threshold of Ra 200 nm (0.2 µm) has been proposed [29,30]. In this study, the surface roughness of all materials was within the optimum surface roughness. Additionally, the Ra value obtained from manual polishing in this present study was consistent with the value obtained from another author [31]. Although 3-YZP exhibited a slightly higher Ra value than IC, the Ra values were not more than the threshold proposed.

The 3-YZP and IC had acceptable tetragonal phase stability. The X-ray diffraction (XRD) test revealed a negligible amount of monoclinic zirconia after sintering [5,11,32]. An increased amount of monoclinic phase zirconia was found when the IC was subjected to accelerated hydrothermal ageing at 124 °C [33]. However, the monoclinic zirconia content after ageing was not exceeded the proposed engineering guidelines for zirconia restoration [34]. The presence of a high level of monoclinic phase is associated with the problem of low-temperature degradation (LTD). The LTD results in surface micro-cracking, increased surface roughening, grains pull-out and degrades the mechanical properties of the dental crown [35]. In a different study [36], where tested zirconia undergone (CIP) produced a tetragonal phase content of 100% and better mechanical properties, higher density and more homogeneous microstructures than zirconia that were not subjected to CIP. Additionally, the pre-sintered block at 1200 °C exhibited the lowest shrinkage (9.0%) among all the samples after the blocks were further sintered to a final temperature of 1500 °C with heating and cooling rates of 3 °C/min and a holding time of 2 h [37].

Recently, studies have incorporated the pro-inflammatory mediator's assessment for cytotoxic changes in cells that directly interact with dental materials [38–40]. The IL-1β was selected in this study as it is a potent pro-inflammatory mediator and is easy to measure. Moreover, the nanomaterials have the potential to trigger the multiprotein complexes and inflammasome, which will result in the secretion of IL-1β [41]. Our results demonstrated that the untreated oral mucosal model released some amount of IL-1β. This was consistent with the findings in previous studies [42–44]. Furthermore, our analysis found a significantly increased amount of IL-1β released when 3D-OMMs were exposed to both 3-YZP and IC. Nevertheless, the difference between both ceramics was insignificant.

The in vitro studies of pro-inflammatory mediators among zirconia restorations, especially utilizing the 3D-OMMs, are limited. In line with our result, a study by Özen et al. [45], who investigated the effects of dental alloys and ceramics on the oral mucosal model, revealed that In-Ceram had no significant influence on IL-1β at 24 h of exposure. However, after 48 h, the amount of IL-1β was about two-fold higher than those released from control cultures. This indicated that the dental ceramic may have caused an inflammatory reaction to the tissue model, but no toxic effect was evident as no significant reduction in cell viability was reported. Another postulation for the upregulation of the IL-1β expression was that the nanomaterials irritated the epithelium of the 3D-OMMs and caused the inflammatory response [46]. The epithelial cells could secrete pro-inflammatory mediators such as IL-1β and IL-6, in response to inflammation or tissue injury. Prior research concluded that most IL-1β has been found in the gingival epithelial [18].

Presently, there is no direct evidence that an increased IL-1β released after exposure to ceramic indicates inflammatory reactions in vivo. The ceramics' immunogenic potential was mainly reported in human clinical studies by estimating the inflammatory mediators in the gingival crevicular fluid (GCF) [47–49]. Therefore, GCF was chosen as an indicator for periodontitis and health. Ariaans et al. [50], who aimed to quantify the inflammatory reaction between lithium disilicate and zirconia, discovered that the gingival reaction between both materials was comparable to the unrestored tooth of periodontally healthy patients. The findings of our study were in agreement with Saravanakumar et al. [51], who found that, after three months, the zirconia crown expressed the lowest amount of IL-1β in the GCF, among other restorations. However, various factors could have influenced human clinical studies; so, comparing their findings with our research is challenging.

In this current research, we assessed the toxicity of the 3-YZP by placing it directly onto the uppermost surface of the oral mucosal models as an experiment by Moharamzadeh et al. [42]. Histological evaluation is currently the gold standard for toxicity assessment of imaging tissue-engineered models [52]. Highly toxic materials can cause discontinuation of the epithelial layer and separation of the epithelium from the basement membrane, some may show marked architectural atrophy and most of the upper cell layers were disintegrated but the basal cells remained intact with connective tissue components [53]. Histological analysis of all models in this study revealed that the epithelial layers were continuous, and the integrity of the connective tissue was preserved. However, only some fibroblasts were seen inside the matrices. Although acellular dermal matrices (ADM) are widely accepted as a scaffold, it suffers from some limitations due to their low porosity, which causes the poor distribution of the fibroblasts inside the connective tissue [54–56]. It is generally accepted that fibroblasts promote epithelial differentiation. However, the dermal matrices are unique as the basement membrane on the epidermal side of the matrices promotes oral keratinocytes adherence better than the collagen matrices.

Our analysis of epithelial thickness revealed that the epithelial thickness was the highest for the untreated models, followed by the 3-YZP-exposed and IC-exposed models. However, the one-way Welch ANOVA failed to demonstrate the statistically significant difference between these groups. Furthermore, the reduction in the epithelial thickness of the model correlated with the increased rate of cell apoptosis [44]. Hence, the thickness of the model can be extrapolated for the quantitative analysis of the histological appearance to determine the material's toxicity. Our result was suggestive that 3-YZP had no toxic effect on the soft tissue, as the model's epithelial thickness was preserved.

With the increasing clinical use of nanoparticles, there is a need to identify risks concerning human health [57]. Currently, the conventional in vitro test employed for cellular biology and toxicology is used to assess nanotoxicity. There are many ways of biological effects can be assessed including cellular attachment and migration, proliferation rates and determination of enzyme activity. However, due to the unique physicochemical properties of nanomaterial, interferences of nanomaterial with conventional toxicity assays such as monolayer cell cultures may have been reported and led to questionable results for nanotoxicity. Notwithstanding, the use of 3D-OMM resembling the physiological environment of the oral cavity and being used for biocompatibility testing could serve as transition testing between monolayers, to preclinical testing. The release of inflammatory cytokines such as interleukin-8 (IL-8) and interleukin-6 (IL-6) can significantly modify the cell viability and enzymic activity of the tissue model [25]. The oxidative imbalance induced by nanosize dental materials zirconia may stimulate apoptosis, immunological, increased expression of oxidative stress [58] and carcinogenic effects in the oral epithelium of 3D-OMM [59,60]. In the oral cavity, the nanozirconia dental crown will be placed in close contact with the gingiva and oral mucosa for prolonged periods, the physiological environment may induce local toxic effects. The nanozirconia dental crown may lead to chemically or pathologically initiated inflammatory diseases such as gingivitis and periodontal disease. Therefore, the re-engineered organotypic model of the oral mucosa will provide indispensable fundamental knowledge in understanding the physiological functions of tissues and the biological response of dental materials. The use of 3D-oral mucosal models could offer more predictable, repeatable and reliable multiple endpoint analyses of nanomaterials in dentistry, which mimic the in vivo morphology and cell behaviour. Moreover, they constitute a cheaper and ethically acceptable alternative to animal testing; therefore, a genotoxicity assessment should be carried out in future, utilizing tissue-engineered equivalents.

5. Strengths and Limitations of the Study

The in vitro biocompatibility assessment is crucial for the clinical validation of dental materials, which allows the evaluation of many samples simultaneously. The evidence regarding the biocompatibility of zirconia on monolayer cells has been discussed extensively in the literature. The use of 3D-OMM could serve as transition testing between monolayers, to preclinical testing, where mucotoxicity and genotoxicity may resemble those in vivo due to multiple cellular interactions that could be observed. Nevertheless, the evidence of zirconia toxicity on oral mucosal equivalent is limited. Using the 3D-OMM would allow the investigation of the inflammatory mediators and the histological evaluation of the changes in soft tissue in response to the toxicity of dental nanomaterials. Additionally, the tissue culture assays will provide a controllable and repeatable method of assessment. Hence, the findings reported from the analysis of the oral mucosal model in this study are more clinically applicable than the monolayer cell culture.

However, this study also had some limitations. The histological analysis of the models was assessed by more than one investigator who was not blinded to the nature of the treatment the tissue had received. This could have potentially caused bias. Furthermore, only one pro-inflammatory cytokine was reported in this current research. The potential use of other interleukins, such as IL-6 [61], IL-8 and tumour necrosis factor-α [62] should be explored in the biocompatibility testing of the newly developed material. The IL-6, the pro-inflammatory cytokine, is also essential for mitogenic and proliferative effects on keratinocytes during wound healing and tissue remodelling [61].

In addition to that, the nanoparticle's size, shape, surface area, agglomeration state, chemical composition and surface charge may influence their toxicity and biological responses. Among the various microscopy method for physicochemical characterization, the scanning electron microscope, transmission electron microscope (TEM) and atomic force microscope are frequently used. With this regard, TEM can be used to evaluate the permeation effects of the cell in contact with nanomaterials. Meanwhile, single-particle ICP-MS can be used for information on the size and size distribution of nanoparticles or the number of leachable elements from the nanozirconia. Even though both the zirconia were stabled following sintering, the oxide bonds of the ceramic could be damaged by the ageing or LTD of the zirconia. A study had shown that some yttrium ions were leaching out from the commercial zirconia in the corrosion test [63]. Nevertheless, the amount of leached yttrium ions as measured from the ICP-MS was relatively low than the level that could potentially be toxic to humans.

6. Conclusions

Within the limitations of this study, the excellent biocompatibility of the 3-YZP, as shown from the biological endpoint analyses of the 3D-OMM, may indicate the potential of its clinical application as a dental restorative material. It was found that 3-YZP supported oral fibroblasts and keratinocytes' cellular attachment and proliferation. There was no cytotoxic damage to the human oral mucosal equivalent, as demonstrated histologically with the preservation of the epithelium layer. However, the 3-YZP had the potential to modulate the secretion of IL-1β, similar to the currently used zirconia (IC).

Author Contributions: Conceptualization, N.A.N. and M.R.; methodology, N.A.N. and M.R.; formal analysis, N.A.N. and W.L.C.; investigation, N.A.N. and M.R.; writing—original draft preparation, N.A.N.; writing—review and editing, M.R., A.M., V.G. and W.L.C.; supervision, M.R., A.M. and V.G.; project administration, M.R.; funding acquisition, A.M. and M.R. All authors have read and agreed to the published version of the manuscript.

Funding: This research is supported by the Universiti Kebangsaan Malaysia Impact Research Grant under code DIP 2019-025.

Institutional Review Board Statement: The study was conducted in accordance with the Declaration of Helsinki and was approved by the Secretariat of Research and Innovation, Faculty of Medicine, Universiti Kebangsaan Malaysia (UKM PPI/111/8/JEP-2020-618), 22nd October 2020.

Informed Consent Statement: Not applicable.

Data Availability Statement: The data presented in this study are available on request from the corresponding author.

Conflicts of Interest: The authors declare no conflict of interest and the funders had no role in the design of the study; in the collection, analyses, or interpretation of data; in the writing of the manuscript, or in the decision to publish the results.

References

1. Amat, N.F.; Muchtar, A.; Amril, M.S.; Ghazali, M.J.; Yahaya, N. Effect of sintering temperature on the aging resistance and mechanical properties of monolithic zirconia. *J. Mater. Res. Technol.* **2019**, *8*, 1092–1101. [CrossRef]
2. Guazzato, M.; Albakry, M.; Ringer, S.P.; Swain, M.V. Strength, fracture toughness and microstructure of a selection of all-ceramic materials. Part I. Pressable and alumina glass-infiltrated ceramics. *Dent. Mater.* **2004**, *20*, 441–448. [CrossRef] [PubMed]
3. Pjetursson, B.E.; Sailer, I.; Makarov, N.A.; Zwahlen, M.; Thoma, D.S. All-ceramic or metal-ceramic tooth-supported fixed dental prostheses (FDPs)? A systematic review of the survival and complication rates. Part II: Multiple-unit FDPs. *Dent. Mater.* **2015**, *31*, 624–639. [CrossRef] [PubMed]
4. Gleiter, H. Nanostructured materials: Basic concepts and microstructure. *Acta Mater.* **2000**, *48*, 1–29. [CrossRef]
5. Hao, C.C.; Muchtar, A.; Azhari, C.H.; Razali, M.; Aboras, M. Fabrication of Y-TZP for dental crowns applications by combining slip casting and cold isostatic pressing. *Malaysian J. Anal. Sci.* **2016**, *20*, 642–650.
6. Schmalz, G.; Hickel, R.; van Landuyt, K.L.; Reichl, F.X. Scientific update on nanoparticles in dentistry. *Int. Dent. J.* **2018**, *68*, 299–305. [CrossRef] [PubMed]
7. Joudeh, N.; Linke, D. Nanoparticle classification, physicochemical properties, characterization, and applications: A comprehensive review for biologists. *J. Nanobiotechnol.* **2022**, *20*, 262. [CrossRef]
8. Agnihotri, R.; Gaur, S.; Albin, S. Nanometals in dentistry: Applications and toxicological implications—A systematic review. *Biol. Trace Elem. Res* **2020**, *197*, 70–88. [CrossRef]
9. Elkassas, D.; Arafa, A. The innovative applications of therapeutic nanostructures in dentistry. *Nanomed. Nanotechnol. Biol. Med.* **2017**, *13*, 1543–1562. [CrossRef]
10. Feng, X.; Chen, A.; Zhang, Y.; Wang, J.; Shao, L.; Wei, L. Application of dental nanomaterials: Potential toxicity to the central nervous system. *Int. J. Nanomed.* **2015**, *10*, 3547–3565. [CrossRef]
11. Chin, C.H.; Muchtar, A.; Azhari, C.H.; Razali, M.; Aboras, M. Influences of the processing method and sintering temperature on the translucency of polycrystalline yttria-stabilized tetragonal zirconia for dental applications. *Ceram. Int.* **2018**, *44*, 18641–18649. [CrossRef]
12. Laiteerapong, A.; Reichl, F.X.; Hickel, R.; Högg, C. Effect of eluates from zirconia-modified glass ionomer cements on DNA double-stranded breaks in human gingival fibroblast cells. *Dent. Mater.* **2019**, *35*, 444–449. [CrossRef] [PubMed]
13. Tabari, K.; Hosseinpour, S.; Parashos, P.; Kardouni Khozestani, P.; Rahimi, H.M. Cytotoxicity of selected nanoparticles on human dental pulp stem cells. *Iran. Endod. J.* **2017**, *12*, 137–142. [CrossRef] [PubMed]
14. Liao, C.; Li, Y.; Tjong, S.C. Bactericidal and cytotoxic properties of silver nanoparticles. *Int. J. Mol. Sci.* **2019**, *20*, 449. [CrossRef]
15. Alzahrani, F.M.; Katubi, K.M.S.; Ali, D.; Alarifi, S. Apoptotic and DNA-damaging effects of yttria-stabilized zirconia nanoparticles on human skin epithelial cells. *Int. J. Nanomed.* **2019**, *14*, 7003–7016. [CrossRef]
16. Ye, M.; Shi, B. Zirconia nanoparticles-induced toxic effects in osteoblast-like 3T3-E1 cells. *Nanoscale Res. Lett.* **2018**, *13*, 353. [CrossRef]
17. Stenken, J.A.; Poschenrieder, A.J. Bioanalytical chemistry of cytokines—A review. *Anal. Chim. Acta* **2015**, *853*, 95–115. [CrossRef]

18. Groeger, S.E.; Meyle, J. Epithelial barrier and oral bacterial infection. *Periodontol. 2000* **2015**, *69*, 46–67. [CrossRef]
19. Dinarello, C.A. Proinflammatory cytokines. *Chest* **2000**, *118*, 503–508. [CrossRef]
20. Faizuddin, M.; Bharathi, S.H.; Rohini, N.V. Estimation of interleukin-1β levels in the gingival crevicular fluid in health and in inflammatory periodontal disease. *J. Periodontal Res.* **2003**, *38*, 111–114. [CrossRef]
21. Nemec, M.; Behm, C.; Maierhofer, V.; Gau, J.; Kolba, A.; Jonke, E.; Rausch-Fan, X.; Andrukhov, O. Effect of titanium and zirconia nanoparticles on human gingival mesenchymal stromal cells. *Int. J. Mol. Sci.* **2022**, *23*, 10022. [CrossRef]
22. Schwarz, F.; Langer, M.; Hagena, T.; Hartig, B.; Sader, R.; Becker, J. Cytotoxicity and proinflammatory effects of titanium and zirconia particles. *Int. J. Implant Dent.* **2019**, *5*, 25. [CrossRef] [PubMed]
23. Salleh, A.; Naomi, R.; Utami, N.D.; Mohammad, A.W.; Mahmoudi, E.; Mustafa, N.; Fauzi, M.B. The potential of silver nanoparticles for antiviral and antibacterial applications: A mechanism of action. *Nanomaterials* **2020**, *10*, 1566. [CrossRef] [PubMed]
24. Rajabi, A.; Ghazali, M.J.; Mahmoudi, E.; Azizkhani, S.; Sulaiman, N.H.; Mohammad, A.W.; Mustafah, N.M.; Ohnmar, H.; Naicker, A.S. Development and antibacterial application of nanocomposites: Effects of molar ratio on Ag2O–CuO nanocomposite synthesised via the microwave-assisted route. *Ceram. Int.* **2018**, *44*, 21591–21598. [CrossRef]
25. Dongari-Bagtzoglou, A.; Kashleva, H. Development of a highly reproducible three-dimensional organotypic model of the oral mucosa. *Nat. Protoc.* **2006**, *1*, 2012–2018. [CrossRef] [PubMed]
26. Chai, W.L.; Moharamzadeh, K.; Brook, I.M.; Emanuelsson, L.; Palmquist, A.; van Noort, R. Development of a novel model for the investigation of implant-soft tissue interface. *J. Periodontol.* **2010**, *81*, 1187–1195. [CrossRef] [PubMed]
27. Khedmat, S.; Sarraf, P.; Seyedjafari, E.; Sanaei-Rad, P.; Noori, F. Comparative evaluation of the effect of cold ceramic and MTA-Angelus on cell viability, attachment and differentiation of dental pulp stem cells and periodontal ligament fibroblasts: An in vitro study. *BMC Oral Health* **2021**, *21*, 628. [CrossRef]
28. Zareidoost, A.; Yousefpour, M.; Ghaseme, B.; Amanzadeh, A. The relationship of surface roughness and cell response of chemical surface modification of titanium. *J. Mater. Sci. Mater. Med.* **2012**, *23*, 1479–1488. [CrossRef] [PubMed]
29. Bollen, C.M.L.; Papaioannou, W.; Van Eldere, J.; Schepers, E.; Quirynen, M.; van Steenberghe, D. The influence of abutment surface roughness on plaque accumulation and peri-implant mucositis. *Clin. Oral Implants Res.* **1996**, *7*, 201–210. [CrossRef]
30. Quirynen, M.; Bollen, C.M.; Papaioannou, W.; Van Eldere, J.; van Steenberghe, D. The influence of titanium abutment surface roughness on plaque accumulation and gingivitis: Short-term observations. *Int. J. Oral Maxillofac. Implants* **1996**, *11*, 169–178.
31. Candido, L.M.; Miotto, L.N.; Fais, L.; Cesar, P.F.; Pinelli, L. Mechanical and surface properties of monolithic zirconia. *Oper. Dent.* **2018**, *43*, E119–E128. [CrossRef]
32. Čokić, S.M.; Vleugels, J.; Van Meerbeek, B.; Camargo, B.; Willems, E.; Li, M.; Zhang, F. Mechanical properties, aging stability and translucency of speed-sintered zirconia for chairside restorations. *Dent. Mater.* **2020**, *36*, 959–972. [CrossRef]
33. Čokić, S.M.; Cóndor, M.; Vleugels, J.; Meerbeek, B.V.; Oosterwyck, H.V.; Inokoshi, M.; Zhang, F. Mechanical properties–translucency–microstructure relationships in commercial monolayer and multilayer monolithic zirconia ceramics. *Dent. Mater.* **2022**, *38*, 797–810. [CrossRef]
34. Lughi, V.; Sergo, V. Low temperature degradation -aging- of zirconia: A critical review of the relevant aspects in dentistry. *Dent. Mater.* **2010**, *26*, 807–820. [CrossRef] [PubMed]
35. Alghazzawi, T.F.; Lemons, J.; Liu, P.R.; Essig, M.E.; Bartolucci, A.A.; Janowski, G.M. Influence of low-temperature environmental exposure on the mechanical properties and structural stability of dental zirconia. *J. Prosthodont.* **2012**, *21*, 363–369. [CrossRef] [PubMed]
36. Aboras, M.; Muchtar, A.; Azhari, C.H.; Yahaya, N.; Mah, J.C.W. Enhancement of the microstructural and mechanical properties of dental zirconia through combined optimized colloidal processing and cold isostatic pressing. *Ceram. Int.* **2019**, *45*, 1831–1836. [CrossRef]
37. Amat, N.F.; Muchtar, A.; Yew, H.Z.; Amril, M.S.; Muhamud, R.L. Machinability of a newly developed pre-sintered zirconia block for dental crown applications. *Mater. Lett.* **2020**, *261*, 126996. [CrossRef]
38. Roffel, S.; Wu, G.; Nedeljkovic, I.; Meyer, M.; Razafiarison, T.; Gibbs, S. Evaluation of a novel oral mucosa in vitro implantation model for analysis of molecular interactions with dental abutment surfaces. *Clin. Implant Dent. Relat. Res.* **2019**, *21*, 25–33. [CrossRef]
39. Soares, D.G.; Sacono, N.T.; Ribeiro, A.P.D.; Leite, M.L.; Duque, C.C.O.; Gallinari, M.O.; Pacheco, L.E.; Hebling, J.; Costa, C.A.S. Pro-inflammatory mediators expression by pulp cells following tooth whitening on restored enamel surface. *Braz. Dent. J.* **2022**, *33*, 83–90. [CrossRef]
40. Barker, E.; AlQobaly, L.; Shaikh, Z.; Franklin, K.; Moharamzadeh, K. Implant soft-tissue attachment using 3D oral mucosal models—A pilot study. *Dent. J.* **2020**, *8*, 72. [CrossRef]
41. Elsabahy, M.; Wooley, K.L. Cytokines as biomarkers of nanoparticle immunotoxicity. *Chem. Soc. Rev.* **2013**, *42*, 5552–5576. [CrossRef]
42. Moharamzadeh, K.; Brook, I.M.; Scutt, A.M.; Thornhill, M.H.; Van Noort, R. Mucotoxicity of dental composite resins on a tissue-engineered human oral mucosal model. *J. Dent.* **2008**, *36*, 331–336. [CrossRef] [PubMed]
43. Mostefaoui, Y.; Claveau, I.; Ross, G.; Rouabhia, M. Tissue structure, and IL-1beta, IL-8, and TNF-alpha secretions after contact by engineered human oral mucosa with dentifrices. *J. Clin. Periodontol.* **2002**, *29*, 1035–1041. [CrossRef]
44. Zingler, S.; Matthei, B.; Diercke, K.; Frese, C.; Ludwig, B.; Kohl, A.; Lux, C.J.; Erber, R. Biological evaluation of enamel sealants in an organotypic model of the human gingiva. *Dent. Mater.* **2014**, *30*, 1039–1051. [CrossRef] [PubMed]

45. Özen, J.; Ural, A.U.; Dalkiz, M.; Beydemir, B. Influence of dental alloys and an all-ceramic material on cell viability and interleukin-1beta release in a three-dimensional cell culture model. *Turk. J. Med. Sci.* **2005**, *35*, 203–208.
46. Aljabali, A.A.; Obeid, M.A.; Bashatwah, R.M.; Serrano-Aroca, A.; Mishra, V.; Mishra, Y.; El-Tanani, M.; Hromic-Jahjefendic, A.; Kapoor, D.N.; Goyal, R.; et al. Nanomaterials and their impact on the immune system. *Int. J. Mol. Sci.* **2023**, *24*, 2008. [CrossRef]
47. Celik, N.; Askin, S.; Gul, M.A.; Seven, N. The effect of restorative materials on cytokines in gingival crevicular fluid. *Arch. Oral Biol.* **2017**, *84*, 139–144. [CrossRef] [PubMed]
48. Cionca, N.; Hashim, D.; Cancela, J.; Giannopoulou, C.; Mombelli, A. Pro-inflammatory cytokines at zirconia implants and teeth. A cross-sectional assessment. *Clin. Oral Investig.* **2016**, *20*, 2285–2291. [CrossRef]
49. Yu, L.; Su, J.; Zou, D.; Mariano, Z. The concentrations of IL-8 and IL-6 in gingival crevicular fluid during nickel–chromium alloy porcelain crown restoration. *J. Mater. Sci. Mater. Med.* **2013**, *24*, 1717–1722. [CrossRef]
50. Ariaans, K.; Heussen, N.; Schiffer, H.; Wienert, A.-L.; Plümäkers, B.; Rink, L.; Wolfart, S. Use of molecular indicators of inflammation to assess the biocompatibility of all-ceramic restorations. *J. Clin. Periodontol.* **2016**, *43*, 173–179. [CrossRef]
51. Saravanakumar, P.; Thallam Veeravalli, P.; Kumar, V.A.; Mohamed, K.; Mani, U.; Grover, M.; Thirumalai Thangarajan, S. Effect of different crown materials on the interleukin-one beta content of gingival crevicular fluid in endodontically treated molars: An original research. *Cureus* **2017**, *9*, e1361. [CrossRef] [PubMed]
52. Moharamzadeh, K.; Franklin, K.L.; Smith, L.E.; Brook, I.M.; van Noort, R. Evaluation of the effects of ethanol on monolayer and 3D models of human oral mucosa. *J. Environ. Anal. Toxicol.* **2015**, *5*, 1. [CrossRef]
53. Vande Vannet, B.; Hanssens, J.L.; Wehrbein, H. The use of three-dimensional oral mucosa cell cultures to assess the toxicity of soldered and welded wires. *Eur. J. Orthod.* **2007**, *29*, 60–66. [CrossRef]
54. Basso, F.G.; Pansani, T.N.; Marcelo, C.L.; de Souza Costa, C.A.; Hebling, J.; Feinberg, S.E. Phenotypic markers of oral keratinocytes seeded on two distinct 3D oral mucosa models. *Toxicol. In Vitro* **2018**, *51*, 34–39. [CrossRef] [PubMed]
55. Maia, L.P.; Novaes, A.B., Jr.; Souza, S.L.; Grisi, M.F.; Taba, M., Jr.; Palioto, D.B. In vitro evaluation of acellular dermal matrix as a three-dimensional scaffold for gingival fibroblasts seeding. *J. Periodontol.* **2011**, *82*, 293–301. [CrossRef]
56. Rodrigues, A.Z.; Oliveira, P.T.; Novaes, A.B., Jr.; Maia, L.P.; Souza, S.L.; Palioto, D.B. Evaluation of in vitro human gingival fibroblast seeding on acellular dermal matrix. *Braz. Dent. J.* **2010**, *21*, 179–189. [CrossRef] [PubMed]
57. Akter, M.; Sikder, M.T.; Rahman, M.M.; Ullah, A.; Hossain, K.F.B.; Banik, S.; Hosokawa, T.; Saito, T.; Kurasaki, M. A systematic review on silver nanoparticles-induced cytotoxicity: Physicochemical properties and perspectives. *J. Adv. Res.* **2018**, *9*, 1–16. [CrossRef] [PubMed]
58. Hamouda, I.M. Current perspectives of nanoparticles in medical and dental biomaterials. *J. Biomed. Res.* **2012**, *26*, 143–151. [CrossRef]
59. Manke, A.; Wang, L.; Rojanasakul, Y. Mechanisms of nanoparticle-induced oxidative stress and toxicity. *Biomed. Res. Int.* **2013**, *2013*, 942916. [CrossRef]
60. Mohammadinejad, R.; Moosavi, M.A.; Tavakol, S.; Vardar, D.; Hosseini, A.; Rahmati, M.; Dini, L.; Hussain, S.; Mandegary, A.; Klionsky, D.J. Necrotic, apoptotic and autophagic cell fates triggered by nanoparticles. *Autophagy* **2019**, *15*, 4–33. [CrossRef]
61. Nosenko, M.A.; Ambaryan, S.G.; Drutskaya, M.S. Proinflammatory cytokines and skin wound healing in mice. *Mol. Biol.* **2019**, *53*, 653–664. [CrossRef]
62. McGinley, E.L.; Moran, G.P.; Fleming, G.J.P. Base-metal dental casting alloy biocompatibility assessment using a human-derived three-dimensional oral mucosal model. *Acta Biomater.* **2012**, *8*, 432–438. [CrossRef] [PubMed]
63. Nowicka, A.; El-Maghraby, H.F.; Švančárková, A.; Galusková, D.; Reveron, H.; Gremillard, L.; Chevalier, J.; Galusek, D. Corrosion and low temperature degradation of 3Y-TZP dental ceramics under acidic conditions. *J. Eur. Ceram. Soc.* **2020**, *40*, 6114–6122. [CrossRef]

Disclaimer/Publisher's Note: The statements, opinions and data contained in all publications are solely those of the individual author(s) and contributor(s) and not of MDPI and/or the editor(s). MDPI and/or the editor(s) disclaim responsibility for any injury to people or property resulting from any ideas, methods, instructions or products referred to in the content.

Article
Cutting Efficiency of Diamond Grinders on Composite and Zirconia

Martin Rosentritt, Thomas Strasser, Maerit-Martha Mueller and Michael Benno Schmidt *

Department of Prosthetic Dentistry, UKR University Hospital Regensburg, 93042 Regensburg, Germany
* Correspondence: michael3.schmidt@ukr.de

Abstract: This in vitro study was carried out to compare the cutting efficiency of diamond grinders on zirconia and resin-based composite materials. Grinders were employed with a special holder for the handpiece to apply a constant load (160 g) for resin-based composite (8 cuts, 40 s each) and zirconia materials (4 cuts, 5 min each; n = 10 for each material and grinder). To assess the efficiency of the grinders, weight measurements of the material were taken before and after the grinding process. Scanning electron micrographs were captured for instrument surfaces before and after testing and for the resulting surface of the materials. In the resin-based composite group, there were significant differences in weight removal between the burs for both the baseline (first cut; $p = 0.009$) and removal after the eighth cut ($p = 0.049$). Statistically significant decreases in weight removal compared to the baseline values were noted for the third, fourth, sixth, and seventh steps ($p \leq 0.046$). For the zirconia group, significant differences existed in weight removal between the burs for the baseline (first cut; $p < 0.001$) and removal after the fourth cut ($p < 0.001$). A significant positive correlation was observed between removal and the number of cuts (Pearson: 0.673; $p < 0.001$). A statistically significant decrease in removal compared to the respective baseline value was found for the fourth step ($p = 0.006$). The initial wear removal and durability significantly differed between the grinders used on resin-based composite and zirconia. Achieving comparable weight removal took five times longer when grinding zirconia compared to the resin-based composite.

Keywords: diamond; grinder; composite; zirconia; cutting efficiency

1. Introduction

Resin-based composite and zirconia are common and widespread as computer-aided design (CAD) and computer-aided manufacturing (CAM) materials for dental applications. With their different material properties, they represent the extreme upper and lower limits of hardness (210 HV vs. 380 HV), modulus (15 GPa vs. 210 GPa), and strength (330 MPa vs. 1200 MPa) of tooth-colored materials and therefore place different demands on handling and grinding [1–7].

These materials are customarily processed with diamond grinders in clinical practice, predominantly to shape the form or to adjust the occlusion [8]. The diamonds are furthermore used to remove, adjust, or polish prosthetic restorations. Extra- or super-coarse (125–180 µm), coarse (100–150 µm), and regular (75–125 µm) diamonds are used for significant material reduction, whereas fine (20–40 µm), super-fine (10–30 µm), and ultra-fine (4–14 µm) diamonds are applied for grinding and polishing [9]. In dental practice the grinders are distinguished between ultra-fine (white, M 4–M 14; 8 µm), extra-fine (yellow, M 10–M 36; 25 µm), fine (red, M 27–D 76; 46 µm), medium (blue, D 64–D 126; 107 µm), coarse (green, D 107–D 181; 151 µm), and very coarse (black, D 151–D 213; 181 µm).

The properties of diamond grinders are determined by certain specifications: They are offered with a high variation in the amount, type, shape, and size of the diamonds, resulting in different cutting efficiencies and lifespans of the bur. Burs should sustain optimal cutting efficiency throughout the treatment. Various metrics can be employed to assess cutting efficiency, for example, changes in the weight of the test substrate over a certain time, volumetric cutting rate, and depth of cut over a fixed time [10–13].

These parameters depend on the design and fabrication of the grinders and can therefore vary greatly. Newer studies with a similar experimental set up to ours showed that a single patient bur is more effective than a multi-patient bur and that diamond burs are more effective for cutting zirconia than tungsten burs [14,15].

Therefore, the purpose of the present study was to compare the cutting efficiency of diamond grinders on zirconia and resin-based composite CAD/CAM materials. The hypothesis of this study was that different types of diamond grinders with different diameters do not show different removal capacity on the materials.

2. Materials and Methods

Specimens of zirconia or resin-based composite were ground with different grinders. The resulting weight removal was determined by measuring the difference in weight (MXX-612, Denver Instrument, Behemia, NY, USA) of the specimens before and after the grinding process. A special holder for the handpiece was developed to ensure a reproducible load (160 g) and grinding process. Due to the different material properties and significantly different removal efficiency, the time and number of grinding steps varied between the two materials. Pretests on the individual materials were performed to determine material dependent grinding time and number of grinding steps. Four cuts were made per side of each blank (Figure 1). Because a grinder lasts significantly longer and is more effective during use on resin-based composite, 8 cuts, 40 seconds each were used for the resin-based material and 4 cuts, 5 min. each for zirconia. All values for the weight removal were statistically compared to the weight removal after the first cut (baseline). Ten specimens were investigated for every material and grinder system. Statistical analysis was performed with one-way ANOVA, Bonferroni, and Pearson comparison (α = 0.05, SPSS, Chicago, IL, USA).

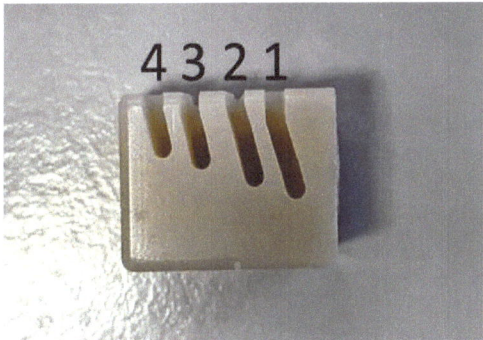

Figure 1. Exemplary grinding steps 1–4 on resin-based composite.

For resin-based composite (Grandio blocs 14L A3.5 HT; VOCO, D), instruments (Z881-016C-FG "ABACUS"; 881-016C-FG; 881-014TC-FG "TURBO"; 881-014C-FG; NTI-Kahla, D; 6881.314.016; 6881.314.014; Komet Dental, D) were used in 8 steps for 40 seconds per step (n = 10, Table 1). Resin-based composite blanks were used as delivered.

For 3Y-TZP zirconia (Cercon base 30 colored; Dentsply, D), instruments (K881-016M-FG "Z-CUT"; 881-016M-FG; all NTI-Kahla, 881.314.016; Komet Dental, D) were used in 4 steps for 5 minutes per step (n = 10, Table 1). 3Y-TZP blanks were cut into cubes (12 mm × 14 mm × 18 mm) and sintered (1350 °C; Cercon heat, Dentsply, D) before testing.

Table 1. Instruments for resin-based composite and zirconia treatment (*: NTI-Kahla; D; °: all Komet Dental, D#; all grinders: l = 8 mm; speed for all: 200,000 rpm).

Material		Diameter [mm]	Type/Diameter		Comment	Comment	Composition/ Properties
Resin-based Composite	Grandio blocs 14L A3.5 HT; VOCO, D	1.6	Z881-016C-FG "ABACUS" *	CS16	Abacus diamond, special coating	8 cuts/40 s per cut	Urethandimethcrylate, dimethycrylate, 86 wt. % filler, flexural strength 220 MPa, E-modulus 18 GPa, Vickers HV 122
			881-016C-FG *	CA16	Diamond, galvanic bond		
			6881.314.016 °	CB16			
		1.4	881-014C-FG *	CA14	Diamond, galvanic bond		
			6881.314.014 °	CB14			
			881-014TC-FG "TURBO" *	CS14	Diamond, spiral form		
	Cercon base 30 colored; DeguDent, D	1.6	K881-016M-FG "Z-CUT" *	ZS16	Special diamond/bond	4 cuts/5 min per cut	Yttriumoxide 5%, hafniumoxide <3%, aluminiumoxide, siliziumoxide, oxide <2%, flexural strength 1200 MPa, E-modulus 210 GPa, Vickers HV1 380
			881-016M-FG *	ZA16	Diamond, galvanic bond		
			881.314.016 °	ZB16			

Scanning electron microscopy (SEM, Phenom, FEI; magnification 500×, working distance ~480 μm) of the instrument surfaces were taken before and after testing. The resulting surfaces on the specimens were also imaged by scanning electron microscopy.

3. Results

3.1. Resin-Based Composite

The measured weight removal for the resin-based composite varied between 0.25 ± 0.05 g (CS16; first step) and 0.09 ± 0.05 g (CB16; eight step). For all instruments, a continuous decrease in weight removal was observed as the number of cuts increased. The baseline removal (first cut; $p = 0.009$) and the removal after the eight cut ($p = 0.049$) were significantly different between the burs. The removal and number of the cuts showed no correlation (Pearson: -0.27, $p = 0.333$). A statistically significant ($p \leq 0.046$) decrease in the weight removal compared to the respective baseline value was shown for the third step (CS16; CS14), fourth step (CA14; CB14), sixth step (CB16) and seventh step (CA16). Figure 2 and Table 2 show the weight removal after the individual cuts. The different diameters in identical groups showed no significant differences ($p = 0.069$) for lower weight reduction.

Table 2. Weight loss [mg] for resin-based composite (mean, standard deviation, statistical comparison ANOVA, Bonferroni, $\alpha = 0.05$).

	Mean	Std	Mean	Std	1st Significant Step to 1st Cut	Bonferoni Comparison (Cut 1:Cut 8)
	1st cut		8th cut			p
CS16	0.21	0.03	0.13	0.05	4	<0.001
CA16	0.25	0.05	0.16	0.05	7	0.023
CB16	0.21	0.06	0.09	0.05	6	0.001
CS14	0.24	0.03	0.12	0.06	3	<0.001
CA14	0.23	0.03	0.13	0.05	4	<0.001
CB14	0.19	0.02	0.11	0.02	4	<0.001
p	0.009		0.049			

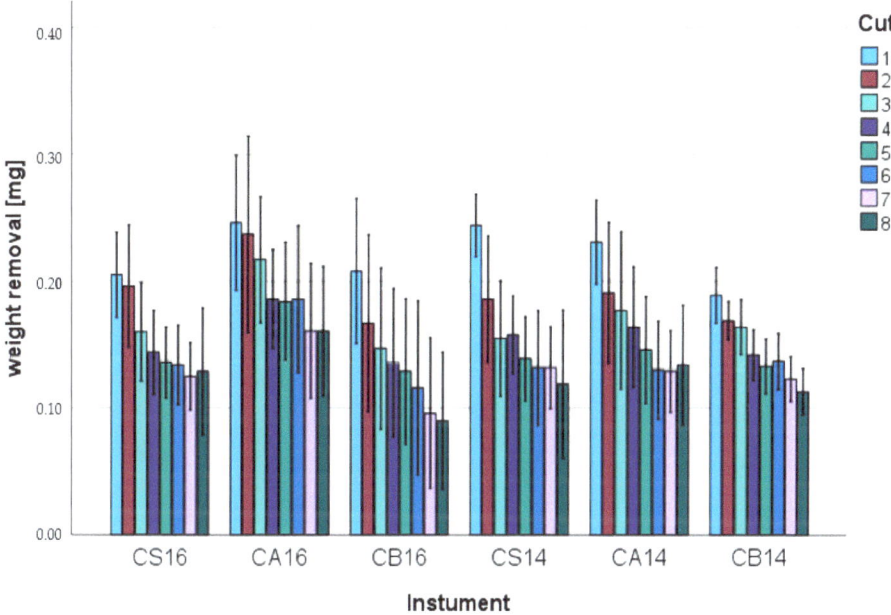

Figure 2. Weight loss [mg] for resin-based composite.

3.2. Zirconia

The weight removal for zirconia varied between 0.21 ± 0.05 g (ZA16; first step) and 0.07 ± 0.01 g (ZS16; third step). For both standard instruments, a continuous decrease in weight removal was observed as the number of cuts increased. The baseline removal (first cut; $p < 0.001$) and the removal after the fourth cut ($p < 0.001$) were significantly different between the burs. The removal and number of cuts showed a significant correlation (Pearson: 0.673; $p < 0.001$). A statistically significant ($p = 0.006$) decrease in the removal compared to the respective baseline value was shown for the fourth step (ZB16). The instruments (ZS16, ZA16) did not show a statistically significant decrease in removal ($p = 1.000$ for ZS16) compared to the baseline value ($p \geq 0.056$ for ZA16). Figure 3 and Table 3 show the weight removal after the individual cuts.

Table 3. Weight loss [mg] for zirconia (mean, standard deviation, statistical comparison ANOVA, Bonferroni, α = 0.05).

	Mean	Std	Mean	Std	1st Significant Step to 1st Cut	Bonferroni
	1st cut		4th cut			p
ZS16	0.08	0.02	0.07	0.01	--	1.000
ZA16	0.21	0.05	0.15	0.04	--	0.056
ZB16	0.20	0.02	0.15	0.04	4	0.006
	$p < 0.001$		$p < 0.001$			

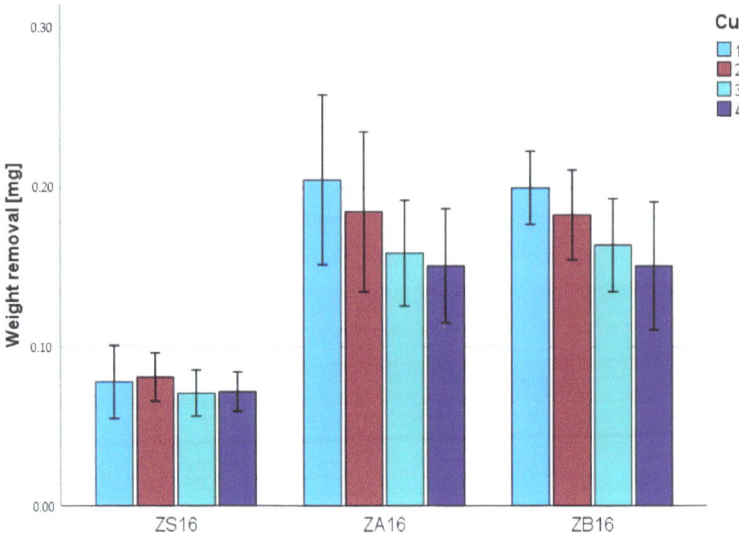

Figure 3. Weight loss [mg] for zirconia.

The scanning electron microscopy (SEM) images showed that the reduced weight removal was primarily due to wear of the diamonds. Rounding of the profile of the individual diamond grains and wear and loss of material along the contours were observed. Only in the case of the ZB16 instrument was a complete loss of diamond particles observed. For the diamonds of instrument ZS16, no superficial wear traces or damage were seen in the SEM images (Figure 4).

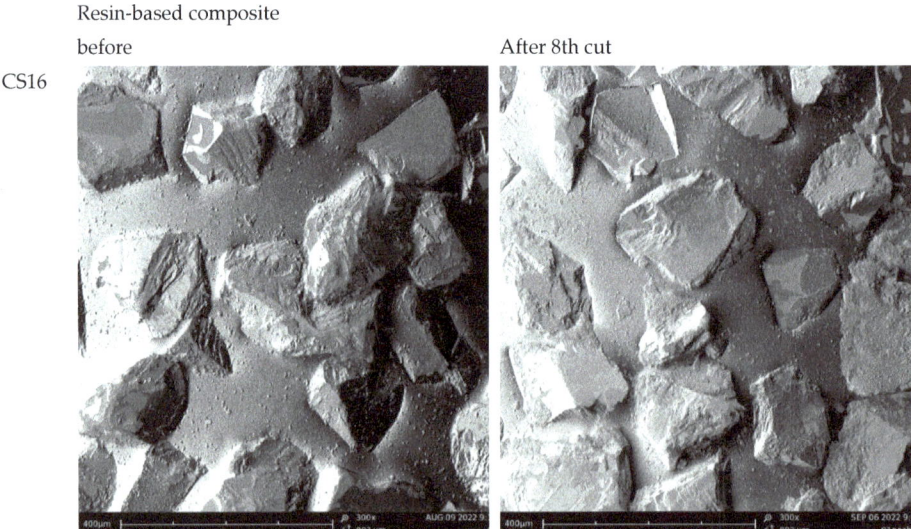

Figure 4. *Cont.*

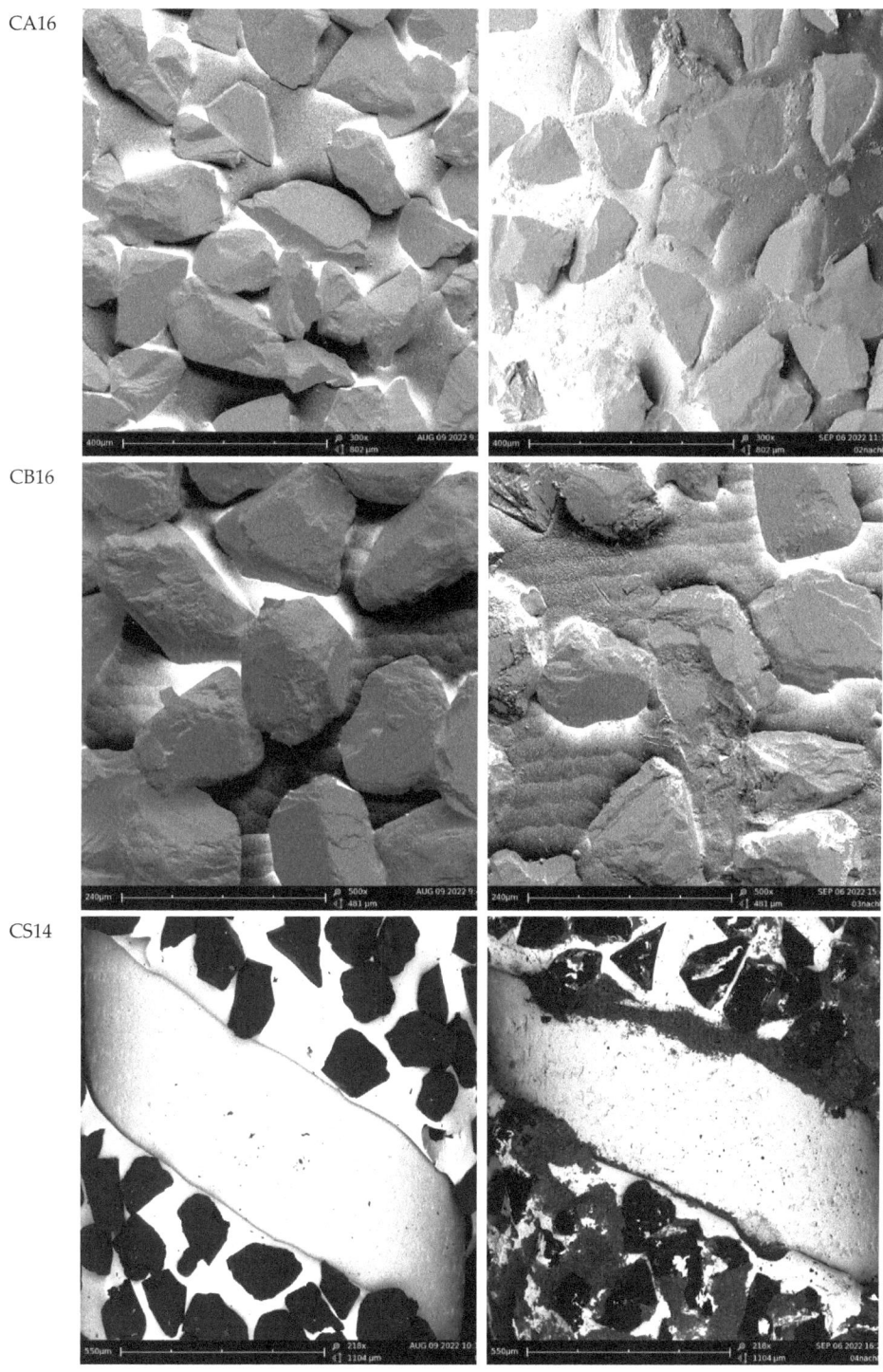

Figure 4. *Cont.*

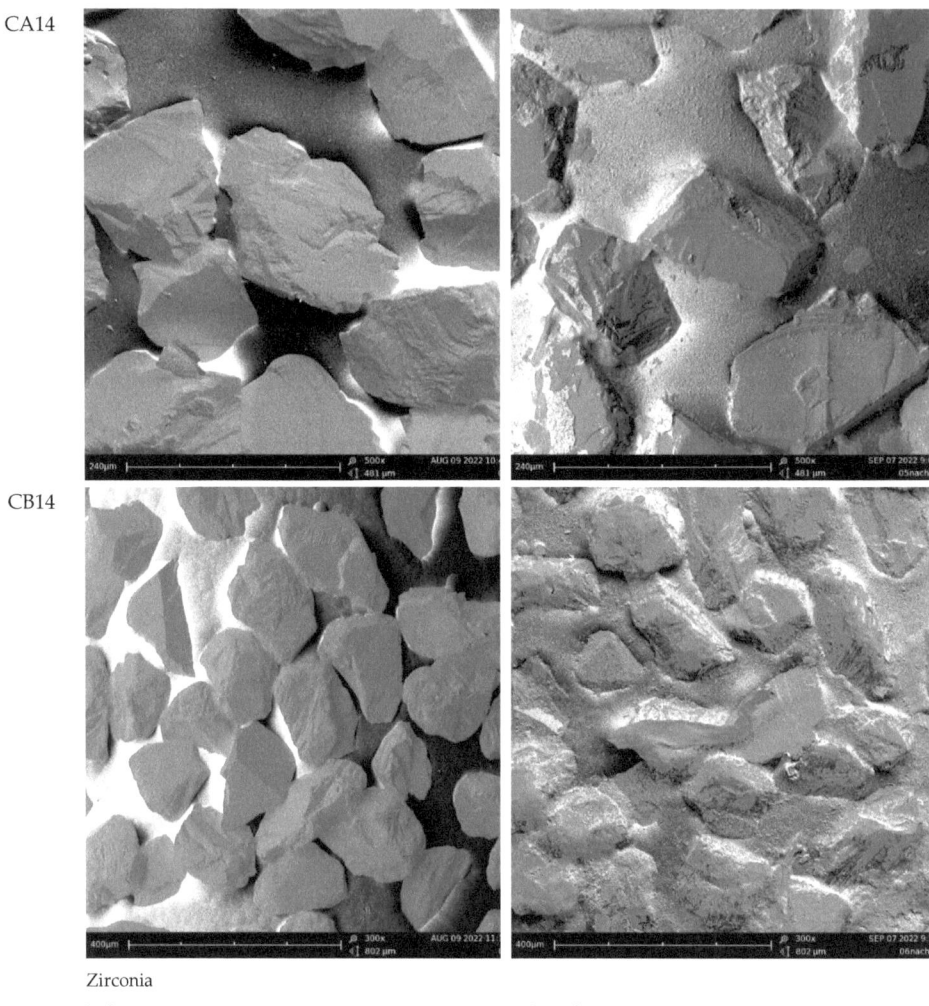

Figure 4. *Cont.*

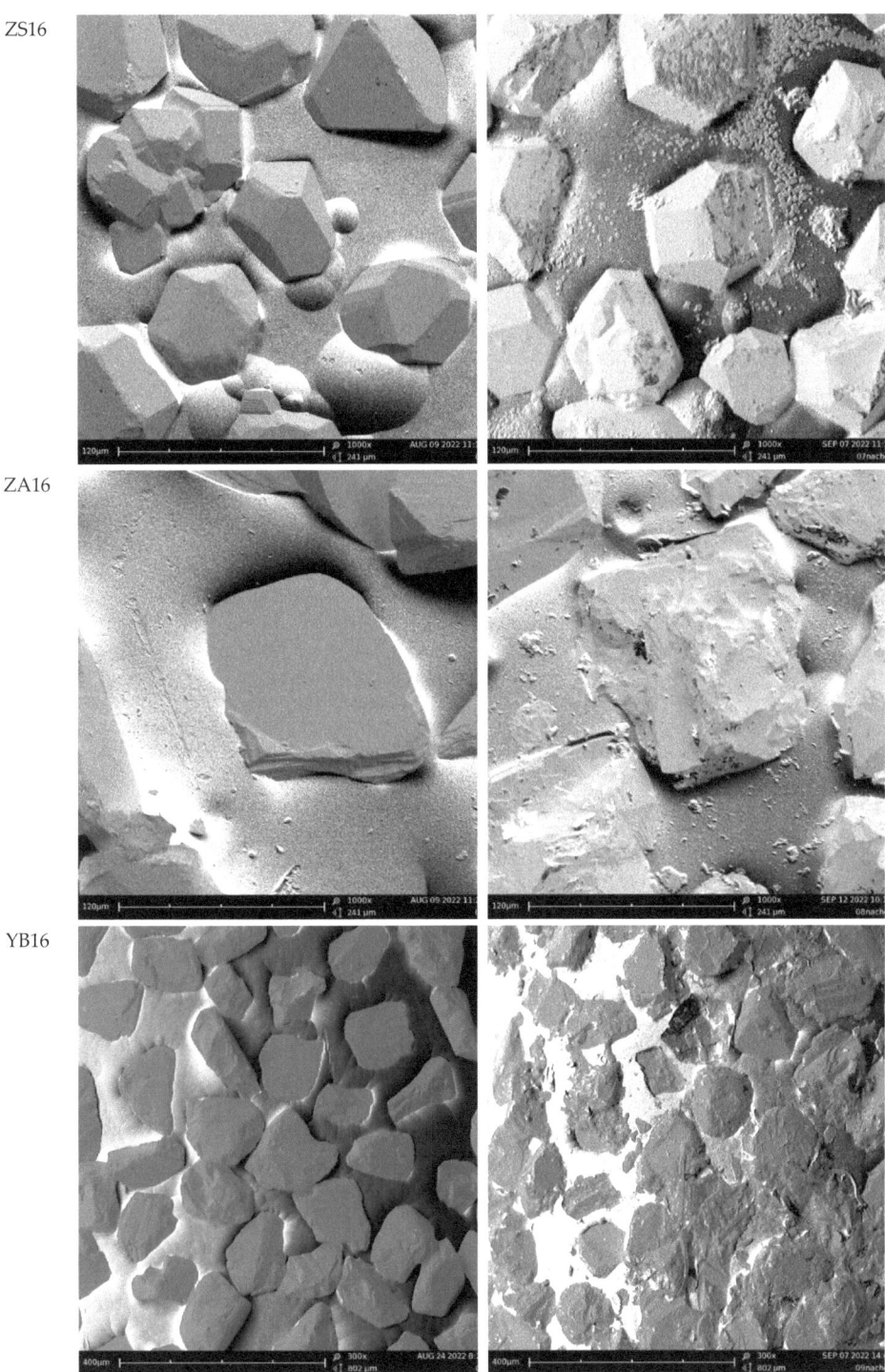

Figure 4. SEM images of the grinder surface before and after use.

4. Discussion

The hypothesis of this study that different types of diamond grinders do not show different removal capacity on the materials considered here could not be confirmed. The weight reduction of the investigated instruments varied significantly between the different grinder systems. The influence of the grinder diameter (1.4 mm vs. 1.6 mm) on the processing of the composite could not be confirmed.

4.1. Resin-Based Composite

The systems examined differed significantly in their initial weight removal for the resin-based composite. The maximal weight reduction was between 0.19 and 0.25 mg for the different diamond systems after the first cut. None of the grinders exceeded eight cuts without a reduction in cutting performance. Similar behavior has already been observed for resin-based composite treatment [16].

However, clear differences could be found: A significant reduction in weight removal, towards the initial weight removal at the first cutting run, was achieved between three and seven cuts. The conventional grinders showed slight advantages over the special grinders. Conventional grinders with larger diameters only showed advantages in the initial cut. One conventional system showed the highest weight results even after eight cuts. The systems examined differed significantly in their final weight removal after eight cuts. For the 1.6 mm grinders, the special coating of the diamonds did not provide any advantages. For the 1.4 mm grinders, the special turbo grinder provided slight advantages in terms of the initial removal but was at the same level as the conventional grinders in the final removal stage. Further studies should be carried out to determine whether such a geometry may have any advantages in terms of a better cooling effect and a more effective removal of the preparation material due to the increased water supply. The SEM images showed undisturbed diamonds, and small amounts of debris were present in the spiral. However, the spiral apparently remained almost free of abraded particles. In contrast to conventional instruments, the special instruments (ABACUS) are diamond-coated using a special process with one matrix (UniMatrix) instead of several matrix steps for conventional systems. The abacus systems have a special layer applied after diamond coating, which is intended to enable the instrument to last longer due to the higher overall hardness. With this technology, the grinder is expected to have a higher diamond density than conventional diamond drills. Further on, this process is supposed to even the grain distribution and define the chip spaces for all diamond grinders. The SEM pictures partly confirm this, showing fewer exposed diamonds in comparison to the conventional coating systems.

4.2. Zirconia

On zirconia, both conventional instruments showed a clear loss in weight removal of about 25% after the fourth cut, which was only significant for one grinder. Conventional diamond burs, which are not specifically marketed for cutting zirconia, sometimes prove to be just as efficient as special diamond burs [17,18]. The weight removal with the first cut was approximately 20 mg and thus clearly higher in comparison to that of the instrument with the special diamonds with approximately half the weight removal. The results confirm the good cutting performance of diamond on zirconia [15]. In contrast, Gonzaga et al. found that the cutting efficiency did not decrease as the number of cuts increased [19]. The SEM images showed clear wear and erosion of the diamonds in the standard systems. Interestingly, however, the removal level for the special grinder remained at the same low level even after four applications. Together with the SEM images, this could be an indication of the good integrity and stability of the special diamond size and nickel coating of the ZS16 system. In contrast to the conventional systems, the structure of the diamonds was completely retained. If the weight removal of this system could be improved, it might be a good option for the sustainable machining of zirconia. The special bond of the Z-Cut instruments in combination with harder diamond grit is supposed to match to the extreme strength of zirconia ceramic to extend service life and improve cutting efficiency. The special character of the diamonds is confirmed by the SEM images, showing a clearly more geometric form of the diamonds. In addition to the special diamonds, all the other diamonds showed clear abrasion due to the cutting steps. Diamond grit fracture was the most dominant wear pattern. As a result of the diamond treatment, the zirconia surfaces were expected to show plastic deformation as evidence of ductile cutting [18]. Zirconia blocks, which were machined with fine grit diamond instruments, showed the least incidence of surface flaws. Consequently, fine-grain diamond instruments showed the lowest number of surface defects [18]. Fine-grit instruments (between 40 and 50 μm) were shown to be most efficient, achieving a high cutting depth without macroscopic damage to the zirconia [20].

The limitations of this study are certainly that only the weight loss criterion was determined. Although it was possible to differentiate between the different amounts of weight removal, the overall level was low. Interestingly, the level of weight loss for the weaker composites was only slightly higher (up to 20%) than that for the significantly harder and stronger zirconia. This could be due to the uniform geometry of the grinders or to a comparable size and arrangement of the diamonds on the surface of the grinder. It was also interesting that the weight loss after four cuts on the zirconia and composite was at a similar level. However, the different grinding times of 40 s (composite) and 5 min (zirconia) must be taken into account. As expected, the processing of zirconia takes considerably longer due to the different material properties [21]. It was shown that hardness, E-modulus, and flexural strength have an influence on grinding performance. Zirconia had to be ground five times longer to achieve the same weight removal as for the resin-based composite.

5. Conclusions

The grinders used on resin-based composite and zirconia provided significantly different initial wear removal and durability. The grinders had comparable durability on the zirconia and resin-based composite. Grinding on zirconia took five times longer to achieve comparable weight removal.

Author Contributions: M.R.: conceptualization, supervision, writing—review and editing; T.S.: conceptualization, supervision, investigation and editing; M.-M.M.: review and editing; M.B.S.: writing, review and editing. All authors have read and agreed to the published version of the manuscript.

Funding: This research received external funding from NTI.

Institutional Review Board Statement: Not applicable.

Informed Consent Statement: Not applicable.

Data Availability Statement: The authors state that they did not use any external data.

Conflicts of Interest: The authors declare no conflicts of interest.

References

1. Yamaguchi, S.; Katsumoto, Y.; Hayashi, K.; Aoki, M.; Kunikata, M.; Nakase, Y.; Lee, C.; Imazato, S. Fracture origin and crack propagation of CAD/CAM composite crowns by combining of in vitro and in silico approaches. *J. Mech. Behav. Biomed. Mater.* **2020**, *112*, 104083. [CrossRef] [PubMed]
2. Karaer, O.; Yamaguchi, S.; Nakase, Y.; Lee, C.; Imazato, S. In silico non-linear dynamic analysis reflecting in vitro physical properties of CAD/CAM resin composite blocks. *J. Mech. Behav. Biomed. Mater.* **2020**, *104*, 103697. [CrossRef] [PubMed]
3. Belli, R.; Wendler, M.; de Ligny, D.; Cicconi, M.R.; Petschelt, A.; Peterlik, H.; Lohbauer, U. Chairside CAD/CAM materials. Part 1: Measurement of elastic constants and microstructural characterization. *Dent. Mater.* **2017**, *33*, 84–98. [CrossRef] [PubMed]
4. Wendler, M.; Belli, R.; Petschelt, A.; Mevec, D.; Harrer, W.; Lube, T.; Danzer, R.; Lohbauer, U. Chairside CAD/CAM materials. Part 2: Flexural strength testing. *Dent. Mater.* **2017**, *33*, 99–109. [CrossRef] [PubMed]
5. Stawarczyk, B.; Liebermann, A.; Eichberger, M.; Guth, J.-F. Evaluation of mechanical and optical behavior of current esthetic dental restorative CAD/CAM composites. *J. Mech. Behav. Biomed. Mater.* **2015**, *55*, 1–11. [CrossRef] [PubMed]
6. Bruhnke, M.; Awwad, Y.; Müller, W.-D.; Beuer, F.; Schmidt, F. Mechanical Properties of New Generations of Monolithic, Multi-Layered Zirconia. *Materials* **2022**, *16*, 276. [CrossRef] [PubMed]

7. Machry, R.V.; Dapieve, K.S.; Cadore-Rodrigues, A.C.; Werner, A.; de Jager, N.; Pereira, G.K.R.; Valandro, L.F.; Kleverlaan, C.J. Mechanical characterization of a multi-layered zirconia: Flexural strength, hardness, and fracture toughness of the different layers. *J. Mech. Behav. Biomed. Mater.* **2022**, *135*, 105455. [CrossRef] [PubMed]
8. Strasser, T.; Preis, V.; Behr, M.; Rosentritt, M. Roughness, surface energy, and superficial damages of CAD/CAM materials after surface treatment. *Clin. Oral. Investig.* **2018**, *22*, 2787–2797. [CrossRef] [PubMed]
9. Hetou, S. Comparison of Cutting Efficiency of Different Rotary Instruments, on Two Different Ceramic Materials Using Electric and Air-Turbine Dental Hand-Pieces. Master Thesis, Nova Southeastern University, Fort Lauderdale, FL, USA, 2018.
10. Watanabe, I.; Ohkubo, C.; Ford, J.P.; Atsuta, M.; Okabe, T. Cutting efficiency of air-turbine burs on cast titanium and dental casting alloys. *Dent. Mater.* **2000**, *16*, 420–425. [CrossRef] [PubMed]
11. Fais, L.M.G.; Pinelli, L.A.P.; Adabo, G.L.; Silva, R.H.B.T.D.; Marcelo, C.C.; Guaglianoni, D.G. Influence of microwave sterilization on the cutting capacity of carbide burs. *J. Appl. Oral Sci.* **2009**, *17*, 584–589. [CrossRef] [PubMed]
12. Pilcher, E.S.; Tietge, J.D.; Draughn, R.A. Comparison of cutting rates among single-patent-use and multiple-patient-use diamond burs. *J. Prosthodont.* **2000**, *9*, 66–70. [CrossRef] [PubMed]
13. Chung, E.M.; Sung, E.C.; Wu, B.; Caputo, A.A. Comparing cutting efficiencies of diamond burs using a high-speed electric handpiece. *Gen. Dent.* **2006**, *54*, 254–257. [PubMed]
14. Keeling, F.L.; Taft, R.M.; Haney, S.J. Bur choice when removing zirconia restorations. *J. Prosthodont.* **2023**, *32*, 347–352. [CrossRef] [PubMed]
15. Peters, O.A.; Du, D.; Ho, M.Y.; Chu, R.; Moule, A. Assessing the cutting efficiency of different burs on zirconia substrate. *Aust. Endod. J.* **2019**, *45*, 289–297. [CrossRef] [PubMed]
16. Ceylan, G.; Emir, F.; Doğdu, C.; Demirel, M.; Özcan, M. Effect of repeated millings on the surface integrity of diamond burs and roughness of different CAD/CAM materials. *Clin. Oral Investig.* **2022**, *26*, 5325–5337. [CrossRef]
17. Hunziker, S.; Thorpe, L.; Zitzmann, N.U.; Rohr, N. Evaluation of diamond rotary instruments marketed for removing zirconia restorations. *J. Prosthet. Dent.* **2022**, *131*, 895–902. [CrossRef]
18. Kim, J.-S.; Bae, J.-H.; Yun, M.-J.; Huh, J.-B. In vitro assessment of cutting efficiency and durability of zirconia removal diamond rotary instruments. *J. Prosthet. Dent.* **2017**, *117*, 775–783. [CrossRef] [PubMed]
19. Gonzaga, C.C.; Spina, D.R.F.; de Paiva Bertoli, F.M.; Feres, R.L.; Fernandes, A.B.F.; da Cunha, L.F. Cutting efficiency of different diamond burs after repeated cuts and sterilization cycles in autoclave. *Indian J. Dent. Res.* **2019**, *30*, 915–919. [CrossRef] [PubMed]
20. van Aswegen, A.; Jagathpal, A.J.; Sykes, L.M.; Schoeman, H. A comparative study of the cutting efficiency of diamond rotary instruments with different grit sizes with a low-speed electric handpiece against zirconia specimens. *J. Prosthet. Dent.* **2023**, *131*, 101.e1–101.e8. [CrossRef] [PubMed]
21. Nakamura, K.; Katsuda, Y.; Ankyu, S.; Harada, A.; Tenkumo, T.; Kanno, T.; Niwano, Y.; Egusa, H.; Milleding, P.; Örtengren, U. Cutting efficiency of diamond burs operated with electric high-speed dental handpiece on zirconia. *Eur. J. Oral Sci.* **2015**, *123*, 375–380. [CrossRef] [PubMed]

Disclaimer/Publisher's Note: The statements, opinions and data contained in all publications are solely those of the individual author(s) and contributor(s) and not of MDPI and/or the editor(s). MDPI and/or the editor(s) disclaim responsibility for any injury to people or property resulting from any ideas, methods, instructions or products referred to in the content.

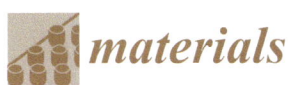

Article

Effect of Sandblasting Parameters and the Type and Hardness of the Material on the Number of Embedded Al$_2$O$_3$ Grains

Beata Śmielak [1,*], Leszek Klimek [2] and Kamil Krześniak [3]

1 Department of Dental Prosthodontics, Medical University of Lodz, ul. Pomorska 251, 92-213 Lodz, Poland
2 Institute of Materials Engineering, Lodz University of Technology, ul. Stefanowskiego 1/15, 90-924 Lodz, Poland; leszek.klimek@p.lodz.pl
3 Pomeranian Medical University, ul. Rybacka 1, 70-204 Szczecin, Poland; kamil.krzesniak@gmail.com
* Correspondence: beata.smielak@umed.lodz.pl

Abstract: Background: Is abrasive blasting accompanied by the phenomenon of driving abrasive particles into the conditioned material? Methods: Three hundred and fifteen cylindrical disks of three types of metal alloy (chromium/cobalt, chromium/nickel, titanium, and sintered zirconium dioxide) were divided into four groups (n = 35) and sandblasted at pressures of 0.2, 0.4, or 0.6 MPa with aluminum oxide (Al$_2$O$_3$), grain size 50, 110, or 250 μm. Then, the surface topography was examined using a scanning microscope, and the amount of embedded grain was measured using quantitative metallography. For each group, five samples were randomly selected and subjected to Vickers hardness testing. In the statistical analyses, a three-factor analysis of variance was carried out, considering the type of material, the size of gradation of the abrasive, and the amount of pressure. Results: The smallest amounts of embedded abrasive (2.62) were observed in the ZrO$_2$ treatment, and the largest (38.19) occurred in the treatment of the Ti alloy. An increase in the gradation and the pressure were a systematic increase in the amount of embedded grain. Conclusions: After abrasive blasting, abrasive particles were found on the surface of the materials. The amount of driven abrasive depends on the hardness of the processed material.

Keywords: abrasive blasting; Cr/Co alloy; Ni/Cr alloy; Ti; ZrO$_2$

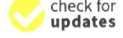

Citation: Śmielak, B.; Klimek, L.; Krześniak, K. Effect of Sandblasting Parameters and the Type and Hardness of the Material on the Number of Embedded Al$_2$O$_3$ Grains. *Materials* **2023**, *16*, 4783. https://doi.org/10.3390/ma16134783

Academic Editors: Lavinia Cosmina Ardelean and Laura-Cristina Rusu

Received: 20 May 2023
Revised: 25 June 2023
Accepted: 30 June 2023
Published: 2 July 2023

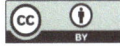

Copyright: © 2023 by the authors. Licensee MDPI, Basel, Switzerland. This article is an open access article distributed under the terms and conditions of the Creative Commons Attribution (CC BY) license (https://creativecommons.org/licenses/by/4.0/).

1. Introduction

Abrasive blasting involves cutting with loose abrasive grain at high speed that generates kinetic energy sufficient to cut. Compressed air, water under pressure (hydro-abrasive treatment), steam, or another medium can be used to set the abrasive grains in motion [1]. Abrasive grains with sharp edges, hitting the treated surface, transfer their impulse completely or partially to a specific area [2,3]. The course of treatment depends on the geometric characteristics of the stream, its energy, and its composition [4]. As a result of abrasive blasting, the obtained surface of the processed material with a different texture. The geometric structure of the surface obtained after machining depends on the variable parameters of the machining process, which include the type of abrasive, the shape and size of abrasive grains, the pressure of the working medium, and the angle of the abrasive stream hitting the surface. The distance of the nozzle from the sandblasted surface can also be a variable. Individual variable process parameters affect the diversification of the surface condition [2–4].

The roughness of the surface increases the adhesion of various types of coatings and, at the same time, increases the strength of the connection with the substrate [5,6]. This is a routine method of cleaning castings made from metal alloys; it allows the creation of mechanical "hooks" for anchoring applied fired ceramic masses. This procedure increases the strength of the bond with the veneering ceramic by developing the surface and increasing the contact area between the phases [2,4]. Properly produced rough surfaces can support the distribution of stresses by increasing the dissipation of energy during the action of breaking forces on the connection of materials [7]. During the machining of metal alloys, weakly attached overhangs and alloy flakes produced in the grinding process are also removed, which ensures better surface wettability and better anchoring of deposited coatings [8,9]. In addition, in the process of abrasive blasting, we obtain a comparable, uniform surface condition, which is also important for the creation of a more durable connection of materials [10–12].

Ceramic forms a stronger bond with Co/Cr and Ni/Cr alloys than with titanium. Many studies have confirmed a two- or three-fold difference in the strength of such connections with Co/Cr or Ni/Cr alloys compared to titanium alloys [13–16]. Other studies have found that the adhesion force of porcelain to titanium alloy was 47–64% of that for Cr/Ni alloy—ceramics [17,18]. However, it should be emphasized that the surface roughness played a major role by creating a better anchorage of the ceramics to the metal substrate. Derand and Herø [13] observed that the use of 250 µm alumina abrasive blasting significantly improved the bonding strength of the ceramic to the titanium alloy compared to 50 µm, which may suggest that the embedded particles have a positive effect. It should be emphasized that this is the only way to increase the strength of the connection in the titanium-ceramic system due to the properties of titanium. Yamada et al. [15] examined the adhesion of ceramics to titanium and revealed that abrasive blasting is a very effective method of surface preparation. The adhesion of ceramics to titanium was almost twice as high as compared to that observed in polished samples [19,20].

However, in the case of some metal alloys, such as stainless steel, copper, or titanium alloys, increasing roughness accelerates corrosion [21–23]. In addition, during abrasive blasting, abrasive particles with high kinetic energy can stick to the workpiece, which can lead to contamination of the surface [14,24]. Derand and Herø [13] found that Al_2O_3 particles could invade up to 10 µm into the treated samples. The contaminated area may hence have less available surface area for connection with ceramics. Gilbert et al. [12] showed that contamination of the titanium surface weakens the mechanical anchoring of dental ceramics, reduces corrosion resistance, and deteriorates the biocompatibility of the material. Additionally, impurities change the topography of the surface, creating a structural discontinuity, which may result in the formation of cracks in the veneering porcelain [25].

Driving abrasive grains with high kinetic energy into the treated surface of prosthetic materials has great practical consequences. Undoubtedly, the particles left in the material contaminate the surface of the treated substrate and reduce the smoothness of the surface [12,21]. With regard to porcelain firing on machined surfaces, the role of embedded particles is not entirely clear. On the one hand, they develop the treated surface, which can improve the quality of the connection; on the other, they can be places where cracks in ceramics can occur [7,21]. There is a strong likelihood that embedded abrasive grains will react with fired ceramics, which may result in the formation of cracks in the veneering porcelain [21]. For example, abrasive blasting may affect the mechanical properties of zirconium oxide [26,27]. Too aggressive action may cause an unfavorable transformation from the tetragonal phase to the undesirable monoclinic (t $\rightarrow$ m) [24–29]. As the transformation phase increases from the surface of the sample to the entire volume of the sample, microcracks, and residual stresses may develop and decrease the bending force [26,27].

Therefore, it is important to determine the number of embedded grains for individual processing parameters. Despite many studies, the combination of ceramics with zirconium oxide and ceramics with titanium alloys is still the weakest point of prosthetic restorations and leads to chipping and fractures.

The aim of the work is to examine the effect of abrasive blasting on the amount of Al_2O_3 abrasive driven into the surface of Cr/Co, Cr/Ni, and Ti alloys and synthesized ZrO_2, as well as to find a relationship between the amount of driven abrasive and the hardness of the materials.

2. Materials and Methods

Three hundred and fifteen cylindrical disks with a diameter of 9 mm and a height of 5 mm from three types of metal alloys: Cr/Co (Heraenium® P, Heraeus Holding GmbH, Hanau, Germany), Ni/Cr (Wiron 99, BEGO USA Inc., Lincoln, RI, USA), Ti (Tritan CpTi 1, DENTAURUM GmbH & Co. KG, Ispringen, Germany), and 315 of the same dimensions of sintered ZrO_2 3TPZ-Y (Cermill, Amann Girrbach AG, Koblach, Austria) were used in the study. The samples were divided into groups (n = 35), and subjected to abrasive blasting with aluminum oxide (Al_2O_3) with grain sizes 50, 110, and 250 μm at pressures of 0.2, 0.4, or 0.6 MPa. To unify the surface of the samples before the test, each surface was ground with SiC sandpapers with grains of 220, 400, 600, and 800, respectively, on a Metasinex grinder with water cooling. Then, the samples were washed in an ultrasonic cleaner (Quantrex 90 WT, L&R Manufacturing, Inc., Kearny, NJ, USA) in ethyl alcohol for 10 min and dried with compressed air. Abrasive blasting was carried out on the Mikroblast Duo device (Prodento - Optimed, Warsaw, Poland). The working distance from the nozzle was 20 mm, the angle of incidence of the abrasive was 45°, and the treatment time was 20 s.

The samples prepared this way were observed in a scanning electron microscope (SEM, HITACHI S3000-N, Hitachi, Ltd., Tokyo, Japan). The surface topography of the samples was obtained with the use of secondary electrons (SE) and the so-called material contrast in the light of backscattered electrons (BSE). Observations conducted in this way, due to the material contrast resulting from the difference in chemical composition, make it possible to determine the areas occupied by abrasive material grains stuck into the surface, which was confirmed in works [12,30,31]. Example photos of samples of metal alloys and zirconium dioxide after abrasive blasting obtained using backscattered electrons BSE are shown in Figure 1. Ten photos were taken at randomly-selected locations of each sample. The surface fraction of the abrasive material particles was determined by quantitative metallography with Mentilo software [22]. From each group, five samples were subjected to Vickers hardness measurements on a KB Prüftechnik hardness tester after a load of 9.81 N (1 kG).

Dark areas appeared on the surface of metal alloy samples after abrasive blasting, indicating a difference in the chemical composition compared to the treated substrate. Quantitative metallography methods with the application of the Metillo program were used to determine the surface fraction of abrasive particles [22,27]. Briefly, the microscope image was loaded into Metillo and subjected to the following procedures: shadow correction, normalisation of the grey-level histogram, and manual binarization. The percentage share of the dark (red) areas of the total abrasive elements embedded in the surface of the sample was then calculated. Figure 2a shows an exemplary microscopic photo presenting the manual binarization of the image of a ZrO_2 sample after abrasive blasting with Al_2O_3 grain size 110 μm and pressure 0.2 MPa. The red areas in Figure 2b are aluminum particles embedded in the surface of the sample.

Statistical analyses of the results were performed using the PQStat statistical package, version 1.8.2.218. A three-factor analysis of variance was carried out comprising the type of material, the size of the gradation of the abrasive, and the amount of pressure. Tukey's test was performed as a post hoc test. Test probability was considered significant for $p < 0.05$ and highly significant for $p < 0.01$.

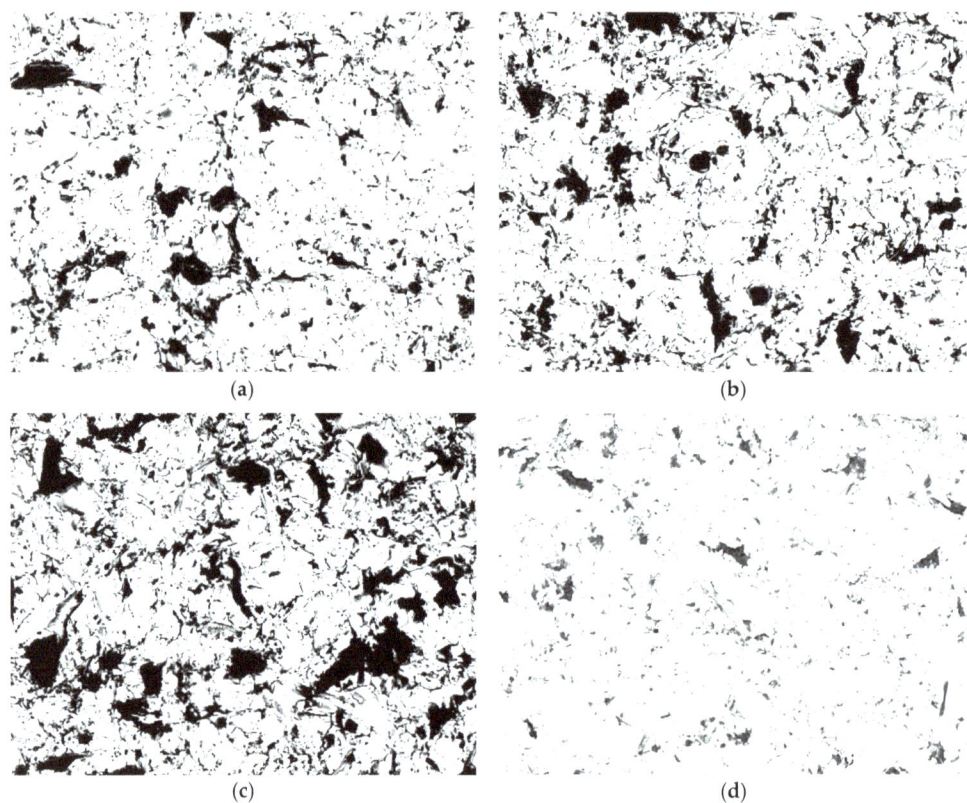

Figure 1. Images obtained using backscattered electrons BSE after abrasion with Al_2O_3 250 μm particles and under the pressure of 0.2 MPa with (magnification 500×): (**a**) Cr/Co alloy, (**b**) Ni/Cr alloy, (**c**) Ti alloy, and (**d**) ZrO_2.

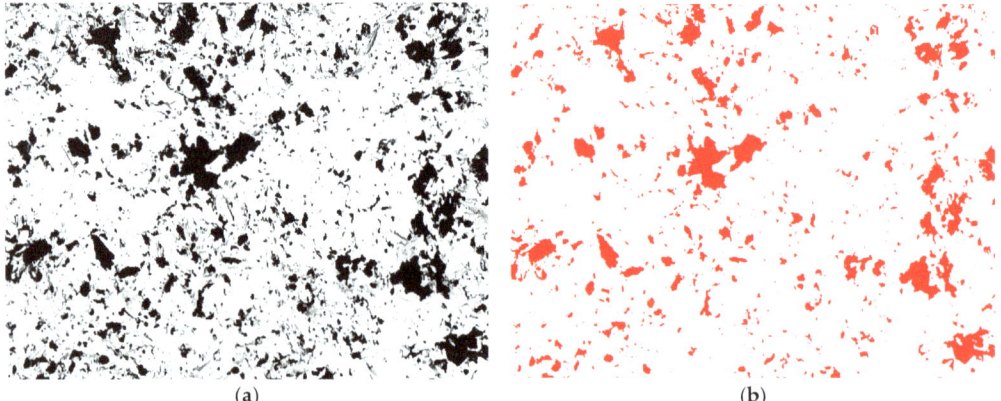

Figure 2. Binarization of the microscopic image: (**a**) initial image and (**b**) image after binarization (for calculations).

3. Results

The amount of driven Al_2O_3 abrasive used for abrasive blasting of four different materials with variable processing parameters is presented in Table 1. The graphical interpretation of the results is shown in Figure 3. The smallest amounts of driven abrasive were observed for ZrO_2 treatment, and among them, the smallest was noted for a value of 250 μm of the abrasive gradation and pressure of 0.6 MPa. In the case of such a combination of factors, the mean value (2.62) of results of the driven abrasive did not differ significantly ($p > 0.05$) from the combination of factors with a pressure of 0.4 MPa (2.88) and 0.2 MPa (3.21). In other words, for ZrO_2 treatment with an abrasive gradation of 250 μm, regardless of the applied pressure, the amount of embedded abrasive was small and constituted a homogeneous group. (Indicated by the letter "a"). Significantly ($p > 0.05$) larger amounts of embedded abrasive were noted for ZrO_2 machining and grain gradation of 110 μm or 50 μm. Then, regardless of the applied pressure, the average amounts of driven abrasive made up another homogeneous group (marked with the letter "b"). All other combinations of factors resulted in significantly ($p > 0.05$) more embedded abrasive than those found for ZrO_2 treatment. Among all the results, the largest amount of grain was embedded in the treatment of the Ti alloy at a pressure of 0.6 MPa and grain gradation of 250 μm. The average amount of embedded grain was 38.19 and was significantly ($p > 0.05$) higher than all other treatment variants.

Table 1. Descriptive statistics of the amount of Al_2O_3 embedded abrasive according to material and airborne-particle abrasion parameters.

Material	Gradation (μm)	Pressure (MPa)	Arithmetic Mean	Standard Deviation	Standard Error of the Mean	Uniform Groups (Tukeys Post Hoc Test)
alloy Ti	50	0.2	23.64	1.71	0.29	lj
		0.4	27.16	1.91	0.32	n
		0.6	31.19	1.88	0.32	p
	110	0.2	23.68	1.76	0.30	ij
		0.4	29.39	1.52	0.26	o
		0.6	33.44	2.06	0.35	r
	250	0.2	26.08	1.43	0.24	lmn
		0.4	31.82	1.91	0.32	p
		0.6	38.19	1.82	0.31	s
alloy Ni/Cr	50	0.2	17.63	4.32	0.73	d
		0.4	18.16	2.00	0.34	de
		0.6	21.11	2.01	0.34	g
	110	0.2	21.35	2.38	0.40	g
		0.4	23.33	1.40	0.24	hi
		0.6	26.67	2.22	0.38	mn
	250	0.2	24.27	1.53	0.26	ijk
		0.4	26.74	1.53	0.26	mn
		0.6	30.48	2.32	0.39	op
alloy Co/Cr	50	0.2	13.51	1.50	0.25	c
		0.4	19.44	2.02	0.34	ef
		0.6	23.69	1.54	0.26	ij
	110	0.2	16.95	1.67	0.28	d
		0.4	21.83	1.81	0.31	gh
		0.6	25.02	1.14	0.19	jkl
	250	0.2	20.79	1.65	0.28	fg
		0.4	20.95	1.66	0.28	fg
		0.6	25.50	1.20	0.20	klm

Table 1. *Cont.*

Material	Gradation (μm)	Pressure (MPa)	Arithmetic Mean	Standard Deviation	Standard Error of the Mean	Uniform Groups (Tukeys Post Hoc Test)
ZrO$_2$	50	0.2	6.52	0.44	0.07	b
		0.4	7.36	0.49	0.08	b
		0.6	6.87	0.35	0.06	b
	110	0.2	6.65	0.45	0.08	b
		0.4	7.58	0.37	0.06	b
		0.6	6.77	0.38	0.06	b
	250	0.2	3.21	0.45	0.08	a
		0.4	2.88	0.40	0.07	a
		0.6	2.62	0.39	0.07	a

Means marked with the same letter did not differ significantly from each other ($p > 0.05$), while if there was no common letter between the two compared means, then the means differed significantly ($p > 0.05$).

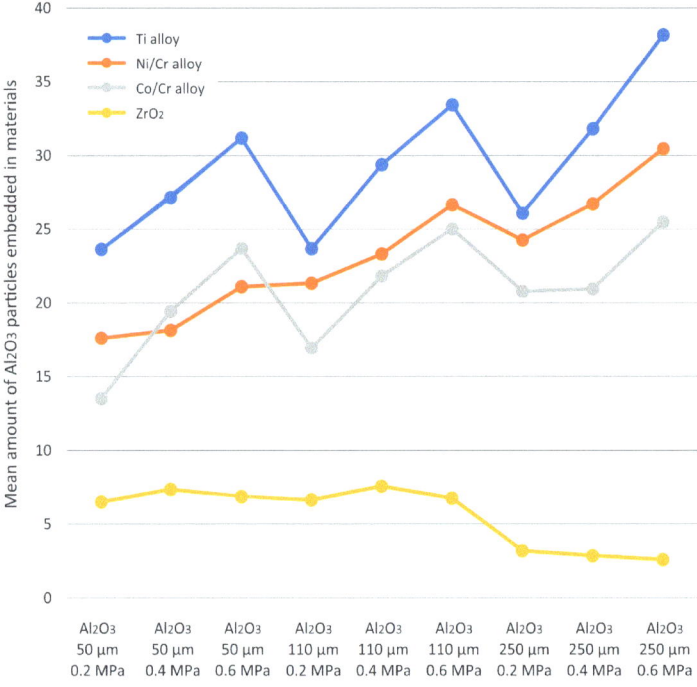

Figure 3. The amount of Al$_2$O$_3$ particles embedded in the four different test materials according to abrasion parameters.

Descriptive statistics of the amount of driven Al$_2$O$_3$ abrasive depending on the main factors and the analysis of the variance table are presented in Table 2. All interactions between the factors were highly significant ($p < 0.0001$). In general, a highly significant ($p < 0.0001$) difference in the amount of embedded abrasive depending on the material subjected to treatment was noted. Highly significant differences ($p < 0.0001$) were observed in each material which was compared with any other material. The smallest amount of embedded abrasive was noted for ZrO$_2$, and the highest amount—for the Ti alloy.

Table 2. Descriptive statistics of the amount of driven Al$_2$O$_3$ abrasive depending on the main factors and the table of the analysis of variance.

		Arithmetic Mean	Standard Deviation	Standard Error of the Mean	Uniform Groups (Tukeys Post Hoc Test)
Material	alloy Ti	29.40	4.87	0.27	d
	alloy Ni/Cr	23.30	4.61	0.26	c
	alloy Co/Cr	20.85	3.97	0.22	b
	ZrO$_2$	5.61	1.99	0.11	a
Gradation [μm]	50	18.02	8.01	0.39	a
	110	20.22	8.74	0.43	b
	250	21.13	11.56	0.56	c
Pressure [MPa]	0.2	17.02	7.75	0.38	a
	0.4	19.72	9.04	0.44	b
	0.6	22.63	11.04	0.54	c
		F	p	Eta-squared partially	
Material		11,312.09	<0.0001	0.9652	
Gradation [μm]		375.41	<0.0001	0.3802	
Pressure [MPa]		1158.38	<0.0001	0.6543	
Material*Gradation		261.33	<0.0001	0.5616	
Material*Pressure [MPa]		170.07	<0.0001	0.4547	
Gradation*Pressure [MPa]		7.27	<0.0001	0.0232	
Material*Gradation*Pressure [MPa]		18.13	<0.0001	0.1509	

Means marked with the same letter did not differ significantly from each other ($p > 0.05$), while if there was no common letter between the two compared means, then the means differed significantly ($p > 0.05$).

A comparison of gradations shows a highly significant difference ($p < 0.0001$) between them. Highly significant differences ($p < 0.0001$) were observed for each gradation which was compared to any other gradation. The lowest amounts of embedded abrasive were observed for 50 μm gradation, and the highest amounts of embedded abrasive were noted at a gradation of 250 μm. This means that the increase in the gradation of the abrasive systematically increased the amount of embedded grain.

A pressure comparison indicated a highly significant difference ($p < 0.0001$) between them. Highly significant differences ($p < 0.0001$) were observed for each pressure compared to any other pressure. The smallest amounts of driven abrasive were observed for a pressure of 0.2 MPa, and the largest amounts of driven abrasive were noted for a pressure of 0.6 MPa. In the case of the metal alloys Ti, Ni/Cr, and Co/Cr, an increase in pressure was associated with a higher number of particles knocked out; however, no such effect was observed for ZrO$_2$.

All factor interactions were highly significant ($p < 0.0001$). In general, a highly significant ($p < 0.0001$) difference in the amount of embedded abrasive depending on the material was found. Highly significant differences ($p < 0.0001$) were observed in each material which was compared with any other material. The smallest amount of driven abrasive was observed during the machining of ZrO$_2$, and the largest—during the machining of the Ti alloy. Comparison of abrasive gradations showed highly significant differences ($p < 0.0001$) between them. A highly significant difference ($p < 0.0001$) was observed for all gradations, which were compared to any other gradations. The smallest amount of embedded abrasive was at 50 μm gradation, and the largest was at 250 μm gradation. This means that the increase in the gradation of the abrasive systematically increased the number of embedded grains. A comparison of pressure values indicated a highly significant difference ($p < 0.0001$) between them. Highly significant differences ($p < 0.0001$) were observed when each pressure was compared to any other pressure. The smallest amounts of driven abrasive were noted for a pressure of 0.2 MPa, and the largest amounts for a pressure of 0.6 MPa. This means that the increase in the pressure systematically increased the amount of embedded abrasive. Results of hardness measurements using the Vickers

HV1 method of individual groups of samples of four different materials used for testing at a load of 9.81 N (1 kG) are presented in Table 3.

Table 3. Results of HV1 hardness measurements of the tested materials.

Material			
Alloy Ti	Alloy Ni/Cr	Alloy Co/Cr	ZrO_2
94	187	405	1410
95	186	400	1405
97	186	396	1410
101	184	422	1399
90	189	393	1432
98	182	402	1416
X mean = 96	X mean = 185	X mean = 403	X mean = 1412
SD = 3.8	SD = 2.4	SD = 10.2	SD = 11.3

ZrO_2 was found to be the hardest substance (mean 1432 HV) and Ti alloy the least (mean 96 HV), with ZrO_2 demonstrating about 15 times greater hardness than the Ti alloy. The mean hardness values were 185 HV for the Ni/Cr alloy and 403 HV for Co/Cr.

4. Discussion

Based on microscopic observations (in backscattered electrons, i.e., material contrast) of the surface of the samples after abrasive blasting, components not belonging to the tested materials were found. Based on previous works, it can be concluded that these are grains of abrasive material embedded in the surfaces of the samples [12,30,31].

When analyzing the phenomena occurring between the grains of the abrasive material and the machined surface, three processes should be considered: grains perform cutting work and bounce off the surface, grains perform cutting work and remain fixed in the surface, or grains stick to the surface without cutting. The grains of the cutting material carried by compressed air carry some energy depending on their mass and speed, which is the result of applied air pressure. The quality of the phenomenon that will occur depends on the energy of the falling grain in relation to the energy needed to perform the cutting work, as well as on its orientation at the moment of contact with the machined surface. It should be emphasized that the abrasive grains are irregular polygons. Therefore, when considering the influence of machining parameters, the type of abrasive grain, its gradation, the applied pressure, and the hardness of the workpiece should be considered.

The amount of embedded abrasive particles was found to depend on the type of material, the abrasive gradation, and the amount of applied pressure. The tested materials were characterized by different hardness, from very soft titanium (97 HV) through a slightly harder Ni/Cr alloy (195 HV), harder Cr/Co alloy (300 HV), to very hard ZrO_2 (1300 HV). It should be emphasized that the hardness of ZrO_2 was close to the hardness of the used abrasive materials. The largest amount of driven abrasive, regardless of the type of abrasive material and processing parameters, was observed on the surfaces of samples made of titanium alloy, followed by Ni/Cr and Co/Cr alloys, and the smallest amount was noted for the surfaces of ZrO_2 samples. Here we can see a clear and most important dependence of the number of driven grains on the hardness of the workpiece—the higher its hardness, the fewer stuck grains with the same machining parameters. The surface occupied by embedded particles can increase many times over. Depending on the parameters used, it ranges from 2.62 to 7.58% for ZrO_2, through 13.51 to 25.50% for the Cr/Co alloy, 17.63 to 30.48% for the Ni/Cr alloy, up to 23.64 to 38.19% for the Ti alloy. This relationship can be explained by the relationship between the grain energy and the energy needed to perform cutting work. We can observe a complete loss of energy by a particle that is stopped at the moment of contact with the treated surface or a partial loss of energy during which the particle bounces off the treated surface. As ZrO_2 is harder than aluminum oxide, fewer particles become embedded. As such, the differences are not as visible. However, it is not obvious how many grains will be driven in, and this has a direct impact on the bond between the framework and the veneering ceramics.

The obtained results are for practical use. As for other parameters, there may also be sandblasting time and particle incidence angle. However, they are of no practical importance. It was found that after several seconds of sandblasting, the condition of the surface did not change. On the other hand, the angle of incidence of the abrasive has an undoubted effect on the amount driven into the surface. However, in prosthetic practice, due to the shape of the processed elements, it is not possible to maintain a constant angle; therefore, we did not consider this parameter.

The size of the abrasive grains used for processing is another parameter influencing the number of embedded particles. The increase in the gradation of the abrasive systematically increased the amount of embedded grain. The change in the size of the abrasive grain was associated with an increase in its weight and resistance to crushing, and thus a change in cutting properties, i.e., also in the geometric structure of the machined surface. Smaller abrasive grains have lower kinetic energy due to their lower mass. The angles of the tops of the abrasive grains also change by changing their geometric dimensions [1,3,4]. It seems that, for example, assuming a similar number of embedded grains, a five-fold increase in the grain size from 50 m to 250 μm should cause a large difference in the area they occupy. However, this did not happen because the accelerated grain cracked and crumbled into smaller parts after its contact with the treated surface. Thus, a fragment of the grain and not the whole of it was driven in, which resulted in a smaller number of grains than expected.

The dependence of the number of embedded grains on the treatment pressure can be explained in a similar way. Increased pressure systematically increased the amount of driven abrasive. However, these relationships were not as clear as in the case of the type and hardness of the material. Increased pressure resulted in greater kinetic energy of the grains and thus also a more intense cutting process [2–4,7]. This will have an undeniable effect on improving the mechanical anchoring and increasing the wettability of the treated surface [6,8,17,27,32]. However, a more accurate explanation of the role of embedded abrasive particles requires further research.

Referring to many studies, it can be stated that the abrasive blasting process has a beneficial effect on most surfaces of materials prepared for bonding with other materials. Additionally, this process is necessary to obtain a surface characterized by parameters that will create a mechanically durable connection. The surface roughness obtained in this way plays a major role in improving the quality of the connection, which can be better anchored in the surface layer of the base material of particles of the applied coating.

While the obtained results have practical significance, sandblasting time and particle incidence angle do not, despite playing a role in embedding. It was found that several seconds of sandblasting did not appear to influence the condition of the surface.

Although the angle of incidence of the abrasive has an undoubted effect on embedding, it is not possible to maintain a constant angle in prosthetic practice due to the shape of the processed elements. Therefore, this parameter was not included in the analysis.

Although sandblasting hardens the surface of the metal, this has no practical significance due to the hardening being negated by the recrystallization that occurs when the ceramic is fired at 900 °C.

5. Conclusions

After abrasive blasting, abrasive particles were found on the surface of treated materials. The amount of driven abrasive depends on the hardness of the processed material, the gradation of the abrasive, as well as the size of the working pressure used during machining. The greater the hardness of the processed material, the smaller the number of grains driven into its surface. In the case of metal alloys: Ti, Ni/Cr, and Co/Cr, an increase in pressure was correlated with an increase in the number of particles knocked out; however, this effect was not observed for ZrO_2. The aim of the work, however, was not to emphasize the advantages of sandblasting but to draw attention to its effect on grain embedding, which may affect any subsequent bond formed with ceramics.

Author Contributions: Conceptualization, L.K. and B.Ś.; methodology, L.K.; software, K.K.; validation, B.Ś., L.K., and K.K.; formal analysis, L.K., B.Ś.; resources, L.K.; data curation, K.K.; writing—original draft preparation, B.Ś.; writing—review and editing, L.K.; visualization, B.Ś.; supervision, L.K.; project administration, B.Ś.; funding acquisition, K.K. All authors have read and agreed to the published version of the manuscript.

Funding: This research received no external funding.

Institutional Review Board Statement: Not applicable.

Informed Consent Statement: Not applicable.

Data Availability Statement: Not applicable.

Conflicts of Interest: The authors declare no conflict of interest.

References

1. Khan, A.A.; Haque, M.M. Performance of different abrasive materials during abrasive water jet machining of glass. *J. Mater. Process. Tech.* **2007**, *191*, 404–407. [CrossRef]
2. Gołębiowski, M.; Sobczyk-Guzenda, A.; Szymański, W.; Klimek, L. Influence of parameters of stream abrasive treatment of titanium surfaces on contact angle and surface free energy. *Mater. Eng.* **2010**, *173*, 978–980.
3. Pietnicki, K.; Wołowiec, E.; Klimek, L. The effect of abrasive blasting on the strength of a joint between dental porcelain and metal base. *Acta Bioeng. Biomech.* **2014**, *16*, 63–68. [PubMed]
4. Gołębiowski, M.; Wołowiec, E.; Klimek, L. Airborne-particle abrasion parameters on the quality of titanium-ceramic bonds. *J. Prosth. Dent.* **2015**, *113*, 453–459. [CrossRef] [PubMed]
5. Białucki, P.; Kozerski, S. Study of adhesion of different plasma-sprayed coatings to aluminium. *Surf. Coat. Technol.* **2006**, *201*, 2061–2064. [CrossRef]
6. Truong, B.; Hu, L.; Jacopo, B.; McKrell, T. Modification of sandblasted plate heaters using nanofluids to enhance pool boiling critical heat flux. *Int. J. Heat Mass Transf.* **2010**, *53*, 85–94. [CrossRef]
7. Lubas, M.; Jasinski, J.J.; Zawada, A.; Przerada, I. Influence of Sandblasting and Chemical Etching on Titanium 99.2–Dental Porcelain Bond Strength. *Materials* **2022**, *15*, 116. [CrossRef]
8. Reyes, M.J.; Oshida, Y.; Andres, C.J.; Barco, T.; Hovijitra, S.; Brown, D. Titanium-porcelain system. Part III: Effects of surface modification on bond strengths. *Biomed. Mater. Eng.* **2001**, *11*, 117–136.
9. Hofstede, T.M.; Ercoli, C.; Graser, G.N.; Tallents, R.H.; Moss, M.E.; Zero, D.T. Influence of metal surface finishing on porcelain porosity and beam failure loads at the metal-ceramic interface. *J. Prosthet. Dent.* **2000**, *84*, 309–317. [CrossRef]
10. Fischer, J.; Zbären, C.; Stawarczyk, B.; Hämmerle, C.H. The effect of thermal cycling on metal-ceramic bond strength. *J. Dent.* **2009**, *37*, 549–553. [CrossRef]
11. Burnat, B.; Walkowiak-Przybyło, M.; Błaszczyk, T.; Klimek, L. Corrosion behaviour of polished and sandblasted titanium alloys in PBS solution. *Acta Bioeng. Biomech.* **2013**, *15*, 87–95. [PubMed]
12. Gilbert, J.L.; Covey, D.L.; Lautenschlager, E.P. Bond characteristic of porcelain fused to milled titanium. *Dent. Mater.* **1994**, *10*, 134–140. [CrossRef] [PubMed]
13. Derand, T.; Herø, H. Bond strength of porcelain on cast vs wrought titanium. *Scand. J. Dent. Res.* **1992**, *100*, 184–188. [CrossRef] [PubMed]
14. Park, W.U.; Park, H.G.; Hwang, K.H.; Zhao, J.; Lee, J.K. Interfacial Property of Dental Cobalt–Chromium Alloys and Their Bonding Strength with Porcelains. *J. Nanosci. Nanotechnol.* **2017**, *17*, 2585–2588. [CrossRef] [PubMed]
15. Yamada, K.; Onizuka, T.; Sumii, T.; Swain, M.V. The effect of Goldbonder™ on the adhesion between porcelain and pure titanium. *J. Oral Rehabil.* **2004**, *31*, 775–784. [CrossRef]
16. Külünk, T.; Kurt, M.; Ural, Ç.; Külünk, Ş.; Baba, S. Effect of different air-abrasion particles on metal-ceramic bond strength. *J. Dent. Sci.* **2011**, *6*, 140–146. [CrossRef]
17. Prado, R.A.D.; Panzeri, H.; Fernandes Neto, A.J.; Neves, F.D.D.; Silva, M.R.D.; Mendonça, G. Shear bond strength of dental porcelains to nickel-chromium alloys. *Braz. Dent. J.* **2005**, *16*, 202–206. [CrossRef]
18. Patel, K.; Mathur, S.; Upadhyay, S. A comparative evaluation of bond strength of feldspathic porcelain to nickel- chromium alloy, when subjected to various surface treat- ments: An in vitro study. *J. Indian Prosthodont. Soc.* **2015**, *15*, 53–57. [CrossRef]
19. Lee, B.A.; Kim, O.S.; Vang, M.S.; Park, Y.J. Effect of surface treatment on bond strength of Ti-10Ta-10Nb to low-fusing porcelain. *J. Prosthet. Dent.* **2013**, *109*, 95–105. [CrossRef]
20. Hjerppe, J.; Närhi, T.O.; Vallittu, P.K.; Lassila, L.V. Surface roughness and the flexural and bend strength of zirconia after different surface treatments. *J. Prosthet. Dent.* **2016**, *116*, 577–583. [CrossRef]

21. Van Niekerk, A.J.; Caputa, T. *Modern Prosthetic Restorations in Art and Craft*, 3rd ed.; Selected Texts; Company Elamed: Katowice, Poland, 2007; pp. 228–234.
22. Szala, J. Application of computer picture analysis methods to quantitative assessment of structure in materials. *Sci. J. Sil. Univ. Technol. Ser. Metall.* **2008**, *82*, 34–42.
23. Pagnano, V.O.; Leal, M.B.; Catirse, A.B.; Curylofo, P.A.; Silva, R.F.; Macedo, A.P. Effect of oxidation heat treatment with airborne-particle abrasion on the shear bond strength of ceramic to base metal alloys. *J. Prosthet. Dent.* **2021**, *126*, 804.e1–804.e9. [CrossRef] [PubMed]
24. Wongkamhaeng, K.; Dawson, D.V.; Holloway, J.A.; Denry, I. Effect of Surface Modification on In-Depth Transformation sand Flexural Strength of Zirconia Ceramics. *J. Prosthodont.* **2019**, *28*, e364–e375. [CrossRef] [PubMed]
25. Ebeid, K.; Wille, S.; Salah, T.; Wahsh, M.; Zohdy, M.; Kern, M. Evaluation of surface treatments of monolithic zirconia in different sintering stages. *J. Prosthodont. Res.* **2018**, *62*, 210–217. [CrossRef] [PubMed]
26. Jain, T.; Porwal, A.; Babu, S.; Khan, Z.A.; Kaur, C.; Jain, R.B. Effect of Different Surface Treatments on Biaxial Flexural Strength of Yttria-stabilized Tetragonal Zirconia Polycrystal. *J. Contemp. Dent. Pract.* **2018**, *19*, 318–323. [CrossRef]
27. Śmielak, B.; Klimek, L. Effect of air abrasion on the number of particles embedded in zirconia. *Materials* **2018**, *11*, 259. [CrossRef]
28. Aurélio, I.L.; Marchionatti, A.M.E.; Montagner, A.F.; May, L.G.; Soares, F.Z.M. Does air particle abrasion affect the flexural strength and phase transformation of Y-TZP? A systematic review and meta-analysis. *Dent. Mater.* **2016**, *32*, 827–845. [CrossRef]
29. Camposilvan, E.; Flamant, Q.; Anglada, M. Surface roughened zirconia: Towards hydrothermal stability. *J. Mech. Behav. Biomed. Mater.* **2015**, *47*, 95–106. [CrossRef]
30. Pruszczyńska, E.; Pietnicki, K.; Klimek, L. Effect of the abrasive blasting treatment on the quality of the pressed ceramics joint for a metal foundation. *Arch. Mater. Sci. Eng.* **2016**, *78*, 17–22. [CrossRef]
31. Czepułkowska, W.; Korecka-Wołowiec, E.; Klimek, L. The Condition of Ni-Cr Alloy Surface after Abrasive Blasting with Various Parameters. *J. Mater. Eng. Perform.* **2019**, *29*, 1439–1444. [CrossRef]
32. Aboushelib, M.N.; Kleverlaan, C.J.; Feilzer, A.J. Microtensile bond strength of different components of core veneered all-ceramic restorations Part II. Zirconia veneering ceramics. *Dent. Mater.* **2006**, *22*, 857–863. [CrossRef] [PubMed]

Disclaimer/Publisher's Note: The statements, opinions and data contained in all publications are solely those of the individual author(s) and contributor(s) and not of MDPI and/or the editor(s). MDPI and/or the editor(s) disclaim responsibility for any injury to people or property resulting from any ideas, methods, instructions or products referred to in the content.

MDPI AG
Grosspeteranlage 5
4052 Basel
Switzerland
Tel.: +41 61 683 77 34

Materials Editorial Office
E-mail: materials@mdpi.com
www.mdpi.com/journal/materials

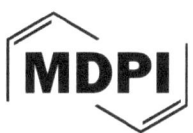

Disclaimer/Publisher's Note: The title and front matter of this reprint are at the discretion of the Guest Editors. The publisher is not responsible for their content or any associated concerns. The statements, opinions and data contained in all individual articles are solely those of the individual Editors and contributors and not of MDPI. MDPI disclaims responsibility for any injury to people or property resulting from any ideas, methods, instructions or products referred to in the content.

www.ingramcontent.com/pod-product-compliance
Lightning Source LLC
LaVergne TN
LVHW072314090526
838202LV00019B/2286

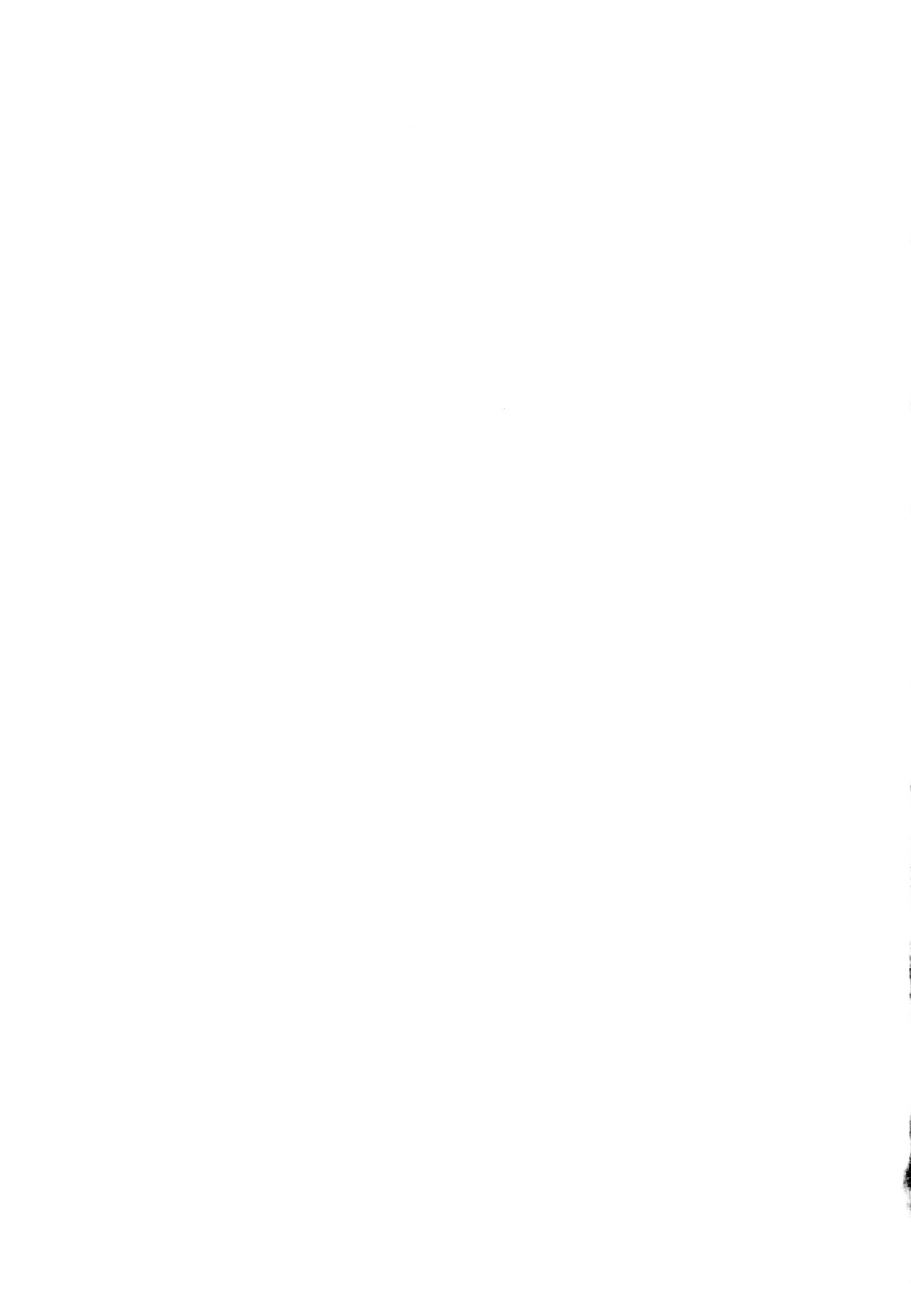